Counseling
Children

NINTH EDITION

Donna A. Henderson
Wake Forest University

Charles L. Thompson, late
The University of Tennessee, Knoxville

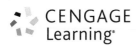

CENGAGE
Learning·

Australia · Brazil · Mexico · Singapore · United Kingdom · United States

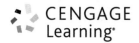
CENGAGE
Learning®

***Counseling Children*, Ninth Edition**
Donna A. Henderson, Charles L. Thompson

Product Director: Jon-David Hague

Product Manager: Julie Martinez

Content Developer: Lori Bradshaw

Product Assistant: Stephen Lagos

Marketing Manager: Margaux Cameron

Art and Cover Direction, Production
Management, and Composition:
Lumina Datamatics, Inc.

Manufacturing Planner: Judy Inouye

Cover Image: ©pjhpix/Shutterstock

Unless otherwise noted, all items
© Cengage Learning

For product information and technology assistance, contact us at
Cengage Learning Customer & Sales Support, 1-800-354-9706

For permission to use material from this text or product,
submit all requests online at **cengage.com/permissions**
Further permissions questions can be emailed to
permissionrequest@cengage.com

Library of Congress Control Number: 2015939480

Student Edition:
ISBN: 978-1-285-46454-1

Cengage Learning
20 Channel Center Street
Boston, MA 02210
USA

Cengage Learning is a leading provider of customized learning solutions
with employees residing in nearly 40 different countries and sales in more
than 125 countries around the world. Find your local representative at
www.cengage.com.

Cengage Learning products are represented in Canada by
Nelson Education, Ltd.

To learn more about Cengage Learning Solutions, visit **www.cengage.com**

Purchase any of our products at your local college store or at our preferred
online store **www.cengagebrain.com**

Printed in the United States of America
Print Number: 02 Print Year: 2016

Counseling Children, Ninth Edition, is dedicated to Charles L. Thompson, who died December 2005. The book mirrors his love for children and his skill in interacting with them. He devoted his working life to sharing that compassion and mastery with his students and to the people who read this book. Hopefully, your reading the text will reveal the smiles and encouraging words that filled his days.

I would also dedicate this volume to my family—J. D., Chris, Amy, and Ella—who teach me daily about love, patience, and the joy of togetherness.

Donna A. Henderson

Contents

CHAPTER 4   Legal and Ethical Considerations for Counselors   110

CHAPTER 7   Gestalt Therapy   214

CHAPTER 8   Behavioral Counseling   241

CHAPTER 11   Individual Psychology   336

CHAPTER 20 Counseling with Children with Disabilities   677

Preface

Counseling Children, Ninth Edition, maintains the focus of earlier editions—putting theory into practice. Video clips of counseling sessions with children accompany this volume. The counselors in those clips demonstrate some techniques, relationship-building skills, and the spirit of working with children. We hope you find these short segments instructive.

The concepts in this book may stimulate seasoned professionals as well as instruct those just beginning their therapeutic work with children and their families. Counselors, psychologists, social workers, and teachers will discover ways to teach children how to meet their needs in ways that do not infringe on the rights of others. The book contains a synthesis of the best ideas from research and practical, current interventions for helping children with specific developmental, educational, personal, social, and behavioral problems. The reader will find suggestions for working with children who have special needs; who are faced with crises such as death, violence, divorce, or substance abuse problems; and who may be victims of abuse or debilitating medical conditions. Particular attention is given to the developmental implications for the theories and interventions discussed.

The ninth edition of *Counseling Children* is based on the principle that people who work effectively with children adapt to the young people they serve. The helpers integrate and adjust interventions and techniques from a variety of theoretical systems into their counseling system in order to both understand and help the child client. A major goal of this book is to present accurate descriptions of a variety of theories from which readers can develop their own approaches to helping.

ORGANIZATION

Each chapter has been updated and many have been expanded with video clips, illustrating concepts from several chapters on theory.

In Part 1, we consider barriers to children's healthy development as well as the resiliency that most children exhibit. We look at the world of the child by discussing some developmental theories—Piaget's stages of cognitive development, Erikson's theory of social development, Freud's psychosexual stages of development, Havighurst's developmental tasks, and Selman's descriptions of changes in perspective taking. We also look at cultural influences on the world of children, focusing on identity development. In the third chapter, we present an overview of the counseling process and universal skills in helping. We explore the practices most likely to contribute to effective counseling as well as the ways helping can be a remedial, preventive, or developmental activity. You will find definitions and dimensions of counseling as well as responses to frequently asked questions and one way to evaluate counseling progress. The final chapter in Part 1 includes legal and ethical considerations in working with minors.

In Part 2, we review counseling theories. This section of the book begins with Chapter 5 on psychoanalytic counseling theory, the stimulus for many other approaches to counseling. Two following chapters cover theories that focus on the emotions. Chapter 6 provides an overview of person-centered counseling and the listening skills necessary for most helping approaches. Gestalt therapy is discussed in Chapter 7 with descriptions of its unique interventions, which are helpful additions to the beginning counselor's repertoire. The next four chapters cover approaches that focus mainly on behaviors—behavioral counseling, reality therapy, brief counseling, and individual counseling. All these chapters offer readers some practical skills for work and field experiences.

The next three chapters incorporate theories that focus on thinking. Chapter 8 contains information about rational emotive behavior therapy. Chapter 9 includes expanded coverage of cognitive-behavioral therapy, an approach to counseling with impressive outcomes for all ages. Transactional analysis is presented so that readers can investigate a way to help others understand how they communicate with other people, how their personality developed, and how life scripts can be rewritten. The systemic approaches of family counseling chapter contains wide choices of ways to work with families, ranging from conjoint family therapy to structural, strategic, and systems approaches to family counseling. Finally, those who work with children often include parents, teachers, and other adults. The chapter on consultation and collaboration discusses skills and models of conducting that work and completes this part of the book.

Part 3 begins with a chapter that includes points about play therapy that have not been covered in the other theories chapters. The topic of the following chapter is working with children in groups. An extended discussion on working with children with special concerns such as divorce, alcoholic families, and grief is contained in Chapter 19. Finally, the particular needs of children with disabilities rounds out the topics covered in Part 3.

Supplements

ONLINE INSTRUCTOR'S MANUAL   The Instructor's Manual contains a variety of resources to aid instructors in preparing and presenting text material in a manner that meets their personal preferences and course needs. It presents chapter-by-chapter suggestions and resources to enhance and facilitate learning.

ONLINE TEST BANK   For assessment support, the updated test bank includes true/false, multiple-choice, matching, short answer, and matching questions.

ONLINE POWERPOINT   These Microsoft® PowerPoint® lecture slides for each chapter assist you with your lecture by providing concept coverage using content directly from the textbook.

COURSEMATE   Available with the text, Cengage Learning's CourseMate brings course concepts to life with interactive learning, study, and exam preparation tools that support the printed textbook. CourseMate includes an integrated e-book, quizzes, videos, downloadable forms, glossaries, flashcards, and Engagement Tracker—a first-of-its-kind tool that monitors student engagement in the course.

ACKNOWLEDGMENTS

No project this big can be completed without encouragement and support. Thanks to colleagues at Wake Forest University who have helped in many ways. I also appreciate the people who provided useful advice in their reviews: Dyanne Anthony, Fontbonne University; Steven Berman, University of Central Florida; Carrie King, Mt. Mary College; Elisabeth Liles, California State University, Sacramento; Poppy Moon, University of West Alabama; and Suzanne Whitehead, Northern State University. I am also so grateful for the support from everyone at Cengage Learning, especially Julie Martinez, Ruth Sakata Corley, Lori Bradshaw, and Sharib Asrar. They and many other fine people at Cengage Learning shepherded this project to completion and were generous with their patience and expertise. A special thanks goes to Inna Fedoseyeva of Cengage, Trevor Buser, Juleen Buser, and Erin Binkley, who developed the video clips that accompany the text. They had the technical expertise of Henry Heidtman, a masterful producer, and of Summit School, which generously donated their space and equipment.

Donna A. Henderson

Author Biographies

Donna A. Henderson is a professor and chair of the Department of Counseling at Wake Forest University in Winston-Salem, North Carolina. She received her bachelor's degree in English from Meredith College, her master's degree from James Madison University, and her Ph.D. degree in counselor education from the University of Tennessee, Knoxville. Donna has held leadership positions in Chi Sigma Iota, the honor society for counselors, the Association for Counselor Education and Supervision, North Carolina Counseling Association, and as a member of the American Counseling Association Governing Council. She is a former teacher and counselor in grades 7 to 12 and is a licensed school counselor and a licensed professional counselor. She holds memberships in the American Counseling Association and has been active in national, regional, and state counseling associations. Her research interests include counseling children, particularly in the school setting, international counseling, and counselor education concerns. She has collaborated with the National Board for Certified Counselors on the Mental Health Facilitators initiative. Donna has co-authored a book on school counseling and has written chapters on legal and ethical issues, developmental issues, creative arts and counseling, and other topics. She has had articles published in *The Journal of Counseling and Development*, *The Journal for Specialists in Group Work*, *Arts in Psychotherapy*, *Journal of Family Therapy*, and *Elementary School Guidance and Counseling*.

Charles L. Thompson was a professor of Counselor Education and Educational Psychology at the University of Tennessee for 39 years. His appointment was in the Department of Educational Psychology & Counseling in the College of Education, Health, & Human Science at the University of Tennessee in Knoxville. He received his bachelor's and master's degrees in science education and educational psychology from the University of Tennessee and did his Ph.D. degree concentration in counselor education, developmental psychology, and counseling psychology at the Ohio State University, where he held NDEA and Delta Theta Tau fellowships. Charles was a former teacher and counselor in grades 7 to 12. He held memberships in the American Counseling Association and the American Psychological Association. He was licensed as a psychologist and school counselor and Board Certified by the National Board of Certified Counselors. He co-authored and authored seven books and over 100 articles in journals, including the *Journal of Counseling & Development*, *Professional School Counseling*, *Journal of Mental Health Counseling*, *Counselor Education & Supervision*, *Journal of Counseling Psychology*, *International Journal of Reality Therapy*, and the *International Journal for the Advancement of Counseling*. Charles was editor of The Idea Exchange Section of the *Elementary School Guidance & Counseling Journal* from 1979 to 1997. Charles Thompson passed away on December 31, 2005.

INTRODUCTION TO COUNSELING CHILDREN

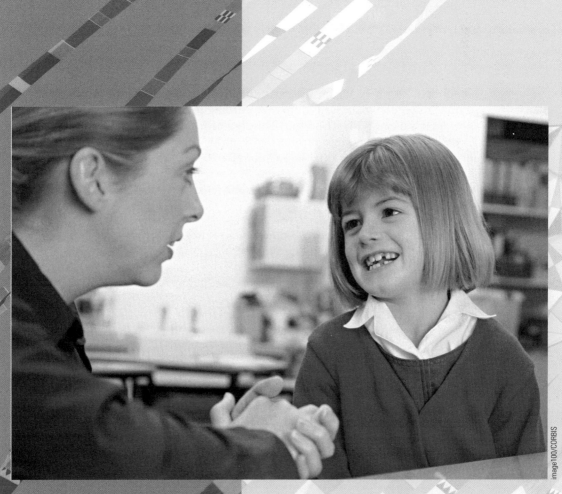

CHAPTER 1

Introduction to a Child's World

The honor of one is the honor of all. The hurt of one is the hurt of all.
—CREEK INDIAN CREED

Childhood is a time to be protected, taught, and nurtured. As the adult caretakers of our future, do we succeed in that? According to the most recent census (Federal Interagency Forum on Child and Family Statistics, 2014), in 2013 there were 73.6 million children under the age of 18 in the United States. That number represents 23.7 percent of the total population. By 2030, that number is projected to be 82 million. This chapter considers some of our responsibilities to young people and the ways our world makes growing up a challenge. After reading this chapter, you should be able to:

- Discuss the state of children in the United States
- Outline the history of children's rights
- List causes of children's problems
- Explain indicators of well-being
- Describe resilience
- Define counseling and its possibilities
- Compare the work of professionals who help children

We pride ourselves on being a child-oriented nation. Laws have been passed to prevent children from being misused in the workplace, to punish adults who exploit children, to provide ways for all children to obtain an education regardless of their mental or physical condition, and to support programs for medical care, food, and clothing for children in need. Politicians continue to debate "save our children" issues such as educational reform, living in poverty, an adolescent girl's right to an abortion without parental consent, family-leave policies in the workplace, and ways of providing a more environmentally safe world for our children's future. Much remains to be accomplished. The Children's Defense Fund (2014) recommends these priorities for elected officials: end child poverty, guarantee health and mental health care for all children, provide high-quality child care options, ensure every child reads on grade level by the fourth grade and guarantee quality education to every child through high school, invest in prevention programs, and stop child exploitation. We can make the world a better place for children and make their well-being a priority.

What could possibly be considered more precious than children? They enrich our lives and contribute to our delight. Certainly the unbounded joy of children frolicking on a playground brings smiles to the eyes of the beholder. Most teachers and other adults who interact often with young people have a storehouse of the humorous sayings and extraordinary wisdom of their charges. Children help us remember the wonder of the world. Many of us have had chances to refine our "mature" views after considering a careful answer to a question stemming from the curiosity of a younger one. Children bring us delight in these and so many other ways.

Furthermore, we know what children need to thrive. They need a place to live, adequate food and clothing, affordable health care, and safety. They need freedom from stress, caring relationships with family and friends, and positive role models. They also need opportunities to succeed in school and at other activities. Children need support and guidance as they move toward adulthood. The Children's Defense Fund (June 2014) calls for adults worldwide to leave no child behind. The mission of that organization, and for all who care for children, is "to ensure every child a *Healthy Start*, a *Head Start*, a *Fair Start*, a *Safe Start*, and a *Moral Start* in life and successful passage to adulthood with the help of caring families and communities" (preface). In addition, McCartney, Yoshikawa, and Forcier (2014) in their volume *Improving the Odds for America's Children* have collected essays that clearly delineate policies and practices needed to do the right things for children.

Yet forces too often impede their opportunities for a childhood of only manageable problems. And for all we do so well in the United States, the status of our children compared to other countries highlights too many failures in protecting childhood.

HOW AMERICA RANKS AMONG INDUSTRIALIZED COUNTRIES IN INVESTING IN AND PROTECTING CHILDREN

1st in gross domestic product

1st in number of billionaires

Second to worst in child poverty rates

Largest gap between the rich and poor

1st in health expenditures

1st in military spending

1st in number of people incarcerated

1st in military weapons exports

24th in 15-year-olds' reading scores

28th in 15-year-olds' science scores

36th in 15-year-olds' math scores

25th in low birth weight rates

31st in infant mortality rates

Second to worst in relative child poverty (ahead of Romania)

Second to worst in teenage birth rates (ahead of Bulgaria)

Worst in protecting our children against gun violence

(Children's Defense Fund, 2014).

Barriers to the well-being of young people contribute significantly to these grim statistics. For example, according to the Addy, Engelhardt, and Skinner (2013) "Children represent 24 percent of the population, but they comprise 34 percent of all people in poverty. Among all children under 18 years of age, 45 percent live in low-income families and approximately one in every five (22 percent) live in poor families." Uninsured children number 7.2 million, or 1 in 10. Furthermore even though school graduation rates have improved in the last few years, more than 8000 students drop out of high school each day in the United States. Life is not always good for too many young people.

Every adult could discover ways to ameliorate those difficulties—ways as distant as casting an informed vote, or as up close and personal as becoming a volunteer Big Brother or Big Sister. Mental health professionals have myriad possibilities for making the world healthier for children and our communities more supportive of positive, productive development. Counselors who work with children must learn to balance an appreciation for the gifts of childhood with the reality of a world of challenges. That world of challenges has changed over time. A brief consideration of the history of children's rights follows.

HISTORY

Children cannot meet their needs without some assistance. Society helps children live normal lives when medical, educational, and psychological resources are accessible and when social policies protect their rights. Those conditions have not been universally available in today's world or in the past. As you will discover, children's rights have improved from earlier times and the treatment of young people by parents and society is more protective now than in earlier times (Aries, 1962).

In early Greek and Roman societies, children were valued as servants of the city-states. Children with handicaps, disabilities, or deformities were abandoned or executed (Mash & Wolfe, 2012). In medieval times, sanitation was scarce and disease widespread. Children worked with their parents in the fields, and childhood was not looked at as a phase of life; children were considered little adults. They were treated harshly and could be punished as adults. Gradually in the Renaissance and Enlightenment, childhood began to be recognized as a special part of life. Berns (2012) referred to the development of the printing press in the 15th century. That invention provoked a new idea of adulthood—being able to read—and of childhood—not being able to read. Before that time, she explained, infancy ended at 7 and adulthood began at once. In the 16th century, schools were formed so that children could learn to read and young ones were considered "unformed adults" (Postman, 1985) which eventually became the idea of childhood—the period between infancy and total dependence and maturity or total independence.

It was not until the end of the 18th century that children's mental health concerns were addressed in professional literature. Mash and Wolfe (2012) explained that during this time the church explained children's distressing behaviors as possession of the devil or other forces of evil. The lack of antibiotics or other treatments for disease resulted in only about a third of children living past their fifth birthday in the 17th and 18th centuries. Radbill (1968) talked about many children being either harshly mistreated or ignored by their parents. Practices that cause us to shudder today such as physical and sexual abuse and neglect were considered an adult's right in the past. Mash and Wolfe discussed that for many years the view of society was that children were the property and responsibility of their parents. Some laws (Massachusetts' Stubborn Child Act of 1654) allowed parents to kill their "stubborn" children and until the mid-1800s children with disabilities could be kept in cages and cellars (Donohue, Hersen, & Ammerman, 2000).

Fortunately, things have improved for children. In the 17th century, John Locke and Jean Jacques Rousseau emphasized the idea that children should be reared with thought and care rather than with indifference and cruelty. However, children were still regarded as the property of their parents. Locke and others influenced expanding the scope of education and other philosophers called for moral guidance and support for children (Mash & Wolfe, 2012). By the late 1800s, children's rights began to be recognized as laws regulating child labor and requiring schooling for children were passed (Child Labor Education Project, n.d.).

LeVine (2007) gave a historical overview of child studies, including the story of Dorothea Dix (1802–1887), the founder of hospitals for the treatment of troubled young people who had previously been confined to cages or cellars. Children were beginning to be recognized as individuals who deserved attention to their needs. A clinic for children having school adjustment problems was founded at the University of Pennsylvania in 1896 and a center for troubled teens was formed in Chicago. In 1905, Alfred Binet finished his first efforts on intelligence testing; his first tests were used for making educational decisions in Paris schools. These efforts built a base for the child guidance movement that focused on a multidisciplinary team for the diagnosis and treatment of children's problems.

A landmark in mental health work with children was Sigmund Freud's writings about Little Hans and his phobia. Freud presented a psychoanalytic explanation of the issues and led the father through the treatment with Hans. In 1926, Anna Freud gave a series of lectures to the Vienna Institute of Psychoanalysis. Her "Introduction to the Technique of Psycho-Analysis of Children" talks provoked interest and established child psychotherapy as a legitimate field (Prout, 2007). In 1932, Melanie Klein introduced concepts of play therapy such as the substitution of play for free association. A positive impact on children's needs being met occurred in 1924, when the American Orthopsychiatric Association of psychologists, social workers, and psychiatrists was formed for the professionals concerned with the mental health problems of children (Prout).

By the mid-1960s, children were considered individuals in their own right and therefore protected by the Bill of Rights. The Supreme Court decision *In re Gault*, 387 U.S. 1 (1967) (United States Courts, n.d.) determined that status. Gault was a 15-year-old who had been arrested for an obscene phone call and incarcerated until the age of 21. Adults convicted of that offense would have been given a $50 fine and 2 months in jail. The dispute about Gault's case reached the Supreme Court. Disputed were facts about the case such as his having no formal hearing or transcript records and no specific charges against him except that he was a delinquent. The court ruled that basic due process rights, such as having a hearing and being represented by counsel, should have been provided. That decision and those of other rulings extended the Fourteenth Amendment protections to minors. While parents still make legal decisions for their children, minors are now protected by the U.S. Constitution (Strom-Gottfried, 2008).

Yet childhood today is still not a time of fantasy, play, freedom from responsibility, and an unfettered freedom to develop (Berns, 2012). Youth face different challenges as they are hurried through childhood. The Children's Defense Fund (2014) admonishes everyone to work harder for children in this world in which both parents work long hours, drugs are easily available, sex can be seen on television or the Internet, and violence is just around the corner. Children are now one of the largest consumer groups and marketing efforts directed at them use provocative temptations in attempts to sell food, clothing, and toys. Sports are more and more competitive, and "play" often happens in front of a computer or play station. Those realities and the societal pressure on parents to provide for all the child wants has contributed to some consequences that influence childhood.

What Causes Our Children's Problems?

The causes of children's problems cannot be isolated to any simple explanation. The intersections of personal factors, family variables, cultural, environmental, and many other influences combine to create situations in which children are floundering and needing help to regain their balance. While reading the following situations, consider whether they sound improbable or all too common:

Tommy is a fifth grader referred for counseling because of "lack of motivation." He is a loner who does not seem to want friends. He appears unenthusiastic about life except his video games. He has begun to exhibit signs of aggressiveness—increased fighting and abusive language. When he isn't fighting, he sits with his head on his desk refusing to participate in anything. His teachers are concerned about this pattern in his behavior.

Maria is a first grader whose parents have recently divorced. Her mother and father have found other partners, and in the excitement of their new lives, they have little time for Maria. She is very confused about whom she can trust. At this very crucial point in her school life, she is floundering in an unstable world. Her school work is poor and she is withdrawing from adults and peers. She cries often and seems lost in any setting.

Stacie's family lives in poverty. Neither of her parents completed high school, and neither has been able to hold a steady job. Stacie's few clothes are too small for her and sometimes not clean. She often does not have lunch or lunch money, and she complains about being hungry at home. At school, she seems to be in her own dream world. She has few friends and is often teased by her classmates.

Carlos, an eighth grader, has been acting out since he was in the first grade, and no adult has been able to work with him effectively. He comes from a family that has obvious wealth, and his parents have tried to provide him with care and loving support. Carlos is constantly in trouble for hitting, lying, and name-calling. He now has begun to fight in class and with children in his neighborhood. There are rumors about spousal abuse in his home, but Carlos refuses to discuss anything about his family life. He is unpleasant to all adults and quick to put everyone on the defensive.

Broken Nose has been diagnosed as having attention-deficit/hyperactivity disorder (ADHD), but his parents refuse to accept his diagnosis. They blame the school for Broken Nose's learning and behavioral problems and insist he has no symptoms at home. Broken Nose is two grades behind in reading and is a constant disruption in his classroom, begging for help but unable to focus for any length of time. His teacher has given up, saying that she cannot help Broken Nose unless his parents cooperate with her educational plan.

A Changing World

Parents often like to think that children are immune to the stressful complexities and troubles of the rapidly changing adult world. They see childhood as a carefree, irresponsible time, with no financial worries, societal pressures, or work-related troubles. Many adults who consider themselves child advocates do not understand children's perceptions. They do not believe a child's concerns matter significantly, and they see children as largely unaware of what is happening politically and economically. Those assumptions are incorrect.

Adults who underestimate children's awareness of the world may also misjudge children in other matters. Our experience in working with children has been that they are effective problem solvers and decision makers when they have the opportunity to be in a nonthreatening counseling atmosphere with a counselor who listens and supports them. Adults who help children discover their own strengths and practice their skills will create the constructive environment needed for reaching their potential.

As you will read in Chapter 2, normal child development involves a series of cognitive, physical, emotional, and social changes. Almost all children at some time experience difficulty in adjusting to the changes, and the accompanying stress or conflict can lead to learning or behavioral problems. Normal child development tasks include achieving independence, learning to relate to peers, developing confidence in self, coping with an ever-changing body, forming basic values, and mastering new ways of thinking and new information. Other circumstances may also heighten stress, including things like changes in home or school locations, death or divorce in the family, and major illnesses. A high degree of stress has been found to be strongly associated with behavior symptoms. Add the stresses and conflicts of a rapidly changing society—which even adults find difficult to understand—to normal developmental concerns, and the child's world looks as complex and difficult as an adult's. However even with that backdrop of challenges, we can encourage a world that supports children's well-being. Next we will consider resources and descriptions devoted to that better situation.

Several authors and organizations collect information on the condition of children. Ben-Arieh, Casas, Frønes, and Korbin (2013) compiled an extensive collection of work on the well-being of children. Weissberg, Walberg, O'Brien, and Kuster (2003) offered a study of the long-term trends in the well-being of children in the United States, an informative volume that details issues in the lives of children and their families. In addition, each year the Children's Defense Fund publishes *The State of America's Children*, which considers the impact of many factors on youth development. An annual collection of trends for those factors can be found in the *Kids Count Data Book* produced by the Annie E. Casey Foundation and the race for results info graphics about progress in building a better world for children. All these sources not only provide data related to children in the United States but also present summaries of successful intervention programs and action guides for child advocates.

Orton (1997) identifies many of those issues in her description of the world as having many faces of poverty, describing these deficiencies as a poverty of resources, a poverty of tolerance, a poverty of time, and a poverty of values. She discusses the poverty of resources, with more than 14 million U.S. children as victims. Hunger, poor housing, unemployment, and homelessness are evidence of this type of poverty. Orton also writes about the poverty of tolerance for each other and for anyone who is dissimilar. Intolerance and the ignorance and fear it engenders reduce the quality of life for each individual in our society. The poverty of time relates to the widespread fatigue of a life moving too fast and of demands too great. Finally, Orton points out what she considers a poverty of values. Her examples include the high incidence of abuse, crime, and violence. Her explanation of these difficulties in the world helps us understand the stresses of childhood.

In summary, mental health professionals need to be prepared to work with issues that significantly impact the lives of young people. They must learn about the things that increase children's vulnerabilities and consider all the environmental stresses that exacerbate normal child development.

The American Home

According to developmental psychologists, children need warm, loving, and stable home environments to grow and develop in a healthy manner. Brazelton and Greenspan (2000) have emphasized that type of home environment as an irreducible need. Hernandez (2003) reminds us that parents are the most important people in a child's world, not only because they provide the day-to-day care and nurturing needed but also because they supply the economic resources needed for shelter, food, health care, and other necessities. In the child's family, the child is socialized to the values, beliefs, attitudes, knowledge, skills, and techniques of their culture. Children also learn their ethnic, racial, religious, socioeconomic, and gender roles in the family with all the inherent behaviors and obligations (Berns, 2012).

In today's society, family constellations include intact families, single-parent homes, teen-parent families, intergenerational families, blended families, same-sex parents, and many other structures. Grandparents may live 3000 miles away and be almost unknown to their grandchildren. Other extended family seldom lives nearby. Parents may work long hours to provide financial security for their families and also may be expected to attend meetings or other community events at night. Mothers still shoulder the primary responsibility for care of the home, so they are often occupied at night with cooking, laundry, cleaning, or helping with homework. Single parents assume the roles of both mother and father, doubling the burden on the parent and too often leaving little free time to spend with their children. Military families often face the deployment of one or both parents to war-torn countries. The pace and stresses of our times may mean that children cannot find someone to listen to them or provide the care and guidance they need, even though adults are present.

Economic issues add to the challenge. Currently, unemployment is high and many workers are underemployed, dissatisfied, or otherwise stressed while trying to provide for a family.

Crime, corrupt public figures, a world full of tension, war, and the threat of terrorism that may strike anywhere at any time also create an environment of uncertainty and fear. Children are as close as a television or Web site to the coverage of our social problems, and without an adult to help them may be overwhelmed by the conditions of our world.

Changing Values

Children are forming values in a rapidly changing world. What is right or wrong seems to change daily or varies with the person. Who has the absolute answer concerning standards of sexuality, cohabitation, alternative lifestyles, or abortion? Are the various liberation movements or tea party politics good or bad? How does a person behave in a world with changing gender roles? Will drugs really harm a person? Should society condone mercy killing? Is capital punishment justified? Adults with mature thinking processes and years of life experience have difficulty making rational judgments on such ethical and moral issues. However, Berns (2012) talked about some basic societal values such as justice, compassion, equality, truth, love, and knowledge. We would add the values of peace, goodness, delight in life, and oneness with humanity. Children will struggle, challenge, and experiment as they try to determine their own value foundations; as teenagers, they will be quick to explain the reasons their choices are the right ones. As adults, we have obligations to be consistent models who exhibit the positive principles of caring for each other.

Summary of Children's Difficulties

No simple answer to what causes our children's problems has emerged. The home, society, and changing values contribute to the well-being and the difficulties of childhood. The most vulnerable children are those who face multiple risk factors. O'Brien, Weissberg, Walberg, and Kuster (2003) identify the most significant indicators of poor long-term outcomes for children as not living with both parents; household headed by a high school dropout; family income below the poverty level; parents who do not have steady, full-time employment; families receiving welfare benefits; and lack of health insurance (p. 23). Finally the largest examination of the correlation between maltreatment in childhood and health as an adult (Center for

Disease Control, Adverse Childhood Experiences [ACE] Study) indicates that certain difficult childhood experiences create risk factors for illnesses and poor health.

No one can deny that every child needs to feel loved and valued at home, at school, and in a community. Some children do enjoy secure childhoods that prepare them to meet the challenges of contemporary society, but many need additional support to navigate the confusing world around them. Although every adult was once a child, as early as the days of Socrates and Aristotle, adults have felt that the younger generation was "going to the dogs." Yet, in spite of the multiple challenges that face children today, there is hope. Let us turn to reasons for being optimistic about our children's future.

World Initiative and Understanding

The world is paying attention to the special care and assistance needed for children. A document titled "The U.N. Convention on the Rights of the Child" has been ratified by all members of the United Nations except the United States and Somalia (which has no legally constituted government). As a rationale for their convention on the rights of the child, UNICEF (1990) recorded these beliefs as fundamental in addressing the needs of children everywhere:

Children are individuals. Children are neither the possessions of parents nor of the state, nor are they mere people-in-the-making; they have equal status as members of the human family.

Children start life as totally dependent beings. Children must rely on adults for the nurture and guidance they need to grow toward independence. Such nurture is ideally found in adults in children's families, but when primary caregivers cannot meet children's needs, it is up to society to fill the gap.

The actions, or inactions, of government impact children more strongly than any other group in society. Practically every area of government policy (e.g., education, public health, and so on) affects children to some degree. Short-sighted policymaking that fails to take children into account has a negative impact on the future of all members of society by giving rise to policies that cannot work.

Children's views are rarely heard and rarely considered in the political process. Children generally do not vote and do not otherwise take part in political processes. Without special attention to the opinions of children—as expressed at home and in schools, in local communities, and even in governments—children's views go unheard on the many important issues that affect them now or will affect them in the future.

Many changes in society are having a disproportionate, and often negative, impact on children. Transformations of the family structure, globalization, shifting employment patterns, and a shrinking social welfare net in many countries all have strong impacts on children. The impact of these changes can be particularly devastating in situations of armed conflict and other emergencies.

The healthy development of children is crucial to the future well-being of any society. Because they are still developing, children are especially vulnerable—more so than adults—to poor living conditions such as poverty, inadequate health care, nutrition, safe water, housing, and environmental pollution. The effects of disease, malnutrition, and poverty threaten the future of children and therefore the future of the societies in which they live.

The costs to society of failing its children are huge. Social research findings show that children's earliest experiences significantly influence their future development. The course of their development determines their contribution, or cost, to society over the course of their lives.

These statements indicate the ratifying governments' written appreciation of the care needed to enact policies to inform practices that support children's well-being. The supportive laws are one component to support healthy development. What else do we know about the things in a child's life that support their reaching their potential?

WELL-BEING

The Center for Disease Control and Prevention (n.d.) has concluded that no one definition of well-being has emerged. However agreement exists that minimally, well-being includes the presence of positive emotions and moods (e.g., contentment, happiness), the absence of negative emotions (e.g., depression, anxiety), satisfaction with life, fulfillment, and positive functioning. Thus well-being can be described as judging life positively and feeling good. Similarly Murphey and his colleagues (July 2014) discuss wellness along the dimensions of illness to no illness and flourishing to struggling. The illness flourishing dimension encompasses functioning well and feeling well.

Moore, Vandivere, Lippman, McPhee, and Bloch (2007) and Moore and other colleagues (2011) have refined indices that display the condition of children in the United States, highlighting specific domains of well-being. They have specific indicators in the physical, psychological, social, and cognitive/educational domains. Their work allows researchers and practitioners to distinguish the causes for concerns from the roots of well-being for children.

Brazelton and Greenspan (2000), a pediatrician and a child psychiatrist, wrote about what they call the "irreducible needs" for a child to grow, learn, and thrive. They list the following components as fundamental for a child's health:

- Continuing, nurturing relationships
- Physical protection and safety with regulations to safeguard those needs
- Experiences tailored to individual differences for each child's optimal development
- Developmentally appropriate opportunities as building blocks for cognitive, motor, language, emotional, and social skills
- Adults who set limits, provide structure, and guide by having appropriate expectations
- A community that is stable, supportive, and consistent.

Murphey and colleagues (n.d.) suggest being well means exercising abilities, forming bonds with other, adapting successfully to challenges, and being happy.

In their policy brief those authors outline a framework for programs and services to promote well-being for children, their parents, and the environments where young people live, learn, play, and grow. They describe the landscape as a world where wellness is a national priority. Those who are not well have access to needed help and milder concerns are addressed in schools, child care settings, or doctor's offices. Parents are supported with more time for maternity leave and visits by professionals who offer guidance on positive parenting. As children grown, parents have access to workshops on relevant developmental issues. Schools and other community institutions provide activities to promote wellness and screen for early signs of illness. Children learn daily habits to build and conserve their own wellness. Schools teach not only cognitive but also social-emotional skills. Teachers know the signs of potential trouble and ways to react appropriately. Caring adults and peers get children to appropriate help. Institutions for young people with troubled lives such as youth shelters, child welfare systems, and the juvenile justice system are dedicated to improving self-efficacy and overall wellness of the youth they serve. We believe counselors have similar ideals for their clients.

The Child Welfare League of America (2013) has published a blueprint for ensuring excellence for children, families, and communities in the United States. The vision states that all children grow up safely in loving families and supportive communities connected to their cultures. The core principles of that vision include children's rights, shared responsibilities, engagement, supports, funding, and resources among other things. That group outlines standards for each principle to raise the bar for children.

Many children pass successfully through the developmental stages of childhood and adolescence and become well-functioning adults. Other children overcome the adversities of their childhoods and go on to lead productive and meaningful lives. These children have the resilience to carry them through health problems, maltreatment, poverty, and other unfavorable conditions.

Resilience

A promising line of research in child counseling revolves around the concept of resiliency, the dynamic process of people who do better than expected in adverse circumstances; they beat the odds (Arbona & Coleman, 2008). Resilience is the ability to handle stress in a positive way.

Rak (2001) explains that counselors often question whether to help clients overcome problems or instead focus on clients' strengths and resiliency. He provides some guidelines for focusing on resilience. In a comprehensive article, Rak and Patterson (1996) define resiliency in children as the ability "to continue to progress in their positive development despite being 'bent,' 'compressed,' or 'stretched' by factors in a risky environment" (p. 368). Benard (2004) summarizes this concept as the capacity all young people have for healthy development and successful living. Masten (2001), who has extensively researched the concept of resiliency, explains:

> What began as a quest to understand the extraordinary has revealed the power of the ordinary. Resilience does not come from rare and special qualities, but from the everyday magic of ordinary, normative human resources in the minds, brains, and bodies of children, in their families and relationships, and in their communities. (p. 235)

According to Benard (2004), Masten (2001), Walsh (2006), and Werner and Smith (2001), our focus needs to be on the strength of people. They consider resilience as a natural drive, a self-righting tendency toward health not limited to any ethnicity, social class, or geographic boundary. Luthar (2006) concluded that as well as personal strength, resilient adaptation requires strong supportive relationships. For more reviews on resilient adaptation, readers can refer to Masten and Obradovic (2006), Masten and Powell (2003), Walsh (2006), and Zolkoski and Bullock (2012).

Benard (2004) states four categories of personal strengths are the positive developmental outcomes of resilience, protective factors that Lee and colleagues (2013) indicated in their meta-analytic approach as the largest effect on resilience. Benard's explanation of those strengths coincides with and summarizes the descriptions of other researchers noted previously. The four categories Benard proposes are social competence, problem solving, autonomy, and a sense of purpose. Characteristics of these qualities are discussed next.

Social competence involves the characteristics, skills, and attitudes needed to form positive relationships and to become attached to other people. The socially competent person has a friendly nature, the ability to elicit positive responses from others, and good verbal skills. These young people can communicate their personal needs in an appropriate way. They show empathy, compassion, altruism, and forgiveness toward others. In addition, resilient children receive affection and support from caregivers.

These young people have "good intellectual functioning" (Masten & Coatsworth, 1998) and are active problem solvers. They are proactive, intentional, and flexible. Resilient children use critical thinking skills and have the capacity to develop meaningful insight.

According to Benard (2004), autonomy concerns developing one's sense of self, one's sense of positive identity, and one's sense of power. Acting independently and having a sense of control over the environment are other characteristics of the autonomous child. Benard also lists the concepts of internal locus of control, initiative, self-efficacy, mastery, adaptive distancing, mindfulness, and humor in this category of personal strengths. Alvord and Grados (2005) and Benzies and Myshasiuk (2009) cite self-regulation as the most fundamental factor in the resilient young person and are confident in their capacity to overcome barriers.

The fourth identified category relates to the sense that life has meaning (Benard, 2004). Resilient youngsters believe in a positive and strong future. That faith in the future has a direct correlation with academic success, positive self-identity, and fewer risky behaviors. Other distinctive attributes within this category are goal direction, creativity, special interest, optimism, and hope.

Benard (2004) argues these resilient characteristics are developmental possibilities of every individual. She supports her line of reasoning in a summary of research from several theoretical models that support these concepts as critical life skills. For example, she has connected the attributes of resilience to the basic needs described by Maslow (1970), to emotional intelligence (Goleman, 1995), to multiple intelligences (Gardner, 1993), and to Erikson's developmental stages (1963).

Resiliency tendencies can be augmented. Some authors (Benson, 1997; Brooks, 2006; Garmezy, 1991; Greenberg, 2006; Hauser, 1999; Lowenthal, 1998; Luthar, 2006; Walsh, 2006; Werner & Smith, 2001) have studied resiliency and developed lists of protective factors or variables that act as buffers for the many children who overcome their difficulties to grow and lead well-adjusted lives. Greenberg integrated neuroscience and prevention research into interventions that promote resilience. He explained those interventions improve the brains' executive functions, inhibitory control, planning, problem solving, emotional regulation, and attention capacities. The PATHS curriculum, a school-based prevention curriculum focused on reducing aggression and problem behavior, includes affective-behavioral-cognitive and dynamic interventions.

Families who enhance resilience have ties with caregivers and associations with friends and others in stable households. Young people in these families are helpful with appropriate domestic responsibilities. Families are warm, structured, and have positive discipline practices. The parents monitor their children, listen, and talk to the child. In addition, families who support resilient behavior have a faith that gives them a sense of coherence, meaning, and compassion (Benzies & Mychasiuk, 2009).

Communities enhance resilience when young people are able to make and keep friends, when the community values education, when there is structure and clear limits, and when there is positive mentoring at school and beyond (Lewis, 2006). Luthar (2006) pointed to the community resources of quality child care, comprehensive family services, relationships outside the family, community cohesion, and participation in community activities as necessary. The environmental characteristics in families and communities that support positive development can be summarized as caring and support, high expectations, and opportunities for participation (Benard, 2004). Lewis further describes these qualities as follows:

- *Caring and support:* A connection with at least one caring adult is the most important variable in fostering positive youth development. Those relationships provide stable care, affection, attention, social networks across generations, a sense of trust, and climates of care and support.
- *High expectations:* Adults recognize the strengths and assets of young people more than the problems and deficits. Adults see a youngster's potential for maturity, responsibility, self-discipline, and common sense. Adults provide structure, order, clear expectations, and cultural traditions. They value young people and promote their chances for social and academic success.
- *Opportunities for participation:* Young people have chances to connect to other people, to their interests, and to valuable life experiences. Youth can participate in socially and economically useful tasks. They have responsibilities for decision making, planning, and helping others as meaningful participants (p. 44).

Rak and Patterson (1996) provide a set of questions to guide counselors in uncovering the patterns of helpful habits that children have. Rak (2001) proposes that the counselor use this set of questions with follow-up responses to develop "an assessment that minimizes judgment, enhances salutogenesis [origins of health], and evaluates the client's life space, support systems, and capacity to endure and overcome" (p. 229). With this understanding of the child's historical pattern of resilience, counselors can provide interventions to reinforce those patterns. The Devereux Early Childhood Assessment (DECA; Naglieri & LeBuffle, 2005) is an assessment for children 2–5, and Ahem, Kiehl, Sole, and Byers (2006) recommend the Resilience Scale (RS) for adolescents.

Counselors can teach or model self-management and effective coping skills for problems and stressors. Rak (2001) notes that counselors who work with resilience in mind do not focus on arriving at solutions or resolving conflicts. Rather, that type of counseling emphasizes the "client's reservoir" of resilient behavior. Some possible ways for counselors to provide support to young people include: (1) role-plays that help young people learn to express themselves; (2) conflict resolution techniques to help young people through interpersonal difficulties; (3) nurturing, empathy, authenticity, realistic reinforcement, and genuine hope from the counselor; (4) models of healthy interactions; (5) peer support interventions; (6) creative imagery; and (7) bibliotherapy (Rak & Patterson, 1996).

The resiliency approach to understanding children provides one example of looking at the positive attributes of human beings. Arbona and Coleman (2008) explained ways African American young people could use resilient adaptation to face discrimination and buffer the inherent negative consequences. Identifying coping mechanisms that lead to protective factors for stress helps counselors promote healthy lifestyles. Likewise, the work of Rogers and Maslow contributes to a view on positive, healthy development that allows counselors to take a perspective focused on strength when working with children, concentrating on what they can rather than what they cannot do (Nystul, 2010). Attachment theory (Ainsworth, 1989; Bowlby, 1988; Ainsworth, 1989) also contributes insights into ways counselors can help children move toward full psychosocial development. A thorough understanding of these strengths-based approaches will support effective counseling practices.

An emphasis on prevention, strengths, and protective factors is gaining favor with policymakers as well. The Institute of Medicine (2009) delivered a report on preventing disorders among young people, the Center for Health and Health Care in Schools (2013) noted lessons from 11 states, and the Affordable Care Act of 2010 (U.S. Department of Health and Human Services, 2014) has provisions to children's mental wellness needs.

Although some children do have the resiliency to survive a poor home environment, extreme adversity threatens them (Masten, 2011). Additionally a growing number of young people have emotional, behavioral, social, and other problems that warrant mental health treatment. Resources for counselors and others who work with children are increasing; however, clinical, agency, and school professionals have felt frustrated because information about specific counseling procedures for developmental, learning, and behavioral problems has been limited and difficult to obtain. This book provides people in clinical, agency, school, and other counseling situations with suggestions for counseling children with specific learning or behavioral problems, as well as ways to support the mental health of children.

COMMUNITY SERVICES

Berns (2012) outlined community services that are available to support children and their families. She categorized the types of services as preventive, supportive, or rehabilitative. Parks, recreation, and education are examples of preventive services that provide for space, socializing, physical activity, and mental stimulation. Boy Scouts and Girl Scouts of America, Boys' and Girls' Clubs, American Red Cross, and the Young Men's Christian Association (YMCA) and the Young Women's Christian Association (YWCA) are examples of preventive services. Schools also fall into that category.

Supportive services have the goal of preserving healthy family life by helping members. The federal Family Preservation and Support Services Program (FPSSP) aims to keep the family safe, to avoid unnecessary placement of children in substitute care, and to improve family functioning. Counseling, education, referrals, assistance, and advocacy are the ways those goals are accomplished. Child welfare agencies are designed to protect the physical, intellectual, and emotional well-being of children. These agencies provide economic and personal help to children living in their own homes, foster care for children who do not have a home or who cannot remain with their families, and institutional care when children cannot go to foster homes and cannot stay with their families. Other supportive services include protective services, child care, and adoption.

Rehabilitation services try to enable or restore a person's ability to participate effectively in the community by correcting behavior, providing mental health services, and responding to special needs. The juvenile justice system attempts to determine causes for children's deviant behavior and what steps need to be taken to effect remediation. Juvenile judges may put children under the supervision of their parents, stipulating family counseling. Judges may choose to place children in foster care or in institutions. Problems like truancy, running away, lying, stealing, vandalism, setting fires, and extreme aggressiveness may result in referrals to clinics that provide medical and psychological examinations and services.

Some programs address services to the poor. One is the Temporary Assistance for Needy Families, a welfare reform program that replaced Aid to Families with Dependent Children. Child nutrition services provide food stamps, school lunches and breakfasts, and other aid for food. Subsidized day care, child health programs, and Medicaid are other supportive programs available for poor children. The professionals, including counselors, in all of these community programs serve the needs of the impoverished community.

WHAT IS COUNSELING?

Earlier the American Psychological Association, Division of Counseling Psychology, Committee on Definition (1956), defined *counseling* as a process "to help individuals toward overcoming obstacles to their personal growth, wherever these may be encountered, and toward achieving optimum development of their personal resources" (p. 283). The following definitions have been adopted by both the American Counseling Association (ACA) and the National Board for Certified Counselors (NBCC):

The Practice of Professional Counseling: The application of mental health, psychological, or human development principles, through cognitive, affective, behavioral, or systemic intervention strategies, that address wellness, personal growth, or career development as well as pathology.

Professional Counseling Specialty: A Professional Counseling Specialty is narrowly focused, requiring advanced knowledge in the field founded on the premise that all Professional Counselors must first meet the requirements for the general practice of professional counseling.

Atkinson (2002) summarizes other explanations of counseling. He identifies counseling as a profession that deals with personal, social, vocational, empowerment, and educational concerns. It is for people who are within the normal range of functioning. Counseling is theory based and structured. In counseling, people learn to make decisions and to find new ways to behave, feel, and think. Counseling includes subspecialties such as career counseling, rehabilitation counseling, and others. Counselors may have roles in prevention, remediation, and positive development. The focus is on intact personalities, personal assets, strengths, and positive mental health, regardless of the severity of the disturbance. Counseling is relatively brief and emphasizes person–environment interactions and the educational and career development of individuals.

How Does Counseling Differ from Psychotherapy?

Distinctions between counseling and psychotherapy may be superficial in that both processes have similar objectives and techniques. Nystul (2010) suggests the main difference involves counseling exploring the conscious processes and psychotherapy examining unconscious processes. In addition, Nystul discusses more specific distinctions between counseling and psychotherapy, underscoring a differentiation in focus, client problems, treatment goals, and treatment approaches. Table 1-1 contains further information about these variations. Although this table summarizes some differences, those features are often lost in the common ground they share. The key question about each process rests with counselors and therapists, who must restrict their practice to their areas of competence.

TABLE 1-1 COMPARISON OF COUNSELING AND PSYCHOTHERAPY

Counseling Is More for	Psychotherapy Is More for
Clients	Patients
Mild disorders	Serious disorders
Personal, social, vocational, educational, and decision-making problems	Personality problems
Preventive and developmental concerns	Remedial concerns
Educational and developmental settings	Clinical and medical settings
Conscious concerns	Unconscious concerns
Teaching methods	Healing methods

WHAT IS OUR WORKING DEFINITION OF COUNSELING?

Counseling involves a relationship between two people who meet so that one person can help the other resolve a problem. One of these people, by virtue of training, is the counselor; the person receiving the help is the client. Some other terms are *helper* and *helpee, child, adolescent, adult,* or *person.* In fact, Carl Rogers (see Chapter 6) refers to his client-centered counseling approach as *person-centered.*

We see counseling as a process in which people learn how to help themselves and, in effect, become their own counselors. Counseling may also be a group process, in which the role of helper and helpee can be shared and interchanged among the group members. The group counselor then functions as a facilitator as well as a counselor.

Coleman, Morris, and Glaros (1987) credit David Palmer of the Student Counseling Center at UCLA with one of the best definitions of counseling we have found:

To be listened to and to be heard

To be supported while you gather your forces and get your bearings

A fresh look at alternatives and some new insights; learning some needed skills

To face your lion—your fears

To come to a decision—and the courage to act on it and to take the risks that living demands (p. 282)

WHAT COUNSELING CAN DO

Mental health incorporates the way we think, feel, and act; how we look at ourselves, our lives, and other people; how we evaluate and make choices; and how we handle stress, relate to others, and make decisions. Mental health exists along a continuum from good to not so good to poor. A person may be more mentally healthy at some times than at other times. At certain times an individual may seek help for handling specific problems. A young person's performance on schoolwork, his or her success in relationships, and his or her physical health may suffer during difficult times. Mental health problems in children and adolescents may lead to school failure, violence, suicide, family distress, drug abuse, and a host of other difficult situations.

Counseling with children is a growing area of interest for mental health professionals. Developmental theorists have studied children's growth and development and the effect of childhood experiences on the adult, whereas child psychiatry has focused on seriously disturbed children. However, children with learning, social, or behavioral problems who are not classified as severely disturbed have been largely overlooked. Counseling can prevent "normal" problems from becoming more serious and resulting in delinquency, school failure, and emotional disturbance. Counselors can work to create a healthy environment to help children cope with the stresses and conflicts of their growth and development. Counseling can also help children in trouble through appraisal, individual or group counseling, parent or teacher consultation, or environmental changes.

The principles of counseling with children are the same as those used with adults; however, as discussed throughout this chapter, the counselor needs to be aware of the world as the child sees it and adjust his or her counseling procedures to suit the child's cognitive level, emotional and social development, and physical abilities. Each child is a unique individual with particular characteristics and needs. Childhood should be a time for healthy growth, for establishing warm and rewarding relationships, for exploring a widening world, for developing confidence in oneself and others, and for learning and experiencing. It should contain some fun and carefree times, and it should also provide a foundation and guidance for the maturing person with many opportunities to stretch.

What Specific Types of Assistance Can Be Expected from the Counseling Session?

Counseling generally involves three areas: (1) the client's thoughts and feelings about life at present, (2) where the client would like to be in life, and (3) plans to reduce any discrepancy between the first and second areas.

The emphasis given to each area varies according to the counseling approach used. Nevertheless, most counseling approaches seem to share the ultimate goal of behavior change, although they may differ in the method used to attain that goal.

Perhaps the most important outcome for counseling occurs when clients learn how to be their own counselors. By teaching children the counseling process, we help them become more skilled in solving their problems and, in turn, they become less dependent on others. In our view, counseling is a process of re-education designed to replace faulty learning with better strategies for getting what the child wants from life. Regardless of the counseling approach, children bring three pieces of information to the counseling session: (1) their problem or concern, (2) their feelings about the problem, and (3) their expectations of the counselor. Failure to listen for these points makes further counseling a waste of time.

Most problems brought to the counselor concerning children can be classified in one or more of five categories:

1. *Interpersonal conflict or conflict with others:* The child has difficulty in relating with parents, siblings, teachers, or peers and is seeking a better way to relate to them.
2. *Intrapersonal conflict or conflict with self:* The child has a decision-making problem and needs some help with clarifying the alternatives and consequences.
3. *Lack of information about self:* The child needs to learn more about his or her abilities, strengths, interests, or values.
4. *Lack of information about the environment:* The child needs information about what it takes to succeed in school or general career education.
5. *Lack of skill:* The child needs to learn a specific skill, such as effective study methods, assertive behavior, listening, or how to make friends.

In summary, counseling goals and objectives can range from becoming one's own counselor to positive behavior change, problem solving, decision making, personal growth, remediation, and self-acceptance. The counseling process for children often includes training in communication, relationship skills, and effective study;

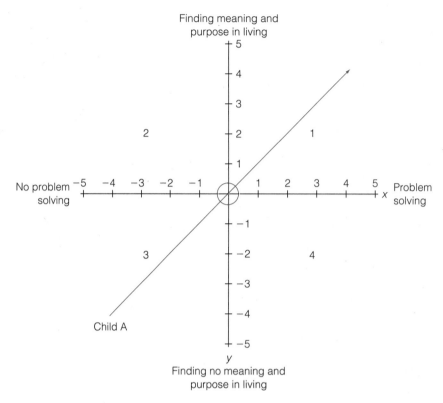

FIGURE 1-1   COUNSELING FOCUS SCALE

however, counselors choose the focus that seems most appropriate for the child and the child's situation. Some counselors prefer to work on developing meaning and purpose in everyday living, whereas others work toward solving specific problems. Of course, many counselors try to accomplish both ends. Conceivably, Child A could start at point –5 on both the x-axis and the y-axis and move toward +5 on both axes.

In counseling children in their middle childhood years (ages 5 to 12), for example, counselors may choose to work with problem areas in any or all of the quadrants represented in Figure 1-1. Some counselors prefer to work with the developmental and personal growth concerns found in Quadrant 1. The children in Quadrant 1 are solving their problems and seem to be finding purpose in living. They are sometimes referred to as stars because they get along well with their friends, teachers, and family. Children in Quadrant 1 seem to have a winner's script for achieving their goals in academic, athletic, social, and artistic endeavors. Working with these children is often a matter of staying out of their way, helping them develop their full potential, and ensuring that they receive the appropriate teaching and parenting necessary for the development of their gifts and talents. This developmental model, emphasizing problem prevention over remediation, was pioneered by Herman J. Peters (Peters & Farwell, 1959), who encouraged counselors to focus on their clients' strengths as a way to facilitate their next steps up the developmental ladder. As we discussed previously, the developmental strengths emphasis continues to be popular in counseling literature.

Children in Quadrant 2 find purpose in life but are not able to solve many of their problems. The counselor's role with these children is remedial in that counseling is directed toward establishing problem-solving strategies. Frequently, these children have good interpersonal relationships but experience problems with academic achievement and self-concept. They lack the success identity found in children in Quadrant 1.

Children in Quadrant 4 do very well with their everyday problem solving but do not seem to find life exciting or challenging. Frequently, these children have little fun and few high points in their lives. If asked to identify successes or celebrations in the past week, they may have difficulty. Counseling plans for this group are more developmental than remedial in that the goals are directed toward building high points for each day of the child's life.

Children in Quadrant 3 represent the toughest counseling cases. They are not solving their problems, and they find little value in living their lives. Children in this group suffer from depression, have a very poor self-concept, and may be potential suicides. Frequently, no one really loves and cares about these children, and they have no one to love and care for in return. These children have experienced a world of failure at home and at school. Counseling with these children is a highly remedial process directed toward encouragement and, as in all counseling, establishing a positive, caring relationship between counselor and child. Once a helpful relationship has been established, the counseling focus can be directed toward building success experiences in the child's life.

Who Are the Professional Caregivers?

Those seeking help for children need to choose the counselor best suited to the child's and family's needs and the particular type of problem. Various people trained in the helping professions—counselors, school counselors, school psychologists, social workers, marriage and family counselors, counseling psychologists, clinical psychologists, rehabilitation counselors, child development counselors—work with children (Table 1-2). Their duties may include individual counseling, group counseling, and/or consultation in a school, agency, clinic, hospital, criminal justice facility, or other institutional setting. These counseling and consulting roles focus on assisting children with their personal, social, developmental, educational, or vocational concerns; collecting and analyzing data (personality, interests, aptitude, attitudes, intelligence, etc.) about an individual through interviews, tests, case histories, observational techniques, and other means; and using statistical data to carry out evaluative functions, research, or follow-up activities. A counselor can serve in an administrative role as the director of a school guidance unit, as the head of an institutional counseling division, or can be engaged primarily in teaching or research. The various types of helpers, the different licensure and degree requirements, the range of skills and responsibilities, as well as the diverse work settings can be found in Table 1-2.

More specifically we include definitions of four professions who help children. Counselors apply "mental health, psychological or human development principles

TABLE 1-2 MENTAL HEALTH PROFESSIONALS

Professional	Minimum Degree Requirement	Work Setting
Human service worker	Baccalaureate	Human service agencies
Juvenile justice counselor	Baccalaureate	Juvenile justice system
Child development specialist	Master's	Community agencies
Community agency counselor	Master's	Private practice Community agencies
Marriage and family therapist	Master's	Private practice Community agencies
Mental health counselor	Master's	Private practice Community agencies
Pastoral counselor	Master's	Churches Counseling centers Private practice
Rehabilitation counselor	Master's	Rehabilitation agencies Hospitals
School counselor	Master's	Elementary, middle, and secondary schools
Social worker	Bachelor's, master's	Private practice Community agencies Hospitals Schools
School psychologist	Educational specialist/doctorate	Schools
Child psychologist	Doctorate	University Private practice Community agencies Hospitals
Clinical psychologist	Doctorate	University Private practice Community agencies Hospitals
Counseling psychologist	Doctorate	University Private practice Industry Community agencies Hospitals
Counselor educator	Doctorate	University Private practice Industry
Psychiatrist	Medical degree	Private practice Hospitals

through cognitive, affective, behavioral, or systematic intervention strategies that address wellness, personal growth, or career development as well as pathology" (www.counseling.org/CareerCenter). Social workers "promote human and community well-being … social work's purpose is actualized through its quest for social and economic justice, the prevention of conditions that limit human rights, the elimination of poverty, and the enhancement of the quality of life for all people" (www.cswe.org). Some psychologists "apply the discipline's scientific knowledge to help people, organizations and communities function better" (www.apa.org/about). A psychiatrist is "a physician who specializes in the prevention, diagnosis, and treatment of mental illness" (www.medterms.com/script/main/art.asp?articlekey=5107).

Accreditation standards outline preparation requirements and state laws govern through certification (protection of title) and licensure (protection of practice) the work of counselors, social workers, psychologists, and psychiatrists. Most require at least a 2-year master's degree, including a supervised practicum or internship. Doctoral programs also require additional supervised practicum and internship experiences.

The Council for Accreditation of Counseling and Related Educational Programs (CACREP), an accrediting body associated with the ACA, recommends a graduate training program, including 60 semester hours of master's degree-level training and competency in such areas as human growth and development, social and cultural foundations, helping relationships, group work, lifestyle and career development, appraisal, research and evaluation, and professional orientation. Its recommendations for doctoral training build on these competencies and include additional internship experiences.

The NBCC administers the National Counselor Examination (NCE) as a component of the NBCC national professional counselor certification program. Special credentialing associations provide information about the recognition of counselors in many specialties, and state licensing boards regulate practice parameters. This look at the state of the counseling profession as outlined by accreditation and credentials will continue to evolve. March (2009) predicts a vastly different delivery system for mentally ill children and adolescents in the year 2030. He proposes more focus on the central nervous system as well as on psychosocial treatments that impact the trajectory of developmental psychopathology. Certainly the scientific advances of neuroscience inform us about the developing brain and about how to influence health. March's conclusion is that treatment will move away from the models of disorders as targets to promoting typical development for each individual. Those who work with troubled children will likely embrace any efficient and effective treatment to facilitate the well-being of all humans.

SUMMARY

Children thrive when adults understand their world and respond appropriately. Recognizing the stresses of everyday life and acknowledging the impact of those problems will allow families, communities, and helping professionals to interact in supporting the mental health and optimal development of all young people.

We know more about the ways to approach the mental health needs of children. Huang et al. (2005) and Prout (2007) and the authors of this book agree that these actions need to be implemented to support children who are struggling:

- Provide comprehensive home- and community-based services and supports
- Create family support and partnerships
- Offer culturally competent care and eliminate disparities in access to resources
- Individualize care for each child
- Use evidence-based practices
- Coordinate services and designate responsibility for wrap-around care
- Deliver multiple prevention activities for groups at risk starting in early childhood
- Expand mental health services in schools

May we all use our energy, knowledge, and skills to build a better world.

INTRODUCTION TO A CHILD'S WORLD VIDEO

To gain a more in-depth understanding of the concepts in this chapter, visit www.cengage.com/counseling/henderson to view short clips of an actual therapist– client session demonstrating a counselor relating to a child's world.

WEB SITES FOR UNDERSTANDING A CHILD'S WORLD

Internet addresses frequently change. To find the sites listed here, visit www.cengage .com/counseling/henderson for an updated list of Internet addresses and direct links to relevant sites.

Annie E. Casey Foundation

Children's Defense Fund (CDF)

Child Welfare League of America (CWLA)

Resiliency in Action (RAND)

REFERENCES

Addy, S., Engelhardt, W., & Skinner, C. (2011). Basic facts about low-income children under 18 years. Retrieved from http://www.nccp.org/publications/pub_1074.html

Ahem, N. R., Kiehl, E. M., Sole, M. L., & Byers, J. (2006). A review of instruments measuring resilience. *Issues in Comprehensive Pediatric Nursing, 29,* 103–125, http://dx.doi .org/10.1080/01460860600677643

Ainsworth, M. D. (1989). Attachments beyond infancy. *American Psychologist, 44,* 709–716.

Alvord, M. K., & Gardos, J. J. (2005). Enhancing resilience in children: A proactive approach. *Professional Psychology: Research and Practice, 36*(3), 238–245.

American Psychological Association, Division of Counseling Psychology, Committee on Definition. (1956). Counseling psychology as a specialty. *American Psychologist, 11,* 282–285.

Arbona, C., & Coleman, N. (2008). Risk and resilience. In S. D.Brown & R. W. Lent (Eds.), *Handbook of Counseling Psychology* (4th ed., pp. 483–499). Hoboken, NJ: Wiley.

Aries, P. (1962). Centuries of childhood: A social history of family life. New York: Knopf.

Atkinson, D. R. (2002). Counseling in the 21st century: A mental health profession comes of age. In C. L. Juntunen & D. R. Atkinson (Eds.), *Counseling across the lifespan* (pp. 3–22). Thousand Oaks, CA: Sage Publications.

Benard, B. (2004). *Resiliency: What we have learned.* San Francisco, CA: WestEd.

Ben-Arieh, A., Casas, R., Frønes, I., & Korbin, J. E. (Eds.). (2013). *Handbook of child well-being: Theories, methods and policies in global perspective.* New York: Springer.

Benson, P. L. (1997). *All kids are our kids.* Minneapolis, MN: Search Institute.

Benzies, K., & Mychasiuk, R. (2009). Fostering family resiliency: A review of the key protective factors. *Child & Family Social Work, 14,* 103–114.

Berns, R. M. (2012). Child, family, school, community: Socialization and support (9th ed.). Belmont, CA: Cengage.

Bowlby, J. (1988). Attachment, communication, and the therapeutic process. In J. Bowlby (Ed.), *A secure base: Clinical applications of attachment theory* (pp. 137–157). London: Routledge.

Brazelton, T. B., & Greenspan, S. I. (2000). The irreducible needs of children: What every child must have to grow, learn, and flourish. Cambridge, MA: Perseus.

Brooks, J. E. (2006). Strengthening resilience in children and youths: Maximizing opportunities in the schools. *Children and Schools, 28*(2), 60–76.

Center for Disease Control and Prevention. (n.d.). Well-being concepts. Retrieved from http://www.cdc.gov/hrqol/wellbeing.htm

Center for Disease Control and Prevention. (n.d.) Adverse Childhood Experiences (ACE) Study. Retrieved from http://www.cdc.gov/violenceprevention/acestudy/about.html

Child Labor Education Project. (n.d.) Child labor in U. S. history. Retrieved from https://www.continuetolearn.uiowa.edu/laborctr/child_labor/about/us_history.html

Child Welfare League of America. (2013). *National blueprint for excellence in child welfare.* Washington, DC: Author.

Children's Defense Fund. (June 2014). Policy priorities. Retrieved from http://www.childrensdefense.org/policy/

Children's Defense Fund. (2014). The State of American's Children. Washington, DC: Author.

Coleman, J., Morris, C., & Glaros, A. (1987). *Contemporary psychology and effective behavior.* Glenview, IL: Scott, Foresman.

Donohue, B., Hersen, M., & Ammerman, R. T. (2000). Historical overview. In M. Hersen & R. Ammerman (Eds.), *Abnormal child psychology* (2nd ed., pp. 3–14). Mahwah, NJ: Erlbaum.

Erikson, E. (1963). *Childhood and society.* New York: Norton.

Federal Interagency Forum on Child and Family Statistics. (2014). America's children at a glance. Retrieved from http://www.childstats.gov/americaschildren/glance.asp

Gardner, H. (1993). Multiple intelligences: The theory in practice. New York: Basic Books.

Garmezy, N. (1991). Resiliency and vulnerability to adverse developmental outcomes associated with poverty. *American Behavioral Scientist, 34,* 416–430.

Goleman, D. (1995). Emotional intelligence: Why it can matter more than I. Q. New York: Bantam Books.

Greenberg, M. T. (2006). Promoting resilience in children and youth: Preventive interventions and their interface with neuroscience. *Annals New York Academy of Sciences, 1094*, 139–150.

Hauser, S. T. (1999). Understanding resilient outcomes: Adolescent lives across time and generations. *Journal of Research on Adolescence, 9*, 1–24.

Hernandez, D. J. (2003). Changing family circumstances. In R. P. Weissberg, H. J. Walberg, M. U. O'Brien, & C. B. Kuster (Eds.), *Long-term trends in the well-being of children and youth: Issues in children's and families' lives* (pp. 155–180). Washington, DC: Child Welfare League of America.

Huang, L., Stroul, B., Friedman, R., Mrazek, P., Friesen, B., Pires, S., et al. (2005). Transforming mental health care for children and their families. *American Psychologist, 60*, 615–627.

Lee, J. H., Nam, S. K., Kim, A., Kim, B., Lee, M. Y., & Lee, S. M. (2013). Resilience: A meta-analytic approach. *Journal of Counseling and Development, 91*, 269–279. doi:10.1002/j.1556-6676.2013.00095.x

LeVine, R. A. (2007). Ethnographic studies of childhood: A historical overview. *American Anthropologist, 109*, 247–260.

Lewis, R. E. (2006). Resilience: Individual, family, school, and community perspectives. In D. Capuzzi & D. R. Gross (Eds.), *Youth at risk: A prevention resource for counselors, teachers, and parents* (4th ed., pp. 35–68). Upper Saddle River, NJ: Pearson.

Lowenthal, B. (1998). The effects of early childhood abuse and the development of resiliency. *Early Child Development and Care, 142*, 43–52.

Luthar, S. S. (2006). Resilience in development: A synthesis of research across five decades. In D. Cicchetti & D. J. Cohen (Eds.), *Developmental psychopathology: Risk, disorder, and adaptation* (2nd ed., Vol. 3, pp. 739–795). Hoboken, NJ: Wiley.

March, J. S. (2009). The future of psychotherapy for mentally ill children and adolescents. *Journal of Child Psychology and Psychiatry, 50*, 170–179.

Mash, E. J., & Wolfe, D. A. (2012). *Abnormal child psychology* (5th ed.). Belmont, CA: Cengage Learning.

Maslow, A. (1970). *Motivation and personality* (2nd ed.). New York: Harper & Row.

Masten, A. (2001). Ordinary magic: Resilience processes in development. *American Psychologist, 56*, 227–238.

Masten, A. S. (2011). Resilience in children threatened by extreme adversity: Framework for research, practice and translational synergy. *Developmental Psychopathology, 23*, 493–506.

Masten, A., & Coatsworth, D. (1998). The development of competence in favorable and unfavorable environments: Lessons from research on successful children. *American Psychologist, 53*, 205–220.

Masten, A. S., & Obradovic, J. (2006). Competence and resilience in development. *Annals of the New York Academy of Sciences, 1094*, 13–27. http://dx.doi.org/10.1196/annals.1376.003

Masten, A. S., & Powell, J. L. (2003). A resilience framework for research, policy and practice. In S.Luthar (Ed.), *Resilience and vulnerability: Adaptation in the context of childhood adversities* (pp. 1–25). Cambridge: Cambridge University Press.

McCartney, K., Yoshikawa, H., & Forcier, L.B. (2014). *Improving the odds for America's children: Future directions in policy and practice.* Cambridge, MA: Harvard Education Press.

Moore, K. A., Mbwana, K., Theokas, C., Lippman, L., Bloch, M., Vandivere, S., & O'Hare, W. (2011). Child well-being: An index based on data of individual children. Retrieved from http://www.childtrends.org/?publications=child-well-being-an-index-based-on-data-of-individual-children

Moore, K. A., Vandivere, S., Lippman, L., McPhee, C., & Bloch, M. (2007). An index of the condition of children: The ideal and a less-than-ideal U.W. example. *Social Indicators Research*, 84, 291–331.

Murphey, D., Stratford, B., Gooze, R., Bringewatt, E., Cooper, P. M., Carney, R., Rojas, A. & Child Trends. (July 2014). Are the children well? A model and recommendations for promoting the mental wellness of the nation's young people. Retrieved from http://www.rwjf.org/content/dam/farm/reports/issue_briefs/2014/rwjf414424

Naglieri, J. A., & LeBuffle, P. A. (2005). Measuring resilience in children. In S. Goldstein, & R. B. Brooks (Eds.), *Handbook of resilience in children* (pp. 107–121). New York: Springer.

Nystul, M. S. (2010). *Introduction to counseling: An art and science perspective* (4th ed.). Upper Saddle River, NJ: Pearson.

O'Brien, M. U., Weissberg, R. P., Walberg, H. J., & Kuster, C. B. (2003). Contributions and complexities of studying trends in the well-being of children and youth. In R. P. Weissberg, H. J. Walberg, M. U.O'Brien, & C. B. Kuster (Eds.), *Long-term trends in the well-being of children and youth: Issues in children's and families' lives* (pp. 3–26). Washington, DC: Child Welfare League of America.

Orton, G. L. (1997). Strategies for counseling with children and their parents. Pacific Grove, CA: Brooks/Cole.

Peters, H., & Farwell, G. (1959). *Guidance: A developmental approach*. Chicago: Rand McNally.

Postman, N. (1985). The disappearance of childhood. *Childhood Education*, 61, 288–293.

Prout, H. T. (2007). Counseling and psychotherapy with children and adolescents: Historical developmental, integrative, and effectiveness perspectives. In H. T. Prout & D. T. Brown (Eds.), *Counseling and psychotherapy with children and adolescents: Theory and practice for school and clinical settings* (4th ed., pp. 1–31). Hoboken, NJ: Wiley.

Rak, C. F. (2001). Understanding and promoting resilience with our clients. In E. R. Welfel & R. E. Ingersoll (Eds.), *The mental health desk reference* (pp. 225–231). New York: Wiley.

Rak, C. F., & Patterson, L. E. (1996). Promoting resilience in at-risk children. *Journal of Counseling and Development*, 74, 368–373.

Radbill, S. X. (1968). A history of child abuse and infanticide. In R. E. Helfer & C. H. Kempe (Eds.), *The battered child* (pp. 3–17). Chicago: University of Chicago Press.

Strom-Gottfried, K. (2008). The ethics of practice with minors: High stakes, hard choices. Chicago: Lyceum.

The Center for Health and Health Care in Schools. (2013). Improving access to mental health care: Lessons from eleven states. Retrieved from http://www.healthinschools.org/School-Based-Mental-Health/Eleven-State-Report.aspx

The Institute of Medicine. (2009). Preventing mental, emotional, and behavioral disorders among young people: Progress and possibilities. Retrieved from http://www.iom.edu/Reports/2009/Preventing-Mental-Emotional-and-Behavioral-Disorders-Among-Young-People-Progress-and-Possibilities.aspx

UNICEF. (1990). Convention on the rights of the child. Retrieved from http://www.unicef.org/crc/index_30167.html

United States Courts. (n.d.) Facts and Case Summary: *In re Gault* 387 U.S. 1(1967). Retrieved from http://www.uscourts.gov/educational-resources/get-involved/constitution-activities/sixth-amendment/right-counsel/facts-case-summary-gault.aspx

U. S. Department of Health and Human Services. (2014). Health Care: About the Law. Retrieved from http://www.hhs.gov/healthcare/rights/

Walsh, F. (2006). *Strengthening family resilience* (2nd ed.). New York: Guilford.

Weissberg, R. P., Walberg, H. J., O'Brien, M. U., & Kuster, C. B. (Eds.). (2003). *Long-term trends in the well-being of children and youth: Issues in children's and families' lives.* Washington, DC: Child Welfare League of America.

Werner, E. E., & Smith, R. S. (2001). *Journeys from childhood to the midlife: Risk, resilience, and recovery.* New York: Cornell University Press.

Zolkoski, S. M., & Bullock, L. M. (2012). Resilience in children and youth: A review. *Children and Youth Services Review, 34,* 2295–2303. doi:10.1016/j.childyouth.2012.08.009

CHAPTER 2

Developmental and Cultural Considerations

To have one's individuality completely ignored is like being pushed quite out of life. Like being blown out as one blows out a light.
—EVELYN SCOTT

The various family, social, and cultural conditions discussed in the introductory chapter can have a profound effect on a child's personal world. The optimal state for any young person would be one of physical and mental health. That requires providing a broad array of activities directly or indirectly to the child's well-being, which the World Health Organization defines as "A state of complete physical, mental and social well-being, and not merely the absence of disease" (http://www.who .int/features/qa/62/en/). Understanding the developmental and cultural variables of childhood will allow adults more opportunities to create an environment in which children can thrive. After reading this chapter, you should be able to:

 ▶ Discuss ways to understand the needs of children
 ▶ Outline theories and other explanations of physical, cognitive, and social development
 ▶ Define culture
 ▶ Demonstrate the knowledge, skills, and awareness of cultural competence
 ▶ Explain ways of working with children of color

THE PERSONAL WORLD OF THE CHILD

Maslow (1970) believed we all have certain basic needs that must be met for us to become "self-actualizing" and reach our potential in all areas of development (Figure 2-1). If our lower-level basic needs are not met, according to Maslow, we will be unable to meet higher-order needs.

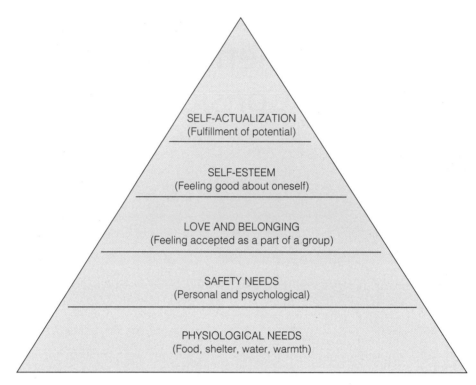

FIGURE 2-1   MASLOW'S HIERARCHY OF NEEDS

The first level of Maslow's hierarchy is physiological needs—food, shelter, water, and warmth. We might be tempted to overlook these needs, believing that children are well fed and have adequate shelter. Yet according to the Child Trends data 22 percent of children under 18 lived in households without food security at some point in the year. That means one in five U.S. children was hungry. Likewise at least 1.1 million children were homeless during the 2010–2011 school year. Obviously the basic needs of many children remain unmet.

Maslow's second level of basic needs refers to safety. Some children feel afraid for their physical safety in their own homes and have cause for that concern. Parents who do not have their own needs adequately met may take out their frustrations on their child through physical or psychological abuse. Some adults who would not think of hurting children physically will psychologically abuse them with demeaning and damaging words. Children may receive similar treatment in school where teachers may use children as a safe target for their personal or professional frustration. Data (Child Trends) indicate that one in 25 students was afraid of being attacked in school or on the way to or from school and one in 20 had been bullied. Also 13 percent live in neighborhoods that are never or only sometimes safe. In addition, media vividly portrays the dangers of natural disasters such as hurricanes, tornados, and earthquakes, as well as other all-too-prevalent acts of violence. Finally, war or the threat of war also seems ever present, and recent acts of terrorism threaten everyone's sense of personal safety. Safety needs exist for many children and youth.

All children's learning and behavior may be influenced by the need to feel loved and to belong—the third-level need that emerges, according to Maslow, after physiological and safety needs have been met. Humans are social beings who want to feel part of a group, a need fulfilled by children's play groups, cliques, gangs, and clubs, as well as the family. Wherever we are, most of us want to be loved and accepted and to be connected to a group. Young people who do not get positive attention from adults or peers may believe they are unlovable and will never be valued, a miserable way to live. Children sometimes hide their feelings of rejection or compensate for the rejection with antisocial behavior; either defense can hurt learning and personal relationships. Sadly many well-meaning adults underestimate the impact their words and actions have on children who may mistake, for example, frustration or impatience for rejection. Young people need to have acceptance, affection, and appreciation to feel loved and connected.

Another hurdle for children involves satisfying their need for self-esteem, an overall sense of self-worth and value—the fourth need in Maslow's hierarchy. Children are often ordered, criticized, and ignored. An adult treated like this feels annoyance, defensiveness, and anger and may rebel or leave the scene. Such responses are not considered acceptable in children. On the other hand, children may also be cosseted, treated like fragile entities, and given no responsibility and never allowed to make choices. All people, adults and children, need to be respected as worthwhile individuals capable of feeling, thinking, and behaving responsibly. Children can be treated with the warmth and respect needed to encourage learning and growth within firm guidelines and expectations. Adults can learn to avoid cruel and thoughtless remarks, reduce criticisms, and increase positive interactions. Adults can provide safe opportunities for children to learn about responsible choices as well as the consequences of mistakes. Feeling respected and worthwhile builds an appropriate, healthy self-esteem.

Satisfaction of needs at the first four levels contributes to achievemenvt of the fifth need in Maslow's hierarchy—self-actualization. Maslow (1970) stated that a self-actualized person is moving toward the fulfillment of his or her inherent potential. Fulfilling this need implies that the child is not blocked by hunger, fear, lack of love or feelings of belonging, or low self-esteem. The child is not without problems but has learned problem-solving skills and can move forward to become all that he or she can be at that stage of life.

According to Glasser (see Chapter 9), society is not meeting our children's needs, and thus children are failing in school and in life, unable to thrive academically and behaviorally. He lists five needs that both mirror and expand Maslow's work: (1) the need to survive and reproduce, (2) the need to belong and love, (3) the need to gain power, (4) the need to be free, and (5) the need to have fun. Glasser states that children's problems relate to their inability to fulfill these needs and emphasizes teaching reality, right and wrong, and responsibility.

Adlerian psychologists (see Chapter 11) believe that children often attempt to meet their needs in a mistaken direction. They suggest that adults examine the goals of misbehavior and redirect the behavior toward achieving more satisfying results.

Behavioral psychologists (see Chapter 8) see academic and behavioral problems as resulting from faulty learning; that is, the child has learned inappropriate ways of behaving through reinforcement or from poor models. Unlearning or extinguishing inappropriate patterns and learning more appropriate behaviors help the child succeed.

Regardless of the factors contributing to children's learning, behavioral, and social problems, parents, counselors, and other professionals must assist and support children as they grow and develop in this complex, changing world. Understanding the process of development helps adults provide that support. Indeed as adults consider children who are struggling, the first question to ask would be "what age is the child," followed by a review of the typical and atypical characteristics of that age. The following section includes a review of some ways of understanding children's maturation process.

DEVELOPMENT

Children and adolescents bound through physical, cognitive, social, and emotional changes almost daily. A critical aspect in defining children's mental health is their successful movement through the normal developmental milestones. As noted earlier, other indicators of success are secure attachments, satisfying relationships, and effective coping skills. Development can be understood as periods of transition and reorganization—a lifelong process of growth, maturation, and change.

One challenge in working with children is the different interpretations of behaviors according to different ages. For example, adults perceive a 3-year-old who has a temper tantrum in the grocery store quite differently than a 14-year-old loudly demanding her favorite cereal. Counselors must be steeped in knowledge of normal development to understand mental health in children. The following sections review just a few of those important concepts.

A CHILD'S PHYSICAL DEVELOPMENT

The Body

Many of the biological aspects of the developing child are visible—they become taller, stronger, and more adult-like as they age. The increase in height and weight of the developing person is greater in the first 2 years of life, is more gradual in the elementary school years, and then changes dramatically during the adolescent growth spurt. That rapid change usually happens earlier in girls, between 11 and 14, than for boys, between 13 and 16. Physical growth is commonly finished by the time a person graduates from high school.

Other aspects of physical development relate to using the body. Motor skills change as children age. New skills develop from those previously learned as children learn coordination and control of their gross motor skills such as running and their fine motor skills like holding a pencil. Vision and eye–hand coordination improve as well. Physical activity is imperative for good health across life as are good nutrition and eating habits.

Other physical changes such as brain development are invisible to the observer but have significant impact on the world of the child. The profession of counseling increasingly turns to neurological findings to determine the best treatment options in particular situations. A discussion of brain development and patterns of physical development will assist counselors in understanding the world of the child.

The Brain

Changes in brain structuring and functioning occur during childhood and adolescence. The connections in the brain become more fine-tuned, and regions of the brain become more efficient. A review of the major parts of the brain from Berger (2014) reminds us of the structure of the brain so that we can better understand the impact of medications and the rapidly increasing knowledge about ways brain topology affects behavior.

The brain contains three main parts: the brain stem, the cerebellum, and the cerebrum. The brain stem, connected to the spinal cord, controls body functions like breathing, circulation, and reflexes. The cerebellum coordinates sensory and motor activities. The cerebrum is the largest part of the brain, and it handles thought, memory, language, emotion, sensory input, and conscious motor control.

The cerebrum is divided into right and left halves, or hemispheres, which have specific purposes. Lateralization refers to that specialization between hemispheres. The left hemisphere contains language and logical thinking functions, and the right hemisphere holds visual and spatial functions. Each hemisphere has sections, or lobes. The *occipital lobe* processes visual stimuli; the *temporal lode*, hearing and language; the *parietal lobe*, touch, spatial information, and eye–hand coordination; and the *frontal lobe*, higher-level functions like speech and reasoning. The cerebral cortex, the outer surface of the cerebrum, is the location of thought and mental processes. The corpus callosum, the tissue that connects the two hemispheres, allows them to share information.

The brain is made of neurons, nerve cells that send and receive information, and glial cells that nourish and protect neurons. Neurons grow axons and dendrites, which are narrow, branching, fibrous extensions. Axons send signals to other neurons and dendrites receive messages. Those messages occur through synapses, the nervous system's communication link. The chemical neurotransmitters bridge the synapses. As the brain matures, neurons multiply and eventually migrate to an assigned location in the brain where they develop connections. At first, the brain has more neurons and synapses than needed but some die because they are not used or they do not function well. That elimination of unneeded synapses continues into adolescence and helps create a more efficient nervous system.

Myelination is the process of the glial cells that provides neural pathways with a fatty substance, myelin. Myelination allows signals to move more quickly and more smoothly toward mature functioning. In early childhood, as the myelination of fibers occurs in the corpus callosum, the young person can transmit information more quickly between the hemispheres of the brain (Toga, Thompson, & Sowell, 2006). That development continues until adolescence and builds coordination of senses, memory, attention, speech, and hearing functions (Lenroot & Giedd, 2006).

Between ages 6 and 13, growth occurs in the connections between the temporal and parietal lobes. Maturation and learning in middle childhood rely on the brain's connections becoming more efficient and the selection of the region of the brain for tasks being fine-tuned. During middle childhood, the density of gray matter in regions of the brain is balanced by an increase in white matter, axons, or nerve fibers that transmit information between neurons to different regions of the brain. The dramatic changes of brains in adolescents have the most impact on the work of counselors because the brain process related to emotions, judgment, organizing behavior, and self-control happens at some point in adolescence. Risk taking seems to be a product of the interaction of a socioemotional network that is sensitive to both social and emotional stimuli and a cognitive-control network that adjusts responses to stimuli. During puberty, the socioemotional network becomes more active. The cognitive-control network develops more gradually as the person reaches early adulthood. Steinberg (2007) suggested these explanations help understanding teenagers' emotional outbursts and risky behaviors as well as provide reasons why unsafe actions often occur in group settings.

Additionally, teens process information about emotions in a different way than adults do. Adolescent brain activity in early teens tends to concentrate in the amygdala, a structure deep in the temporal lobe involved in emotional and instinctual reactions. In that study of brain imaging, older teens tended to use the frontal lobe, which has the functions of planning, reasoning, judgment, emotional regulation, and impulse control. Younger adolescents did not use that part of the brain; consequently, their mental processes did not have the more accurate, reasoned, adult-like pattern. The immature brain development of the adolescent may allow emotions to override reason and lead to unwise decisions in spite of warnings that would deter adults (Blakemore, 2008; Dreyfuss, 2014; Sowell, Thompson, & Toga, 2007). The lack of development in the frontal cortical systems linked to motivation, impulse, and addiction may also explain teens' seeking thrills and novelty and being unable to focus on long-term plans (Bijork et al., 2004; Chambers, Taylor, & Potenza, 2003; Steinberg, 2008). In fact Laurence Steinberg, an expert on adolescent thinking, captures this phenomenon in his explanation that it is not that decision making is deficient, in many cases with young teens it is nonexistent. When they think about risks, adolescents assess danger more accurately than children (Pfeifer, Dapretto, & Lieberman, 2010); the critical problem is they may not think but allow emotions, the group and the excitement dictate their actions. The balance among the parts of a teenage brain may be off kilter, the brain itself is not (Casey, Jones, & Somerville, 2011).

Teens continue to have an increase in white matter in the frontal lobes and a reduction of gray matter so that by mid- to late-adolescence teens have fewer but stronger, smoother, and more efficient neural connections (Kuhn, 2006). The activities and experiences of teenagers greatly influence their cognitive growth. Teens who learn to organize their thoughts, understand abstractions, and control their impulses will be poised for a healthy life. However, the implications of substance abuse and other risky behavior that may create damage will be difficult to reverse. Counselors must be aware of the rapidly increasing information about brain development and the implications for working with children of all ages. Hopefully in the near future the research on teenage brains will guide prevention efforts to protect adolescents from their impulsive, too often dangerous choices. A helpful resource for professionals and parents can be found on the Internet at the Public Broadcasting Systems (PBS) Web site where the *Frontline* series "Inside the Teenage Brain" can be accessed.

MATURATION

The timing of maturation, for example, puberty earlier or later than his or her peers, may lead to adjustment problems. Early-maturing girls may be unprepared for the social pressures and experiences related to sexual maturity, leading to anxiety and depression (Compian, Gowen, & Hayward, 2009). They may also become involved with older boys, a connection that increases the risk of substance use, eating disorders and being a victim of relational violence (DeRose, Shiyko, Foster, & Brooks-Gunn, 2011). Early maturation for boys once may have positive effects on their social development (Taga, Markey, & Friedman, 2006), but for the past few decades, early-maturing boys engage in more aggressive, illegal, and alcohol-abusing behavior than later-maturing boys (Biehl, Natsuaki, & Ge, 2007; Lynne, Graber, Nichols, Brooks-Gunn, & Botvin, 2007). Late maturation may make young men targets of teasing, bullying, and other belittling behaviors. They may be more anxious, depressed, and more afraid of sex than other boys (Lindfors et al., 2007). Early or late maturity increases the likelihood of problems in adolescence.

The impact of the timing of puberty depends on how the adolescent and others perceive the changes. If the teen is much more or less developed than peers, the effects are more likely to be negative. Other situations that create negative response to early or late maturation are when the changes are not seen as advantages and when there are other simultaneous stressors. Ethnicity, school, and neighborhood also make a difference (Woolfolk & Perry, 2012).

Patterns in physical development, particularly the adolescent growth spurt and the implications of timing for puberty, are important considerations for counselors in understanding the world of a young person.

GENES

Brain and body development cannot be understood without an appreciation of genetics (Wilmshurst, 2014). Genetics refers to the study of the ways humans and other species obtain their unique traits as well as the ways those inherited traits interact with the environment to impact development. The investigations decode cells, chromosomes, genes, and DNA. Specifically the Human Genome Project (http://www.genome.gov/10001772) and other studies have uncovered similarities and differences between the genes of humans and other species, allowing professionals to expand their understanding of genes and their effects on children's growth. Of particular interest to helping professions is the growing knowledge base about both genes and environment contributing to temperament and personality as well as to psychological disorders (Burt, 2009; Gagne, Vendlinski, & Goldsmith, 2009). Recently scientists learned of common genetic factors in five mental disorders: autism, attention-deficit/hyperactivity disorder (ADHD), bipolar disorder, major depression, and schizophrenia (National Institute of Mental Health, 2014).

We are learning more about the ways children may inherit tendencies to develop particular traits or problems. Their experiences interweave with their genetic makeup as their lives unfold in adjusted or maladjusted ways. However, genes do not operate in any simple, predetermined fashion; they are affected by nutrition, stress, and other environmental factors. A person may have a greater likelihood of a condition with the genetic marker for that condition; however, many other factors affect whether or not the condition will occur.

Informed counselors will monitor the continuing research on genetic predispositions to better serve children. The clear messages about gene and environment interactions should guide adults in making allowances for individual differences and to respect the influence of environmental factors on all aspects of development.

A CHILD'S COGNITIVE WORLD

Cognitive development refers to the thinking skills of the child. According to Jean Piaget (Piaget & Inhelder, 1969), children move to increasingly sophisticated thought processes as they progress through four stages (Table 2-1). These distinct patterns of thought occur in the stages of sensorimotor (birth to age 2), preoperational (ages 2–7), concrete operations (ages 7–11), and formal operations (after age 11).

TABLE 2-1 PIAGET'S FOUR STAGES OF COGNITIVE DEVELOPMENT

Stage	Type of Development	Age	Cognitive Traits
Infancy	Sensorimotor	0–2	Children: • Learn through their senses by touching, hitting, biting, tasting, smelling, observing, and listening • Distinguish between "me" and "not me" world • Learn about invariants in their environment (e.g., chairs are for sitting) • Form language • Develop habits • Begin to communicate symbolically • Can distinguish self and other objects • Have the ability to think about things and engage in purposeful behavior • Achieve a sense of object permanence • Begin trial-and-error problem solving
Childhood	Preoperational	2–7	Children: • Are not able to conserve in problem solving • Have greatest language growth • Are trial-and-error problem solvers who focus on one stimulus at a time • Can classify objects more than one way (i.e., by shape, color, size, texture) • Have trouble with reversible thinking • Prefer to learn things in ascending rather than descending order • Are egocentric thinkers • Are able to use mental images, imagination, and symbolic thought • Are capable of understanding simple rules—regarded as sacred and unchangeable

(continued)

TABLE 2-1 *(Continued)*

Stage	Type of Development	Age	Cognitive Traits
Preadolescence	Concrete	7–11	Children: <ul><li>Have conversation skills</li><li>Can do reversible thinking</li><li>Have difficulty with abstract reasoning</li><li>Can appreciate views of others</li><li>Need concrete aids for learning</li><li>Move toward logical thought</li><li>Are less egocentric</li><li>See rules as more changeable</li><li>Can distinguish reality from fantasy</li><li>Have greater capacity for concentration, attention, and memory</li><li>Are capable of understanding that distance equals rate times time</li></ul>
Adolescence through adulthood:	Formal	11+	Children: <ul><li>Have no need to manipulate objects to solve problems</li><li>Are capable of abstract thought and scientific experimentation</li><li>Are capable of understanding and applying ethical and moral principles</li><li>Are capable of self-reflective thought and high levels of empathic understanding</li><li>Have a sense of what is best for society</li></ul>

The work of Piaget and Inhelder (1969) establishes that children from ages 5 to 12 may function in as many as three stages of cognitive development. Although age is no guarantee of a child's stage of development, 5- and 6-year-old children are on the verge of moving from the preoperational to the concrete stage of cognitive development, and 11-year-old children are moving into the formal stage. The counselor must know the child's level of cognitive development, particularly the degree to which a child is able to engage in abstract reasoning, a characteristic of the formal thinking stage. Children in the concrete thinking stage need explicit examples, learning aids, and directions. For example, the concrete thinker can walk through a series of directions but cannot draw a map of the same route.

Counseling methods need to be matched with the child's cognitive ability if counseling is to be effective. Piaget characterized the preoperational child's behavior and thinking as egocentric; that is, the child cannot take the role of or understand the viewpoint of another. Preoperational children believe that everyone thinks the same way and does the same things they do. As a result, preoperational children never question their own thoughts; as far as they are concerned, their thoughts are the only thoughts possible and consequently must be correct. When they are confronted with evidence that is contradictory to their thoughts, they conclude that the evidence must be wrong because their thoughts cannot be wrong. Thus, from the children's point of view, their thinking is always logical and correct. This egocentrism of thought is not egocentric by intent; children remain unaware that they are egocentric and consequently see no problem in need of a resolution.

Wadsworth (2003) adds that not until about age 6 or 7, when children's thoughts and those of their peers clearly conflict, do children begin to accommodate others and their egocentric thoughts begin to give way to social pressure. Peer group social interaction and the repeated conflict of the child's own thoughts with those of others eventually jar the child to question and seek verification of his or her thoughts. The very source of conflict—social interaction—becomes the child's source of verification. Thus, peer social interaction is the primary factor that acts to dissolve the cognitive egocentrism of the preoperational child.

The Roots of Empathy (ROE), an exemplary school-based intervention program, is designed to build empathy, emotional understanding, and concern for others. Over 500 classrooms across Canada and in several U.S. locations are implementing this program that involves adopting an infant for the school year. The infant and mother visit once a month and provide the impetus for discussions about interpreting nonverbal communication and responding to the needs of others. Evaluations of the program indicate that children increase their understanding of the needs and emotions of infants which is translated into more prosocial and less aggressive behavior with peers (Schonert-Reichl, Smith, Zaidman-Zait, & Hertzman, 2012).

Adolescents enter the formal operational level when they have the ability to think abstractly. They then have a more flexible way to manipulate information. In Piaget's stage of formal operations, young people can think logically, rationally, and abstractly (Woolfolk & Perry, 2012). Teenagers can combine facts and ideas to build an argumentative case, as well as multiple reasons to invalidate any contradictions. Elkind (1994) discusses adolescent egocentrism, a self-centered nature of adolescent thinking that may make communication processes difficult. Another characteristic of adolescent thinking is the "imaginary audience," a concept involved in teenagers' self-consciousness that results from their belief that they are always at the center of everyone's attention. The assumption that they are constantly watched as well as their often heightened emotions can make public criticism devastating to a teenager. Another characteristic of the adolescent work is the "personal fable"; that is, the belief that leads teenagers to feel invincible and immune from harm. Leading to exaggerated expectations for self and unwise risk taking, the personal fable and brain development significantly impact decision making in teen years. Counselors need to recognize these tendencies when working with adolescents.

Selman (1980) offers explanations of a child's and an adolescent's perspective taking; that is, the capacity to imagine what someone else may be thinking and feeling. This ability supports important social skills needed to build and maintain friendships. In the first stage (ages 3–6), children have undifferentiated perspective taking. They may recognize that other people can have different thoughts and feelings from their own, but they confuse the separation. In social-informational perspective taking (ages 4–9), children comprehend that other people may have different information and therefore different perspectives. Self-reflective perspective taking (ages 7–12) involves children being able to step into another person's views and see their own thoughts, feelings, and actions from the other person's perspective. They also recognize that other people have the same ability. For third-party perspective taking (ages 10–15), children move beyond the two-person situation and can imagine how they and others are seen from the view of a third, impartial party. With the last type, societal perspective taking (age 14 to adult), people understand that third-party perspective taking can be influenced by systems of societal values. Thus, children move from a limited idea of what others might be thinking to a more differentiated view of the thoughts and feelings of others. A summary of these stages of friendship and perspective taking can be found in Table 2-2.

Vygotsky (1978), a Russian psychologist, proposed a sociocultural theory of cognitive development in which social and cultural processes significantly impact

TABLE 2-2 SELMAN'S STAGES OF FRIENDSHIP AND PERSPECTIVE TAKING

Stage	Description	Example
Stage 0: Momentary playmates (ages 3 to 7)	On this *undifferentiated* level of friendship, children are egocentric, have trouble considering another person's point of view, think only about what they want from a relationship. These young children define their friends in terms of physical closeness and value them for material or physical attributes.	"She lives on my street" or "He has the Xbox."
Stage 1: One-way assistance; social-informational perspective (ages 4 to 9)	On this *unilateral level*, a "good friend" does what the child wants the friend to do; can understand people have different information and different views.	"She's not my friend anymore, because she wouldn't go with me when I wanted her to" or "He's my friend because he always says yes when I want to borrow his eraser."
Stage 2: Two-way fair-weather cooperation; self-reflective perspective (ages 6 to 12)	This *reciprocal level* overlaps Stage 1. It involves give-and-take but still serves many separate self-interests, rather than the common interests of two friends. Children can step into another person's views and see their own thoughts from the other person's perspective.	"We are friends; we do things for each other" or "A friend is someone who plays with you when you don't have anyone else to play with."
Stage 3: Intimate, mutually shared relationships; third-party perspective (ages 9 to 15)	On this *mutual level*, children view a friendship as having a life of its own. It is an ongoing, systematic, committed relationship that incorporates more than doing things for each other. Friends become possessive and demand exclusivity. Children can imagine how a third, impartial person could view them.	"It takes a long time to make a close friend so you really feel bad if you find out that your friend is trying to make other friends too."
Stage 4: Autonomous interdependences; societal perspective taking (beginning at age 12)	In this *interdependent* stage, children respect friends' needs for both dependency and autonomy. People can understand systems of social values influence perspective taking.	"A good friendship is a real commitment, a risk you have to take; you have to support and trust and give, but you have to be able to let go too."

Papalia, D. E., Olds, S. W., & Feldman, R. D. (2009). *Human development* (11th ed, p. 338). Boston: McGraw-Hill. Reprinted with permission.

growth. Piaget emphasizes the child's active engagement with environment, a solitary mind incorporating information about the world. Vygotsky considered cognitive growth as a collaborative process or the acquisition of knowledge through social interaction. Skills are learned through shared activities which are then internalized. According to Vygotsky, adults or advanced peers direct and organize a child's learning. He discussed the zone of proximal development as the gap between what children are already able to accomplish and what they are not quite ready to do by themselves. With the right kind of guidance, children can move from cannot to can. An example would be a child learning to ride a bicycle with a parent supporting the bike and then letting go as the child balances by herself or himself. Scaffolds are the way of teaching, a temporary support given to a child who is trying to complete a task until the child can do it alone (Woolfolk & Perry, 2012). Counselors who focus on the child's potential and give the child the guidance needed to work on their problems will find Vygotsky's work valuable.

The information-processing approach to cognition analyzes the ways people make sense of incoming information and perform tasks effectively. Attention, memory, planning strategies, decision making, and goal setting are processes within this framework. This approach compares the work of the brain to a computer with sensory information as the input and behaviors the output. Some researchers have used flowcharts to illustrate the steps used to gather, store, retrieve, and use information. Information-processing proponents do not suggest stages of development but do recognize age-related speed, complexity, and efficiency as well as the amount and variety of material that can be stored in memory (Woolfolk & Perry, 2012). The mind works on information by paying attention to it, holding it in "working memory," putting it into long-term storage, organizing, and drawing conclusions from it (Sigelman & Rider, 2012). Cognitive development is the growth of short-term memory capacity, long-term knowledge, and strategies for acquiring knowledge (McDevitt & Ormrod, 2012). Teachers and counselors can help children learn strategies for building short- and long-term memory capacity and retrieval.

THE CHILD'S WORLD OF SOCIAL DEVELOPMENT

Psychosocial development relates to the attitudes and skills needed to become a productive member of society. Erikson (1963, 1968) and Havighurst (1961) have written extensively about these stages of human development. Erikson describes eight stages of human development from birth through adulthood beyond the age of 50. Havighurst, in a similar vein, describes expectations and developmental tasks over the life span. Effective counselors are well informed about human development and know how to incorporate this knowledge into their work with children and adults.

Using Erikson's (1963, 1968) and Havighurst's (1961) systems as a frame of reference, counselors can compare expectations, human needs, and developmental tasks across the childhood years. Table 2-3 shows developmental tasks and necessary interventions for each of the eight stages of human development. The two basic tasks are: (1) coping with others' demands and expectations that conflict with an individual's own needs and (2) meeting these demands with the limited abilities individuals have in each developmental stage. Newman and Newman (2011) have

TABLE 2-3 DEVELOPMENT TASKS AND INTERVENTIONS FOR THE EIGHT STAGES OF HUMAN DEVELOPMENT

STAGE I: BIRTH TO AGE 1½

Basic Trust versus Basic Mistrust

Task:
- Develop trust in their parents and environment
- Learn the world is safe, consistent, predictable, and interesting

Interventions:
- Children need responsive, affectionate, consistent caregivers who meet their basic needs in order to bond with others

---

STAGE II: AGES 1½ TO 3

Autonomy versus Shame and Doubt

Task:
- Gain a sense of self-control as well as control over their environment

Interventions:
- Children have gained trust, need to experience success in doing things for themselves
- Overly restrained or overly punished children develop a sense of shame and doubt

---

STAGE III: AGES 3 TO 6

Initiative versus Guilt

Task:
- Develop a sense of initiative as opposed to feelings of guilt about never doing anything right

Interventions:
- Children begin to set goals and take leadership roles in carrying out projects
- Parents should empower children by giving them choices and allowing them to participate in family activities
- Unacceptable behavior is corrected in a loving, caring manner
- Discipline is based on logical consequences
- Expectations are realistic in order to prevent guilt and anxiety

---

STAGE IV: AGES 6 TO 12

Industry versus Inferiority

Task:
- Learn range of academic, social, physical, and practical skills needed in an adult world

Interventions:
- Encouragement and praise will help children achieve competence and be productive
- Nurturing can help children develop special talents and abilities

---

STAGE V: AGES 12 TO 18

Identity versus Role Confusion

Task:
- Develop a self-image, know who they are, and how their roles will fit into their future

Interventions:
- Adults should make teens feel accepted as they develop their identity through group activities, work, or play
- Key questions are: "Who am I?" and "Where am I going?"
- Period of exploration for further education, training, jobs, career, and marriage

---

(continued)

TABLE 2-3 (*Continued*)

STAGES VI, VII, AND VIII	

Adult Stages

Tasks:
- Achieve intimacy through sharing a close friendship or love relationship in young adulthood
- Middle adulthood tasks are proper care of children and productive work life
- Older adults are concerned with ego integrity—acceptance of past life, a search for meaning in the present, and continued growth and learning in the future

Interventions:
- Must match young adult's counseling to his or her learning style
- Adults may use concrete or abstract thinking in problem solving
- Issues in counseling often center on relationships, careers, and the search for meaning and purpose in life

extended Erikson's eight stages of human development to include three additional stages: prenatal, from conception to birth; later adolescence, from ages 18 to 22; and old age, from age 75 until death. They point out that theories of human development emerge and change because development is shaped by biological and psychosocial evolution within the context of cultural, environmental, and genetic influences.

To become a contributing member of the world, a person must build relationships. A way of understanding that ability has been provided by some other developmental theorists. John Bowlby (1969) introduced the concept of attachment when studying the bond between a mother and her infant. Attachment refers to a lasting emotional connection. Bowlby and Ainsworth (1989) discussed attachments beyond infancy and related caregiving relationships to future friendships, kinship bonds, and intimate relations, suggesting the pattern of early attachment forms the basis for later relationships. Attachment to another gives us pleasure and joy when we interact, as well as comfort in being near to that loved one when we are stressed. Out of the experiences infants have with their caretakers, children build a set of expectations about the availability of attachment figures and the likelihood that those figures will provide support.

Those expectations guide close relationships through childhood, adolescence, and the adult years (Bretherton, 1992; Kline, 2008). For example, Simpson, Collins, Tran, and Haydon (2007) followed 78 people from infancy to their 20s. These researchers linked a secure early attachment to good peer relationships in elementary school, intimate friendships in adolescence, as well as positive romantic relationships in early adulthood. These authors continue to inform about the impact of early attachment to adult relationships (Simpson & Overall, 2014; Simpson & Rholes, 2010).

Three models explain different types of attachments. People who report *secure* attachment had parents they described as warm, loving, and supportive. The adults considered themselves likable and easy to get to know. They were comfortable with intimacy and rarely worried about being abandoned or about someone getting too close to them. They talked about loving relationships in terms of trust, happiness, and friendship. Mothers who were securely attached to their mothers or who understood why they were insecurely attached can recognize and respond encouragingly to their babies' attachment behaviors. Peers of people with secure attachments talked about competent, charming, cheerful, and likable young adults (Sigelman & Rider, 2012).

The two types of insecure attachments are described as avoidant and resistant. People who reported avoidant attachment described their parents as demanding, disrespectful, and critical. As adults, they mistrusted partners and had anxiety about people getting too close to them. They downplay their need for love and their belief they will be abandoned. They believe that others did not like them and that love is elusive. Their intimate relationships were apt to include jealousy, emotional distance, and lack of acceptance. They avoid relationships due to their discomfort over intimacy and being dependent. Finally adults who discussed resistant attachment characterized their parents as unpredictable and unfair. They worried about intense feelings overwhelming them and about being abandoned by those they love. Their relationships included jealousy, emotional highs and lows, and desperation. They think little of themselves and others and have a confused, unpredictable array of neediness and fear of closeness (Sigelman & Rider, 2012).

Bowlby (1988) suggests that a therapist becomes an attachment figure who inspires trust in a client. That relationship then would become a secure base for clients to explore themselves and their relationships with others. Lopez and Brennan (2000) suggest that counseling provides a place to learn ways to lessen negative attachment patterns and cope more effectively. Mohr, Gelso, and Hill (2005) looked at the mix of client and counselor attachment styles in therapy sessions and ways those combinations help or hurt the counseling process, conclusions that supported Meyer and Pilkonis (2001) hypothesis that client's and counselor's reported attachments influenced both the process and the outcome of counseling. Lynch (2013) proposed a multilevel model to understand attachment and emotional security. Finally, Corcoran and Mallinckrodt (2000) reporting on correlates of attachment style concluded that, when clients experienced success, their functioning improved.

Connections with other people also impact a child's well-being. Children must build relationships with siblings and peers, as well as with adults. These bonds also change over time. Because toddlers have few social skills, time with others involves playing side by side. As children mature, they learn the give-and-take of relationships. Children who can form close friendships have highly developed social skills. They can interpret and understand other children's nonverbal cues. They can respond appropriately to what other children say. They use eye contact and the other person's name and may touch the other person to get attention. If they disagree with a peer, they can explain why their plan is a good one. They are willing to forgo their desires to reach a compromise and may even change their stated belief. When they are with strange children, they observe until they have a sense of the group. Children without these skills tend to be rejected. They are withdrawn, do not listen well, and give few reasons for their wishes. They rarely praise others and have trouble participating in cooperative activities (Rubin, Coplan, Chen, Buskirk, & Wojslawowica, 2005; Woolfolk & Perry, 2012). Research has overwhelmingly supported positive social skills as critical for healthy social development. Child Trends (www.childtrends.org) has a database of experimentally evaluated, effective program interventions designed to address positive skills. Child Trends and the Tauck Foundation have also partnered to produce a measurement of elementary students' social-emotional skills of self-control, persistence, mastery orientation, academic self-efficacy, and social competence. The instrument has potential for researchers and practitioners to measure and monitor these critical skills.

Children with relationship difficulties may have a negative sense of self. Broderick and Blewitt (2014) explain two main domains of self-concept: academic and nonacademic. Academic self-concept is divided into specific school subjects such as math, science, social studies, and English. Nonacademic self-concept includes a person's sense of self in the social, emotional, and physical realms. Different areas of self-concept emerge at different times in life. For children, the scholastic competence, athletic ability, physical appearance, peer acceptance, and behavioral conduct are the most important dimensions. People who have great discrepancies between their adequacy in a dimension and the importance of that domain experience a negative impact on their self-concept.

These brief descriptions of a child's cognitive, personal, and interpersonal development illustrate the multiple factors that must be taken into account in constructing healthy environments. Developmental psychology also provides a base for understanding the range of normal and abnormal behaviors at various times in life. Many professionals in the mental health field rely on those areas of knowledge as they work with children. Too many young people have mental health problems so we will now consider ways to understand that aspect of their lives.

Children's Mental Health

The Surgeon General (2000) discusses principles necessary for understanding children's mental health. First, professionals must acknowledge the complexity of all of these dynamics: the interactions within the child (biological, psychological, and genetic factors), the child's environment (parents, siblings, family relations, peers, as well as neighborhood, school, community, and national factors), and the way these factors interact.

Therefore, the history of the child is crucial. Second, the report identifies the child's innate abilities to adapt. These "self-righting" and "self-organizing" tendencies allow a child to cope with the world. Third, the importance of age and timing in a professional's understanding of normality is stressed. Crying after separation from a caretaker seems normal for a 2-year-old and perhaps a disturbing symptom in a 10-year-old child. Table 2-4 contains information about normal achievements, common behavior problems, and clinical disorders in childhood. A final point is that the difference between mental health and mental illness often involves only differences in degrees. Mash and Wolfe (2012) explained that children's psychological disorders have different symptoms but share a common ground of being an indication of failing to adapt and the lack of mastering or progressing to a developmental milestone.

Children with psychological disorders are different from other children their age in some aspect of normal development. That failure cannot be credited to a single cause but results from the ongoing interaction between the person and environmental conditions. The American Psychological Association (2009) convened a

TABLE 2-4 DEVELOPMENTAL PERSPECTIVES

Approximate Age	Normal Achievements	Common Behavior Problems	Clinical Disorders
0–2	Eating, sleeping, attachment	stubborn, temper, toileting difficulties	Mental retardation, feeding disorders, autistic spectrum disorder
2–5	Language, toileting, self-care skills, self-control, peer relationships	Arguing, demanding attention, disobedience, fears, over activity, resisting bedtime	speech and language disorders, problems stemming from child abuse and neglect, some anxiety disorders, such as phobias
6–11	Academic skills and rules, rule-governed games, simple responsibilities	Arguing, inability to concentrate, self-consciousness, showing off	ADHD, learning disorders, school refusal behavior, conduct problems
12–20	Relations with opposite sex, personal identity, separation from family, increased responsibilities	Arguing, bragging	Anorexia, bulimia, delinquency, suicide attempts, drug and alcohol abuse, schizophrenia, depression

Mash, E. J., & Wolfe, D. A. (2010). *Abnormal child psychology* (4th ed., p. 34). Belmont, CA: Wadsworth. Reprinted with permission.

summit with the goal of increasing recognition and providing support for efforts to improve the state of child mental health in the United States. That group identified the importance of mental health for normal child development and prevention and treatment options for responding to childhood mental, emotional, and behavioral disorders. These guidelines help professionals by identifying factors for recovery, thus reducing a tendency to oversimplify the complexity of the child's concerns. The guidelines also offer perspectives of multiple targets for intervention and highlight windows of opportunity during a child's development. Counselors will be well served to take advantage of those possibilities.

One of the most disturbing as well as promising research paths has been the Adverse Childhood Experiences (ACEs) study conducted by the Center for Disease Control and the Kaiser Foundation. Adverse childhood experiences were defined as childhood abuse, neglect, and exposure to traumatic stressors. Each of the 17,000 study participants completed a confidential survey about childhood maltreatment and family dysfunction, as well as their current health status and behaviors. This information was combined with the results of their physical examination to form the baseline data for the study which will assess the connections between ACEs, health care use, and causes of death.

So far the researchers have concluded that ACEs are common. Almost two-thirds of our study participants reported at least one ACE, and more than one of five reported three or more ACEs. The short- and long-term outcomes of these childhood exposures include a multitude of health and social problems such as suicide, unintended pregnancies, and substance abuse. The ACE Study uses the ACE

Score, which is a total count of the number of ACEs reported by respondents. The ACE Score is used to assess the total amount of stress during childhood and has demonstrated that as the number of ACE increases, the risk for the health and mental problems increases (Center for Disease Control, n.d.). One positive outcome of these findings outlines the ways communities and individuals can attack these risks to protect young people by developing safe, strong, and nurturing relationships, a goal in which counselors can play a big role.

The preceding discussion has highlighted the individual's development, but throughout life the interaction between the person and the world affects health and all other aspects of life. Bronfenbrenner (1993) helps us understand that interaction with his proposal of an ecological or contextual theory of human development. He proposes that physical and psychological development from child to adult is shaped by many factors and systems. Family is the primary source of socialization and has the predominant impact on the growing child. However, occupations, schools, government, societal norms, and the passage and events of time are also variables to be considered.

Bronfenbrenner's (1993) bio-ecological model categorizes the complex system within which a person exists and grows. Any person lives within nested rings or levels of influence, with each level signifying a different kind of impact on the child. The levels include an immediate environment with expanding connections beyond the home, school, and other settings. Thus, the model ranges from the very personal to the very broad. Therefore, to understand a person, we must consider those multiple environments.

Bronfenbrenner (1993) calls the closest level of the environment the microsystem, which is the activities and interactions in a child's immediate surroundings, the level in which the child has the most contact. He emphasizes that all interactions are bidirectional; for example, the parent's child-rearing practices affect the child, and the child's temperament affects parenting practices. The next ring is the mesosystem and refers to the connections between the immediate environment (family) and other systems that support the child; for example, the parent's workplace or school or place of worship. The exosystem, the next level, relates to social settings, such as health policy and unemployment, which are yet another step removed from the individual. The child is indirectly affected by this system; for example, neighborhood stresses caused by unemployment may affect the child. The final, outermost level of this model is the macrosystem, which is not a specific context but rather the laws, customs, and resources of the society in which the child lives. Bronfenbrenner delivers a comprehensive look at the many factors that influence childhood, as well as a way to categorize those variables. Culture, a complex, encompassing factor, blankets all of those interacting levels. Thus, in order to understand the world of the child we need to investigate the culture of the child.

CULTURE

Herskovits (1948) reportedly defined culture as "the man made part of the environment" (as cited in Draguns, 2008, p. 22). That pithy definition encompasses things that comprise a group's way of life, including customs, traditions, laws, knowledge, shared meanings, norms, and values—all the behavior and attitudes that are learned, shared, and transmitted among group members (Papalia, Olds, & Feldman, 2009). Lefley (2002) more specifically says culture is "a set of shared beliefs, values, behavioral norms, and practices that characterize a particular group of people who share a common identity and the symbolic meanings of a common language" (p. 4). Goodenough (1981) explains that culture has these aspects:

- Ways people perceive their experiences
- Beliefs people use to explain events
- Principles for dealing with people and for accomplishing goals
- Value systems for defining purposes and staying focused on purpose

Children have a culture among themselves that can be observed by adults who probably have limited ability to understand all of the language, rationales, humor, and priorities that young people do not have to explain to each other. Recognizing and accepting that childhood world is one of the joys of working with youngsters as well as a reminder that we encounter different cultures daily.

Vontress (2009) simplifies the concept of culture as the support system for human beings, a way of life transmitted from one generation to another. Often that transmission occurs for children in caregiving relationships as well as by peers, institutions, and the media. Young people are shaped by their interactions with all these systems of influence as Bronfenbrenner (1993) explained. Similarities exist across those interacting spheres. As Maslow (1970) stated people need shelter, food, love, and other essentials to sustain life. Vontress calls this *universal culture* "the biological construction of human beings" and states that each person adjusts to and maintains the physical and mental being of existence—a similarity for all humans. Another system includes the location where a person lives. The language, laws, customs, and other variables that set the nation apart from others form the *national culture*, which may include a *regional culture* specific to certain locations within the nation, such as the Southwest or North in the United States. Free public education is a prominent example of a national culture that greatly impacts children. Finally people may reside in *racioethnic cultures*, which segregate along racial, ethnic, or religious lines. Together these interacting spheres contain many people, places, things, and situations that build the multidimensional world in which we exist.

Jones and McEwen (2000) provided another conceptual model of the multiple dimensions of identity that considers both identity dimensions and contextual influences on identity development. The core variables are personal attributes, characteristics, and identity. Dimensions in the model consist of sexual orientation, race, culture, gender, religion, and social class. Those six dimensions and the core variables are influenced by family background, sociocultural conditions, current experiences, and planning for the future. All these variables coexist in intersecting circles that represent an ongoing construction of identity.

Lee and Diaz (2009) state that counselors must concurrently acknowledge the similarities in humans while celebrating the differences. Counselors work from a stance of acknowledging individuals as unique while understanding the common experiences of humans such as development, school, and family. Choudhuri, Santiago-Rivera, and Garrett (2012) propose a way to understand clients that "neither generalizes identity nor ignores its many dimensions" (p.24). This discussion will focus on concepts and practices to better prepare helpers to accomplish that.

Counselors will always have opportunities to work with children who live with cultural practices and beliefs that the counselors do not know. Baruth and Manning (2012) list the challenges counselors may face in those situations. Counselors may have communication difficulties and may misunderstand the culture and the impact of the culture on the process of counseling. Mental health professionals may hold mistaken assumptions about cultural assimilation and acculturation. The counselor and the client may have different social class values and orientations, and the counselor may be working from stereotypical generalizations. Counselors may make an assumption of cultural bias and may not be able to understand the worldview of the client.

Pedersen (2008) includes other cautions that follow: cultural beliefs influence diagnosis and treatment; diagnoses differ across cultures; clients express symptoms differently across cultures; diagnoses may vary according to categories found most often in the majority populations; and finally, most counselors are members of the majority population, whereas most clients are members of groups underrepresented in the profession.

As noted previously all counselors in some ways work with culturally diverse people. Rather than be daunted by the challenges, we recommend counselors make a commitment to continuous renewal and vigilance in increasing their awareness of self, as well as to refining and deepening the knowledge and skills needed to be an effective counselor in an increasingly pluralistic world.

As a caution we want to point out that some of the terms used to refer to ethnic groups such as black or Hispanic oversimplify the complexities of their culture and any attempt to capture the richness of culture in a few words is inadequate. Papalia et al. (2009) used the term *ethnic gloss* to define the overgeneralization that blurs the variations in different groups but Pedersen, Draguns, Lonner, and Trimble (2008) reminded us that the field of multicultural and cross-cultural counseling has evolved to the extent that our attention must be focused on the between- and within-group variations of populations and the challenges they present to counselors. This chapter section is intended only as an overview of some considerations necessary in counseling across cultures. We use the terms *diversity, cross-cultural, multicultural*, and *pluralistic* as synonyms for the concept of working with someone who has a cultural heritage different from the counselor.

DEFINITION

Sue and Torino (2005) offered a definition of *multicultural counseling* as a helping role and process that utilizes techniques and defines goals that are consistent with the experiences and values of the client. Personal identities are recognized as having individual, group, and universal dimensions. Counselors advocate both universal and culture-specific strategies and roles in the healing process and balance the importance of individualism and collectivism in assessment, diagnosis, and treatment of the client and client systems. That definition broadens the roles counselors play and expands therapy skills. It also calls for inclusive understanding of identity and interventions for both the individual and the context within which the person exists.

Baruth and Manning (2012) explain that counseling professionals may have different descriptions of multicultural counseling but the definitions agree on these key parts:

- Interventions should be sensitive to clients' backgrounds, time of life, gender perspectives, and sexual orientation.
- Counselors plan for differences during the counseling process.
- Counseling is culturally based, both the counselor and the client have their own worldviews and cultural perspectives.
- Clients bring their concerns based on their cultural and ethnic backgrounds, as well as their life period, gender, and sexual orientation perspectives.
- Counselors and clients may have different perceptions of the counseling process and of the outcomes of treatment.

Clearly multicultural counseling must be mastered for one to be an effective counselor in our pluralistic world.

Lee (2013) explains the cross-cultural encounter as a helping space in which a metaphorical wall that may help or hurt counseling. If the counselor is culturally incompetent, unintended cultural regard or disrespect may occur. If the counselor has greater cultural competence, the possibility of building a successful working alliance increases and thus a greater likelihood of resolving a problem and building decision making for the client. He discusses the goal being acknowledging the wall and decreasing the cultural distance between the counselor and the client.

COMPETENCE

Culturally competent counselors are active in the process of becoming aware of their own values, biases, preconceived notions, limitations, and ideas about human behaviors. Second, they actively work to understand the other person's worldview. Third, culturally competent healers constantly develop and practice appropriate, relevant, and sensitive intervention strategies and skills in their counseling (Sue & Sue, 2013). Holcomb-McCoy and Chen-Hayes (2011) explain that counselors with multicultural competence know that child–counselor cultural differences and similarities are important variables in the counseling relationship. In contrast, counselors with low multicultural competence ignore those critical variables.

The areas of awareness, knowledge, and skills have been identified as the main areas of multicultural counseling competence (Sue, Arredondo, & McDavis, 1992). Awareness refers to the understanding of personal worldviews, including that of the counselor. Knowledge relates to the importance of understanding the worldview of culturally different clients. The skills dimension includes the process of developing and practicing strategies for working with culturally different people. Let us now consider more detailed information about counseling competencies.

MULTICULTURAL COUNSELING COMPETENCIES

Multicultural counseling competencies, based on this model of knowledge, awareness, and skills, were articulated by Arredondo and her colleagues (Arredondo et al., 1996). They clearly outline the attitudes and beliefs, knowledge, and skills into

34 competencies that counselors should develop in becoming aware of their own cultural values and biases, their clients' worldviews, and appropriate intervention strategies. The competencies deserve intense study and ongoing practice. Lee (2001) suggests that counselors who succeed with clients from a variety of ethnic backgrounds use a perspective that "acknowledges human differences and celebrates human similarities" (p. 583). Multicultural counseling competencies guide counselors in achieving that perspective and the resulting skills.

Awareness

Self-awareness involves gaining an understanding of the specific things that influence one's psychological, emotional, and cultural attributes. Baruth and Manning (2012) and Lee (2001) suggest that counselors investigate their own cultural background and the impact it has on their beliefs, attitudes, and values. Sue and Sue (2013) explain that counselors who possess the awareness of cultural competency have moved from being culturally unaware to being aware and sensitive to their own heritage and to valuing differences in others. Those counselors know their own values and biases and the ways they may affect diverse clients. Culturally aware counselors are comfortable with the differences between themselves and their clients in terms of age, gender, sexual orientation, and other sociodemographic variables. They recognize the harm that their own racist, sexist, heterosexist, or other damaging attitudes, beliefs, and feelings may cause.

Counselors who are members of the dominant culture, which currently in North American culture is white European American, must begin by becoming aware of their own racial identity. The goals of that growing awareness are the development of a healthy white racial identity and the elimination of intentional or unintentional racism and other biases. Helms (1994) proposed the White Racial Identity Development Model that contains six stages moving from racial obliviousness to commitment to racial equity. The stage of *contact* is one of unawareness of racial identification with minimal acknowledgment of the benefits that one's ethnicity has granted him or her. In the *disintegration* stage, people begin to challenge earlier beliefs but also deny the existence of racism. As people move to the *reintegration* phase, they either overtly or covertly express white superiority. *Pseudoindependence* incorporates an intellectual acceptance of racism but unacceptance of any responsibility of perpetuating the oppression. If they reach the *immersion/emersion* stage, people learn about being white and develop a positive racial identity; and in the *autonomy* phase, they welcome relationships with many ethnic groups and are committed to continuing growth as an ethnic person. Understanding and engaging in this process will help white counselors work with others from different backgrounds. Sue and Sue (2012) integrated Helms' model into a white racial identity development that moves from naïve stage to conformity, dissonance, resistance and immersion, introspection, integrative awareness, and commitment to antiracist action. Counselors must recognize their own racial identity development status and move toward a positive, integrative awareness that embraces growth.

As well as knowledge of self, counselors must develop extensive awareness of racism, sexism, and poverty; individual differences; other culture(s); and diversity (Locke & Parker, 1994). Building an understanding of how culture influences

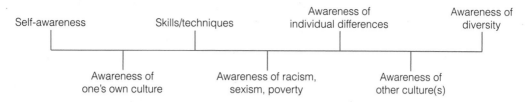

FIGURE 2-2 CROSS-CULTURAL AWARENESS CONTINUUM

Pedersen & Carey, *Multicultural Counseling in Schools: A Practical Handbook*, Second Edition. Published by Allyn and Bacon, Boston, MA. Copyright © 2003 by Pearson Education. Reprinted by permission of the publisher.

educational opportunities, cognitive development, and the interpretation of history (Arredondo et al., 1996) is another desired outcome of the awareness process. Locke (2003) proposes a cross-cultural awareness continuum, a linear illustration that has levels of awareness building on previous levels. He explains that competence in cross-cultural relationships must be a lifelong process of growing self-awareness and developing cultural skills (Figure 2-2). The process of awareness is flexible with absolute mastery elusive. Nevertheless, counselors must undertake the challenge to be helpful in cross-cultural interactions. Locke states that counselors must begin with self-understanding that includes intrapersonal and interpersonal dynamics. Counselors must explore their own culture, and they must understand the effects of racism, sexism, and poverty on themselves and others. Locke continues by explaining that people must be recognized as both individuals and members of their particular cultural group. Those four levels form the foundation for exploring other cultural groups.

Knowledge

Pedersen (2008) explains that people learn behaviors that are always displayed within cultural contexts. He states that a counselor who considers the cultural context will be able to measure behavior more accurately, define personal identity more clearly, understand problems more fully, and counsel more meaningfully. Baruth and Manning (2012) point out that culture should not be considered as fixed but as fluid. As stated earlier, we must recognize the impact of the world where a child lives as we build and maintain a helpful counseling relationship.

Lee (2013) proposes various knowledge bases needed for planning, delivering, and evaluating counseling services. Counselors should understand the impact of economic, social, and political systems on ethnic groups. Counselors should accumulate information about the history, customs, and values of various groups in an effort to understand the intersection of ethnic contexts with the person. He suggests counselors use media, the Internet, and personal experiences with diverse groups to gain the knowledge needed.

Sue and Sue (2013) detail the knowledge needed by culturally competent healers. Counselors need to have information and understanding of culturally diverse groups, especially those with whom the counselor works. They must be familiar with the sociopolitical system of the United States, particularly as it impacts marginalized groups in society. Counselors proficient in cultural work need to have mastered the generic characteristics of counseling. They must also know the barriers that prevent some diverse clients from accessing mental health services.

Among some of the important terms in the field of cross-cultural counseling that counselors need to understand are *race, ethnicity, worldview, ethnic identity development*, and *acculturation*. The following paragraphs provide explanations for these terms.

Thomas, Solórzano, and Cobb (2007) explained that *race* refers to a concept from anthropology and biology used for classifications of people according to physical and genetic characteristics. The term has social meaning, political implications, and stereotypes. Mio, Trimble, Arredondo, Cheatham, and Sue (1999) define race as a classification system that is scientifically meaningless while Baruth and Manning (2012) state race refers to the way a group of people defines itself or is defined as being different due to assumed innate physical qualities. Choudhuri and colleagues (2012) like Thomas enlighten with their explanations of race as a biological construct that groups populations by differences on biological variables such as features such as skin pigmentation and build. Race as a social construct according to those authors incorporated the historical groupings of people into a societal mechanism of classification. However credited, the concept of race and the emotion related to that concept must be understood and accounted for in counseling.

Ethnicity refers to a population with members that have a shared social and cultural identity and heritage (Thomas et al., 2007). Using these definitions, Lee (2001) stated that the "Personality characteristics among people that become reinforced through association over time…these long-standing dynamics of thinking, feeling, and behaving that form the cultural basis of *ethnicity* or an *ethnic group*" (p. 582). He suggested using terminology that captures the realities of ethnic group membership such as Irish American, Korean American, Lakota, and Jamaican American.

Worldview, according to Koltko-Rivera (2004), consists of sets of beliefs and assumptions that describe reality for that person. Worldview constitutes the source of personal values, beliefs, and assumptions, or one's dominant cognitive framework (Baruth & Manning, 2012). It affect the way a person sees self, others, and the world as well as the ways a person thinks and feels. Thus a person's worldview is the source of contact with and assumptions about the world, its meaningfulness, and purpose. Some authors (Grieger & Ponterotto, 2001; Ibrahim, Roysircar-Sodowsky, & Ohnishi, 2001) assert that worldview is the most important variable in multicultural counseling.

In their theoretical model Kluckhohn and Strodbeck (1961) recognize different cultural values in worldviews. They discuss ways cultures address *time* as precise with lives scheduled or variable in which lives are in tune with seasons and weather rather than a clock. Cultures differ in value dimensions related to human nature, relationship to nature, sense of time, activity, and social relationships. The continuum of ways different cultures think of the *nature of humans* ranges from good, bad, or a combination of both. *Relationships between humans and nature* refer to how powerful humans consider nature and want either of mastery over it, harmony with it or suppression of nature. *Time orientation* indicates what aspect of time is foremost—past, present, or future. *Activity* orientation relates to how self-expression occurs—personal achievement focused (doing), personal growth and development focused (becoming), or carefree and spontaneous (being). *Social relationships* refer to three categories related to hierarchy and group focus: lineal-hierarchical (like traditional cultures with hierarchal positions (typically patriarchal); collateral-mutual (such as collectivistic focus), and individualistic (needs of the groups are secondary to those of individuals). These dimensions interact for a system of group norms that shape worldview.

Sue (1978) adds *locus of control* (the degree of control individuals perceive they have over their mastery of the environment) and *locus of responsibility* (what system is accountable for things that happen to the individual) to the categories of worldview. Locus of control and locus of responsibility can be either internal or external. Finally Hofstede (2001) includes *individualism* (individuals are loosely connected and expected to be independent) and *collectivism* (people are part of collective group, protected by the group, and work on behalf of the group) to ways to understand worldview.

Ethnic identity development compounds one's sense of self. Ho (1992) explains the difference between ethnicity and ethnic identity. Ethnicity refers to the person's sense of membership in a group and the associated thoughts, feelings, and behavior; that is, ethnicity denotes group patterns. Ethnic identity refers to the person's incorporation of those patterns and the acceptance of the beliefs, feelings, and actions as one's own. Ethnic identity would shape beliefs about mental health and illness, styles, coping, and help seeking. Lee (2001) calls this the "interior vision," a foundation of social practices and personality dimensions. Robinson-Wood (2009) refers to ethnicity as commonality that includes characteristics of shared group image and identity; shared political, social, and economic interests; and shared involuntary membership.

Ethnic identity development models have been proposed for biracial individuals (Poston, 1990), Asian Americans (Sodowsky et al., 1995), Latinos (Ferdman & Gallegos, 2001), American Indian acculturation (Trimble, 2010), African Americans (Cross, 1995), and whites (Helms, 1995).

The Racial/Cultural Identity development model (Sue & Sue, 2013) describes five phases of change people experience as they come to understand themselves in terms of their own culture, the dominant culture, and the relationships between cultures. Those stages of ethnic identity development are conformity, dissonance, resistance and immersion, introspection, and integrative awareness. Sue and Sue suggest that people move from a stage of *conformity*, in which the dominant group is considered superior to the ethnic group, to a stage of *dissonance*, in which people begin to question their previous beliefs, struggle with discrimination experiences, and have more positive perceptions of their own ethnic group. In the *resistance* and *immersion* stage, people have developed an appreciation for their own ethnic group and a diminished valuing of the dominant group. Stage 4 of the identity development model, *introspection*, refers to more flexibility with both the birth and the dominant culture that leads to the *integrative awareness* stage. That fifth stage represents the time in which individuals realize that both their birth culture and the dominant culture have positive and negative aspects.

Helms (2003) proposes three interacting components that influence a person's ethnic identity: personal, affiliative, and reference group. The personal component relates to self-concept, "Who am I?" The affiliative component relates to the degree to which the person believes that he or she shares whatever happens to other members of his or her ethnic group. The reference group component includes the person's level of conforming to the norms of the group. Helms explains that young children probably reflect the identity climate of their home. During the school years, their understandings become more complex and they may struggle with exclusion in their schools and communities. To help meet these challenges, Washington et al. (2003) have detailed a developmental group process that helps young people recognize their cultural identity group and develop confidence and pride. Ethnic identity can be considered a protective factor for young people's identity (Greig, 2003; Yasuri, Dorham, & Dishion, 2004; Zaff, Blount, Phillips, & Cohen, 2002). High levels of ethnic identity predict positive social and emotional adjustment in adolescents as well as higher self-esteem and better mental health for teens.

Acculturation is the process of adopting cultural traits or social patterns of another group (Vontress, 2009). Ramirez (1999) explains that when children are born into a culture different from the dominant culture, they acquire, at some degree, the second culture. One way of understanding that concept is to think of a continuum with strong connections to the birth culture at one end and strong connections to the dominant culture on the other end (Phinney, 1990). Acculturation can cause changes in a child's original cultural values as the dominant society's values and traditions become internalized (Robinson-Wood, 2009).

Garrett (1995) describes levels of acculturation. In the *traditional* level, a person embraces traditional beliefs and values of the home culture. A person in the *transition* level holds on to the traditional mores as well as those of the dominant culture. This person may not accept all of either culture. At the *bicultural* level, the person accepts and is accepted by both the dominant and the traditional cultures. The fourth type of acculturation is *assimilation*—that is, accepting only the dominant cultural beliefs and values. Ho (1992) suggests that group counseling is most appropriate for minority children who are experiencing difficulties related to acculturation, ethnic identity, and/or bicultural skills.

Counselors working with children will want to acknowledge and assess the impact of *race, ethnicity, worldview, ethnic identity development*, and *acculturation* on the lives and concerns of the young client.

Skills

At its best counseling leads to less distress, resolved problems, balance between person and environment, and an enhanced quality of life (Draguns, 2008). Culturally competent counselors have skills to accomplish this in a way that is consistent with their clients' cultures. Sue and Sue (2013) outlined the skills of cultural competence. Culturally skilled counselors provide a wide variety of both verbal and nonverbal helping responses. They communicate accurately and appropriately in their interactions. As well as their work with individuals, culturally proficient counselors implement institutional interventions on behalf of their clients when needed. They know the impact of their helping styles and realize their limitations in working with culturally diverse people. Culturally skilled counselors are able to perform their roles as active systemic change agents that work for environmental interventions.

Diller (2004) explained that interventions with culturally diverse children require attention to an expanded definition of family, structure, and process; resiliency as a treatment goal; and the reality of biculturalism in the children's lives. Strengthening the personal characteristics in the child will allow enhanced coping without using methods that encourage the child to accept negative environmental situations. Children can learn about underutilized resources and help-seeking strategies. An additional challenge for counselors is monitoring the child's ability to deal with inconsistencies between home and school.

Ho (1992) looked closely at the process of selecting appropriate counseling interventions in a counseling context. According to Ho, the identified skills and guidelines for interventions are necessary when preparing for counseling, when identifying and specifying the problem, when forming goals, solving problems, and ending the counseling relationship. The needed counseling intervention skills for working with children of color are summarized in the Table 2-5.

TABLE 2-5 GUIDELINES FOR INTERVENTIONS WITH CHILDREN OF COLOR

Counseling Phase	Counseling Skills—The Abilities to
Preparation	Recognize the child's ethnic reality, including the effects of racism and poverty
	Understand the child's ethnicity, race, language, social class and differences in status such as refugees, immigrants, and native born
	Use professional culture (counseling, social work, psychology) to work for the child
	Be sensitive to the child's fear of prejudiced orientation
Problem identification	Comprehend the child's cultural dispositions, behaviors, and family structures
	Discuss openly racial/ethnic differences and respond to culturally based cues
	Adapt to the child's interactive style and language
	Understand the child's help seeking, idea of the problem, and ways it can be solved
Problem specification	Identify environmental sources of the child's problems
	specific links between the systemic problems and the individual concerns
	Consider the implications of what is being suggested in relation to the child's reality of personality, strategies, and experiences
Goal formation	Formulate goals consistent with the child's emphasis
	Differentiate and select from three goal categories: situational stress (e.g., social isolation, poverty); cultural transition (e.g., school-family conflict in practices), and transcultural patterns (e.g., friendship skills, future planning)
	Engage the child in determining a goal that is focused on growth, structured, realistic, concrete, practical, and easily achieved
Problem solving	Encourage the child's existing life skills and coping strategies
	Express the change in traditional, culturally acceptable language
	Suggest a new strategy as an expansion of the "old" response
	Apply new strategies consistent with the child's needs and problems, degree of acculturation, motivation for change, and comfort in responding to the counselor's directives
Termination	Determine whether therapeutic goals have been achieved within the child's cultural milieu
	Reconnect and restore the child to the larger world
	Assist the child in incorporating changes into life strategies
	Consider the child's concepts of time and space in a relationship and be sure termination is natural and gradual

Adapted from Ho., M. (1992). *Minority children and adolescents in therapy* (pp. 28–9). Los Angeles: Sage Publishing.

General guidelines for multicultural counselors that Kincade and Evans (1996) suggest include the following:

- Make no assumptions—gather information and re-evaluate your biases often
- Learn about your client's culture from sources other than the client; that is, the library, tapes, brochures, novels, poems, other literature
- Admit your ignorance about your client's culture—be willing to ask questions and learn
- Look for similarities in order to connect—find common ground to share
- Be sensitive to client expectations and needs—together define what counseling is and is not

Thomas et al. (2007) advocated for an interpersonal, multidimensional, systemic approach for culturally responsive counseling. The interpersonal perspective highlights the alliance between counselor and child as the most effective tool in helping. The multidimensional approach involves having several counseling methods that have empirical and clinical support such as solution-focused and cognitive-behavioral theory. It also includes the active involvement of the counselor. Flexibility is essential. Working in a systemic framework means gathering a number of resources in addressing a child's problems such as extended family, schools, medical, and social services. The foundations for cultural sensitivity, according to Thomas et al., are accurate empathy, respect, and genuineness. To become culturally competent, counselors should participate in community activities. Most importantly, counselors reject prejudice and racism and speak out against those practices.

Atkinson (2004) presents a three-dimensional model that includes several roles that counselors can take. He suggests counselors select roles and strategies after considering three variables. Each of the variables exists on a continuum. Counselors determine the client's level of acculturation to the dominant society (ranges from high to low), the locus of the problem origin (external to internal continuum), and the goals of helping (prevention, which includes education/development, to remediation). The appropriate counselor role may change within and between sessions as the professional works to determine how to think and act for the client's well-being. The possible roles that intersect with the factors above include the counselor's being:

- **Adviser**—when the client is *low* in acculturation, the problem is *externally* located, and *prevention* is the treatment goal.
- **Advocate**—when the client is *low* in acculturation, the problem is *external*, and the goal of treatment is *remediation*.
- **Facilitator of indigenous support systems**—when the client is *low* in acculturation, the problem is *internal* in nature, and *prevention* is the goal of treatment.
- **Facilitator of indigenous healing systems**—when the client is *low* in acculturation, the problem is *internal*, and *remediation* is the treatment goal.
- **Consultant**—when the client is *high* in acculturation, the problem is *external* in nature, and *prevention* is the goal.
- **Change agent**—when the client is *high* in acculturation, the problem is *external* in nature, and *remediation* is the treatment goal.
- **Counselor**—when the client is *high* in acculturation, the problem is *internal* in nature, and *prevention* is the primary goal in treatment.

The forgoing overview of the components of multicultural counseling competencies provides some guidance for practicing with clients from a culture different from the counselor's. The following sections contain information more specific to working with children from cultures different than the counselor's.

CHILDREN OF COLOR

Children's lives reflect the culture in which they are raised. The rich, varied landscape of the United States includes a constellation of kinship systems, parenting practices, spiritual traditions, and many other ways of being in the world that influence child rearing. When young people enter school, they encounter other children who have family structures, housing arrangements, and other lifestyle differences. Sometimes as the awareness of those disparities increase, tension builds as children struggle to reconcile life at home with life at school.

Children who have ethnic or social class backgrounds different from those of the mainstream population may face challenges related to not being accepted, receiving unfair treatment, being ridiculed, and being subjected to lower expectations. The socioeconomic status of a family contributes sometimes favorably and sometimes unfavorably to the activities, friends, educational attainment, lifestyle, occupational aspirations, and social roles of the family members. All of those variables may also create stressors for children. For counselors working with children from diverse cultural backgrounds, Kottman (2010) recommends choosing from the following questions to investigate the facts about the child and family:

1. What is the country of origin and cultural identity of the child and his or her family?
2. Which generation of family emigrated?
3. What languages are spoken? Where are the languages spoken?
4. What English knowledge do the parents have? Can they understand the written word? Spoken word? How adequately can they express themselves in English?
5. What are the sleeping and eating patterns at home?
6. What are the expectations for children in the culture?
7. What is the level of acculturation?
8. Which holidays, celebrations, and cultural responsibilities are important?
9. What is the attitude of the family about play?
10. Who are playmates of the child at home and in the community?
11. With what materials does the child play? What are the child's play activities?
12. What are family members' attitudes toward discipline?
13. What are the patterns of discipline?
14. What responsibilities and expectations does the child have at home?

Bernal, Knight, Garza, Ocampo, and Cota (1993) have explained a model of children's ethnic identity development. Although the five components were discussed in terms of Hispanic children, the model can be used to help understand the process as it occurs with other children.

1. *Ethnic self-identification:* Children categorize themselves as members of an ethnic group.
2. *Ethnic constancy:* Children develop knowledge that their ethnic characteristics are constant across time and place.
3. *Ethnic role behavior:* Children take part in behaviors that reflect cultural values, customs, and language.
4. *Ethnic knowledge:* Children understand that some role behaviors, traits, styles, traditions, and language are relevant to their ethnic group.
5. *Ethnic feelings and preferences:* This represents children's emotional response to their ethnic group.

In agreement with other researchers we have discussed earlier, we emphasize the importance of assessing cultural identity and level of acculturation before deciding on interventions with children of color. The child client's cultural frame of reference and mode of communication are essential considerations in working with ethnic children.

Ho (1992) suggested individual counseling when the child's problem is related to stresses of immigration and acculturation, developmental tasks, past traumatic reactions, self-identity, and serious behavioral issues. The goals of the individual therapy would involve strengthening the child's self-image, helping the child acquire coping skills in a bicultural world, improving the child's interpersonal relationships, and modifying inappropriate behavioral patterns. He recommended short-term supportive therapy, cognitive-behavioral therapy, music therapy, and play therapy for intervention choices. Ho stated that group therapy would be beneficial for minority youth who are struggling with the acculturation process, their ethnic identity, bicultural socialization skills, and feelings of isolation. Those suggestions provide a helpful variety of choices for working with children who identify with all cultures.

Similarly Baruth and Manning (2012) suggest that children of color may experience problems that warrant counseling interventions. They may not have developed a strong cultural identity. They may be subjected to the adverse effects of racism and inappropriate value judgments. They may be unable to overcome the perception of being "problem children" in schools and communities. Interpersonal relations, autonomy, academic performance, and future plans may also be concerns young people bring to counselors. Fusick and Bordeau (2004) remind us to focus also on the strengths and potential of all children. We remind counselors to begin with those assets as the helping relationship unfolds and to return to those positives and build upon them often.

Counselors need to avoid being influenced or biased by overly generalized descriptions of individuals and groups and see the child as unique and special. Children who have been reared in American cultures have a great deal in common with one another and with other cultures; however, counselors should not overlook possible differences between cultures and should work to understand both the similarities and the differences, the multidimensionality of the world where we and our child clients exist.

SUMMARY

Children are not miniature adults. As they age, they pass through physical, cognitive, and social changes toward more adult-like bodies, thoughts, and relationships. Counselors must be familiar with those normative changes and the range of accomplishments at different stages of childhood. Additionally, those individual patterns of growth will be affected by the environment in which the child exists. The family, school, community, and many other variables enhance or impede a child's well-being. A critical factor of a child's world is culture. Some of the awareness, knowledge, and skills needed to be a culturally competent counselor are included in this chapter.

Liu and Clay (2002) suggest a decision-making model to use when working with children from diverse backgrounds. They advise counselors first to evaluate which, if any, cultural variables are relevant. Counselors must decide the level of skills and knowledge needed for them to provide competent treatment. The helping professional must assess how much, when, and how to pull in cultural issues. Counselors should always examine the cultural implications of all possible treatments and choose strategies that focus on cultural strengths. The model proposed by Atkinson (2004) provides a means for making those decisions. The number of minority group members living in the United States will continue to grow. Counselors must be prepared to bridge cultural gaps and adopt techniques and procedures to meet the needs of many different children and families.

WEB SITES FOR CULTURAL AND DEVELOPMENTAL FACTORS IN COUNSELING CHILDREN

Internet addresses frequently change. To find the sites listed here, visit www.cengage.com/counseling/henderson for an updated list of Internet addresses and direct links to relevant sites.

Child Trends

American Children and Families (CACF)

Healthy Children

National Center for Children in Poverty (NCCP)

Southern Poverty Law Center Teaching Tolerance

REFERENCES

Ainsworth, M. D. (1989). Attachments beyond infancy. *American Psychologist, 44,* 709–716.

American Psychological Association. (2009). Report of healthy development: A summit on young children's mental health. Retrieved from http://www.apa.org/pi/families/summit-report.aspx

Arredondo, P., Toporek, R., Brown, S. P., Jones, J., Locke, D. C., Sanchez, J., & Stadler, H. (1996). Operationalization of the multicultural counseling competencies. *Journal of Multicultural Counseling and Development, 24*(1), 42–78.

Atkinson, D. R. (2004). *Counseling American minorities: A cross-cultural perspective* (6th ed.). New York: McGraw-Hill.

Baruth, L. G., & Manning, M. L. (2012). *Multicultural counseling and psychotherapy: A lifespan perspective* (5th ed.). Upper Saddle River, NJ: Merrill.

Berger, K. S. (2014). *Invitation to the life span* (2nd ed.). New York: Worth Publishing.

Bernal, M. E., Knight, G., Garza, C., Ocampo, K., & Cota, M. K. (1993). *Ethnic identity: Formation and transmission among Hispanics and other minorities.* Albany, NY: State University of New York Press.

Biehl, M. C., Natsuaki, M. N., & Ge, Z. (2007). The influence of pubertal timing on alcohol use and heavy drinking trajectories. *Journal of Youth and Adolescence, 36,* 153–167.

Bijork, J. M., Knutson, B., Fong, G. W., Caggiano, D. M., Bennett, S. M., & Hommer, D. W. (2004). Incentive-elicited brain activities in adolescents: Similarities and differences from young adults. *Journal of Neuroscience, 24,* 1793–1802.

Blakemore, S. (2008). Development of the social brain during adolescence. *The Quarterly Journal of Experimental Psychology, 61,* 40-49.

Bretherton, I. (1992). The origins of attachment theory: John Bowlby and Mary Ainsworth. *Developmental Psychology, 28,* 759–775.

Broderick, P. C., & Blewitt, P. (2014). *The life span: Human development for helping professionals* (4th ed.). Upper Saddle River, NJ: Merrill.

Bronfenbrenner, U. (1993). The ecology of cognitive development: Research models and fugitive findings. In R. H. Wozniak & K. W. Fischer (Eds.), *Development in context* (pp. 3–44). Hillsdale, NJ: Erlbaum.

Bowlby, J. (1969). *Attachment and loss: Attachment* (Vol. 1). London: Hogarth.

Bowlby, J. (1988). Attachment, communication, and the therapeutic process. In J. Bowlby (Ed.), *A secure base: Clinical applications of attachment theory* (pp. 137–157). London: Routledge.

Burt, S. A. (2009). Rethinking environmental contributions to child and adolescent psychopathology: A meta-analysis of shared environmental influences. *Psychological Bulletin, 135,* 608–637.

Casey, B. J., Jones, R. M., & Somerville, L. H. (2011). Braking and accelerating of the adolescent brain. *Journal of Research on Adolescence, 21,* 21–33.

Center for Disease Control. (n.d.). Injury and prevention control: Adverse child experiences (ACE) study. Retrieved from http://www.cdc.gov/violenceprevention/acestudy/

Chambers, R. A., Taylor, J. R., & Potenza, M. N. (2003). Developmental neurocircuitry of motivation in adolescence: A critical period of addiction vulnerability. *American Journal of Psychiatry, 160,* 1041–1052.

ChildTrends.(2014).Measuringelementaryschoolstudents'socialandemotionalskills.Retrieved from http://www.childtrends.org/?publications=measuring-elementary-school-students -social-and-emotional-skills-providing-educators-with-tools-to-measure-and-monitor -social-and-emotional-skills-that-lead-to-academic-success&utm_source=E-News% 3A+Measuring+the+Social+Genome&utm_campaign=enews+8%2F7%2F14&utm _medium=email

Child Trends Databank. (n.d.) Bullying. Retrieved from http://www.childtrends.org/databank /indicators-by-topic-area/education/

Child Trends Databank. (n.d.). Food insecurity. Retrieved from http://www.childtrends.org /databank/indicators-by-topic-area/poverty/

Child Trends Databank. (n.d.). Homeless children and youth. Retrieved from http://www .childtrends.org/databank/indicators-by-topic-area/poverty/

Child Trends Databank. (n.d.). Neighborhood safety. Retrieved from http://www.childtrends.org/?indicators=neighborhood-safety

Child Trends Databank. (n.d.). Unsafe at school. Retrieved from http://www.childtrends.org/databank/indicators-by-topic-area/education/

Choudhuri, D. D., Santiago-Rivera, A. L., & Garrett, M. T. (2012). *Counseling & diversity.* Belmont, CA: Brooks/Cole.

Compian, L. J., Gowen, L. K., & Hayward, C. (2009). The interactive effects of puberty and peer victimization on weight concerns and depression symptoms among early adolescent girls. *Journal of Early Adolescence, 29,* 357–375.

Corcoran, K. O., & Mallinckrodt, B. (2000). Adult attachment, self-efficacy, perspective-taking, and conflict resolution. *Journal of Counseling and Development, 78,* 473–483.

Cross, W. E. (1995). The psychology of Nigrescence: Revisiting the Cross model. In J. G. Ponterotto, J. M. Casas, L. A. Suzuki, & C. M. Alexander (Eds.), *Handbook of multicultural counseling* (pp. 93–122). Thousand Oaks, CA: Sage.

DeRose, L. M., Shiyki, M. P., Foster, H., & Brooks-Gunn, J. (2011). Associations between menarcheal timing and behavioral developmental trajectories for girls from age 6 to age 15. *Journal of Youth and Adolescence, 40,* 1329–1342.

Diller, J. V. (2004). *Cultural diversity: A primer for the human services* (2nd ed.). Belmont, CA: Thomson.

Draguns, J. (2008). Universal and cultural threads in counseling individuals. In P. B. Pedersen, J. G. Draguns, W. J. Lonner, & J. E. Trimble (Eds.), *Counseling across cultures* (6th ed., pp. 21–36). Los Angeles: Sage.

Dreyfuss, M. (2014). Teens impulsively react rather than retreat from threat. *Developmental neuroscience.* doi: 10.1159/000357755

Elkind, D. (1994). *A sympathetic understanding of the child: Birth to sixteen* (3rd ed.). Boston: Allyn & Bacon.

Erikson, E. (1963). *Childhood and society.* New York: Norton.

Erikson, E. (1968). *Identity, youth, and crisis.* New York: Norton.

Ferdman, B. M., & Gallegos, P. I. (2001). Racial identity development and Latinos in the United States. In C. Wijeyesinghe & B. Jackson III (Eds.), *New perspectives on racial identity development: A theoretical and practical anthology* (pp. 32–66). New York: New York University Press.

Fusick, L., & Bordeau, L. C. (2004). Counseling at-risk Afro-American youth. *Professional School Counseling, 8,* 102–115.

Gagne, J. R., Vendlinski, M. K., & Goldsmith, H. H. (2009). The genetics of childhood temperament. In Y-K Kim (Ed.), *Handbook of behavior genetics.* New York: Springer.

Garrett, M. W. (1995). Between two worlds: Cultural discontinuity in the dropout of Native American youth. *The School Counselor, 42,* 186–195.

Goodenough, W. H. (1981). *Culture, language, and society.* Menlo Park, CA: Benjamin/Cummings.

Greig, R. (2003). Ethnic identity development: Implications for mental health in African-American and Hispanic adolescents. *Issues in Mental Health Nursing, 24,* 317–331.

Grieger, I., & Ponterotto, J. G. (2001). A framework for assessment in multicultural counseling. In J. G. Ponterotto, J. M. Casas, L. A. Suzuki, & C. M. Alexander (Eds.), *Handbook of multicultural counseling* (2nd ed., pp. 357–374). Thousand Oaks, CA: Sage.

Havighurst, R. (1961). *Human development and education* (2nd ed.). New York: David McKay.

Helms, J. E. (1995). An update of Helms's White and People of Color racial identity models. In J. G. Ponterotto, J. M. Casas, L. A. Suzuki, & C. M. Alexander (Eds.), *Handbook of multicultural counseling* (pp. 181–198). Thousand Oaks, CA: Sage.

Helms, J. E. (2003). Racial identity in the social environment. In P. B. Pedersen, & J. C. Carey (Eds.), *Multicultural counseling in schools: A practical handbook* (2nd ed., pp. 44–58). Boston: Allyn & Bacon.

Herskovits, M. J. (1948). *Man and his works: The science of cultural anthropology.* New York: Knopf.

Ho, M. K. (1992). *Minority children and adolescents in therapy.* Thousand Oaks, CA: Sage.

Hofstede, G. (2001). *Cultures consequences: Comparing values, behaviors and organizations across nations* (2nd ed.). Thousand Oaks, CA: Sage.

Holcomb-McCoy, C., & Chen-Hayes, S. F. (2011). Culturally competent school counselors: Affirming diversity by challenging oppression. In B. Erford (Ed.), *Transforming the school counseling profession* (3rd ed., pp. 90–109). Upper Saddle River, NJ: Pearson.

Ibrahim, F. A., Roysircar-Sodowsky, G., & Ohnishi, H. (2001). Worldview: Recent developments and needed directions. In J. G. Ponterotto, J. M. Casas, L. A. Suzuki, & C. M. Alexander (Eds.), *Handbook of multicultural counseling* (2nd ed., pp. 425–456). Thousand Oaks, CA: Sage.

Kincade, E., & Evans, K. (1996). Counseling theories, process and intervention in a multicultural context. *Multicultural counseling competencies: Implications for training and practice.* Alexandria, VA: Association for Counselor Education and Supervision.

Kline, K. K. (Ed.). (2008). *Authoritative communities: The scientific case for nurturing the whole child.* New York, NY: Springer.

Kluckhohn, F. R., & Stodtbeck, F. L. (1962). *Variations in value orientations.* Evanston, IL: Row, Patterson.

Koltko-Rivera, M. E. (2004). The psychology of worldviews. *Review of General Psychology, 8,* 3–58.

Kottman, T. (2010). *Play therapy: Basics and beyond* (2nd ed.). Alexandria, VA: American Counseling Association.

Kuhn, D. (2006). Do cognitive changes accompany developments in the adolescent brain? *Perspectives on Psychological Science, 1,* 59–67.

Lee, C. C. (2001). Defining and responding to racial and ethnic diversity. In D. C. Locke, J. E. Myers, & E. L. Herr (Eds.), *The handbook of counseling* (pp. 581–588). Thousand Oaks, CA: Sage.

Lee, C. C. (2013). The cross-cultural encounter. In C. C. Lee (Ed.), *Multicultural issues in counseling: New approaches to diversity* (4th ed., pp. 13–17). Alexandria, VA: American Counseling Association.

Lee, C. C., & Diaz, J. M. (2009). The cross-cultural zone in counseling. In C. Lee, D. A. Burnhill, A. L. Butler, C. P. Hipolito-Delgado, M. Humphrey, O. Muñoz, H. Shin (Eds.), *Elements of culture in counseling* (pp. 95–104). Upper Saddle River, NJ: Pearson.

Lefley, H. P. (2002). Ethical issues in mental health services for culturally diverse communities. In P. Backlar & D. L. Cutler (Eds.), *Ethics in community mental health care: Commonplace concerns* (pp. 3–22). New York: Kluwer Academic/Plenum Publishers.

Lenroot, R. K., & Giedd, J. N. (2006). Brain development in children and adolescents: Insights from anatomical magnetic resonance imaging. *Neuroscience and Biobehavioral Reviews, 30*(6), 718–729. doi:10.1016/j.neubiorev.2006.06.001

Lindfors, K., Elovainio, M., Wickman, S., Vuorinen, R., Sinkkonen, J., Dunkel, L., & Rappana, A. (2007). Brief report: The role of ego development in psychosocial adjustment among boys with delayed puberty. *Journal of Research on Adolescence, 17*(4), 601–612. doi:10.1111/j.1532-7795.2007.00537.x

Liu, W. M., & Clay, D. L. (2002). Multicultural counseling competencies: Guidelines in working with children and adolescents. *Journal of Mental Health Counseling, 24*, 177–187.

Locke, D. C. (2003). Improving the multicultural competence of educators. In P. B. Pedersen & J. C. Carey (Eds.), *Multicultural counseling in schools: A practical handbook* (2nd ed., pp. 171–189). Boston: Allyn & Bacon.

Locke, D. C. & Parker, L. D. (1994). Improving the multicultural competence of educators. In P. Pedersen & J. C. Carey (Eds.), *Multicultural counseling in schools: A practical handbook* (pp. 39–58). Boston: Allyn & Bacon.

Lopez, R. G., & Brennan, K. A. (2000). Dynamic processes underlying adult attachment organization: Toward an attachment theoretical perspective on the healthy and effective self. *Journal of Counseling Psychology, 47*, 283–300.

Lynch, M. F. (2013). Attachment, autonomy, and emotional reliance: A multilevel model. *Journal of Counseling & Development, 91*(3), 301–312. doi:10.1002/j.1556-6676.2013.00098.x

Lynne, S. D., Graber, J. A., Nichols, T. R., Brooks-Gunn, J., & Botvin, G. J. (2007). Links between pubertal timing, peer influences, and externalizing behaviors among urban students followed through middle school. *Journal of Adolescent Health, 40*(2), 181.e7–181.e13. doi:10.1016/j.jadohealth.2006.09.008

Mash, E. J., & Wolfe, D. A. (2012). *Abnormal child psychology* (5th ed.). Belmont, CA: Cengage.

Maslow, A. (1970). *Motivation and personality* (2nd ed.). New York: Harper & Row.

McDevitt, T. M., & Ormond, J. E. (2012). *Child development and education* (5th ed.). Upper Saddle River, NJ: Pearson.

Meyer, B., & Pilkonis, P. A. (2001). Attachment style. *Psychotherapy, 38*, 466–472.

Mohr, J. J., Gelso, C. J., & Hill, C. E. (2005). Client and counselor trainee attachment as predictors of session evaluation and countertransference behavior in first counseling sessions. *Journal of Counseling Psychology, 52*(3), 298–309. doi:10.1037/0022-0167.52.3.298

National Institute of Mental Health. (2014). Five major mental disorders share genetic roots. Retrieved from http://www.nimh.nih.gov/news/science-news/2013/five-major-mental -disorders-share-genetic-roots.shtml

Newman, B. M, & Newman, P. R. (2011). *Development through life: A psychosocial approach* (11th ed.). Belmont, CA: Cengage.

Papalia, D. E., Olds, S. W., & Feldman, R. D. (2009). *Human development* (11th ed.). Boston: McGraw-Hill.

Pedersen, P. B. (2008). Ethics, competence, and professional issues in cross-cultural counseling. In P. B. Pedersen, J. G. Draguns, W. J. Lonner, & J. E. Trimble (Eds.), *Counseling across cultures* (6th ed., pp. 5–20). Los Angeles, CA: Sage.

Pedersen, P. B., Draguns, J. G., Lonner, W. J., & Trimble, J. E. (Eds.), (2008). *Counseling across cultures* (6th ed., pp. 113–138). Los Angeles: Sage.

Pfeifer, J. H., Dapretto, M., & Lieberman, M. D. (2010). The neural foundations of evaluative self-knowledge in middle childhood, early adolescence, and adulthood. In P. D. Zelazo, M. J. Chandler, & E. Crone (Eds.), *Developmental social cognitive neuroscience* (pp. 141–164). New York, NY: Psychology Press.

Piaget, J., & Inhelder, B. (1969). *The psychology of the child*. New York, NY: Basic Books.

Poston, W. S. C. (1990). The biracial identity development model: A needed addition. *Journal of Counseling and Development, 69*, 152–155.

Robinson-Wood, T. (2009). *The convergence of race, ethnicity and gender: Multiple identities in counseling* (3rd ed.). Upper Saddle River, NJ: Merrill.

Rubin, K. H., Coplan, R., Chen, X., Buskirk, A. A., & Wojslawowica, J. C. (2005). Peer relationships in childhood. In M. H. Bornstein & M. E. Lamb (Eds.), *Developmental science* (pp. 469–512). Mahwah, NJ: Erlbaum.

Schonert-Reichl, K. A., Smith, V., Zaidman-Zait, A., & Hertzman, C. (2012; 2011). Promoting Children's prosocial behaviors in school: Impact of the "Roots of empathy" program on the social and emotional competence of school-aged children. *School Mental Health, 4*(1), 1–21. doi:10.1007/s12310-011-9064-7

Selman, R. L. (1980). *The growth of interpersonal understanding.* New York, NY: Academic Press.

Sigelman, C. K., & Rider, E. A. (2012). *Life-span human development* (7th ed.). Belmont, CA: Wadsworth.

Simpson, J. A., Collins, W. A., Tran, S., & Haydon, K. C. (2007). Attachment and the experience and expression of emotions in romantic relationships: A developmental perspective. *Journal of Personality and Social Psychology, 92*(2), 355–367. doi:10.1037/0022-3514.92.2.355

Simpson, J. A., & Overall, N. C. (2014). Partner buffering of attachment insecurity. *Current Directions in Psychological Science, 23*(1), 54–59.

Simpson, J. A., & Rholes, W. S. (2010). Attachment and relationships: Milestones and future directions. *Journal of Social and Personal Relationships, 27*(2), 173–180. doi:10.1177/0265407509360909

Sowell, E. R., Thompson, P. M., & Toga, A. W. (2007). Mapping adolescent brain maturation using structural magnetic resonance imaging. In D. Romer & E. F. Walker (Eds.), *Adolescent psychopathology and the developing brain: Integrating brain and prevention science* (pp. 55–84). Oxford, UK: Oxford University Press.

Steinberg, L. (2007). Risk taking in adolescence: New perspectives from brain and behavioral science. *Current Directions in Psychological Science, 16*, 55–59.

Sue, D. W. (1978). World views and counseling. *Personnel and Guidance Journal, 56*, 458–462.

Sue, D. W., Arredondo, P., & McDavis, R. J. (1992). Multicultural counseling competencies and standards: A call to the profession. *Journal of Counseling and Development, 70*, 477–486.

Sue, D. W., & Sue, D. (2013). *Counseling the culturally different: Theory and practice* (6th ed.). New York: John Wiley & Sons.

Sue, D. W., & Torino, G. C. (2005). Racial-cultural competence: Awareness, knowledge and skills. In R. T. Carter (Ed.), *Handbook of racial-cultural psychology and counseling* (pp. 3–18). Hoboken, NJ: Wiley.

Taga, K. A., Markey, C. N., & Friedman, H. S. (2006). A longitudinal investigation of associations between boys' pubertal timing and adult behavioral health and well-being. *Journal of Youth and Adolescence, 35*, 401–411.

The Surgeon General. (2000). Children and mental health (pp. 124–220). In Mental health: A report of the Surgeon General. Retrieved from http://profiles.nlm.nih.gov/ps/retrieve /ResourceMetadata/NNBBHS

Thomas, A. R., Solórzano, L., & Cobb, H. C. (2007). Culturally responsive counseling and psychotherapy with children and adolescents. In H. T. Prout & D. T. Brown (Eds). *Counseling and psychotherapy with children and adolescents: Theory and practice for school and clinical settings* (4th ed., pp. 64–93). Hoboken, NJ: Wiley.

Toga, A. W., Thompson, P. M., & Sowell, E. R. (2006). Mapping brain maturation. *Trends in Neurosciences, 29*, 148–159.

Trimble, J. E. (2010). Bear spends time in our dreams now: Magical thinking and cultural empathy in multicultural counselling theory and practice. *Counselling Psychology Quarterly, 23*(3), 241–253.

Vontress, C. E. (2009). A conceptual approach to counseling across cultures. In C. Lee, D.A. Burnhill, A.L. Butler, C.P. Hipolito-Delgado, M. Humphrey, O. Muñoz, & H. Shin (Eds.), *Elements of culture in counseling* (pp. 19–30). Upper Saddle River, NJ: Pearson.

Vygotsky, L. (1978). *Mind in society: The development of higher psychological processes*. Cambridge, MA: Harvard University Press.

Wadsworth, B. (2003). *Piaget's Theory of Cognitive and Affective Development: Foundations of Constructivism* (Allyn & Bacon Classics Edition) (5th ed.). Boston: Allyn & Bacon.

Washington, E. D., Crosby, T., Hernandez, M., Vernon-Jones, R., Medley, R., Nishamura, B., & Torres, D. (2003). Cultural identity groups and cultural maps: Meaning making in groups. In P. B. Pedersen & J. C. Carey (Eds.), *Multicultural counseling in schools: A practical handbook* (pp. 26–43). Boston: Allyn & Bacon.

Wilmshurst, L. (2014). *Child and adolescent psychopathology* (3rd ed.). Los Angeles, CA: Sage.

Woolfolk, A., & Perry, N. E. (2012). *Child and adolescent development*. Upper Saddle River, NJ: Pearson.

World Health Organization. What is mental health? Retrieved from http://www.who.int/features/qa/62/en/

Yasuri, M., Dorham, C. L., & Dishion, T. J. (2004). Ethnic identity and psychological adjustment: A validity analysis for European American and African American adolescents. *Journal of Adolescent Research, 19*, 807–825.

Zaff, J. F., Blount, R. L., Phillips, L., & Cohen, L. (2002). The role of ethnic identity and self-construal in coping among African American and Caucasian American seventh graders: An exploratory analysis of within-group variance. *Adolescence, 37*, 751–773.

CHAPTER 3

The Counseling Process

We shall not cease from exploration
And the end of all our exploring
Will be to arrive where we started
And know the place for the first time.
—T. S. ELIOT, *FOUR QUARTETS*

The type of help counselors offer children may vary according to the model of counseling used. In simple terms, theories provide a way to organize and use information. Theories help counselors understand patterns of personalities and causes of difficulties. Theories explain behavior change and provide details about relationship factors, counseling goals, techniques, processes, and hoped-for outcomes. Counselors use theory to make sense of their observations and to organize information (Gladding, 2013). The following chapters provide an overview of counseling theories and the building of a helping relationship. Counseling theories often differ more in name and description than in actual practice. However, some counseling situations and some children are better suited to one approach than to another. Counseling is basically a learning situation, and individuals have their own favorite ways of learning. After reading this chapter, you should be able to:

- Discuss counseling effectiveness
- Talk about ways to classify counseling theories
- Demonstrate universal counseling skills
- Answer some common questions about the counseling process
- Outline the stages of counseling
- Explain managed care and evidence-based practices

WHICH APPROACHES TO COUNSELING ARE EFFECTIVE?

Years of research support the correlation between counselor's interpersonal skills and counseling effectiveness. According to many sources (Greenberg, Watson, Elliott, & Bohart, 2001; Lambert & Barley, 2001; Lambert & Cattani-Thompson, 1996; Muran & Barber, 2010; Orlinsky, Grawe, & Parks, 1994; Rimondini et al., 2010; Seligman & Reichenberg, 2012), these characteristics, attitudes, and approaches lead to successful outcomes:

- Communicating empathy and understanding
- Being personally and psychologically mature and well
- Having high ethical standards
- Being authoritative and freeing rather than authoritarian and controlling
- Using strong interpersonal skills; showing warmth, care, respect, and acceptance with a helping, reassuring, affirming, protecting attitude
- Handling emotions, asking about emotions, and focusing on emotions
- Being nondefensive; having a capacity for self-criticism and awareness of limitations but not being discouraged; always looking for the best way to help
- Empowering and supporting clients' autonomy and use of resources
- Being tolerant of diversity, ambiguity, and complexity
- Being open-minded and flexible
- Being self-actualized, self-fulfilled, creative, committed to self-development, responsible, and able to cope effectively with stress
- Being authentic, genuine, and having credibility
- Focusing on people and processes, not on rules
- Being optimistic and hopeful, having positive expectation, and being able to encourage those feelings in clients
- Being actively engaged with and receptive to clients and providing structure and focus to treatment
- Establishing a positive alliance early on and maintaining the alliance throughout treatment; addressing ruptures as they occur and managing negative processes effectively

Thus, according to Seligman and Reichenberg, the findings suggest that the emotionally healthy, active, optimistic, expressive, and straightforward, yet supportive, counselor who encourages responsibility on the part of the client is much more likely to have positive outcomes in counseling. Orlinsky, Grawe, and Parks (1994) and Shirk and Karver (2003) found a positive association between the quality of the counseling relationship and treatment effectiveness. They conclude that the counseling relationship is the best predictor of counseling outcome and is critical to its success and effectiveness. Nevertheless, the therapeutic approach to counseling also impacts the outcome.

More than 400 therapy approaches exist (Seligman & Reichenberg, 2012). However, these various systems can generally be classified into intervention categories: thoughts, actions, emotions, systems, and some combination of categories, referred to as eclectic or integrative systems. In comparison studies of the different systems of counseling and psychotherapy, no one approach has emerged as consistently most effective although increasing researchers are learning more about which intervention is more likely to work for a particular problem or client. Generally various counseling approaches based on different theories and emphasizing different methods have been found to be effective for a wide range of people and their problems. Carr (2009) expressed this succinctly by stating that "all approaches to psychotherapy when averaged across different populations, problems and studies lead to moderate to large effect sizes, and benefits for two-thirds to three-quarters of treated cases" (p. 49).

How do we know if counseling is working? We know because the client changes, which is the ultimate goal of counseling and the penultimate outcome. The child may think differently (cognition), feel differently (affect), or act differently (behavior). Therefore, counseling helps a person learn and do something differently.

In his explanation of a large body of research on the effectiveness of therapy, Lambert (2013) concludes that looking either at broad summaries or at the outcome of specific disorders and specific treatment, the evidence remains that therapy is highly beneficial. People who are treated have more positive outcomes than those untreated. While investigators will continue to assess whether counseling is effective, they now also consider what supports to those positive outcomes.

What contributes to that change occurring? That question concerns the process of counseling—what kind of things can counselors do so that clients improve? Seligman and Reichenberg (2012) state that all successful treatments have the following common ingredients:

- A helping relationship that is based on collaboration, trust, a mutual commitment to the counseling process, respect, genuineness, positive emotions, and a holistic understanding of the client
- A safe, supportive, therapeutic setting
- Goals and direction
- A shared understanding of the concerns that will be addressed and the process to be used in working on them
- Learning
- Encouragement
- Clients' improved ability to name, express appropriately, and change their emotions
- Clients' improvement in identifying, assessing the validity of, and changing their thoughts
- Clients' increased ability to gauge and change their actions, as well as acquire new, more effective behaviors to promote coping, impulse control, positive relationships, and sensible emotional and physical health (p. 20)

Seligman and Reichenberg also note that effective counseling promotes feelings of mastery, self-efficacy, realistic hope, and optimism. We will now turn to another explanation of effective treatment.

Corsini (2008) described his search for the critical elements in the counseling process necessary for change. His compilation of nine factors of change hinges on three categories of cognitive, affective, and behavioral factors as outcomes for the client. He summarizes those categories as "know yourself," "love your neighbor;" and "do good works." Fuller descriptions of these basic mechanisms for change follow. More specifically these factors unfold according to the following explanations.

Cognitive Factors

Universalization: People get better when they understand that they are not alone, that other people have similar problems, and that suffering is universal.

Insight: When people understand themselves and gain new perspectives, they improve.

Modeling: People profit from watching other people.

Affective Factors

Acceptance: Receiving unconditional positive regard from a significant person, such as the counselor, builds a person's acceptance of self.

Altruism: Change can happen when a person recognizes the gift of care from the counselor or others or from the sense of giving love, care, and help to others.

Transference: This factor implies the emotional bond created between the counselor and the client.

Behavioral Factors

Reality testing: People can change when they can experiment with new behavior and receive support and feedback.

Ventilation: Having a place to express anger, fear, or sadness and still be accepted promotes change.

Interaction: People improve when they can admit something is wrong.

The incorporation of those factors into a therapeutic relationship leads to the affirmation that counseling works because clients improve.

Kazdin and Weisz (2003) reviewed meta-analyses of child and adolescent therapy. They concluded that treatment appears to be better than no treatment, and the positive effects with children and adolescents are equivalent to the benefits obtained with adults. The documentation of effective intervention and prevention programs for young people has also been compiled by the American Psychological Association Task Force on Evidence-Based Practice for Children and Adolescents in 2008. A special edition of the *Journal of Clinical Child & Adolescent Psychology* includes articles about treatment for depression (David-Ferdon & Kaslow, 2008), disruptive behavior (Eyberg, Nelson, & Boggs, 2008), phobia and anxiety (Silverman, Viswesvaran, & Pina, 2008), substance abuse (Waldron & Turner, 2008), and other disorders.

Lambert and Cattani-Thompson (1996) likewise found that counseling is more effective than no treatment, that the positive effects are lasting, and that improvement can occur relatively quickly. Those and other authors (Kazdin & Weisz, 2003; Sexton & Whiston, 1996; Smith, Glass, & Miller, 1980) have found little evidence for specific techniques being consistently more effective than others. Lambert (2013) categorizes the broad categories of change agents and proportional effects on counseling as the following:

A. *Client variables* (40 percent): These include elements like the problem type and the number of problems being experienced, the maturity and strength of the client, and the motivation for change. Other factors such as the support system and the world in which the client lives impact therapy.

B. *Common factors* (30 percent): These are factors that strengthen the counseling relationships such as empathy, warmth, respect, acceptance, and encouragement of risk taking. Obviously these directly relate to the counselor. A welcome resource for delineation of relationship elements that strengthen counseling has been compiled by Norcross (2011).

C. *Expectations for change* (15 percent): These variables involve the sense of hopefulness and awareness of being treated. Fraser and Solovey (2007) state that restoring hope is the ultimate goal of counseling and the thread across all interventions.

D. *Therapy models and techniques* (15 percent): This small but important contribution to change refers to models of counseling (e.g., behavior therapy, child-centered therapy) and interventions (e.g., role-plays, life scripts). The models organize and provide direction to counseling (Lambert, 2013; Slattery & Park, 2011).

Counselors therefore have options about what they do to help clients change. In fact, Carr (2009) and Imel and Wampold (2008), like Seligman and Reichenberg (2012), support the notion that common factors across counseling approaches contribute to effectiveness. According to those authors the elements of change are present in all theories and change happens because counselors attend to those elements regardless of their theoretical stance, or as Lambert (2013) contends, learning ways to engage the person in a collaborative effort is central to effective counseling. Therefore, effective counseling involves an alliance of the client and counselor in:

- Exploring and rethinking problems
- Giving a credible reason for counseling
- Generating hope for improvement
- Mobilizing the person to resolve the problem

Counselors accomplish that process by providing *support factors*, *learning factors*, and *action factors* (Lambert & Cattani-Thompson, 1996; Lambert & Ogles, 2004). Support factors include variables such as the counselor building a positive relationship, developing a working alliance, and demonstrating warmth, empathy, and trust. As the supportive environment grows, the counseling process moves to the client learning to see the problem in new ways. Some of the learning factors the counselor generates are corrective emotional expression, affective experiencing, reframing, and assimilating problem experiences. Next, the counselor uses interventions to promote behavior change. Some examples of the third category, action factors, are gaining cognitive mastery, facing fears, interpersonal risk taking, practicing new behaviors, and regulating behaviors. understanding those common factors can help counselors build essential skills. Their theoretical knowledge will allow them to use those skills wisely as they determine what theory should guide their practice.

Our position is that counselors should understand a range of theories, and training counselors in a variety of approaches has considerable support. Thompson and Campbell (1992), in a phenomenological study, surveyed 500 people on what type of self-help interventions they chose to alleviate mild depression. These interventions were spread fairly equally across affective, behavioral, cognitive, and eclectic categories, with a slight but significant preference for affective remedies. The authors attributed these results to the preponderance of women in the sample and to their expressed preference for affective interventions. Men, by contrast, tended to favor cognitive interventions. The study indicates that effective counselors should be able to adapt to the client's preferred learning style rather than expecting the client to adapt to the counselor's preferred counseling style.

Corsini (2008) states that good counselors take an eclectic stance or integration of theories. That is possible only when the counselor can draw on a vast array of theories and techniques in an integrated approach and is not bound by any single theory. However, Gladding (2013) cautions that if the counselor is not completely familiar with all parts of the theories involved, the results can be harmful. Two approaches to integrative counseling are outlined next.

Lazarus (2008) recommends a multimodal, or comprehensive, eclectic framework for counseling that can be adapted to meet the needs of individual children. Lazarus developed his BASIC ID model based on a social learning model to describe seven ways people experience their world and some of the problem areas related to his categories that are often treated in counseling. The BASIC ID model is as follows:

Behavior: This includes habits, responses, and reactions that can be observed. Examples of counseling problems in this modality would be concerns such as fighting, crying, inappropriate talking, stealing, and procrastination.

Affect: This arena refers to a variety of emotions and moods. Some of the resulting counseling concerns would be expressions of anger, anxiety, phobias, depression, loneliness, and feelings of helplessness.

Sensation/School: This includes the basic senses of seeing, hearing, touching, tasting, and smelling. The negative aspects include difficulties such as headaches, backaches, dizziness, and stomachaches; perceptual or motor difficulties; and for children, concerns about school failure or lack of achievement.

Imagery: This category incorporates fantasies, mental pictures, and dreams, as well as images from auditory or other senses. Related counseling problems would be things such as nightmares, low self-esteem, negative body image, fear of rejection, and excessive daydreaming and fantasizing.

Cognition: This category incorporates thoughts, ideas, values, and opinions. Children may come to counselors with problems such as irrational thinking, difficulty in setting goals, decision-making problems, problem-solving difficulties, or thoughts of worthlessness.

Interpersonal relationships: An area devoted to the way one interacts with family, friends, peers, teachers, and others. Related counseling concerns may be withdrawing from others (shyness), conflict with adults, conflict with peers, family problems, or difficulties with others.

Drugs/Diet/Biology: The final category focuses on health and medical concerns. Examples of problems counselors may work with include hyperactivity, weight-control problems, drug abuse, and addictions.

The Lazarus BASIC ID model covers most of the problems that counselors working with children, adolescents, or adults are likely to encounter and provides a well-defined eclectic approach to understanding and working with people seeking help. Lazarus (2008) says this model answers "What works?" "For whom?" and "Under what conditions?" The selection of treatment strategies involves matching the intervention to the client, problem, and situation (Lazarus). Counselors must have a sound knowledge of the theories, an integrative view of behavior that brings the different theories together, and a flexible way of fitting the approach to the client. Counselors must also be sensitive to knowing what approach to use as well as when, where, and how (Gladding, 2013).

Lazarus (2008) explained a scale to assess the person's BASIC ID modality preferences. He provided a seven-point rating scale that can provide a profile of the person's reports of behavior, affect, sensation, imagery, cognition, interpersonal, and drugs/biology. He also outlined a helpful formula for outcome evaluations by listing the particular gains of counseling in each modality:

Behavior:	Less withdrawn; less compulsive; more honest
Affect:	More feelings of joy, less hostile; less depressed
Sensation:	Enjoys more; less anxious; more relaxed
Imagery:	Fewer nightmares; better self-image
Cognition:	Less self-criticism; more positive self-statements
Interpersonal:	More or deeper friendships; states wishes and preferences
Drugs/biology:	Has reduced bad habits; sleeps well; active (p. 390)

After identifying the problem areas, counselors design interventions to strengthen weak areas before those areas become more serious problems.

Another eclectic approach is the integrative model (Norcross & Beutler, 2014). These authors base treatment decisions on client characteristics such as diagnosis, coping style, resistance, and patience preferences. They incorporate outcome research, specific contributions of system of therapy, and matching methods in their approach. A critical part of this model is the client's readiness to change, which they describe as a set of tasks needed for movement to the next step. *Precontemplation* refers to the client who has no intention to change—children who are referred to counseling will most often be in this stage because they are unaware or under aware of what others see as a problem. *Contemplation* is the stage in which people know a problem exists and are seriously considering overcoming the concern, but they have not yet made a commitment to action. *Preparation* combines intent with behavioral criteria. People mean to do something in the near future, but they have not reached the level of change that is desired. *Action* is the phase in which people change behavior, experiences, or setting in order to overcome their problems. Finally, *maintenance* is the stage in which people work to avoid reverting to the previous behavior and to incorporating their progress into their lives. Those change stages are critical to any form of counseling. The counseling approaches presented in this book offer possibilities for helping counselors work with one or more of the seven areas presented in the BASIC ID model and the processes in the integrative approach to counseling.

CLASSIFYING COUNSELING THEORIES

One way to classify counseling theories is to examine how the practitioners of each theory encounter their clients. As noted previously some counselors focus on the client's feelings, whereas others intervene with thinking or behavior. Change in any one of these three areas is likely to produce change in the other two. The outline of change mechanisms articulated by Norcross and Beutler (2014) and explained earlier supports that assumption. Therefore, rather than a two-dimensional continuum, we propose a model showing the interwoven relationship that exists among thoughts, feelings, and behaviors as shown in (Figure 3-1).

Counselors may also choose to work beyond the individual on a systemic level. At that level, counselors may intervene with families, institutions, teachers, health care professionals, communities, or other systems that have an impact on the lives

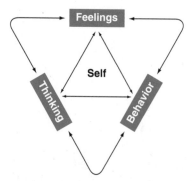

FIGURE 3-1 CLASSIFICATION OF COUNSELING APPROACHES

of children. We focus on the point of intervention, classifying the theories and interventions presented in this book as follows:

Affective (feeling)
> Person-centered counseling
> Gestalt therapy

Behavior (behaving)
> Behavioral counseling
> Reality therapy
> Brief counseling
> Individual psychology

Cognitive (thinking)
> Rational Emotive Behavior Therapy
> Cognitive behavioral therapy
> Psychoanalytic counseling
> Transactional analysis

Systemic interventions
> Family therapy
> Consultation and collaboration

Our intention is not to isolate feeling, thinking, behaving, or systems. Failure to integrate feelings, thoughts, and behaviors is a symptom of schizophrenia, a diagnosis that describes a loss of contact with the environment, a split from reality, and a disintegration of personality. Rather, we attempt to describe how effective intervention in one of the three areas helps the individual maximize the other two areas into a more fully functioning lifestyle.

Counseling theories can also be classified as belonging to one of two broad categories. The first category focuses on observable events and data: behavior, antecedents to behavior, consequences of behavior, behavioral goals, and plans. The second category focuses on the unobservable events and data surrounding counseling: feelings, thoughts, motivation, and causes of behavior (Figure 3-2).

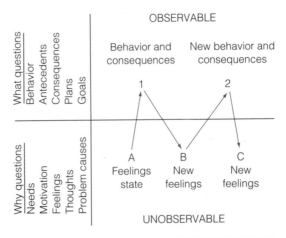

FIGURE 3-2   FOCUS POINTS FOR COUNSELING INTERVENTIONS

Category 1 counselors believe that if you feel bad at Point A (see Figure 3-2), the only way to feel better at Point B is to make a positive change in your behavior, which, in turn, leads to better feelings at Point B. Additional positive change in behavior leads to even better feelings at Point C.

Category 2 counselors believe just the opposite. If you feel bad at Point A, you need to work through these feelings and/or thoughts with your counselor until you have sufficient strength to make a behavioral change at Point A. You then examine the resulting thoughts and feelings at Point B for meaning and significance, which helps you to gather sufficient strength to tackle the next behavioral change.

Classifying the various approaches to counseling creates a framework for examining their similarities and differences. These approaches have a variety of techniques adaptable to learning style differences. The cognitive, affective, and behavioral classifications should help counselors provide children with appropriate counseling methods.

Attending to the points of intervention helps counselors make treatment plans for their young clients. Counselors also need to pay attention to particular skills to allow the counseling process to succeed. Erdman and Lampe (1996) and Van Velsor (2004) have identified critical adaptations to basic counseling skills when working with children. They urge counselors to attend to the following issues:

- Understanding the child's level of cognitive and emotional development
- Presenting information in a way that matches that understanding
- Using concrete examples, hands-on activities, details about rules if they are necessary, and careful explanation of consequences
- Recognizing that the egocentric child will be unable to see another point of view and will not question his or her own thoughts or reasons
- Realizing children do not have clear ideas about time, amount, and frequency
- Knowing that memories and expectations of the child may be distorted
- Acknowledging the reality that children often lack control over many aspects of their existence
- Understanding that reluctance to change may be expected and may involve crying, silence, laughing, fidgeting, and fighting

To address these characteristics in counseling settings, counselors work to establish appropriate physical environments, build trust in the relationship, maintain a helpful attitude, and use questions appropriately (Erdman & Lampe, 1996; Van Velsor, 2004).

Counselors have a repertoire of universal verbal skills to use as they work with children and others. Those skills help build rapport and encourage discussion, help in gathering data, and add depth and support to the counseling process.

Counselors encourage children to talk and interact with active-listening skills. First, counselors pay attention with their bodies. Their posture, gestures, facial expressions, and general demeanor denote an open, friendly presence that invites communication. The foundations of active listening are empathy, reflections of feelings, and reflections of meaning. Chapter 6 has extended discussions and exercises related to those skills. Explanations of other universal skills follow.

Minimal encouragers are brief responses to show you are listening. Counselors can use murmurs, like "umm-hmm," repeat a word or phrase or nod, motion with the hand, or give other indications for the child to continue.

Minimal encourager:

CHILD: I have a new friend that just moved here.

COUNSELOR: Umm-hmm.

Other active-listening skills are *restating* and *paraphrasing*, the act of giving back the thoughts or feelings the child has mentioned. Restatement uses the exact words, and paraphrase changes the words the child uttered.

Restatement:

CHILD: I really want to go to that dance and be with Ken and have time just for us.

COUNSELOR: You want to go.

Paraphrase:

CHILD: I really want to go to that dance and be with Ken and have time just for us.

COUNSELOR: You want to be there to spend time with him.

Another useful skill is *summarizing*, which pulls together a group of statements, giving back information children have shared in a concise way. You can use summarizing to review, highlight, or give the child a chance to hear what has been shared.

Summary:

COUNSELOR: You've told me about your new friend, your teacher, and reasons you want to go to that dance. You have lots of plans for next week.

Counselors also use their responses to gather more information about the person and situation. *Clarifying* strategies allow the child to explain something in more detail.

Clarifying:

CHILD: My mom says if I'm really, really good she'll let me go.

COUNSELOR: What do you do to be really, really good?

Counselors use *perception checks* to determine if they have understood what has been said.

Perception check:

COUNSELOR: Let me see if I understand—you do your homework, help with the dishes, and go to bed without complaining—is that it?

Counselors use *behavioral tracking* to reflect what the child is doing and to communicate their attention when children are playing.

Tracking:

COUNSELOR: You're stacking that.

Short descriptions of those and some other skills, purposes, and ways to use them are included in Table 3-1. In the sections following, we will indicate at what stage of the counseling process the skills might be most useful. Included in the following sections are considerations for counseling such as preparing for the interview, working with resistance, a model of counseling, and questions that are often asked.

PREPARING FOR THE INTERVIEW

Effective counselors create a relaxed counseling environment and build rapport with their clients. The counseling environment should contribute to a client's feelings of comfort and ease. A cluttered, stimulating, busy room can distract children, whose attention is easily drawn to interesting objects in the room and away from the counseling interaction. Restless, distractible children may be affected by brightly colored objects, mobiles, ticking clocks, outside noise, or even darting fish in an aquarium. Inasmuch as counselors are part of the environment, you should also check yourself for distracting jewelry, colorful ties, or patterns in clothing that may affect children. We recommend a room with warm colors, soft seats, and a place to sit on the floor and play.

The furniture in the counseling room should be comfortable for both adults and children. We suggest that the counselor not sit behind a desk or table that can act as a barrier between child and counselor. Children see people sitting behind desks as authority figures, such as teachers, principals, and caseworkers. Children prefer chairs that are low enough to allow them to keep their feet on the floor.

Counseling seems to work better if children can control the distance between themselves and the counselor. Adults are often too aggressive in trying to initiate conversations with children. Children prefer to talk with adults at the same eye level; thus, some care needs to be given to seating arrangements that allow for eye-to-eye contact and feet on the floor. Of the various possible seating arrangements (Figure 3-3), two seem to be *least* effective: (1) having a desk between the counselor and the child, and (2) having no barrier at all between counselor and child. The third arrangement, which uses the corner of a desk or table as an optional barrier that allows the child to retreat behind the desk or

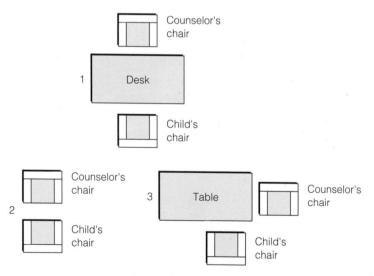

FIGURE 3-3   SEATING ARRANGEMENTS FOR COUNSELING CHILDREN

table corner or to move out around the corner when he or she feels comfortable doing so, is the preferred seating arrangement.

A thick carpet, comfortable chairs, floor pillows, puppets, dollhouses, and other toys to facilitate communication are also recommended for the counseling room. Many counselors conduct all of their interviews with children on the carpet in a play therapy room (see Chapter 17). Play media have developed a relaxed atmosphere with younger children, and older children and adolescents will find clay and other manipulatives relaxing to hold. Some counselors employ large, friendly dogs as icebreakers, with child and counselor sitting on a rug and playing with the dog during the session. Animal-assisted therapy has been well addressed by several authors (Dugatkin, 2009; Fine, 2010; King, 2007).

Counselors should be models of promptness for scheduled sessions. Children (and adult clients) dislike being kept waiting. Tardiness may be interpreted as lack of interest or cause restlessness, fatigue, or irritability. The counselor should be free from distracting worries and thoughts and ready to devote full attention to the child. Children are extremely sensitive to adult moods and can recognize insincerity or lack of concern quickly. Many counselors reschedule appointments when they do not feel well rather than risk hurting the counseling relationship. If you have a cold, headache, or other minor ailment, you may want to admit to the child that you are not feeling up to par rather than have the child misinterpret your behavior as a lack of interest.

WHAT ARE SOME THINGS TO CONSIDER DURING THE FIRST INTERVIEW?

Children's Resistance to Counseling

Children who are clients are still children, with their own feelings, behaviors, problems, and expectations of counselors. Like adults, children have fear of the unknown. To be frightened of new faces in new places with new activities and mystery outcomes is very natural. Children may not know why they are being taken to a counselor's office. In fact, parents or teachers may have given them misinformation that could result in mistrust of the counselor who does not meet a child's expectations. Questions children may have about counseling include:

- What is counseling, and why do I have to go there?
- Did I do something wrong? Am I being punished?
- Is something wrong with me?
- Do Mom and Dad (or teacher) think something is wrong with me? Do they love me?
- Will my friends think something is wrong with me? Will they make fun of me if they find out?
- Will it hurt? Is it like going to the doctor?
- How long does it take? When will I get to go home or back to class?
- If I don't like it, will I have to come back?
- What am I supposed to say and do? What if I say something wrong?
- Should I tell bad things about my family?
- Will the counselor tell anybody what I say?

Effective counselors understand the full range of fears, misunderstandings, and questions children might have about visiting a counselor's office for the first time. In addition, children, as well as adults, naturally resist situations in which they might lose their freedom to choose what they would like to say and do. When children are forced to do things, they become angry, resistant, and oppositional in an attempt to regain control. Children may also get angry because they view the trip to the counselor's office as unfair. They may think they are being blamed for the family's or someone else's problems.

Children generally are not motivated to seek counseling. Children are drawn to pleasurable thoughts, feelings, and behaviors and tend to avoid negative feelings, thoughts, and activities. Until they reach adolescence, they are seldom self-reflective and prefer simple answers to connect to something they know well. A first visit to the counselor would ordinarily not be a favorite activity. However, in those elementary and middle schools that are fortunate enough to have talented counselors who lead regular group meetings with all of the students, children will have a stronger trust and understanding of counseling. Often in those inviting environments children refer themselves to these trusted counselors.

Children do many of the same things adult clients do to resist counseling, such as:

- Refuse to talk, refuse to share anything of importance, deny there is a problem, and/or talk about irrelevant topics
- Avoid any type of connection with the counselor such as eye contact or thoughtful interaction
- Come late for or miss their appointments
- Exhibit negative body language and make hostile comments
- Act out and refuse to cooperate (e.g., hide behind the furniture or sit with arms crossed and eyes on the floor)

The above list is certainly not exhaustive. People can be very creative in devising ways to resist anything, and counselors should rely on their own feelings as indicators of client resistance. Frustration and anger are common reactions counselors have toward uncooperative clients. Counselors need considerable patience and high levels of frustration tolerance to work with difficult children. Their major task is to get on the same team with their child clients and try to help these children find better ways to get what they want and need. Remember that resistant children are reacting normally, as anyone would do, to a strange situation and to someone who is trying to change them in ways they do not understand. Many children are not self-referred, and counselors are often viewed as extensions of the system that has been unhelpful and even painful to them. Resistant children are protecting themselves from the counselor's agenda, which they are unwilling or afraid to follow.

Steps to Overcoming Children's Resistance

The first step in the successful application of all counseling theories is the development of a good counseling relationship, a therapeutic alliance between counselor and client. The relationship-building process begins with the counselor as a person. *Friendly, warm, interested, genuine,* and *empathic* are the key descriptive words used to define successful counselors. For children, such a person truly listens and understands how they think and feel about things. The counselor does not rush the child, bombard the young one with questions, or smother the child with perhaps well-meaning but disrespectful pity. Children view effective counselors as caring, protective, safe, and on their side. "On the child's side" means being the child's advocate rather than best friend. However, taking the role of a child's advocate does not excuse the counselor from maintaining the empathy/objectivity balance necessary for successful counseling. Effective counselors are also able to strike a healthy balance between adult–adult and parent–child activities in the counseling session. From transactional analysis (see Chapter 14), adult–adult activities are the problem-solving and decision-making parts of counseling; the parent–child activities are the nurturing and relationship-building parts of counseling. Finally, the counselor should offer children as many choices as possible to restore to them some of the control children might have thought they lost by coming to counseling; for example, allowing them to choose where to sit or what to discuss gives them a sense of mastery.

As a second step, as mentioned earlier, the counselor's office should seem like a friendly, comfortable, relaxed, safe place to be. Children find security in consistency, limits, and predictability. Counseling appointments should be regularly scheduled for the same time and day. Counseling time is the child's time. The appointment should begin on time and not be interrupted by phone calls or knocks on the door or any other disruption. Attention to these scheduling details makes children feel worthy and important, a person who is getting undivided attention. Counselors should set behavioral limits that can be enforced with logical consequences; for example, "the sand must stay in the sandbox, and sand play has to stop until the sand is swept up and put back in the box." Misbehavior is handled best by redirecting it to appropriate activity; for example, "People are not for hitting; punching bags are for hitting."

Third, children need to understand what counseling is and what they can expect from it. Some counselors prefer to ease the anxiety of the initial meeting by engaging in general conversation with the child for a few minutes. After initial introductions, the counselor may start to talk with the child about home, school, friends, hobbies, or other interests. For nonverbal or extremely anxious children, the first session or two may include play therapy. Through these methods the counselor can begin to build a good relationship with the child while learning something about the child's world. Other counselors prefer to go directly to the problem; for example, "Would you like to tell me why you have come to see me?" During the initial interview, the counselor should explain to the child the process of counseling and the counselor's expectations for their relationship. The following is sample dialogue between a counselor and a child of middle school age:

COUNSELOR: Do you know what counseling is?

CHILD: No. [If the child answers yes, the counselor might say, "Tell me your ideas about what counseling is."]

COUNSELOR: Well, at some time during our lives, most of us have things that worry or upset us— things we would like to talk to someone about. It could be something that's going on at school, like another student in our class or our teacher; or it could be something at home, brothers or sisters, or maybe parents who don't really understand how we feel. It could be that we are having trouble with friends or we're confused about how things are going. We may have some thoughts or feelings that would be helpful to discuss with someone. A counselor listens and tries to help the other person work out these things. A counselor tries to think with that person about ways to solve these worries. Your job is to tell me whatever is bothering you. My job is to listen carefully and try to help you find ways to solve these problems.

The preceding statement is too long and wordy for children younger than 7 years. Counselors should adjust their explanations of the process to the developmental level of the child and use sentences with fewer words.

For children whom others have referred for counseling, the counselor can begin with a statement such as "Mrs. Jones told me that you were very unhappy since you moved here and that you might want to talk to me about it," or "Mr. Clifford told me that you would be coming by," and wait for the child to respond to tell what the trouble is.

In the first example, the counselor has informed the child that he or she is aware of the problem and is ready to discuss it. In the second example, the counselor is less directive, provides less structure, and allows the child to explain the problem, which may or may not be the one for which the child was referred. The counselor will want to consider the child's age; culture; and cognitive, social, and emotional development; as well as the type of presenting problem, before deciding which type of opening statement to use. The younger the child, chronologically and developmentally, and the more specific the problem, the greater the probability that the child will respond more readily to a structured approach.

In a more direct approach for counseling "other-referred" children, a counselor might say, "Let me tell you what your teacher shared with me that led to your being asked to see me." The counselor states the teacher's concern in a way that lets the child know that the counselor is there to help and not to punish. The counselor could say, for example, "Mr. Thompson is concerned about your behavior in class. He is afraid you will not learn all you need to know if you don't change what you are doing." Carlson (1990) believes that counseling needs to be defined for "other-referred" children in language they can understand. For example, "Counseling is a time when you can talk to me about things that bother you. We can also talk about what we need to do to make things better."

Children need to know how much of what they say in counseling is confidential and what is not. Counselors are required by to report any evidence of homicidal or suicidal ideation, child sexual or physical abuse, and child neglect. Counselors may say something such as "What we talk about is confidential or just between you and me unless I have to stop someone from getting hurt. I'll tell you if I have to talk to someone if you say something like that, and I will not tell anybody about anything else unless you say it is okay to tell something." These examples of what counselors might say can be modified to fit the situation, the age and maturity level of the child, and the counselor's personality. Of course, counselors may divulge any of the content of counseling that child clients give them permission to report.

First Interview Goals and Observations

Children begin counseling in an exploratory way (Van Velsor, 2004). Counselors should focus on building the relationship with their child client by building trust. Defining the counselor's role and the child's expectations provides the structure for an ongoing counseling relationship. During the first session, the counselor's main task is to build bridges between the child's world and the counseling office. Friendly, confident counselors who seem in control help children feel safe and secure in the new counseling environment. Counselors can begin by asking children what name they want to be called. Fun activities are helpful in getting the first session off to a relaxed start. A child who feels anxious about separating from a parent can have the parent join the activity. Serving a snack, reading a favorite story, and playing a game are good ways to reach the child. A parent may be included in all of these introductory activities. Some children, having been told not to speak to strangers, need assurance from their parents that the counselor can be trusted and that it is all right to speak to him or her.

For children who can read, counselors should have an engaging brochure that outlines the counseling process and other things the child needs to know to understand what will happen during your time together. The child and counselor can review this document as the informed consent process that is mentioned in Chapter 4.

Children differ from adults in several ways that affect counseling and play therapy. For example, the following are differences:

1. Children, lacking elaborate adult defenses, regress quickly and easily into spontaneous and revealing play activities.
2. Children have rich fantasy lives that reveal their thoughts, feelings, and expectations.
3. Lacking adults' formal thinking skills, insight, and verbal skills, children communicate through acting out their fantasies in their stories or play activities.

Once the relationship is established, the counselor can focus on how children conduct themselves in the counseling session. The counselor's work is to evaluate the climate of each counseling session. Was it happy, sad, pleasant, neutral, stormy, or productive? What seemed to set the tone? Next, counselors should look for patterns in the child's behavior or play. Children with ADHD act out with disorganization and impulsive behavior. Obsessive-compulsive children, by contrast, are rigid and structured in their play activities. Counselors observe those patterns and all other clues to the world of the child.

Children's choices of toys provide another rich area of data for counselors. Toys can be classified as passive or aggressive, masculine or feminine, and constructive or destructive; however, many toys may be neutral. Counselors will want to observe what the child does with each toy. Counselors search for themes in children's behavior and play therapy activities in the effort to learn the motivation directing their behavior. Some themes that may arise in the counseling process include aggression/power/control, nurturing/healing, boundary/intrusion, violation/protection, anger/sadness, loyalty/betrayal, adjustment/change, fear/anxiety, rejection/abandonment, relationships, loss/death, loneliness, and safety/security/trust (Benedict & Mongoven, 1997; Halstead, Pehrsson, & Mullen, 2011).

As important as the themes uncovered in counseling is the intensity with which these themes are played out in the sessions. The play themes of well-adjusted children vary from those of disturbed children in frequency and intensity.

Counselors' accurate reflection of content, feelings, expectations, and behavior helps focus children's attention on their actions and stimulates the self-observation needed to gain insight about their lifestyle and incentive to change. As you review the skills listed in Table 3-1, you will find verbal responses to increase the child's sense of being understood. Play therapy methods are presented in detail in Chapter 17. The following six-step counseling model combines the best of reality planning with person-centered, active listening for children receiving general counseling or a combination of counseling and play therapy.

A GENERAL MODEL FOR COUNSELING

Counselors work to create an environment in which helping relationships can be formed. The works of Rogers (1957), Egan (2010), and Truax and Carkhuff (1967) support the concept of core conditions that set the stage for effective counseling. Those conditions include empathic understanding, respect and positive regard, genuineness and congruence, concreteness, warmth, and immediacy. Gross and Capuzzi (2006) also include cultural awareness as a critical condition of counseling. Empathic understanding refers to the ability to understand a child's feelings, thoughts, ideas, and experiences through the child's frame of reference. Respect and positive regard concern the counselor's unwavering belief in the innate worth and potential of each person and the counselor's ability to communicate that belief. Genuineness and congruence refer to the ability to be authentic rather than artificial in the relationship. Concreteness refers to the counselor's ability to infer complete pictures from a child's incomplete view of the situation. This ability helps clarify vague issues, focus on specific topics, and reduce ambiguity (Gross & Capuzzi, 2006). Warmth relates to being able to demonstrate caring and concern for the young person. Another core condition, immediacy, refers to dealing with things that emerge in the helping relationship such as the child being angry at the counselor. Finally, cultural awareness relates to counselors being open and motivated to understand their own culture, as well as the cultural diversity young people bring to their relationships. Gross and Capuzzi contend that the core conditions are universal and, when used with cultural sensitivity, are applicable to all children. Using these core conditions will increase the likelihood of success for the counseling process.

Counseling with children has a beginning, middle, and end. At first, children explore, trying to decide if they can trust. During the middle stage, children begin to face their concerns and move to directly or indirectly solving their problems. In the final stage, the child works through the issues for the present (Van Velsor, 2004). We propose the following steps for that process.

Step 1: Defining the Problem through Active Listening

The way the counselor listens to the child is important in building rapport. An open, relaxed body posture is the best way to invite a child to talk. It is often helpful to suggest a time limit for your interview, which should vary according to the attention span of the child. For example, saying, "Jimmy, we have 20 minutes today to talk about anything you'd like to discuss" sets an open tone and clear expectation.

In fact, several 20-minute periods might be used to build a friendship with Jimmy. individualizing the counseling process to fit each child you counsel is important.

When the child wishes to discuss a concern or problem with you, it is necessary to listen for three significant points: (1) a problem that has not been solved, (2) feelings about the problem, and (3) expectations of what the counselor should do about the problem. The counselor can assume the role of student and let the child teach these three topics because people learn best when they teach something to another person.

Counselors have the responsibility of letting the child know what they have heard and learned as their clients teach them. For example, the counselor should periodically respond with a statement, such as "In other words, you are feeling _____ because _____, and you want _____." This feedback to the child is referred to as *active listening*; it promotes better communication and lets the child know you are paying attention. The active-listening process continues throughout the interview, but it is most important in helping to clarify the nature of the child's problem. When the child confirms your response as an accurate understanding of the problem, counseling can move to the next phase (see Chapter 6 for a detailed explanation of the active-listening process and Table 3-1 for short descriptions of reflections of feeling, meaning, and empathy).

TABLE 3-1 UNIVERSAL COUNSELING SKILLS

Universal Skill	Purpose	Description	Examples
Minimal encouragers	To encourage the client to continue	Words or phrases to help client continue talking	"Uh huh," "hmmm," "I see," "continue," "right."
Paraphrase	To give back the message in a different way	Use a few words of the client to repeat the message	"You have lots going on right now."
Reflection of feeling	To show awareness of emotional parts of the story	Highlight what has been said with a feeling word	"You are afraid to talk to him or her."
Reflection of meaning	To show understanding of the meaning of the story	Listen to the story and reduce to the core meaning	"No one takes time to help you with your homework."
Summary	To capture the content of the discussion across time	Make a statement to sum up what has been said	"Let's see—you talked about your classmates, your dog, and your soccer team and how you take care of things with all them."
Empathy	To use words or actions to show understanding	Reflect back the deeper meaning of what has been said	"It must have been awful to watch your cat die."
Prompts	To help the child add to the story or continue with more detail	Encourage by highlighting or asking for more about the story	"Please tell me more about when you are happy."
Closed questions	To get specific information	Ask a question that can be answered with one or two words	"Did you go to the sleepover?"

(continued)

TABLE 3-1 (*Continued*)

Universal Skill	Purpose	Description	Examples
Open questions	To promote discussion	Ask a question to get more details	"How did you get everything done?"
Scaling question	To identify the intensity of a situation	Ask the client to put something on a scale such as 10 to 1	"Help me understand this hope you have about your parents getting back together. On a scale of 10 to 1 with 10 being certain, where are you?"
Defining the problem	To help direct the discussion to the problem and its management	Highlight what the client wants help with	"You want me to help you decide which high school to choose?"
Defining goals/objectives/outcomes	To highlight what the client wants out of counseling	State or ask what you think the client wants from counseling	"Talk to me about what we can accomplish in our time together."
Reframing	To take the deeper meaning of what's been said and state it more positively	Take the gist of what's been said and move from a negative to more hopeful	"You help out at home a lot."
Exploring alternatives	To help the client see other possibilities	Ask the client to consider different perspectives	"What else could be going on?" "What other ways could you do that?"
Identifying/building strengths	To highlight the strengths and assets of the client	Focus on unrecognized strengths	"You seem to be so quick to understand other people."
Exploration	To connect resources to the goals of counseling	Ask about resources, meanings, or allies	"Who will be someone to encourage you when you try this?"
Affirmation	To encourage	Highlight strengths and positive insights	"You seem to be trying harder to get along with your teacher."
Providing information	To provide facts	State the information that is pertinent	"You have to have 4 years of English to graduate."
Logical consequences	To give the client a chance to explore what might happen as a result of change	Help the client assess the pros and cons of actions	"If you decide to leave the team, what will happen?"
Role-playing	To have the client practice behaviors	Ask the client to act out what they want to see happen	"Show me how you will act when you ask her to the dance."
Homework	To promote practice after sessions	Give an assignment to practice something related to counseling goals	"Between now and when we meet again, keep a count of how many times you say hello to people."

Adapted from McHenry, B., & McHenry, J. (2007). *What therapists say and why they say it: Effective therapeutic responses and techniques.* Boston, MA: Allyn and Bacon.

Step 2: Clarifying the Child's Expectations

Counselors also need to let children know whether they can meet their expectations for counseling. For example, the counselor probably cannot have an unpopular teacher fired. However, counselors can inform children and their parents what they are able to do and let them determine whether they want to accept or reject the supportive, realistic problem solving counselors can provide. If the service is rejected, the counselor may want to explore other alternatives with the family about where or how the child can obtain other help. Counselors can refer to Table 3-1 for skills of clarification, structuring, probing, and questioning that can aid in clarifying the child's expectations.

Step 3: Exploring What Has Been Done to Solve the Problem

Counselors need to know about past attempts to solve the problem. Open-ended questions generally elicit the best responses. Counselors should avoid closed questions that yield one-word answers such as *yes, no,* and *maybe.* As noted in this text, many approaches to counseling avoid heavy questioning, and others rely on a predetermined series of questions. Statements often work better than questions; they empower the client by letting the client maintain the pace and direction of the interview. For example, rather than asking the child, "What have you done to solve the problem?" the counselor would say, "Tell me what you have already tried to solve the problem." Counselors may ask the client to list what has already been tried; if the child cannot write, he or she can dictate the answers to the counselor. The list becomes important if the child does make a commitment to stop behaviors that are not helping to solve the problem. It is helpful to explore the possible rewards or payoffs the child derives from ineffective or unhelpful behaviors. Change is facilitated when both the pluses and the minuses are examined. A "profit-and-loss" statement can be prepared to determine whether the behavior is actually worth the cost the child is paying. If it is not, the child may discard the behavior in favor of a more productive alternative. Many of the skills listed in Table 3-1 will help this and the next step of counseling.

Step 4: Exploring What New Things Could Be Done to Solve the Problem

The next step could be a brainstorming session in which the counselor encourages the child to develop as many problem-solving alternatives as possible. Counselors encourage children to generate as many alternatives as possible and to withhold judgment until the list is finished. Quantity of ideas is more important than quality in this first step. Thompson and Poppen (1992) recommended drawing empty circles on a sheet of paper and then seeing how many circles the child can fill with ideas. If children are blocked from thinking of possible new ideas, the counselor can fill two circles with ideas as a way of encouraging the child to get started. After the brainstorming list is complete, children are asked to evaluate each alternative in light of its expected success in helping them get what they want.

Step 5: Obtaining a Commitment to Try One of the Problem-Solving Ideas

After the possibilities have been listed and their viability considered, the client can decide on a plan of action. Building commitment to try a new plan may be difficult because the child may be quite discouraged by his or her previous failures to solve the problem. We suggest that the child not set impossible goals in this first attempt; the first plan should be achievable. Children do better if they are asked to report the results of their plan to the counselor. When plans do not work, the counselor helps the child write new ones until the child achieves success. Homework and encouragement are useful skills (see Table 3-1) in this counseling step.

Step 6: Closing the Counseling Interview

A good way to close the interview is to invite the child to summarize or review what was discussed in the session; for example, the summary might include what progress was made and what plans were developed. Summarizing by the child is also helpful when the interview becomes mired and the child cannot think of anything to say. Because the process seems to stimulate new thoughts, summarizing at the close of the interview should be limited to 2 to 4 minutes. We also recommend asking the child to summarize the last counseling interview at the start of each new interview.

These counselor requests to summarize teach children to pay attention in the session and to review counseling plans between sessions; they have the effect of an oral quiz without the threat of a failing grade. The summary also helps counselors evaluate their own effectiveness. Finally, the counselor and the child make plans for the next counseling interview or for some type of maintenance plan if counseling is to be terminated.

QUESTIONS COUNSELORS ASK

What Does the Counselor Need to Know about Counseling Records?

Most counselors keep some record of interviews with their clients. Notes that summarize the content of sessions and observations the counselor makes can assist in recalling previous information. Before deciding on a method of taking notes, counselors are wise to become knowledgeable about their state's laws regarding privileged communication and the regulations contained in the Buckley Amendment (the federal Family Rights and Privacy Act of 1974), which gave parents and young people of legal age the right to inspect records, letters, and recommendations about themselves. Personal notes do not fall under these regulations in some states; however, for their own protection, counselors in institutional settings should become aware of the full requirements of the law. A wise maxim is that notes should always be written as though others will read them.

Recording counseling sessions may be common practice. This procedure not only provides a record of the interview but also aids counselors in gaining self-understanding and self-awareness. Counselors can listen to or watch their tapes with another counselor and continue to grow and learn by evaluating their own work. In addition, listening to and discussing some sessions with the client may promote growth. Written permission to record counseling sessions should be obtained from the child and the parents before any taping is done Tapes, like notes, should be stored in secure locations inaccessible to others. Digital audio recorders do not typically have the option for password protection or data encryption and are therefore not secure means of keeping recordings. In all cases if you record sessions either leave your recording device safely under lock and key at your work setting or ensure that any client audio files are completely removed from the device before leaving the workplace.

When introducing a recording system to children, show them the recorder, perhaps allow them to listen to themselves for a minute, and then place the equipment in an out-of-the-way place. Occasionally, children are unable to talk when they are being recorded; most, however, quickly forget the equipment. However, if circumstances indicate that recording is inhibiting the counseling process, the counselor may choose to remove the equipment. At the other extreme, some children become so excited and curious about the taping equipment that counseling becomes impossible. Again, the counselor may prefer to remove the equipment, or a contract may be made with the child, such as "After 30 minutes of the counseling work, Mickey may listen to the tape for 5 minutes." It is usually best to give as little attention to the recorder as possible after a brief initial explanation of its purpose and uses. Counselors who choose to use their computers or phones as recording devices must assess the security of those media.

How Much Self-Disclosure Is Appropriate for the Counselor?

Children are often interested in their counselors as people. They ask counselors their age, where they went to school, where they live, and whether they have children, and counselors are faced with the perplexing problem of how much personal information to share. Counselors who refuse to answer any personal questions run the risk of hurting the counseling relationship or being viewed as a mysterious figure, bringing forth more questions. If counselors answer all personal questions, however, the interview time may center on the counselor rather than the client.

A general guideline might be to share some personal information (favorite sport or TV show, number of children) and, when the questions become too personal or continue too long, reflect to the child, "You seem to be very interested in me personally," and explore the child's curiosity. Understanding the child's interest in the counselor could promote understanding of the child as a person. Questioning the counselor can be a defense for children who wish to avoid discussing their own problems.

A second problem concerning self-disclosure relates to the counselor's feelings and emotions. Counselor training programs are founded on the assumption that people are unique, capable of growth, and worthy of respect. These programs focus on listening and responding to clients with empathic understanding and respect. The programs also emphasize being genuine; however, genuineness is often interpreted as showing only genuine *positive* emotions and feelings. Counselor trainees are sometimes quite surprised when their supervisors encourage them to admit to the client their negative feelings, such as frustration or anger. Obviously, admitting emotions does not mean attacking and degrading the client; rather, it means admitting that the counselor is a person with feelings and is frustrated or angry over what is occurring ("I am upset when you call me mean names.").

The counselor's proper level of self-disclosure is a controversial issue in the profession. Some feel comfortable being completely open and honest about their feelings (high levels of self-disclosure); others think such openness interferes with the counselor–client relationship and prefer low levels of self-disclosure. However, most counselors agree that self-disclosure is not "true confessions." Poppen and Thompson (1974) have summarized the arguments on both sides of the issue. The principal arguments in favor of high levels of self-disclosure are as follows:

1. Counselors who are open and honest about their thoughts and feelings encourage similar behavior by their clients.
2. Knowing that the counselor has had similar adjustment problems helps clients feel more at ease to discuss their own problems.
3. Children learn by imitation and can learn to solve their own problems through hearing about the experiences of others.
4. Counselors could be models for behavior.

On the other side of the issue, those opposing high levels of self-disclosure have the following points:

1. Clients are in the counselor's office for help with their problems, not to hear about the counselor's problems.
2. Counseling could become a time for sharing gripes or problems, rather than a working session for personal growth.
3. Counselors can lose objectivity if they identify too strongly with the child's concerns.

According to Poppen and Thompson (1974), self-disclosure is more beneficial when it takes a here-and-now focus—that is, when self-disclosure becomes an open and authentic expression of the counselor's or student's (child's) thoughts and feelings experienced at a particular time. Self-disclosure, when examined in the here-and-now context, means much more than dredging up the dark secrets of the past (p. 15).

Yalom (2009) describes three types of disclosure in counseling. He discusses disclosure about the process and mechanics of counseling as one type. Another disclosure involves the expression of the here-and-now feelings the counselor is having during the session. The third kind of disclosure is about the personal life of the counselor. He proposes that disclosure exists on a continuum from the first type, the least risky, to the third type, the one with the most potential to not be useful. His guidelines state counselors should have complete transparency about the mechanism of therapy, openness about the present as it serves the welfare of the client, and discussions of personal life only as much as the therapist is comfortable with the caveat that the therapist inquire about the client's interest as part of the process. Those ideas may help a counselor determine how much disclosure is appropriate.

What Types of Questions Should the Counselor Use?

Adults often think they must ask children several questions to get the "whole story." Usually, these questions are of the "who," "what," "when," "where," and "what did you do next" variety. These questions may or may not be asked for the purpose of helping the child or for clarification; too often they arise out of general Curiosity. Some questions may even be irrelevant and interrupt or ignore the child's thoughts and expressions. Questions can also be used to judge, blame, or criticize. For example:

CHILD: The teacher called me a dummy in front of the whole class today!

ADULT: (sarcastically) What did you say this time to make him call you that?

At that particular moment, the important fact is not what the child said, but that the child was embarrassed, hurt, and possibly angered. By listening and understanding feelings and expressions rather than probing for details of who said what and when, the adult will get the whole story eventually and maintain a much friendlier relationship with the child. Counselors who listen and respond with understanding often learn the child's important thoughts or problems. In other words, questions rephrased as statements work better. Some counselors, in their efforts to help the child, take over the counseling interview.

Counselors who direct the interview risk missing important feelings and thoughts. The counselor may guide the conversation in a totally meaningless direction. For example:

CHILD: I hate my brother.

COUNSELOR: Why do you hate your brother?

CHILD: Because he's mean.

COUNSELOR: How is he mean?

CHILD: He hits me.

COUNSELOR: What do you do to make him hit you? [in accusing tone]

CHILD: Nothing.

COUNSELOR: Come on, now. Tell me about when he hits you—and what your mother does when he hits you.

This example sounds more like an inquisition than a counseling session. The hitting and what the mother does may or may not be what is really troubling the child. What could be more important is the feeling that exists between the child and her brother. Is it really "hate" because he hits her, or could there be other problems in the relationship that the counselor will miss by focusing on hitting rather than listening to the child tell about her relationship with her brother? It is also possible that "hating her brother" could have been a test problem to determine whether the counselor really would listen and be understanding. A counselor who guides the interview by questions could overlook the true problem entirely.

In the preceding example, the child answered the counselor's questions but offered no further information. Children easily fall into the role of answering adults' questions and then waiting for the next question. Rather than being a listener and helper, the counselor assumes the role of inquisitor. Once this pattern has been established, the interview may die when the counselor runs out of questions.

Obviously, there are times in counseling when direct questions should be asked. The counselor may need factual information or clarification. However, counselors can probably get more information from children with open-ended questions. An open-ended question does not require a specific answer. It encourages the child to give the counselor more information about the topic, but it does not restrict replies or discourage further communication in the area. Suppose a counselor was interested in learning about a child's social relationships. Rather than asking the direct, closed question "Do you have friends?" the counselor might elicit more information about the child's social relationships by saying, "Tell me what you like to do for fun—things that you enjoy doing in your free time." In this way, the counselor could learn not only about friends but possibly also about the child's sports interests, hobbies, and other activities (or lack of activities).

Another open-ended question that might help the counselor understand what is going on in the child's life is "Tell me about your family," out of which could come answers to such unasked questions as " Do both your mother and father live in the home?" "How many people live in the household?" "What are your feelings about various members of the household?" One further point should be made about questioning in counseling. Adults should be careful about the use of "why" questions with youth because they are associated with blame; "Why did you do that?" is often interpreted in the mind of a child as "Why did you do a *stupid thing* like that?" These questions put people on the defensive; when asked why we acted a certain way, we feel forced to find some logical reason or excuse for our behavior. Glasser (see Chapter 9) suggests that a better question might be a "what" question. Most of us are not really sure *why* we behaved a certain way, but we can tell *what* occurred. A "what" question does not deal with possible unconscious motives and desires but rather focuses on present behavior; the client and counselor can look at what is happening now and what can be done.

Garbarino and Stott (1992) remind counselors that effective questions must be appropriate for the developmental level of their clients. They make the following suggestions for interviewing preschoolers and probably most elementary school-aged children:

- Use sentences that do not exceed by more than five words the number of words in a sentence the child uses.
- Use names rather than pronouns.
- Use the child's terms.
- Do not ask, "Do you understand?" Ask the child to repeat your message.
- Do not repeat questions children do not understand because they may think they have made errors and attempt to "correct" their answers. Rephrase the question instead.
- Avoid time-sequence questions.
- Preschoolers, being very literal, may give us answers that are easy to over-interpret.
- Do not respond to every answer with another question. A short summary or acknowledgment encourages the child to expand on his or her previous statement.

In summary, counselors learn more by listening and summarizing than by questioning. The habit of questioning is difficult to break. When tempted to question, counselors might first ask themselves whether the questions they ask will (1) contribute therapeutically to understanding the child and the child's problems, or (2) inhibit the further flow of expression. Our suggestion is for counselors to use as few questions as possible, a skill most will need to refine.

How Can Silences Be Used in Counseling?

Most of us are uncomfortable with silence. We have been socially conditioned to keep the conversation going; when conversation begins to ebb, we search through our thoughts for a new topic of interest to introduce to the group. Although silences can be very productive in a counseling interview, counselors may rush to fill the pauses. However, a child may need a few moments of silence to sort out thoughts and feelings. The child may have related some very emotional event or thought and may need a moment of silence to think about this revelation or regain composure. The child or the counselor may have behaved or spoken in a confusing manner, and sorting things out may take time and silence.

Silences can be used for problem solving, and therefore be productive, but how long should the counselor allow the silence to last? Obviously, an entire session of silence between child and counselor is not likely to be helpful. The child may spontaneously begin to speak again when ready. Children's nonverbal behavior may provide counselors with clues that they are ready to begin. The counselor may test the water by making a quiet statement reflecting the possible cause of the silence; for example, "You seem a little confused about what you just told me." The child's response to this reflection should indicate whether he or she is ready to proceed.

Should Counselors Give Advice?

The role of a counselor has often been interpreted as an advice giver, and some counseling theorists advocate giving advice to clients. Their rationale is that the counselor, who is trained in helping and is more knowledgeable, should advise the less knowledgeable client.

We prefer to view the role of the counselor as using skills and knowledge to assist another person in solving his or her own problems or conflicts. Counselors who believe in the uniqueness, worth, dignity, and responsibility of the individual and who believe that, given the right conditions, individuals can make correct choices for themselves are reluctant to give advice on solving life's problems. Instead, they use their counseling knowledge and skills to help clients make responsible choices of their own and, in effect, learn how to become their own counselor. An illustration of the difference between giving advice and assisting in problem solving may clarify the point. Consider the following example: Tony was threatened by neighborhood bullies who were going to beat him up on the way home from school. Tony confided his fear of fighting to the counselor, who advised him to talk this over with his parents. Even though Tony was reluctant to talk to his parents, the counselor persuaded him they would understand and help. Tony returned later to relate that his father lectured him for being a "sissy" and instructed him to "go out and fight like a man." Tony was more terrified than ever because neither his parents nor the counselor understood his dilemma or could be counted on to support him. In this case, the counselor, not considering the client's home and culture, gave advice that intensified the problem. The counselor might have been more helpful by assisting Tony to think of ways of solving the problem—ways that Tony would choose.

Another possible disadvantage of counselors' advice is the problem of dependency. Counselors want their clients to become responsible individuals capable of solving their own problems. Children have a multitude of adults telling them how and when to act, but only a few assist them to learn responsible problem-solving behavior. In counseling, children learn the problem-solving process; they learn that they do not have to depend entirely on adults to make all their decisions for them. The process can develop confident, mature, and independent individuals moving toward self-actualization.

This conflict is analogous to the typical adolescent struggle for independence. Because many people see the counselor's role as that of advice giver, some clients may become frustrated and angry when counselors will not give advice. Talking about the role of the counselor and working with the client to negotiate realistic expectations may ease the tension and assist in building a working alliance with the client.

When asked what they think they could do to work out the conflict or problem, children typically are unable to think of possible solutions. It is a new experience for many children to be involved in solving their own problems. When pressed to give advice, a counselor could reflect the feeling that the child is not sure what to do and would like to have an answer, and then suggest again that they explore possibilities together. If the child is persistent and demands an answer, the counselor may wish to explore the reasons for this demand. Another way to stimulate ideas might be the counselor asking the child what advise the child would give to a good friend facing a similar situation.

We need to point out, however, that counselors have a duty to protect their clients from any harm they might do to themselves, as well as to prevent them from harming others. Therefore, counselors may need to give advice in emergency situations and to act on the advice they give.

Should Counselors Give Information?

Beginning counselors, believing that giving information is the same as giving advice, often give neither. Clients need good information to make good decisions, and counselors help clients by sharing what good information they have. For example, counselors should inform their clients of community and school resources where clients can receive assistance. The decision to seek assistance should be the client's. In other words, advice often takes the form of a suggestion to perform a certain behavior or to take some course of action.

Giving information, however, means providing facts, general knowledge, and to some extent, alternatives.

Two primary causes of problems are lack of information about oneself and the environment. The counselor's role is to help clients find the information they need to solve their problems. Once again, we believe the more actively clients seek their own information, the better their learning experience.

How Does the Counselor Keep the Client on Task During the Counseling Session?

Children soon discover that the counselor is a good listener who gives them undivided attention. Because many children are not listened to by adults, they often take advantage of the counseling situation to talk about everything except the reason for coming to counseling. With the least suggestion, the counselor may find the child rambling on about a TV show, last night's ball game, a current movie, tricks a pet dog can do, or any number of other irrelevant topics. Children, like adults, can ramble excessively when they wish to avoid a problem. Talkativeness then becomes a diversionary tactic either to avoid admitting what is troubling them or to avoid coping with the conflict. The conflict could be too traumatic or painful to face.

Another possible reason for losing focus in a counseling session is that children do not understand their role in the counseling interview. If the purpose of counseling and expectations of the people involved are clearly defined in the initial interview, pointless chatting is less likely.

Counselors who discover themselves being led into superficial or rambling conversations may want to bring the conversation back to the problem at hand by reflecting to the child, "We seem to be getting away from the reason for our time together. I wonder if you could tell me more about…." If a child consistently wanders, state that you notice the wandering and then explore possible reasons for the avoidance. A recording can be an excellent means of determining when, how, and why the distractions occur. A contract might be drawn up, such as "[The counselor] and I will work on [the problem] for 25 minutes. I can talk to [the counselor] about anything else for the last 5 minutes." The skills of summarizing, focusing, and clarifying may help (see Table 3-1).

What Limits Should Be Set in Counseling?

In their preparation programs, most counselors are taught to be empathic, respectful, genuine, accepting, and nonjudgmental—characteristics that writers such as Carl Rogers and Robert Carkhuff define as essential for a facilitative counseling relationship and skills also known as common factors in counseling. Being accepting and nonjudgmental can be challenging for some counselors around some issues, especially regarding moral and ethical differences. Counselors have their own attitudes, values, and beliefs. Remaining open minded enough to really hear the client's entire story is difficult if the client's values and those of the counselor conflict.

Being nonjudgmental involves withholding those judgments we ordinarily make and allowing clients to tell the whole story without the young person being threatened by the counselor's condemnation or disgust. Counselors refrain from blaming, accusing, criticizing, and moralizing. They also attempt to teach responsible, reality-oriented behavior to their child clients. The counselor does not tell children they are wrong; the counselor's job is to help children explore the consequences, advantages, and disadvantages of their choices and, perhaps, discover better methods of resolving the conflict. For instance based on the previous example, rather than sermonizing to Tony that fighting is wrong, the counselor might be more helpful by thinking with him about what would happen if he challenged the bully to a fight and whether he could gain his father's acceptance and respect in other ways. Of course not having given advice to Tony would have avoided that situation altogether.

In summary, accepting and nonjudgmental attitudes are essential for good counseling, as those attitudes show respect for the rights of others, the reality of the situation, and responsibility for one's own behavior.

What about the Issue of Confidentiality?

Early in their training counselors learn that whatever is said in a counseling interview should remain confidential unless there is danger to the client or to another person or if there is suspicion of child abuse. As noted earlier, counselors explain the principle of confidentiality to their clients during the first interview. If information indicating danger to a person is revealed during later interviews, counselors remind children of the counselor's obligation to report such danger to the proper authorities. Privileged communication in their counselor–client relationships is a legal right authorized by a state regulatory board. Counselors' records can be subpoenaed, and counselors can be called to testify in court proceedings should the information they possess be deemed necessary for a court decision. If counselors think that revealing the information required in their testimony could harm the child, they can request a private conference with the judge to share both the information and their reasons for wanting to keep the information confidential. See Chapter 4 for more information on confidentiality and privileged communication.

Some counselors maintain that children and adults should be encouraged to communicate more openly and that the counselor can facilitate this process in the family counseling interview. They further contend that parents and other adults can provide insight and needed information about the child; the significant adult in the child's life can become a co-counselor. A signed contract with the parents to protect the confidentiality of the child's counseling sessions, although not legally binding, may establish the privacy of the communication. Talking with the parent about the counseling relationship may also allow the counselor opportunities to involve the parent in the out-of-session activities of the client, such as homework assignments or information gathering.

Careful evaluation of the child's presenting problem and the adults involved may help the counselor decide whether strict confidentiality should be maintained or others should be included. The decision to include others or share information should always be discussed with the child to avoid misunderstandings and to maintain the trust necessary for the counseling relationship. The child may agree and, in fact, lead the discussions.

Is This Child Telling Me the Truth?

Another counseling problem is whether the child is telling the counselor the truth or enhancing or exaggerating to get attention or sympathy. Children may tell their counselors about extraordinary events such as seeing people shoot one another, raging fires, and robberies. Unfortunately, many of these stories are true; however, children have vivid imaginations, and it is sometimes difficult to know how much to believe.

Children may feel they have to tell of major difficulties to keep the counselor interested. Counselors can ask for more details of the incident (e.g., by saying, "Tell me more"), which might clarify whether the story is truth or fiction. When asked to give specifics, children may admit they were "only kidding" or "making it up." Counselors might also admit their genuine concerns: "I am really having trouble with this because I have never heard anything like it." An admission of this sort by a counselor expresses a genuine feeling and avoids labeling the child a liar or possibly denying a true story. It also provides the child with an opportunity to change the story while saving face.

Counselors should also be aware that children may think they need to please the counselor, so try to give answers or details the children believe the counselor would want to hear. Clever counselors will acknowledge this motivation and provide other opportunities for the young person to give more accurate information. Likewise some children may decide to keep the counselor's attention by saying exactly what might offend the counselor as the child may assume the counselor, like other adults, will give up on such a despicable human—again the smart counselor will not be pulled into this game of the supposedly unlovable child.

What Can Be Done When the Interview Process Becomes Blocked?

In some counseling sessions the child does not feel like talking. It is possible that things have been going well for the past few days and the child really has nothing to discuss. Child clients may need a lull before new material is introduced. One way to avoid these unexpected empty periods is to be prepared for a session. Some counselors have general goals for their client (for instance, to increase social skills) and also define specific short-term goals for each session as counseling proceeds. Regardless of whether the counselor prefers to define objectives, notes from the previous session can be reviewed and a tentative plan made for the coming interview. Obviously, this plan is subject to change according to the content of the interview.

When the child seems highly distracted, a short summary by the counselor or child of the previous conversation may stimulate further communication. If the child does not seem to want to talk, the techniques of play therapy (drawing, clay, games) may be beneficial. At certain times (e.g., because of illness, extreme excitability, or apathy), ending the session short of the designated time is best. The length of counseling sessions can vary from a few minutes to an hour, depending on the client's age and presenting problem.

When sessions become blocked, evaluate what is happening. Reviewing recordings of sessions assists in assessing the lack of progress. A blocked session may be a sign that the child is ready for the counseling to conclude. It could also be resistance on the part of the child. It could come from the counselor's inadequate skills or lack of planning in which case the counselor would want to seek supervision to rectify ineffective practices. Unproductive sessions occur occasionally with all counselors, but frequent periods of nonproductivity should signal the counselor to investigate what is happening.

When Should Counseling Be Terminated?

How does a counselor decide when to end counseling? Does the counselor or the client decide? How does either party know the client is ready to stand alone? If the counselor and client have clearly defined the problem brought to counseling and the goal to be accomplished, the termination time will be evident—when the goal is accomplished. The counselor may also want to look for any of the following signs suggested by Landreth (2012):

- Is the child more open?
- Does the child accept responsibility for feelings and actions?
- Is the child more tolerant of self and others?
- Is the child more independent and self-directing?
- Is the child less fearful, less unhappy, and less anxious than when the counseling relationship began?

Termination may be difficult for children, who usually find the sessions to be a time when a caring adult gives them undivided attention. Mutual attachments may be formed between counselor and child, and the child (and possibly the counselor) does not wish to end this pleasant relationship. To ease the break, client and counselor can discuss a possible termination date several weeks ahead of time and together do a countdown until the designated day. Plans can be made and rehearsed about how the child will react should problems recur. The child learns that the counselor still cares and will be available should trouble arise. Counselors may even consider building in a follow-up time when they ask their child clients to drop them a note or call to let them know how things are going. The counselor may want to schedule a brief follow-up visit. Any informal method of showing the child that a counselor's caring does not end with the last interview can signal the counselor's continued interest in the child's growth and development. Most successful counselors use a plan for maintaining the gains their clients have achieved during counseling. Such maintenance plans require periodic follow-up contacts, for example, 30 days or 6 months.

How Can Counseling Be Evaluated?

Accountability has become a high priority because of budgetary pressures. Counselors are being asked to demonstrate their effectiveness in specific and measurable outcomes. In addition, providers of mental health services working with clients enrolled in managed care plans are under pressure to deliver services in the most cost-effective way possible (Steenbarger & Smith, 1996). Certainly attention to the results of counseling benefits clients. Seligman (1995) suggested three areas for assessment: (1) "How much did treatment help with the specific problem?" (2) "How satisfied was the consumer with services received?" and (3) overall, "How much did the client improve?"

Steenbarger and Smith (1996) recommend using similar measures. They propose a measure evaluating the degree to which clients feel they have received services that are convenient and useful. These authors acknowledge several scales designed to measure satisfaction. Unfortunately, most scales that have been validated and have established reliability are constructed for adults. The instruments would have to be adapted for the developmental age of the child client, and validity and reliability would need to be re-established.

A second measure suggested by Steenbarger and Smith (1996) would be to complete outcome measures at two or more points. Outcome measures are related to the goals of counseling and are statements about the counselors' and clients' expected outcomes from counseling written in measurable terms. Measures could be evaluated by both client and counselor and by parents or other significant adults. Again, most published measures are for adults and usually assess symptoms that are indicative of pathology, rather than growth and development, and they may not be individualized to the clients' particular goals. The Youth Outcome Questionnaires (Y-OQ) (Burlingame et al., 1996) is one instrument counselors can use for parents to indicate their child's progress. Other assessment measures such as the Achenbach System of Empirically Based Assessment (Achenbach & Rescorla, 2001) and the Conners' 3 (Conners, 2013) can be used at the beginning of treatment for a baseline reading, during treatment for progress, and at the end of counseling for outcome measures.

Chorpita, Weisz, and others (Chorpita et al., 2010; Weisz et al., 2011) have developed an ongoing, frequent feedback sequence for young clients. The Brief Problem Checklist (Chorpita et al.) is a 12-item method for young people and caregivers to report on the severity of the young person's problems during the week. The other measure is Youth Top Problems (Weisz et al.), a three-item method through which young people and caregivers identify, before treatment, the three most important problems and then rate the severity of the problems weekly as treatment progresses. Those weekly rating systems provide updates on the youth's response to treatment.

Steenbarger and Smith (1996) and Ahn and Wampold (2001) also report that standards of care can be used as measures of effectiveness if professionals agree on the *best practices* of the profession and *common factors*, including the healing context, working alliance, and rationale of the treatment. Counselors would be required to document in their notes how and when they engaged in these practices. The writers conclude that professionals in counseling need to assess and document client satisfaction, outcomes, and counselor performance on selected criteria to demonstrate effectiveness. The challenge for counselors working with children is to develop age-appropriate satisfaction scales, to develop outcome measures from initial goals set early in counseling, and to work with other professionals to establish *best practices* and *common factors* for highly effective care.

Goal attainment scaling (Kiresuk, Smith, & Cardillo, 1994), another method for evaluation of counseling outcomes, allows counselor and client the opportunity to establish counseling goals cooperatively. The counselor's task is to help the child clarify these goals in measurable terms as a way of evaluating the distance between "What I have" and "What I would like to have." The counselor and child create a five-point scale or continuum with a range from the most to the least desirable treatment outcomes for each goal. Each level should be written in measurable terms so the counselor and the child can monitor where the child is on the scale and thereby determine progress during their work. Chang, Scott, and Decker (2009) use the acronym MAPS for goals or expected outcomes. Rather than general goals, clients and counselors need to identify *Measurable, Attainable, Positive, and Specific (MAPS)* goals that will provide clarity and detail to desired outcomes.

Generally one to five goals are set, with five levels of attainment defined for each goal (Table 3-2). In addition, each goal is given a weight to represent its importance to the client. Clients establish priorities for their goals and assign weights to the most important and least important. For instance, Goal 1 may be three times more important than Goal 2. Intermediate goals are assigned weights representing their relative importance to the client. For example, if the most important goal is three times as important as the least important goal, it would receive a weight of 30 compared with a weight of 10 for the least important goal. Goals are then weighed on a scale of 10, 20, or 30, depending on their relative importance to the client. Marson, Wei, and Wasserman (2009) present a study on the reliability of those scales.

Levels of attainment for each goal range from a "+2" for the best anticipated success to a "−2" for the least favorable outcome. A "0" value is assigned for the middle level or expected outcome success. Values of "+1" and "−1" represent "more than" and "less than" expected levels of success, respectively.

As stated earlier, the goals are defined in measurable and observable terms, with the level of entry checked on the goal attainment follow-up guide. After counseling, an asterisk is placed on the guide indicating where the client is after counseling. Follow-up data can also be recorded periodically on the chart.

Goal attainment scaling (Dowd & Kelly, 1975) can be graphed to show weekly progress (Figure 3-4). The graph also can be used to chart the results of periodic follow-up checks on the maintenance of counseling gains.

TABLE 3-2 GOAL ATTAINMENT SCALE

Scale Attainment Level	Scale 1: On Task $W_1 = 20$	Scale 2: Behavior $W_2 = 30$	Scale 3: Punctuality $W_3 = 10$	Scale 4: Relationships $W_4 = 30$	Scale 5: Grade Improvements $W_5 = 10$
a. Most unfavorable counseling outcome expected (−2)	Daydreams, leaves desk; ignores assignments [	Breaks classroom rules 4 or more times/day [	Late to class 4 times/week [	Child gets into three fights/week [	Child continues to fail [
b. Less than expected success with counseling (−1)	Completes one assignment per day	Breaks rules 3 times/day [	Late to class 3 times/week	Child gets into at least one fight/week	Child demonstrates D work
c. Expected level of counseling success (0)	Completes two assignments per day	Breaks rules 2 times/day	Late to class 2 times/week	Child avoids all fights	Child demonstrates C work
d. More than expected success with counseling (+1)	Completes three assignments per day φ	Breaks rules 1 time/day φ	Late to class 1 time/week	Child develops one new friend φ	Child demonstrates B work
e. Most favorable Counseling outcome expected (+2)	Completes four assignments per day	Follows all rules	Late to class 0 time/week φ	Child develops three new friends	Child demonstrates A work

NOTE: Level at intake: [; level at follow-up: φ .

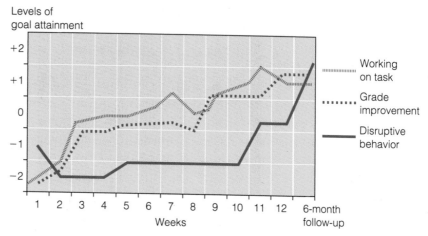

FIGURE 3-4   WEEKLY GOAL ATTAINMENT SCALE

Goal attainment scaling has been effective in many settings with young people (Compton, Galaway, & Cournoyer, 2005; Donnelly & Carswell, 2002; Kleinrahm et al., 2013; Ruble, McGrew, & Toland, 2012; Shogren et al., 2012), such as institutional settings, hospitals, and special education programs. Roach and Elliott (2005) have applied goal attainment scaling as an approach to monitor student academic and social behavior performance. This scale allows counselors and children to check progress across many domains.

How Do Professional Counselors Work with Managed Health Care?[*]

Several important trends in mental health care have emerged with the growth of managed care. Ringel and Sturm (2001) conclude that the majority of children who could respond favorably to mental health care do not receive the needed services. They also found that primary care medical settings provide a substantial amount of mental health care for children. In a policy statement made by the American Academy of Pediatrics, this last trend is seen as a barrier because "pediatricians often are professionally unprepared and usually have inadequate appointment time to address the mental health needs of children and adolescents" (Taras & Young, 2004, p. 1839).

The public sector also has seen significant changes as a result of managed care. Medicaid is the primary insurer of 52 million low-income, elderly, and disabled citizens, and it provides insurance for approximately one in four children in the United States (Heflinger & Saunders, 2005). One critical multisite study (Cook, Heflinger, Hoven, Kelleher, Mulkern, & Paulson, 2004) found that when compared with traditional fee-for-service care, three of four levels of

---

[*] We appreciate Dr. Laura Veach, Wake Forest University, for her help with this section.

care (inpatient/residential, psychiatric medication, and nontraditional services) in Medicaid-funded managed care were much less utilized. The authors cite that less utilization of these levels of care contributed to reducing the probability for children to receive "the full spectrum of services comprising the system of care approach" (p. 401). The major findings also cite "factors other than children's service needs are influencing their receipt of mental health care, which may be cause for concern if needed services are denied because of attempts to control costs" (p. 399).

In 2008 mental health parity legislation was passed and in 2010 health care reform was mandated. The 2008 federal legislation bans insurers from charging differently for out-of-network providers, hopefully overcoming the previous barriers built with the necessity of being in a network of approved providers to receive equal reimbursement for services. The 2010 reform offers parity of medical coverage for both mental health and addiction care (Garfield, Lave, & Donohue, 2010; Welfel, 2013). Hopefully both these acts will improve access to quality care.

Clarke, Lynch, Spofford, and DeBar (2006) emphasize a growing trend of improving the quality of care in the delivery of mental health services. Accountability for performance is evident in The Centers for Medicare and Medicaid Services working with 12 states to create pay-for-performance programs (Lichtenberg, Goodyear, & Genther, 2008). More information about those initiatives with home health care and physician care can be found at the http://cms.hhs.gov/ website.

Another significant trend is the current emphasis on evidence-based practice (EBP)—"the integration of the best available research with clinical expertise in the context of patient characteristics, culture, and preference" (APA Task Force on Evidence-Based Practice, 2006, p. 273). Evidence-based practice can be understood as practice or policy guidelines. Practice guidelines outline treatment for a disorder, condition, or life problem. The recommended treatment assumes the same intervention is needed for any person who has the problem, or a suggestion of the best treatment approach for the average person (Spring, 2007). This push for EBP arose from the desire to assure treatment interventions had been tested in controlled experimental research with results that indicated what worked and what did not.

Pope and Wedding (2008) discussed the challenges associated with generalizing studies to individuals, cultures, and situations; defining effectiveness; and the messiness of trying to capture the interactive, multidimensional practice of counseling. However, Norcross, Hedges, and Prochaska (2002) predict the use of empirically supported therapies, a component of evidence-based practices, will eventually be required by managed care companies. The National Guideline Clearinghouse maintains a compilation of guidelines for review (www.guideline.gov). The APA Presidential Task Force on Evidence-Based Practice (2006) defined EBP as the "integration of the best available research with clinical expertise in the context of patient characteristics, culture, and preferences" (p. 273). Additionally, Dr. Spring (2007) has developed training modules for learning about evidence-based behavioral practice process inform-ing the delivery of counseling. Those modules are available at www.ebbp.org.

In summary, professional counselors need to be highly accountable for quality and cost, whether they choose to work with or without the managed health care systems. Evidence-based practice will provide some guidelines to ensure a sound start to decision making about treatment options.

Davis (1998) summarizes six steps for developing effective treatment plans that meet managed care organization (MCO) specifications. These steps are explained in the next section. The steps are taken from a presentation by Judy Stone, manager of training and development for Value Behavioral Health.

STEP ONE: *PROBLEM IDENTIFICATION*   Concentrate on those problems that are within the realm of managed care's short-term treatment focus. Describe client problems with descriptor words for behaviors that occur with excessive or defi-cient intensity, frequency, and duration. Examples include the terms *acting out, compulsive drinking,* and *physically assaultive.* Descriptor words for frequency and duration include *prolonged excitement, daily worry,* and *consistent dread.* Examples of behavioral deficits include the terms *social withdrawal* and *lack of concentration.*

STEP TWO: *PROBLEM DEFINITION*   After identification of the problem, the counselor needs to define the problem in terms that are consistent with the *Diagnostic and Statistical Manual, Fifth Edition,* (DSM-V). Definitions should include the cognitive process that motivates the problem behaviors of the client and a description of the history of the problem. For example, for an anger management problem, the report could read that the client has a history of explosive, aggressive behaviors dispro-portionate to any precipitating stressors leading to assaultive acts and destruction of property.

STEP THREE: *GOAL DEVELOPMENT*   Write broad goals that are more general in scope and may be long term. For example, "stabilized mood" or "sustained abstinence" are broad goals that help focus on the overarching, larger picture for which the client aims.

STEP FOUR: *MEASURABLE OBJECTIVES*   As mentioned earlier, substeps or objectives need to be developed for each goal with projected time lines for meeting them. Objectives help the client and counselor have specific, brief, measurable steps to reach the broad goal. For example, if a client had attempted suicide, objectives leading to the overall goal of preventing future attempts could be the development of future plans to build relationships with others and to find a job. These steps could be broken down into joining an organization such as a church to meet people and the development of a résumé to use in job applications. Again, the goal attain-ment scale described in this chapter is an excellent instrument for meeting managed care guidelines. It is important to have goals for which small steps in progress can be charted.

STEP FIVE: *CREATING INTERVENTIONS*   Develop at least one intervention for every outcome objective. Regardless of one's personal orientation to counseling, it is important that treatment plans include specific, well-defined steps that are understood by Managed Behavioral Healthcare Organization (MBHO) personnel. For example, a counselor practicing reality therapy would list how the reality therapy steps were to be used to get the client to explore better alternatives to meet personal needs, the intervention frequency, and the duration of the intervention. For example, "individual counseling once per week for 8 weeks" and re-evaluate as needed.

STEP SIX: *DIAGNOSING*   Diagnoses must fit the DSM-V, ICD system if treatment is to be reimbursed by MBHOs.

SUMMARY

Shapiro, Friedberg, and Bardenstein (2006) recommend that counselors see both the forest and the trees. Children who come to counseling should receive the best possible care. Research indicates that counseling is as effective for young people as it is for adults. Therefore, the forest that contains meta-analysis and other research compilations supports the general effectiveness of counseling. Yet counselors work with the child and family—to extend our analogy, the trees. In this chapter, we have reviewed ways to classify that counseling into affective, cognitive, behavioral, or systemic categories. We have also provided an overview of the process of counseling. We have considered some frequent concerns and some universal skills as well as some answers to typical questions from counselors. Finally, the practical considerations of managed care and evidence-based practice were discussed. This overview of the practice of counseling should provide the underpinning to our look at theories and other topics.

THE COUNSELING PROCESS VIDEO

To gain a more in-depth understanding of the concepts in this chapter, visit www.cengage.com/counseling/henderson to view a short clip of an actual therapist–client session demonstrating the counseling process.

WEB SITES FOR THE COUNSELING PROCESS

Counseling is a challenging field because the world is changing so rapidly. The need for new information about how to handle counseling cases confronts counselors on an almost daily basis. There are hundreds of Web sites with specific kinds of information available to help counselors with these challenges. Internet addresses frequently change. To find the sites listed here, visit www.cengage.com /counseling/henderson for an updated list of Internet addresses and direct links to relevant sites.

American Counseling Association (ACA)

American Psychological Association (APA)

American School Counselor Association (ASCA)

Evidence-Based Behavioral Practice (EBBP)

Mental Health America (MHA)

Mental Health Patient's Bill of Rights National Alliance on Mental Illness (NAMI)

National Coalition of Mental Health Professionals and Consumers (NCMHPC)

REFERENCES

Achenbach, T. M., & Rescorla, L. A. (2001). *Manual for the Achenbach System of Empirically Based Assessment (ASEBA)*. Burlington, VT: ASEBA.

Ahn, M., & Wampold, B. (2001). Where oh where are the specific ingredients? A meta-analysis of component studies in counseling and psychotherapy. *Journal of Counseling Psychology, 48*, 251–257.

American Psychological Association Task Force on Evidence-Based Practice for Children and Adolescents. (2008). *Disseminating evidence-based practice for children and adolescents: A systems approach to enhancing care*. Washington, DC: American Psychological Association.

APA Task Force on Evidence-Based Practice. (2006). Evidence-based practice in psychology. *American Psychologist, 61*, 271–285.

Benedict, H. E., & Mongoven, L. B. (1997). Thematic play therapy: An approach to treatment of attachment disorders in young children. In H. G. Kaduson, D. Cangelosi, & C. E. Schaefer (Eds.), *The playing cure: Individualized play therapy for specific childhood problems* (pp. 277–315). Northvale, NJ: Aronson.

Burlingame, G. M., Wells, M. G., Hoag, M. J., Hope, C. A., Nebeker, S. R., Konkel, K., et al. (1996). *Manual for the youth outcome questionnaire*. Stevenson, MD: American Professional Credentialing Service.

Carlson, K. (1990). Suggestions for counseling "other-referred" children. *Elementary School Guidance and Counseling, 24*, 222–229.

Carr, A. (2009). *What works with children, adolescents, and adults? A review of research on the effectiveness of psychotherapy*. New York, NY: Routledge.

Chang, V., Scott, S., & Decker, C. (2009). *Developing helping skills: A step-by-step approach*. Belmont, CA: Brooks/Cole.

Chorpita, B. F., Reise, S., Weisz, J. R., Grubbs, K., Becker, K. D., Knull, J. L., & the Research Network on Youth Mental Health. (2010). Evaluation of the brief problem checklist: Child and caregiver interviews to measure clinical progress. *Journal of Consulting and Clinical Psychology, 78*, 526–536.

Clarke, G., Lynch, F., Spofford, M., & DeBar, L. (2006). Trends influencing future delivery of mental health services in large healthcare systems. *Clinical Psychology: Science and Practice, 13*, 287–292.

Compton, B., Galaway, B., & Cournoyer, B. (2005). *Social work processes* (7th ed.). Belmont, CA: Thomson.

Conners,. C. K. (2013). *Manual for the Conners' 3*. North Tonawanda, NJ: Multi-Health Systems.

Cook, J. A., Heflinger, C. A., Hoven,. C. W., Kelleher, K. J., Mulkern, V., & Paulson, R. I. (2004). A multi-site study of Medicaid-funded managed care versus fee-for-service plans' effects on mental health service utilization of children with severe emotional disturbance. *Journal of Behavioral Health Services & Research, 31*(4), 384–402.

Corsini, R. J. (2008). Introduction. In R. J. Corsini & D.Wedding (Eds.), *Current psychotherapies* (8th ed., pp. 1–14). Belmont, CA: Thomson.

David-Ferdon, C., & Kaslow, N. (2008). Evidence-based psychosocial treatments for child and adolescent depression. *Journal of Clinical Child & Adolescent Psychology, 37*(1), 62–104. doi:10.1080/15374410701817865

Davis, J. (1998). Managed care forum offers counselors advice on how to gain the competitive edge. *The Advocate, 21*, 5, 9, 12.

Donnelly, C, & Carswell, A. (2002). Individualized outcome measures: A review of the literature. *Canadian Journal of Occupational Therapy, 69*, 84–94.

Dowd, E., & Kelly, F. (1975). The use of goal attainment scaling in single case study research. *Goal Attainment Review, 2*, 11–21.

Dugatkin, L. A. (2009). *Principles of animal behavior* (2nd ed.). New York, NY: Norton.

Egan, G. (2010). *The skilled helper* (9th ed.). Belmont, CA: Cengage.

Erdman, P., & Lampe, R. (1996). Adapting basic skills to counsel children. *Journal of Counseling and Development, 74*, 374–377.

Eyberg, S., Nelson, M., & Boggs, S. (2008). Evidence-based psychosocial treatments for children and adolescents with disruptive behavior. *Journal of Clinical Child & Adolescent Psychology, 37*(1), 215–237. doi: 10.1080/15374410701820117

Fine, A. H. (2010). *Handbook on animal-assisted therapy: Theoretical foundations and guidelines for practice* (3rd ed.). Boston,MA: Elsevier/Academic Press.

Fraser, J. S., & Solovey, A. D. (2007). *Second-order change in psychotherapy: The golden thread that unifies effective treatments*. Washington, DC: American Psychological Association.

Garbarino, J., & Stott, F. (1992). *What children can tell us*. San Francisco, CA: Jossey-Bass.

Garfield, R. L., Lave, J. R., & Donohue, J. M. (2010). Health reform and the scope of benefits for mental health and substance use disorder services. *Psychiatric Services, 61*, 1081–1086.

Gladding, S. T. (2013). *Counseling: A comprehensive profession* (7th ed.). Upper Saddle River, NJ: Merrill.

Greenberg, L. A., Watson, J. C., Elliott, R., & Bohart, A. (2001). Empathy. *Psychotherapy, 38*, 380–384.

Gross, D. R., & Capuzzi, D. (2006). Helping relationships: From core dimensions to brief approaches. In D. Capuzzi & D. R.Gross (Eds.), *Counseling and psychotherapy: Theories and interventions* (4th ed., pp. 2–25). Upper Saddle River, NJ: Merrill.

Halstead, R. W., Pehrsson, D., & Mullen, J. A. (2011). *Counseling children: A core issues approach*. Alexandria, VA: American Counseling Association.

Heflinger, C. A., & Saunders R. C. (2005). Physical and behavioral health of Medicaid children in two southern states. *Southern Medical Journal, 98*(4), 429–435.

Imel, Z. E., & Wampold, B. E. (2008). The importance of treatment and the science of common factors in psychotherapy. In S. D. Brown & R. W. Lent (Eds.), *Handbook of counseling psychology* (4th ed., pp. 249–266). Hoboken, NJ: Wiley.

Kazdin, A., & Weisz, J. (2003). *Evidence-based psychotherapies for children and adolescents.* New York: Guilford Press.

King, L. M. (2007). *Animal-assisted therapy: A guide for professional counselors, school counselors, social workers, and educators.* Bloomington, IN: Author House.

Kiresuk, T., Smith, A., & Cardillo, J. (1994). *Goal attainment selling: Applications, theory, and measurement.* Hillsdale, NJ: Erlbaum.

Kleinrahm, R., Keller, F., Lutz, K., Kölch, M., & Fegert, J. M. (2013). Assessing change in the behavior of children and adolescents in youth welfare institutions using goal attainment scaling. *Child and Adolescent Psychiatry and Mental Health*, 7(1), 33. doi:10.1186/1753-2000-7-33

Lambert, M. (2013). The efficacy and effectiveness of psychotherapy. In M. J. Lambert (Ed.), *Bergin and Garfield's handbook of psychotherapy and behavior change* (6th ed.). Hoboken, NJ: John Wiley & Sons.

Lambert, M. J., & Barley, D. E. (2001). Research summary on the therapeutic relationship and psychotherapy outcome. *Psychotherapy*, *38*, 357–361.

Lambert, M., & Cattani-Thompson, K. (1996). Current findings regarding the effectiveness of counseling: Implications for practice. *Journal of Counseling and Development*, *74*, 601–608.

Lambert, M. J., & Ogles, B. M. (2004). The efficacy and effectiveness of psychotherapy. In M. J. Lambert (Ed.), *Bergin and Garfield's handbook of psychotherapy and behavior change* (5th ed., pp. 139–193). Hoboken, NJ: Wiley.

Landreth, G. (2012). *Play therapy: The art of the relationship* (3rd ed.). New York, NY: Routledge.

Lazarus, A. (2008). Multimodal therapy. In R. J. Corsini & D. Wedding (Eds.), *Current psychotherapies* (8th ed., pp. 368–401). Belmont, CA: Thomson.

Lichtenberg, J. W., Goodyear, R. K., & Genther, D. Y. (2008). The changing landscape of professional practice in counseling psychology. In. S. D. Brown & R. W. Lent (Eds.), *Handbook of counseling psychology* (4th ed., pp. 21–37). Hoboken, NJ: Wiley.

Marson, S. M., Wei, G., & Wasserman, D. (2009). A reliability analysis of goal attainment scaling (GAS) weights. *American Journal of Evaluation*, *30*(2), 203–216. doi:10.1177/1098214009334676

Muran, J. C., & Barber, J. P. (2010). *The therapeutic alliance: An evidence-based guide to practice.* New York, NY: Guilford Press.

Norcross, J. (Ed.). (2011). *Psychotherapy relationships that work: Evidence-based responsiveness* (2nd ed.). New York, NY: Oxford University Press.

Norcross, J. C., & Beutler, L. E. (2014). Integrative psychotherapies. In D.Wedding & R. J.Corsini (Eds.), *Current psychotherapies* (10th ed., pp. 499–532). Belmont, CA: Thomson.

Norcross, J. C. Hedges, M., & Prochaska, J. O. (2002). The face of 2010: A Delphi poll on the future of psychotherapy. *Professional Psychology: Research and Practice*, *33*, 316–322.

Orlinsky, D. E., Grawe, K., & Parks, B. K. (1994). Process and outcome in psychotherapy. In A. E.Bergin & S. L.Garfield (Eds.), *Handbook of psychotherapy and behavior change* (pp. 270–378). New York: John Wiley.

Pope, K. S., & Wedding, D. (2008). Contemporary challenges and controversies. In R. J. Corsini & D. Wedding (Eds.), *Current psychotherapies* (8th ed., pp. 512–540). Belmont, CA: Thomson.

Poppen, W., & Thompson, C. (1974). *School counseling: Theories and concepts.* Lincoln, NE: Professional Educators.

Rimondini, M., Del Piccolo, L., Goss, C., Mazzi, M., Paccloni, M., & Zimmermann, C. (2010). The evaluation of training in patient-centered interviewing skills for psychiatric residents. *Psychological Medicine, 40,* 467–476.

Ringel, J. S., & Sturm, R. (2001). National estimates of mental health utilization and expenditures for children in 1998. *Journal of Behavioral Health Services and Research, 28,* 319–334.

Roach, A. T., & Elliott, S. N. (2005). Goal attainment scaling: An efficient and effective approach to monitoring student progress. *Teaching Exceptional Children, 37,* 8–17.

Rogers, C. R. (1957). The necessary and sufficient conditions of therapeutic personality change. *Journal of Consulting Psychology, 21,* 95–103.

Ruble, L., McGrew, J. H., & Toland, M. D. (2012). Goal attainment scaling as an outcome measure in randomized controlled trials of psychosocial interventions in autism. *Journal of Autism and Developmental Disorders, 42*(9), 1974–1983. doi: 10.1007/s10803-012-1446-7

Seligman, L., & Reichenberg, L. W. (2012). *Selecting effective treatments: A comprehensive, systematic guide to treating mental disorders.* Hoboken, NJ: Wiley and Sons.

Seligman, M. (1995). The effectiveness of psychotherapy. *American Psychologist, 50*(12), 965–974.

Sexton, T. L., & Whiston, S. C. (1996). Integrating counseling research and practice. *Journal of Counseling and Development, 74,* 588–589.

Shapiro, J. P., Friedberg, R. D., & Bardenstein, K. K. (2006). *Child and adolescent therapy: Science and art.* Hoboken, NJ: Wiley.

Shirk, S. R., & Karver, M. (2003). Prediction of treatment outcome from relationship variables in child and adolescent therapy: A meta-analytic review. *Journal of Consulting and Clinical Psychology, 71,* 465–481.

Shogren, K. A., Palmer, S. B., Wehmeyer, M. L., Williams-Diehm, K., & Little, T. D. (2012). Effect of intervention with the self-determined learning model of instruction on access and goal attainment. *Remedial and Special Education, 33*(5), 320–330. doi: 10.1177/0741932511410072

Silverman, W., Viswesvaran, C., & Pina, A. (2008). Evidence-based psychosocial treatments for phobic and anxiety disorders in children and adolescents. *Journal of Clinical Child & Adolescent Psychology, 37*(1), 105–130. doi: 10.1080/15374410701817907

Slattery, J. M., & Park, C. L. (2011). *Empathic counseling.* Belmont, CA: Brooks/Cole.

Smith, M. L., Glass, G. V., & Miller, T. I. (1980). *The benefits of psychotherapy.* Baltimore, MD: Johns Hopkins University Press.

Spring, B. (2007). Evidence-based practice in clinical psychology: What it is, why it matters; what you need to know. *Journal of Clinical Psychology, 63,* 611–631.

Steenbarger, B., & Smith, H. (1996). Assessing the quality of counseling services: Developing accountable helping systems. *Journal of Counseling & Development, 75*(2), 145–150.

Taras, H. L., & Young, T. L. (2004). Policy statement: School-based mental health services. *Pediatrics, 113*(6), 1839–1845.

Thompson, C., & Campbell, S. (1992). Personal intervention preferences for alleviating mild depression. *Journal of Counseling and Development, 71*(1), 69–73.

Thompson, C., & Poppen, W. (1992). *Guidance activities for counselors and teachers.* Knoxville, TN: Authors.

Truax, C. B., & Carkhuff, R. R. (1967). *Towards effective counseling and psychotherapy: Training and practice.* Chicago: Aldine.

Van Velsor, P. (2004). Revisiting basic counseling skills with children. *Journal of Counseling & Development, 82,* 313–318.

Waldron, H., & Turner, C. (2008). Evidence-based psychosocial treatments for adolescent substance abuse. *Journal of Clinical Child & Adolescent Psychology, 37*(1), 238–261. doi: 10.1080/15374410701820133

Weisz, J. R., Chorpita, B. R., Frye, A., Ng, M. Y., Lau, N., Bearman, S. K., and the Research Network on Youth Mental Health. (2011). Youth top problems: Using idiographic, consumer-guided assessment to identify treatment needs and track change during psychotherapy. *Journal of Consulting and Clinical Psychology, 79,* 369–380.

Welfel, E. R. (2013). *Ethics in counseling & psychotherapy* (5th ed.). Belmont, CA: Brooks/ Cole.

Yalom, I. (2009). *The gift of therapy: An open letter to a new generation of therapists and their patients.* New York, NY: Harper Publishing.

CHAPTER 4

Legal and Ethical Considerations for Counselors

May you live your life as if the maxim of your actions were to become universal law.
—IMMANUEL KANT

Legal, ethical, moral, and professional guidelines combine in many of the issues counselors face every day. Counselors' frustration may be fueled by the lack of unequivocal answers from ethical or legal guidelines for the dilemmas created in their practice. Working with children creates particular challenges for counselors because the rights of minors are more ambiguous than some other points of law and ethics. This chapter highlights issues that often arise in counseling children and contains a survey of some of the writers in this area of counseling. Counselor education programs provide courses that incorporate a foundational understanding of legal and ethical issues, but this practice area often changes. Therefore, anyone who counsels is advised to commit to an ongoing study of legal and ethical considerations. After reading this chapter, you should be able to:

▶ Define ethical, professional, and legal issues in counseling
▶ Discuss principle and virtue ethics
▶ Explain competence, consent, confidentiality, privileged communication, and child abuse reporting
▶ Use an ethical decision-making model

ETHICAL, PROFESSIONAL, AND LEGAL ISSUES

Ethics is a branch of philosophy that focuses on morals and morality in their relationship to making decisions. Cottone and Tarvydas (2007) explained that ethics refers to theories of what is acceptable behavior and morality relates to the application of ethical principles. Some authors (Francis & Dugger, 2014;

Herlihy & Corey, 2015) explain ethics as the communication to the public and practitioners, the customs, mores, standards, and accepted practices of a profession. Ethical standards refer to "the profession-relevant directives or guidelines that reflect the best ethical practice of professions" (Cottone & Travydas, 2007, p. 29). Thus, ethical guidelines educate professionals about principled conduct in practice, provide a means of accountability in practice, and create ways to improve the profession (Herlihy & Corey, 2015). The most important ethical codes serve as a protection to the public by delineating the boundaries within which counselors should practice.

The codes of ethics are written in broad terms and serve as starting points for making decisions (Welfel, 2013). Counselors may refer to a number of ethical codes that inform their practice. Examples include those codes of the American Counseling Association (2014), National Board of Certified Counselors (2012), American School Counselor Association (2010), American Association for Marriage and Family Therapy (2012), American Psychological Association (2010), and National Association of Social Workers (2008). All those documents address some common issues such as competence of the practitioner, responsibilities to the person being counseled, confidentiality, cultural diversity, and potentially harmful relationships. Many of the latest editions also provide guidelines to the use of technology.

Professional issues are technical, procedural, or cultural standards that members of the profession are expected to accept as part of their practice. For example, Daniels (2001) provides a summary of the ways managed care affects professional issues, such as fair billing practices, advertising, and access to your place of visit.

Finally, laws impact counseling practices. Laws are sets of rules that have been enacted by federal, state, and local legislative bodies (Wheeler & Bertram, 2014). According to Fischer and Sorenson (1996), laws are the minimum standard that society will accept. Dahir and Stone (2013) explain that laws require that counselors act as a "reasonably competent professional would" (p. 301). That guideline refers to the "standard of care" target that may guide decisions about whether a course of action would meet that criterion (Dahir & Stone, 2013). Someone who does not follow the law faces greater punitive sanctions or penalties for not complying than for not following ethical and/or professional standards. All three sets of standards exist to guide behavior for professionals. If the standards appear contradictory in a particular situation, the counselor is left to determine the most prudent action to protect the best interest of the client. With children, those decisions become complex. Some scholars provide fundamental concepts to help practitioners make the best possible decisions.

Meara, Schmidt, and Day (1996) have written that a code of ethics cannot contain everything one needs to know and that codes and their interpretations change due to a changing society, technology, rules, and public policy. For these reasons, these authors argue that professionals need to be aware of principle ethics but must also possess "virtue ethics," or character ethics. According to the authors, "Proponents of virtue ethics believe that motivation, emotion, character, ideals, and moral habits situated within the tradition and practices of a culture or other group present a more complete account of moral life than actions based on prescribed rules or principles of practice ..." (p. 24).

Nystul (2010) agrees and states that virtue ethics relate to exceeding obligations and striving toward the ideals of a profession. Cottone and Tarvydas (2007) explained that virtue ethics relate not to what is to be done but rather who we should be, the being and character of the therapist (Jungers & Gregoire, 2013). Virtue ethics, therefore, have two goals. One is for the counselor to reach and maintain professional competence and the second is to strive for the common good. Another critical component of virtue ethics involves being sensitive to cultural issues in any decision making. The focus of principle ethics has been on duty, laws, rules, obligations; the focus of virtue ethics, in contrast, is on the human character.

Welfel (2013) lists the following five virtues as those most commonly cited: *integrity, acting consistently on personal values; prudence, acting with discernment and restraint; trustworthiness, acting and following through on commitments even in the face of difficulty; compassion, deep concern for a person's welfare; and respectfulness, avoiding action that diminishes a person's dignity or rights.* Meara, Schmidt, and Day (1996) describe the virtuous counselor as one who is motivated to do good, able to discern ethical elements of clinical situations, tolerant of ambiguity, self-aware and growth oriented, willing to face one's shortcomings and biases, and open to using knowledge about cultural context in counseling. They urge the integration of principle and virtue ethics to assist professionals in making difficult decisions and in more fully developing the ethical character of the profession.

Cottone and Tarvydas (2007), Remley and Herlihy (2014), and Welfel (2013) suggest that professional practice is built on certain basic elements. One foundation is intentionality—that is, wanting to do the right thing for those being served. Another element consists of the moral principles of the helping profession. Those shared beliefs that guide our ethical reasoning include the following:

- Autonomy (respecting freedom of choice; allowing self-determination and decision making)
- Nonmaleficence (doing no harm)
- Beneficence (being helpful; doing good; benefiting the client)
- Justice (being fair and egalitarian)
- Fidelity (being faithful or loyal)
- Veracity (being honest and keeping promises)

Other aspects these authors discuss include the knowledge of ethical, legal, and professional standards and the skills to apply that knowledge. These authors recommend having a decision-making model to help when encountering dilemmas. Finally, these ethicists challenge counselors to have the courage of their convictions to function in an ethical and professional manner.

Decision-Making Models

Many scholars propose models of ethical decision making. Counselors may find useful suggestions for approaching ethical choices in the work of these authors: Cottone (2001); Cottone and Tarvydas (2007); Forester-Miller and Davis (1995); Garcia, Cartwright, Winston, and Borzuchowska (2003); Kitchener (1984); Meara, Schmidt, and Day (1996); Rave and Larsen (1995); Stadler (1986); and Tarvydas (1987).

A synthesis of these and other models that Remley and Herlihy (2014) and Welfel (2013) discuss may be helpful as counselors encounter ethical dilemmas. Those steps of decision making include the following:

1. Develop ethical sensitivity to the moral dimensions of counseling.
2. Identify and define the problem. Clarify facts, who has a stake in the situation, and the sociocultural context of the case.
3. Think about your own emotional reactions to the situation.
4. Apply fundamental ethical principles and theories to the situation (autonomy, nonmaleficence, beneficence, justice, fidelity, veracity). Define the central issues in the dilemma and possible options.
5. Refer to professional standards, relevant laws and regulations, and current ethics literature.
6. Consult with colleagues or experts.
7. Involve the client in the decision-making process.
8. Identify desired outcomes and actions to achieve those outcomes.
9. Consider different courses of action.
10. Choose and act.
11. Reflect on the actions taken (Remley & Herlihy, 2014, pp. 14–17; Welfel, 2013, pp. 29–55).

After resolving an ethical dilemma, Remley and Herlihy (2014) suggest applying four self-tests. The first is the test of justice; you ask yourself if you would treat other people the same in this situation. A second test of universality means you ask yourself whether you would recommend the course of action you followed to other counselors in similar situations. Third is the test of publicity and the question is whether you would be willing to have your actions known by others. Finally, you can check for moral traces or lingering feelings of doubt, discomfort, or uncertainty. Those unpleasant feelings may be a warning that your decision placed you on an ethical slippery slope or what happens when you begin to compromise your principles and you find it easier and easier to slide down the slope and diminish your moral principles.

An example using the proposed decision-making model can be found later in this chapter. some tips from the American School Counselor Association (n.d.) may also serve as guidelines to all choices made by counselors. Following is a summary of those hints:

- Always act in the best interest of the client.
- Always act in good faith and without malice.
- Be aware of your personal values, attitudes, and beliefs.
- Alert clients to the possible limitations on the counseling relationship before beginning counseling.
- Be culturally aware.
- Function within the boundaries of personal competence. Be aware of personal skill levels and limitations.
- Be able to fully explain why you do what you do. A theoretical rationale should undergird counseling strategies and interventions.
- Encourage family involvement, where possible, when working with minors in sensitive areas that might be controversial.

- Follow written job descriptions. Be sure what you are doing is defined as an appropriate function in your work setting.
- Read and adhere to the ethical standards of your profession. Keep copies of ethical standards on hand, review them periodically, and act accordingly.
- Consult with other professionals (colleagues, supervisors, counselor educators, professional association ethics committee, etc.). Have a readily accessible support network of professionals.
- Join appropriate professional associations. Read association publications and participate in professional development opportunities.
- Stay up-to-date with laws and current court rulings, particularly those pertaining to counseling with minors.

Strom-Gottfried (2008) offered a condensed decision-making framework that can be easily remembered—as she says, it is as simple as the ABCs. She explained that decision-making models have differences in the level of detail but that all have similar steps of understanding the dilemma, coming up with options, talking with others, and recording and assessing the actions that were taken. Her framework is a five-part process, but rather than steps, these parts can occur in any order. she suggested practitioners facing an ethical dilemma:

A—Assess the options

B—Be mindful of the process

C—Consult

D—Document

E—Evaluate

In assessing the model, the practitioner would look at the situation from many sides and generate as many responses to the dilemma as possible. At the same time, the counselor can evaluate the benefits and disadvantages of each response. According to Strom-Gottfried, the mnemonic ELVIS can help the mental health professional assure the variables that must be considered are covered in the assessment. E refers to the *ethical principles* involved; L refers to the *laws and policies* that are relevant; V stands for the *values*, the beliefs about how things should be and what is preferable or right; I refers to *information* or the facts of the situation; and S means paying attention to ethical *standards* and practice standards. Considering all these factors in assessing the ethically troubling situation helps the counselor with the other variables in this framework.

Being mindful of the process means counselors think beyond what actions to take to also consider how the decisions will be enacted. For example, if a counselor decides to breach confidentiality of a teen client, what steps will be taken with the teen and others so that the damage can be minimized and the benefits increased?

Counselors consult with other professionals as they try to determine the resolution of the dilemma. Strom-Gottfried (2008) explained that extra ears, eyes, and minds can open new possibilities. Documents should contain the factors considered in the decision, the resources and people consulted, the decision itself, and the basis for the decision. Information about the outcomes should also be part of these notes which should be kept. Documentation should be done as the decision unfolds rather than waiting for the conclusion of the situation so that as things occur, counselors

TABLE 4-1 AN ETHICAL DECISION-MAKING MODEL

Assess options
    Ethical theories and principles
    Laws and policies
    Values
    Information
    Standards
Be mindful of process
Consult
Document
Evaluate

Strom-Gottfried, K. (2008). *The ethics of practice with minors: High stakes, hard choices* (p. 35). Chicago, IL: Lyceum. Reprinted with permission.

can capture them to create a comprehensive entry. The decision must be evaluated so that the results can be considered, improved for the next time, and the professional learns what works, why it works, and under what conditions it may or may not work in the future. Strom-Gottfried's model is summarized in Table 4-1.

Mental health professionals need to memorize an ethical decision-making model and practice the process in order to be prepared for dilemmas that will come their way.

Counseling Minors

Salo and Shumate (1993) and Salo (2015) write that "Counseling minor clients is an ambiguous practice" (p. 1). They suggest that absolute guidelines are difficult to determine because statutes and court decisions do not always agree. In addition, conflicts arise between codes of ethics and state and federal laws. An example of the variation in state laws is the different "ages of majority," that is, the age at which a minor becomes an adult. In some states, that age is 18, in others, 19, and still others, 21 (see state law survey). Koocher (2008) emphasized that practitioners working with children in mental health services will encounter ethical concerns that do not arise with adult clients.

Hussey (2008) and Lawrence and Kurpius (2000) have traced the history of children's rights and crucial court cases that have set precedents for the interpretation of those rights. Those authors conclude that safeguarding basic rights for children involve balancing three social systems:

1. The state that must accept the imperative of maintaining the safety and rights of citizens, including children
2. The parent or family, interested in their freedom to raise their children without interference
3. The minor child "whose vested interest has been self-protection from perceived harm, preservation of privacy, and maintenance of personal dignity" (Lawrence & Kurpius, 2000, p. 132)

Lawrence and Kurpius conclude that, currently, parents and others in positions of authority over children have the balance of power. Thus, although most adults agree on the worth and dignity of children, it must be recognized that legally minors have fewer rights than adults. several sources help monitor the rights children do have in each state. For example, both the National District Attorneys Association (2013) and a state law survey have identified minors' rights to ask for health care and other services. English, Bass, Boyle, and Eshragh (2010) have generated a state-by-state description of the legal status of minors in their book *State Minor Consent Laws: A Summary, 3rd Edition.* Information in that volume outlines minors' rights to request health services. The book includes data about minors' health privacy and confidentiality statutes, disclosure to parents, and other laws that affect young people. The Guttmacher Institute (www.guttmacher.org) publishes policy briefs and summaries of laws that pertain to young people. Their report on minor consent for health care is contained in Figure 4-1.

Prout and Prout (2007) summarizes the key right for children and parents as these:

Children in counseling have the right:

- To be respected and told the truth
- To know about the evaluation process, rationale, and results in understandable terms
- To be told about the interventions and reasons for them in clear language
- To receive information about confidentiality and its limits
- To be involved with the counselor and/or parents in decision making and goal setting
- To control the release of their personal information
- To be released from treatment if unsuccessful
- Not to be the scapegoat in a dysfunctional family

Parents' rights and responsibilities include:

- Providing for the child's welfare
- Having access to information that pertains to the child's welfare
- Seeking treatment for their child
- Participating in therapy decisions and goal setting for their child
- Giving permission for treatments
- Releasing confidential information about their child

The overlap in these rights highlights some of the unique concerns that arise when counseling children. A fundamental issue for counselors is to determine who is the client—the child, the family, the school, the community, the court, or some other child support system. The identification of the person or group who is the "client" will enlighten some of the dilemmas of working with minors. Lawrence and Kurpius (2000) and Remley and Herlihy (2014) identify counselor competence, parental permission, confidentiality, and child abuse reporting as ethical issues that consistently emerge when counseling children.

The ACA *Code of Ethics* (2014) outlines the responsibilities of counselors toward their clients, colleagues, workplace, and self. Most basically, the Code calls for counselors to "facilitate client growth and development in ways that foster the interest and welfare of client …" (p. 4). The purpose is to guide counselors through the most common problems in practice, as well as to communicate the goals of the profession.

MINORS MAY CONSENT TO:

STATE	CONTRACEPTIVE SERVICES	STI SERVICES	PRENATAL CARE	ADOPTION	MEDICAL CARE FOR MINOR'S CHILD	ABORTION SERVICES
Alabama	All[†]	All[*]	All	All	All	Parental Consent
Alaska	All	All	All		All	▼ (Parental Consent)
Arizona	All	All		All		Parental Consent
Arkansas	All	All[*]	All		All	Parental Consent
California	All	All	All	All		▼ (Parental Consent)
Colorado	All	All	All	All	All	Parental Notice
Connecticut	Some	All[*]		Legal counsel	All	All
Delaware	All[*]	All[*]	All[*]	All	All	Parental Notice[‡]
Dist. of Columbia	All	All[*]	All	All	All	All
Florida	Some	All	All		All	Parental Notice
Georgia	All	All[*]	All	All	All	Parental Notice
Hawaii	All[*,†]	All[*,†]	All[*,†]	All		
Idaho	All	All[†]	All	All	All	Parental Consent
Illinois	Some	All[†]	All	All	All	Parental Notice
Indiana	Some	All		All		Parental Consent
Iowa	All	All				Parental Notice
Kansas	Some	All[*]	Some	All	All	Parental Notice
Kentucky	All[*]	All[*]	All[*]	Legal counsel	All	Parental Consent
Louisiana	Some	All[*]		Parental consent	All	Parental Consent
Maine	Some	All[*]				All
Maryland	All[*]	All[*]	All[*]	All	All	All
Massachusetts	All	All	All		All	Parental Consent
Michigan	Some	All[*]	All[*]	Parental consent	All	Parental Consent
Minnesota	All[*]	All[*]	All[*]	Parental consent	All	Parental Notice
Mississippi	Some	All	All	All	All	Parental Consent
Missouri	Some	All[*]	All[*]	Legal counsel	All	Parental Consent
Montana	All[*]	All[*]	All[*]	Legal counsel	All	▼ (Parental Notice)
Nebraska	Some	All				Parental Notice
Nevada	Some	All	Some	All	All	▼ (Parental Notice)
New Hampshire	Some	All[†]	Some	All[Ω]		
New Jersey	Some	All[*]	All[*]	All	All	
New Mexico	All	All	All	All		▼ (Parental Consent)
New York	All	All	All	All	All	
North Carolina	All	All	All			Parental Consent
North Dakota		All[*,†]	ξ[*]	All		Parental Consent
Ohio		All		All		Parental Consent
Oklahoma	Some	All[*]	All[*]	All[†]	All	Parental Consent and Notice
Oregon	All[*]	All	All[*,Φ]			
Pennsylvania	All[†]	All	All	Parental notice	All	Parental Consent
Rhode Island		All		Parental consent	All	Parental Consent
South Carolina	All[◊]	All[◊]	All[◊]	All	All	Parental Consent
South Dakota	Some	All				Parental Notice
Tennessee	All	All	All	All	All	Parental Consent
Texas	Some	All[*]	All[*]			Parental Consent and Notice
Utah	Some	All	All	All	All	Parental Consent and Notice
Vermont	Some	All		All		
Virginia	All	All	All	All	All	Parental Consent
Washington	All	All[†]	All	Legal counsel		
West Virginia	Some	All	Some	All		Parental Notice
Wisconsin		All				Parental Consent
Wyoming	All	All		All		Parental Consent and Notice
TOTAL	**26+DC**	**50+DC**	**32+DC**	**28+DC**	**30+DC**	**3+DC**

▼ Enforcement permanently or temporarily enjoined by a court order; policy not in effect.

Notes: "All" applies to minors 12 and older unless otherwise noted. "Some" applies to specified categories of minors (those who have a health issue, or are married, pregnant, mature, etc.) The totals include only those states that allow all minors to consent.

* Physicians may, but are not required to, inform the minor's parents.

† Applies to minors 14 and older.

‡ Applies to minors younger than 17.

Ω A court may require parental consent.

ξ A minor may consent to prenatal care during the 1st trimester and for the first visit after the 1st trimester. Parental consent is required for all other visits during the 2nd and 3rd trimesters.

Φ Applies to minors 15 and older.

◊ Applies to mature minors 15 and younger and to minors 16 and older.

The State Policy in Brief series is made possible in part by support from The John Merck Fund.

FIGURE 4-1   MINOR CONSENT LAWS

Counselors have the ethical code to guide them on ways to maintain professional be-havior, to practice with the best interest of the client in mind, and to practice within the limits of their competence. The following sections review the particular challenges of counseling children based on the ACA Code. Koocher (2008) echoes other authors in the summary of challenges for providing mental health services to children as four *c* words: competence, consent, confidentiality, and competing interests.

Competence

The fundamental purpose of professional competence is to protect clients from harm (Wheeler & Bertram, 2014). Koocher (2008) explained that competence refers to possessing adequate or better ability to complete some task physically, intellectu-ally, emotionally, or otherwise. Welfel (2013) proposes a summation of competence that occurs when a person demonstrates knowledge, skill, and diligence. Knowledge includes mastering information about the history, theory, and research of the field and awareness of the limits of current understanding. Pope and Vasquez (2010) report that in the mental health field, competence begins with the completion of an appropriate program of study and often a licensing examination. In order to main-tain their knowledge base, mental health professionals continue to study. Welfel sug-gests that about half of what is learned in schooling will be obsolete within a decade of graduation. Counselors need particular areas of skills to work with children rather than assuming they can generalize from their coursework on adults. Clinical skills, for example, refer to the use of basic interviewing procedures and technical skills in using specific interventions. Counselors need to use those abilities diligently and to modify their language, sentence structure, and process for working with chil-dren as noted in Chapter 3. Diligence, the third variable in competence, refers to ongoing attentiveness to the needs of the client, or working hard to help the person who is struggling. Practitioners should participate in coursework in child counsel-ing before working with young people. Counselors must be thoroughly familiar with child and adolescent development, developmental tasks, family dynamics, and interventions designed for a particular age and stage (Weiner & Robinson Kurpius, 1995). Thus to be competent to counsel children, counselors must participate in specialized education, training, and supervised practice.

Detailed information can be found in the ACA *Code of Ethics* (2014), Section C.2.b: **Professional Competence.** Counselors practice in specialty areas new to them only after appropriate education, training, and supervised experience. While developing skills in new specialty areas, counselors take steps to ensure the competence of their work and protect others from possible harm.

While following those guidelines will help a counselor develop and maintain professional competence, Corey, Corey, and Callanan (2010) define competence as a continuing process instead of something that is ever achieved completely, so compe-tent counselors commit to lifelong learning.

Informed Consent/Assent

A primary goal of the counseling relationship is the creation of a climate of safety and trust. Also, people have a right to know what is going to happen in counseling and to decide whether or not they want that experience (Remley & Herlihy, 2014).

Professionals therefore provide information to build a climate of trust and to ensure that counseling is what the client wants. Part of the explanation to counseling involves the client's right to privacy and confidentiality, something that becomes complicated with minors. Informed consent, the ethical way to begin a counseling relationship, presents the first complication.

Children need to know about the nature, potential outcomes, and limitations of counseling (Wagner, 2008). The formal permission given by a client for the beginning of counseling is known as informed consent. In effect, that permission constitutes a contract that allows treatment. Two central parts of informed consent are important. One is the disclosure of information the client needs to make a reasoned decision about whether to begin counseling, and the second is free consent which means the decision is made without coercion or undue pressure (Welfel, 2013). Lawrence and Kurpius (2000) note "Informed consent must be given voluntarily with sufficient knowledge of the treatment and its consequences, and the person must be competent to give it, that is, able to understand the consequences and implications of the choices being made" (p. 133). The ACA (2014) *Code of Ethics* reads as follows:

> When counseling minor clients or adult clients who lack the capacity to give voluntary, informed consent, counselors protect the confidentiality of information received in the counseling relationship as specified by federal and state laws, written policies, and applicable ethical standards. (Section B.5.a)

Welfel (2013) explains that legally minors usually cannot give their informed consent for counseling services; at least one parent or guardian must provide permission instead. If parents share custody after a divorce, Welfel suggests getting consent from both parents. The impact of developmental factors relative to cognitive maturity, ethical guidelines, and legal requirements points to counselors getting the assent of minors to counseling. Assent can be described as a general agreement to counseling that does not have a minimum legal age (Wagner, 2008). Therefore, any child can give assent but not consent. Welfel defines assent as involving children in decisions about their own care and in an agreement to participate in counseling. In any case, children who are unable to understand counseling and who are not committed to it would probably not be capable of working toward a treatment goal. Assent is supplemental to parental consent.

Consequently, parental permission may be necessary for children to receive treatment. Remley and Herlihy (2014) explain that unless a federal or state law exists that requires otherwise, school counselors do not have an obligation to attain parent's permission for counseling services. Counselors outside of school do need a parent or guardian's consent for a minor to receive counseling. Lawrence and Kurpius (2000) have discussed some situations that are exceptions to this practice. One exception is court-ordered treatment. Another exception involves a *mature* minor, an older adolescent capable of understanding the consent. These authors note that, in some states, minors can give consent to treatment in an emergency when waiting would endanger their lives or health. A minor who is legally emancipated, such as being the head of a household, being employed, being in the armed forces, or married, may also be an exception (Welfel, 2013). Finally, a court order can be used to waive parental consent. The writers also caution care when working with a minor of divorced parents to obtain consent from the custodial parent. Dahir and Stone (2013) caution counselors to check the rights on the noncustodial parent who has rights as a psychological guardian even without having legal custody.

Informed consent can be made more concrete when written statements such as a disclosure letter or brochure are prepared. At the beginning of counseling, the client should receive documents that explain confidentiality, privileged communication, and limits to either. The information should be written in simple, informal language appropriate for the age of the child. Green, Duncan, Barnes, and Oberklaid (2003) explained that when giving information to children, adults should use everyday words, short sentences, active voice, and no technical language. Hussey (2008) stated that children should have access to their records, be allowed to take part in treatment decisions, and be told of any risks associated with counseling.

Glosoff and Pate (2002) explain that informed consent is an ongoing and clarifying part of the counseling relationship. They recommend that counselors remind young people of the contents throughout their work. Counselors may have a simple disclosure statement for the minor client and another statement with more details for parents or guardians.

Remley and Herlihy (2014) outline what to include in a disclosure statement or counseling brochure. The document should have a short description of the counselor's education, training, degrees, and work experiences. An explanation of the theory and treatment approach most often used should be included, as well as the benefits and limitations of service (Welfel, 2013). As stated earlier, a definition of confidentiality and its limits, such as danger to others; reporting child maltreatment; and any agency policies that conflict with confidentiality, such as filing for insurance benefits. Procedural details such as guidelines about appointments, how to contact the counselor, and approximate number of sessions can also be listed. Remley and Herlihy state that counselors should give clients their diagnosis, proposed treatment for the problem, probability of success, and possible alternative treatments.

The requirements of the Health Insurance Portability and Accountability Act (HIPAA) require informed consent be verified by the client's signature. That federal law and its regulations require that the informed consent document must also have other information, such as an explanation that the client's personal information may be used and disclosed to complete treatment, and that information may be given to health care companies who pay for services. The text should have a written description of procedures the counselor will follow for keeping or disclosing personal information of the clients and a statement that tells the clients how to access a fuller description of their procedures. Clients have the right to review that complete description before they sign the consent form. The paper must cite ways the client can restrict access to their personal information. The brochure or statement explains that clients have the right to revoke their previous consent in writing. The form should be kept for at least 6 years (Remley & Herlihy, 2014). The Web site for the Centers for Medicare and Medicaid Services has information that will help in determining whether you are a covered entity under HIPAA regulations (Wheeler & Bertram, 2014). Additionally, the Health Information Technology for Economic and Clinical Health Act (2009) has privacy and security compliance requirements to protect client's records.

Confidentiality

Wheeler and Bertram (2014) clarify the terms *privacy, confidentiality,* and *privileged communication.* They explain that the right to privacy ensures that people may choose what others know about them. Confidentiality refers to the professional responsibility to respect and limits access to clients' personal information. Issues of confidentiality are frequently encountered ethical problems meaning that counselors should be extremely careful to apprise their clients of their limits of confidentiality at the very beginning of counseling.

Privileged communication is a legal term used to describe the privacy of the counselor–client communication. It exists because a law has been written that refers to a client's right to prevent a court from requiring a mental health professional to disclose material covered in a professional relationship (Younggren & Harris, 2008). The privilege belongs to the client, who always has the right to waive the privilege and allow the counselor to testify with no legal grounds for withholding the requested confidential information. The limits of privileged communication are determined by federal, state, and local mandates and vary in existence and parameters accordingly. Wheeler and Bertram (2014) explained that for privilege to apply the communication must be made "in confidence, with the indicated desire that it remain so" (p. 78). Glosoff, Herlihy, and Spence (2000) found 44 states that included licensed counselors in privileged communication statutes. Some states have exceptions to privilege law because the interests of justice are greater than the privacy of records. Therefore, counselors must know local, state, and federal laws to understand how privileged communication applies. In most states, the legal concept of privileged communication does not extend to groups, couples, or family counseling, nor does it cover disclosures made in the presence of third parties not specified under the umbrella of privileged communication.

Exceptions to the privileged communication right in which professionals must disclose information include the following situations:

- The professional is fulfilling a court-ordered role, such as expert witness.
- A court mandates the release of information considered to be privileged communication.
- A lawsuit against the professional is initiated by the client (e.g., malpractice).
- The client uses his or her mental condition as a defense in a lawsuit.
- A professional determines the client needs hospitalization because of a mental disorder.
- A client discloses intent to commit a crime or is assessed to be dangerous to self or others.
- A client is a minor and has been or is suspected of being the victim of a crime such as child abuse (Remley & Herlihy, 2014; Welfel, 2013).

Counselors and their clients may not have the legal protection of privilege but confidentiality is a cornerstone of the counseling relationship and so must be maintained to the greatest extent possible. One assumption on which counseling proceeds is that the promise of confidentiality helps create trust and safety both with adults and children. For example, Welfel (2013) notes that counselors may not share child client information with anyone other than parents or guardians, records must be secure, and child client identity must be protected. She notes that respect for the dignity and autonomy of clients has no age limit. The work setting of the counselor impacts the types of confidentiality concerns that arise with minors (Salo, 2015) so that private practice therapists may encounter fewer issues with confidentiality than school counselors.

Welfel (2013) has reviewed the writing of ethics scholars and concludes that "The degree to which confidentiality can be honored is directly related to the age and maturity of the minor ... the closer the young person is to the age of maturity, the greater the likelihood that he or she can be granted a fuller measure of confidentiality" (p. 143). Fundudis (2003) and Wheeler and Bertram (2014) stated these factors should be considered to determine a minor's competence:

- Chronological age, which includes developmental history and maturational progress
- Cognitive level, which includes language, memory, reasoning ability, and logic
- Emotional maturity with factors such as temperament, stability of mood, attachment, educational adjustment, and attitudinal style
- Sociocultural factors such as family values and religious beliefs

However, children may have parents or guardians who want to know the contents of counseling sessions, and those adults probably have a legal right to know (Remley & Herlihy, 2014). Stone (2005) captures the dilemma when she talked about counselors being caught between protecting the client's privacy and the parent's right to know what is happening in their child's life. Salo and Shumate (1993) contend, "When a child approaches a counselor without parental knowledge or consent, immediate tension arises between the child's right to privacy and the parent's right—on the child's behalf—to provide informed consent for the counseling" (p. 10). Obtaining parental consent is good practice for counselors unless potential danger to the minor exists. The authors point out that early communication with parents concerning the purpose of counseling can prevent later problems. The law generally supports parents who forbid counseling of their minor children unless there are extenuating circumstances. Counselors must balance offering privacy to minors with not only the rights of parents but also the therapeutic goal of engaging parents in helping children. Remley and Herlihy suggest that counselors consider these facts about children and privacy:

- Younger children have little understanding of confidentiality or a need for privacy. Huey (1996) concurs and states that young children often are much less concerned about confidentiality than is the counselor. The children may not need the reassurances about confidentiality (Corr & Balk, 2010).
- Preadolescents and adolescents, in contrast, may have a heightened need for privacy due to their developmental stage.
- Some children may want their parents or guardians to know what has occurred in the counseling session(s).
- Children will sometimes disclose something to an adult hoping that the adult will intervene with other adults.
- Children's reasoning capacity may limit their ability to make decisions in their best interest.

Other authors have suggestions as well. Welfel (2013) proposes that parents will be reassured when they know that counselors will not practice outside other competence, will make reasonable efforts to meet parents' requests, and will respect family values. She thinks that having handbooks or brochures with information about the counseling practice will help build a climate of cooperation and open communication. Koocher (2008) suggests having in-depth discussions with families and the child about "necessary secrets" before counseling begins. Huey (1996) reminds us that parents can be valuable allies in work with children. Parents are entitled to general information from the counselor about the child's progress and short updates will meet that request (Stromberg and colleagues, as cited in Corey et al., 2010). Zingaro (1983) advises that when it is in the best interest of the child for an adult to have information, the counselor could let the adult know ways to help the minor rather than revealing specific information. Corey et al. admonish counselors to be cautious in both the kind and extent of information that is released.

To safeguard against confidentiality becoming a possible ethical or legal problem, counselors should inform the client during the first and subsequent interviews (as applicable) about confidentiality and its limits. When possible, have parents and guardians, as well as the minor, present in the first session so that all understand the parameters of therapy and limits of confidentiality. Those limits should be clearly disclosed and explained, and should include examples of legally and ethically mandated breaches of confidentiality. As noted above, this disclosure should be done both verbally in language easily understood by the client and in a written professional disclosure statement that should be signed by the child client, parents, and the counselor. All parties should keep a copy of the professional disclosure statement.

Remley and Herlihy (2014) suggest ways to cope with requests when parents want to know about counseling and the minor client has strong feelings about the disclosure not happening:

1. Discuss the request with the child and ask if the minor is willing to talk to the adult. If the child refuses, proceed with the next step.
2. Try to convince the adult that the nature of the counseling relationship and the importance of confidentiality work for the best interests of the child. Assure the adult that information concerning any danger to the child will be disclosed. If that does not convince the adult, move to the next step.
3. Hold a session with the child and the adult and act as a mediator hoping that one or the other will acquiesce. Failing that, proceed according to Step 4 or 5.
4. Inform the child beforehand, and then tell the content of the counseling session to the adult who has requested the information. Or, proceed to Step 5.
5. Refuse to disclose the information after having informed your supervisor.

Mitchell, Disque, and Robertson (2002) encourage counselors to use empathic skills to give parents an opportunity to express concerns. Counselors should show respect for the parents' fears. Counselors can explain the dilemma and the role confidentiality plays in the counseling relationship. These authors recommend that children be told about the inquiry. They also encourage counselors to prepare procedures and alternatives for responses in advance of the problem situations.

Files

Access to files presents another concern involving confidentiality. The 1974 federal Family Education Rights and Privacy Act (FERPA) provided parents and students of legal age the right to inspect their records and to protect unlimited access to their records. The act governs education records and regulates ways written information about a student will be handled and distributed in order to protect the student and family (Alexander & Alexander, 2011; Fischer & Sorenson, 1996; Stone, 2005). Also known as the Buckley Amendment, the act applies to all educational records collected, maintained, or used by a school the student has attended. FERPA legislation also allows for parents (including noncustodial parents) to ask for corrections to the records in order to alter information that is incorrect or may be misleading. Parents must be given due process so they can protest when they disagree on the accuracy of the records (Stone, 2005).

Personal logs, treatment records, and directory information are excluded. Personal logs are defined as records of instructional, supervisory, administrative, and associated educational personnel. The records must be in sole possession of the individual and must not have been shared. Treatment records include the records of a physician, psychiatrist, psychologist, or other recognized professional acting in the professional role. The records can be used only in conjunction with the treatment of the student. Koocher (2008) recommends keeping notes about contact with the child separate from notes about contacts with others. However, Wheeler and Bertram (2014) caution counselors in schools that the interpretation that their counseling records are sole possession notes and therefore being exempt may be incorrect. Those authors noted the U.S. Department of Education opinion that states a school counselor's notes are generally part of the education record. School counselors should be cautious about notes they keep and should talk to their school system's attorney or their own attorney if they are asked to reveal confidential information to parents or other people. Directory information includes the demographic information, grade, or field of study; participation in extracurricular activities; physical descriptions; and dates of attendance (Alexander & Alexander, 2011; Family Educational Rights and Privacy Act, 1974; and U.S. Department of Education, n.d.). The Individuals with Disabilities Education Act (IDEA) (1997) also mandates that parents have access to student files in a form they can understand. A useful resource about protecting student privacy and possible changes in laws can be found at this Web site http://www2.ed.gov/policy/gen/guid/fpco/ferpa/safeguarding-student-privacy.pdf

The U.S. Department of Education (n.d.) has clarified that schools need written permission from the parent to release information, except as follows:

- School officials with legitimate educational interests
- School to which a student is transferring
- Officials for auditing or evaluation purposes
- In conjunction with financial aid requests
- Organizations conducting research on behalf of the school
- Accrediting bodies
- To comply with a judicial order or subpoena
- Appropriate officials in cases of emergency
- State and local authorities in a juvenile justice system (p. 2)

Keeping Records

Welfel (2013) reminds us that records of a counseling session benefit clients and professionals in providing services. she said that records help counselors to be reflective and prepared. Wheeler and Bertram (2014) said that records are now the standard of care and the failure to keep them could be a basis for a claim of professional malpractice. Wheeler and Bertram said that client records and documentation of counseling services serve four purposes. The first is to manage treatment and provide quality care. The second involves legal implication for the client should the documents be needed if the client become involved in a judicial process such as divorce or child custody. A third reason for documentation is to protect health information according to HIPAA guidelines, and the fourth is a risk management strategy for counselors to protect them from complaints and lawsuits.

The ACA *Code of Ethics* (Section B.6 Records and Documentation) explains maintaining, storing, and disposing of records. For the counselor's notes, Remley (1990) suggests that factual information concerning actual occurrences in the session should be kept separate from the subjective section in which the counselor records diagnoses and develops future treatment plans. Remley also recommends writing notes carefully, with the thought in mind that they could become public one day and that counselors may want to document questionable or controversial information. Clinical case notes may follow the *SOAP* notes format (Remley & Herlihy, 2014)

Subjective: information provided by the client

Objective: results of counselor's tests and other assessments

Assessment: the counselor's impressions generated by the data

Plans: diagnosis and treatment plan, as well as any modifications to them.

The American Psychological Association (2007), Drogin and colleagues (2010), and Mitchell (2007) have details on the types of information for counseling records: identifying information; assessment data; treatment plans; case notes; termination summary; and miscellaneous information such as consent forms, correspondence, and releases. Medication information is another component of client records required by the HIPAA (Welfel, 2013). HIPAA protects personal health information that may be used for treatment or payment purposes and protects electronic communication systems from unauthorized access. Health care officials obtain a signature on the Notice of Privacy Practices document that signifies permission to send information to third parties for payment, to provide treatment, and to keep ordinary operation proceedings (Welfel).

Breaching Confidentiality

In court cases in states where the clients of counselors and psychologists (or other helpers) are not protected by a licensure law providing for privileged communication, counselors have no recourse except to reveal information if subpoenaed. Some courts are more tolerant than others, allowing the counselor to share the privileged information with the judge in private to determine whether the information is necessary to the proceeding or whether public disclosure would be too hurtful to those involved, such as children who are a part of the case.

Examples of legally and ethically mandated breaches of confidentiality include the following situations:

- The client is younger than 18 years (or the recognized age of majority in that jurisdiction). (The parent or legal guardian then has a legal right to the child's counseling records and to be informed of the counseling content, progress, and other information.)
- The client expresses an intent to harm self, others, or property. (Court decisions such as *Tarasoff v. Regents of the University of California* [1974] have delineated the counselor's duty to warn and to protect others at the expense of breaking client confidentiality.) Kachgian and Felthous (2004) report that in cases of clients who are dangerous, courts in many states view a breach of confidentiality as an obligation. Wheeler and Bertram (2014) explained the immunity law that protects mental health professionals in reporting the threat of harm.
- The client discloses acts (either past or present) of verbal, physical, or sexual abuse toward a child, or the counselor has reasonable suspicion that such acts occurred or are occurring.
- The counselor is court ordered to break confidentiality or to provide counseling notes or records subpoenaed or requested by the court.
- An adult client willingly provides written informed consent requesting the counselor to breach confidentiality or to release counseling records.
- The counselor is a student or is being supervised for licensure. The client's written consent to record counseling sessions must be obtained to provide the student counselor with professional supervision or consultation with treatment teams. In these cases, student counselors should disclose only as much confidential information as is required or is necessary for professional supervision or consultation.

If breaking of confidentiality is necessary, it is suggested that the counselor discuss with the client his or her intention to do so and ask the client for assistance with deciding on the best process. The counselor should explain why confidentiality must be broken, summarize what has to be done or said, and then ask the client to help resolve the dilemma. The child client might prefer to take the lead by calling parents or other authorities or by taking whatever appropriate action is necessary.

Duty to Warn/Duty to Protect

The duty to protect refers to a counselor's responsibility to protect intended victims of a client or others who may be at risk of harm. Duty to warn is the counselor's responsibility to inform an endangered person when the counselor believes a client poses a serious, imminent danger to an identifiable, potential victim (Cottone & Tarvydas, 2007). Both of those duties require breaching confidentiality, a duty that may occur when a counselor has a dangerous client and requires extreme care. ACA *Code of Ethics*, Section B.2.a: Serious and Foreseeable Harm and Legal Requirements reads as follows:

> The general requirement that counselors keep information confidential does not apply when disclosure is required to protect clients or identified others from serious and foreseeable harm or when legal requirements demand that confidential

information must be revealed. Counselors consult with other professionals when in doubt as to the validity of an exception.

Wheeler and Bertram (2014) explained that the questions for counselors are these: How can I fulfill my legal and ethical duties to protect human life, act in the best interest of my client, and be protected from potential liability for malpractice? Welfel (2013) provides specifics about legal guidelines. She says that 23 states have either a duty to protect or a duty to warn statute, 9 states have a common law duty that resulted from court cases, 10 states allow the breach of confidentiality to warn potential victims but do not require it, and 10 states have not ruled. Benjamin, Kent, and Sirikantraporn (2009) have a comprehensive chapter on these laws and cases.

DANGEROUS CLIENTS   Isaacs (1997) suggested that the Tarasoff case, case law in other jurisdictions, legal requirements, and ethical guidelines can confuse counselors on ways to proceed with dangerous clients. She proposes counselors develop protocols for consistency in handling crisis situations. James and Gilliland (2013) concur and state that every school system needs a written formal policy for emergencies.

Among other things, those protocols should include:

- Current standards of care
- List of treatment alternatives
- Full informed consent
- Consultation guidelines with parents, attorneys, school officials, and other counselors
- School and/or agency policy

Isaacs (1997) concludes that establishing protocols will prepare counselors to recognize the issues, identify their options, and have ready access to needed information. Welfel (2013) explains that legal duty requires the counseling professional to take steps to protect an identifiable victim from harm such as informing the third party, notifying police, and assessing the risk for violence. That risk assessment includes client attitudes that support violence, client capacity to carry out violence, having means to complete the violent act, the intention in contrast with the idea of acting violently, responses of others to the client's plan, and the degree of client compliance with recommendations to reduce the risk. Welfel suggests consultation with other professionals when counselors are trying to determine the predictability of danger, something Wheeler and Bertram (2014) see as almost impossible.

School counselors may have systemic imperatives for reporting the threat of violence. Some school districts have policies requiring any school employee to report a student if illegal acts are being considered or if the student has destructive impulses (Sandhu, 2000). Counselors who report any thoughts of violence may find students no longer willing to reveal anything which reduces the opportunity to reduce the risk (Welfel, 2013). Remley and Herlihy (2014) recommend discussing policies with school administrators to lessen the barriers to counseling such policies may create.

SUICIDAL CLIENTS   James and Gillilard (2013) make clear that suicide is a more prevalent and lethal problem than many others facing children. When a young person is at risk for suicide, the counselor's primary responsibility is to protect the child from that self-destruction (Jobes & O'Connor, 2009). Using the therapeutic relationship to help reduce the impulse is a good first step but prudent, immediate action must be taken. Corey et al. (2010) and Welfel (2013) explain that working with suicidal clients can be considered the most stressful part of counseling. Suicide risk assessment provides some measure of the level of danger. Becoming competent in suicide risk assessment is critical because of the high likelihood practitioners will face suicidal risk in their work (Wagner, 2008). Counselors need to be trained and supervised to become competent in this type of assessment. Granello and Granello (2007) provide a comprehensive explanation of risk factors, assessment options, and treatment interventions for suicide.

Wheeler and Bertram (2014) note that the moral principles of autonomy, self-determination, and beneficence, promoting good for the client, are at odds when counselors confront people who are suicidal. Counselors determine the thoughts, plans, and means of the client to decide whether the person should be protected from him- or herself. Berg, Hendricks, and Bradley (2009) discuss the ethical issues involved in counseling suicidal adolescents. Remley and Herlihy (2014) offer an action plan for responding to the crisis situation that occurs when a client's life may be in danger. The parents or guardians of a minor MUST be notified if the child is suicidal (Capuzzi, 2002) and school officials have a legal obligation to take action (Maples et al., 2005).

LESBIAN, GAY, BISEXUAL, AND TRANSGENDERED YOUNG PEOPLE   McFarland and Dupuis (2001) admonish counselors to protect gay, lesbian, bisexual, and transgendered (LGBT) students from violence by educating others, advocating for safe schools, and implementing prevention efforts. These authors cite emerging case law as mandating this protection for LGBT students. The National School Boards Association has published a resource document for school personnel about legal issues with students' sexual orientation and gender identity. The Center for Effective Collaboration and Practice (http://cecp.air.org/center.asp) (1999) and the American Civil Liberties Union (ACLU) have materials to help make schools safer for all students, particularly those at severe risks, such as LGBT youth (e.g., Center for Disease Control, 2014). Counselors must be very careful not to impose their values about gender, race or ethnicity, or sexual orientation onto young clients. That caution has particular relevance when the client is an adolescent, the time when young people are shaping their unique identities (Remley & Herlihy, 2014). Welfel (2013) provided some strategies for combating harassment and violence in schools. She talked about using inclusive, nonsexist language; challenging antigay and anti-anything comments; educating students and staff about harassment and homophobias; and having appropriate referral sources.

Confidentiality in Groups

Corey et al. (2010) and Crespi (2009) have particular concerns about confidentiality in counseling groups for minors. They urge group leaders to instruct members, in language they can understand, about the nature, purposes, and limitations of confidentiality in the group setting. Leaders need to remind members to discuss their concerns about confidentiality whenever they need to do so. With complete information about the limits of confidentiality, members can decide how much they want to disclose. Salo and Shumate (1993) also note that "groups, by their very nature, negate the presumption of privacy" (p. 34). They advise counselors to inform all group members about the necessity for confidentiality, but also to point out that privileged communication may not apply to group discussion. Welfel (2013) states that even though group counselors cannot guarantee confidentiality, they encourage it. Having children practice keeping group communication private by role-playing situations may eliminate some complications. Crespi (2009) examines ethical dilemmas involved in holding group counseling in schools and provides helpful tips.

Child Abuse Reporting

All states have statutes that require adults who have responsibility to care for and treat children to report suspected abuse of children (Lawrence & Kurpius, 2000). Foreman and Bernet (2000) provide clarification on state laws relative to child abuse reporting, such as whether reported suspicions of abuse or incidences of abuse are mandated. Lawrence and Kurpius state that not reporting suspected abuse is one of the most common breaches of ethical and legal standards. They hypothesize that counselors think reporting may harm the therapeutic relationship and may destabilize the family. Remley and Herlihy (2014) added other reasons counselors may be reluctant to report child maltreatment. Counselors may want to avoid betraying the child's trust. They may be afraid the child protective services investigation will be mishandled, and they may fear retaliation from the accused. Also, counselors may hope to maintain the relationship with the family so they can teach better parenting skills. The need to protect the abused child outweighs those concerns and the mandatory reporting laws of the states attest to that legal requirement.

Wagner (2008) summarized the case of *Phillis P. v. Clairmont Unified School District* (1986). School officials were found accountable for their failure to report suspected child abuse. The case involved an 8-year-old girl who was being sexually molested by another child at school. Her teacher, school psychologist, and principal knew about the abuse but did not file a report as state law required. The mother sued the district and the court agreed with her that the school had not protected the child. Small, Lyons, and Guy (2002) explain civil and criminal liability for mental health professionals reporting suspected cases of child maltreatment. Their article listed penalties for failing to report or falsely reporting in each state with case examples for illustration. For readers who would like more information about reporting statutes, we recommend the Small, Lyons, and Guy summary article.

Counselors need to know the exact language of their state law, the categories of people who must report, and whether past abuse must be reported. Counselors also need to know when the report should be made—immediately, within 24 or 48 hours, or some other time frame—whether an oral or written report is made, what information is required, and which suspected abusers must be named. Information on child abuse reporting laws may be found at the Child Welfare Information Gateway at www.childwelfare.gov. That material is updated often.

After a report has been made, counselors have to judge whether to tell the child a report has been made, how to interact with the child, parents, or guardians, and whether to let the alleged perpetrator know a report has been made. None of those are easy decisions.

Rokop (2003) suggests that counselors can reduce damage to the counseling relationship by developing a strong alliance with the child, communicating clearly about the law, expressing empathy with the client's distress, and offering support after the report is done. Lawrence and Kurpius (2000) suggest that counselors confer with professional colleagues and get legal advice before a decision is made to refrain from reporting child abuse. Welfel (2013) suggests the "well-lit room standard" in which counselors consider whether they would be proud to communicate their decision to their professional peers and expect approval of their position. That standard applies across many of the legal and ethical decisions counselors must make.

Competing Interests

Child abuse reporting is one incident of what Koocher (2008) identified as one of competing interests. He explained that counseling with children and adolescents forces multiple relationships with the family. Counselors have a child, identified as the client, but complications are inherent. Other people probably forced the child into treatment; have responsibility for the cost of counseling; may have different outcome goals for the child; and may have legal authority to make decisions for the child. Additionally, during the course of counseling, a parent may ask for individual counseling for himself or herself. As well as dealing with that type of request, counselors may be drawn into divorce proceedings and custody battles. Koocher suggests counselors be clear throughout their work that the child is the client and that unless the treatment contract involves custody evaluations, the practitioner cannot make a recommendation in those cases. If called as a witness or if therapy records are requested for custody decisions, Koocher proposes asking the judge to appoint a guardian ad litem to oversee the child's rights in the proceedings. Counselors may find themselves in the middle of competing interests when working with children and need procedures to protect their client, the child. Koocher provides some examples to be added to consent forms that may clarify those points:

Who Is My Client? Talking to parents or guardians is a vital part of counseling children, and I will have a professional relationship with all of you. Sometimes parents will have concerns as they talk to me as their child's counselor. I will listen to those concerns and help to the degree I can; however, my primary role is as the counselor to your son/daughter. If your own difficulties require some professional help, I will give you the names of some trusted colleagues or agencies.

Confidentiality Counseling works best when children can trust their counselors to treat concerns confidentially. Parents or guardians also have a need to know how counseling with their child is progressing. I will ask you to respect the privacy of your child's treatment records, but I will plan to have regular meetings with you to keep you posted on your child's progress with me. I will contact you immediately if I think your child's behavior constitutes a risk to himself/herself or to others. We should talk about any concerns you have about specific risky behavior before treatment starts.

Legal Proceedings Requiring discussion of a child's counseling in court or legal proceedings can undermine the counseling relationship and may be harmful to the child. As I start counseling your child, we all need to agree that my work will not involve any evaluation relevant to legal matters. Your signature on this form means that you agree that you will not call me as a witness to testify in any child custody matter or other legal proceeding. (p. 610)

Those additions to consent for counseling forms may prevent some of the conflicts that arise from competing interests.

Technology

The virtual world also complicates counseling practices and the recently published *ACA Ethical Standards* (2014) includes Section H that outlines responsibilities in distance counseling, technology and social media, and ways those resources may be used to serve clients as well as the concerns related to them. The use of distance counseling technology and/or social media requires the development of knowledge and skills in the technical, ethical, and legal arenas. Particular attention must be given to the informed consent and disclosure process and multiple safeguards to confidentiality must be in place. Encryption standards on Web sites and technology-based communications should meet legal standards with counselors taking precautions with any information transmitted electronically. Clients need to know how electronic records are maintained and how long they are stored. Additionally if counselors want to maintain a professional and personal social media presence, pages and profiles should be created to clearly distinguish between the two different types of virtual presence. Counselors should respect the privacy of their client's virtual presence and should avoid disclosing confidential information through public media sites. Obviously stringent guidelines must be used to protect clients in the world of technology.

Civil Liability and Licensure Board Complaints

Wheeler and Bertram (2014) provide a useful summary of the legal and ethical practices of counselors. They explain that counselors must provide *due care* in their counseling relationships or face potential liability for failing to perform their duties. Counselors can be sued for acting wrongly toward a client or for failing to act when they had a recognized duty and when the action or inaction causes injury. *Negligence* is the *unintentional* violation of an obligation one person owes another. The four elements of negligent action that must exist are a legal duty, that the duty has been breached, there is a causal connection between the breach and the injury (Stone, 2005), and injury has occurred such as physical harm, exacerbated problems, or negative changes in life circumstances. *Malpractice* as applied to counselors is based on negligence in performing professional responsibilities or duties. Remley and Herlihy (2014) define malpractice as professional misconduct or unreasonable lack of skill. Situations in which malpractice may be found include things like using a procedure that was not an accepted professional practice, using a technique for which the counselor was not trained, failing to follow a procedure that would have been more helpful, failing to warn and/or protect others from a violent client, not obtaining informed consent to treatment, and failing to explain the possible consequences of the treatment. Fischer and Sorenson (1996) listed some activities that may increase a school counselor's vulnerability to a malpractice suit: administering drugs; giving birth control advice; providing abortion-related advice; making statements that could be defamatory; assisting in searches of student lockers, cars, or other property; and violating confidentiality and records privacy. Counselors may also be charged with intentional torts such as invasion of privacy, defamation of character, assault, battery, inflicting emotional distress, or other intentional violations of protected interests.

Other than civil or criminal lawsuits, complaints against counselors may be filed in several places, but they are most commonly filed with licensure boards. Wheeler and Bertram (2014) looked at a history of complaints made to the ACA Insurance Trust. Claims involved included negligence, sexual misconduct, breach of confidentiality, unprofessional conduct, boundary issues, and defamation/libel/slander. Besides those complaints, which included both civil suits and licensure board complaints, reported state licensure complaints involved these: misrepresentation of credentials; failure to check credentials of employed therapists; failure to make fees and charges clear to clients; boundary violations; alteration of records; making a recommendation about child custody when a thorough evaluation was not completed; violating confidentiality; practicing outside the scope of experience, education, training, and licensure; and filing an insurance claim in the name of a psychologist or psychiatrist without noting the counselor who performed the work.

To protect yourself from those complaints, Wheeler and Bertram (2014) recommend these steps. Keep current copies of all statutes, regulations, ethical codes, and standards of practice. Represent your credentials accurately. Draft your informed consent and/or professional disclosure statements carefully and specify your charges in writing. Take part in continuing education regularly. Be particularly careful to avoid harmful co-occurring relationships. Have a resource network of colleagues and an attorney for consultation. Document actions you have taken or rejected and your reasons for those decisions. All those risk management strategies help counselors be effective.

AN ETHICAL DECISION-MAKING PROCESS

Many situations have no *right* solution; the final answer depends on your counseling setting, the philosophy of your practice, the interpretation of the law by your local or state authorities, potential advantages or disadvantages of the solution, and the risks to the counselor and client. Variations in situations create nuances that impact any decision. We suggest you generate some possible ethical dilemmas and practice the process we outline in the following section. Our example from the model based on Remley and Herlihy (2014) and Welfel (2013) may be a workable way to think through ethical decision making.

1. *Develop ethical sensitivity to the moral dimensions of counseling.* Felicity, the counselor involved, took an ethics course in her degree program and has

attended several educational sessions since graduation. She also followed the advice of Welfel (2013) and has added a question about potential ethical issues to her intake form and to the outline she uses for case notes.

2. *Identify and define the problem. Clarify facts, who has a stake in the counseling outcome, and the sociocultural context of the case.* Felicity has a 15-year-old female client, Cyndi, who has reported having an ongoing sexual relationship with an older man (Lewis), the husband of her best friend's (Janet) sister. Cyndi's parents have abandoned her, and she is staying with Janet who lives with the sister and Lewis. Cyndi loves that arrangement because she has no rules to follow. She says she wants to stay with them until she can establish herself as an emancipated minor, but she also talks often about reconciliation with her parents. Cyndi's present concern is that if Janet finds out about the sexual encounters with Lewis, the girls' friendship will end.

Felicity does not know how old Lewis is, although she believes he was in high school about 4 years ago. She also is confused about what adult is currently responsible for Cyndi's well-being. Cyndi had been in foster care earlier in her life but is not in that system now. Felicity's concerns include: Is the situation one that should be reported as sexual abuse or rape or another legal duty? Depending on those answers, does the need to maintain confidentiality outweigh the potential concerns for Cyndi's safety? Felicity is uncertain whether this complex situation meets the "serious and foreseeable harm" criteria in the *Code of Ethics.*

Felicity needs information about the legal aspects and the ethical standard of what constitutes serious harm. She wants to understand more about the cultural norms of the community in which this is happening. She is familiar with other members of Cyndi and Janet's circle of friends and knows some of them are sexually active. In this situation, Felicity sees these people as stakeholders: Cyndi, Cyndi's parents, Janet, Lewis, and his wife. She recognizes that her decisions should center on Cyndi and her well-being.

3. *Think about your own emotional reactions.* Felicity recognizes that her immediate reaction is anger at all the adults involved—the parents for turning their daughter out and Lewis for exploiting Cyndi's situation.

4. *Apply fundamental ethical principles and theories to the situation (autonomy, nonmaleficence, beneficence, justice, fidelity, veracity). Define the central issues in the dilemma and possible options.* Felicity believes in this situation the moral principles of autonomy and beneficence conflict. Her understanding of autonomy would lead her to respect Cyndi's choice of living arrangements and sexual partner. However, she thinks that her understanding of the principle of beneficence would encourage intervening in this situation to protect Cyndi's health and safety.

Felicity has identified the options of calling Cyndi's parents and asking about the possibility of Cyndi's moving back home, speaking with the police, or waiting to see what happens next.

5. *Refer to professional standards, relevant laws and regulations, and current ethics literature.* Felicity uncovered an informative article in *Counseling Today* titled "The End of 'Clear and Imminent Danger'" (Kaplan, 2006). She also found

an article on the legal aspects of rape and sexual abuse helpful (Mitchell & Rogers, 2003). The information from her particular state on the age of majority, emancipated minors, and minors' rights also helped clarify some of the murky guidelines.

6. *Consult with colleagues or experts.* Felicity talked about this case during her weekly supervision session. She conferred with two other people in her practice, and she asked a friend on the police force about a "hypothetical" situation that had similar characteristics. She has found the state standard requires a 6-year age difference to meet the state mandated criteria of statutory rape of a person who is 13, 14, or 15, and the ages of the people in this situation are not separated by 6 years. The legal criteria for sexual abuse has also not been met, so Felicity does not have to wrestle with whether to report to the legal system or child protective services because those guidelines have been clearly defined for her.

7. *Involve the client in the decision-making process.* The next time Felicity met with Cyndi she began, "You told me last week about you and Lewis having intercourse. You were worried about what Janet would think if she found out. Cyndi, I'm worried about you and how this affair with an older man might lead to some dangerous complications. I'd like to ask you some questions that will help me understand things better, and then together we can figure out what needs to happen to protect your health and safety."

8. *Identify desired outcomes and actions to achieve those outcomes.* Felicity and Cyndi arrived at a list of desired outcomes. First, Cyndi had to have a safe place to stay. They decided to use some local resources to find Cyndi somewhere to sleep and eat until the rest of this situation could be unraveled. Cyndi agreed to contact her parents and ask them to come with her to Felicity's office to talk about the possibilities of her returning home. Cyndi did not agree to break off the affair with Lewis even though she promised she would not stay at his house again.

9. *Consider different courses of action.* Felicity sees the crux of the problem as a minor having an affair with an adult. As discussed earlier, Felicity had determined that she had no legal obligation to report this as child abuse or statutory rape. She felt she had honored the ethical principle of autonomy by helping Cyndi create a plan of action for her own well-being. Felicity decided she would see what transpired before taking any further steps.

10. *Choose and act.* Felicity has chosen to wait another week before doing anything else.

11. *Reflect on the actions taken.* As she reviews what has happened, Felicity is satisfied with the research she has done and the consultation she has sought. She has learned from the readings and the conversations. She has based her decisions on the moral principles of autonomy and beneficence as she confronted Cyndi with her concerns and helped Cyndi develop her own plan for removing herself from Lewis's environment. Felicity will continue to be directive and probing as she monitors Cyndi's living arrangements.

SUMMARY

One of the few certainties in practicing counseling is that you will be faced with situations in which ethics, the law, and what is best for the child client do not seem to align. The pressures of having to make critical, timely decisions may overwhelm any professional so having a clear process for deliberating and a current understanding of standards of care are necessary. One way to prevent as well as face these difficult circumstances is to follow the practices Lawrence and Kurpius (2000) propose as guidelines for counseling with minors:

1. Practice within the boundaries of your competence as defined by your education, training, and supervised practice.
2. Know state laws regarding privilege. Privileged communication does not exist unless the state has mandated it.
3. Explain your policies on confidentiality with both the child and parents at the beginning of the counseling relationship and ask them for cooperation. Provide a written informed consent that everyone signs.
4. Should you decide to work with a minor without the consent of the parent or guardian, ask the child to give informed consent in writing (Hendrix, 1991), and recognize the legal risks involved.
5. Maintain accurate and objective records.
6. Purchase adequate professional liability insurance.
7. Confer with colleagues and have access to professional legal advice when you are uncertain about how to proceed (Lawrence and Kurpius, 2000, p. 135).

WEB SITES FOR LEGAL AND ETHICAL CONSIDERATIONS FOR COUNSELORS

Internet addresses frequently change. To find the sites listed here, visit www.cengage.com/counseling/henderson for an updated list of Internet addresses and direct links to relevant sites.

ACA *Code of Ethics*—Frequently Asked Questions

APA Ethical Principles of Psychologists and Code of Conduct

Child Welfare Information Gateway

U.S. Department of Education

Department of Education Office for Civil Rights (OCR)

National Board for Certified Counselors (NBCC)

REFERENCES

Alexander, K., & Alexander, M. D. (2011). *American public school law* (8th ed.). Belmont, CA: Thomson West.

American Association for Marriage and Family Therapy. (2012). *AAMFT code of ethics*. Retrieved from http://www.aamft.org/iMIS15/AAMFT/Content/Legal_Ethics/code_of_ethics.aspx

American Civil Liberties Union. Library: LGBT Youth and Schools. Retrieved from https://www.aclu.org/lgbt-rights_hiv-aids/library

American Counseling Association. (2009).

American Counseling Association. (2014). *Code of ethics and standards of practice*. Alexandria, VA: Author.

American Psychological Association, W., DC, & American Psychological Association. (2007). Record keeping guidelines. *The American Psychologist, 62*(9), 993–1004. doi: 10.1037/0003-066X.62.9.993

American Psychological Association. (2010). *Ethical principles of psychologists and code of conduct*. Retrieved from http://www.apa.org/ethics/code/index.aspx

American School Counselor Association. (n.d.). *Ethical tips for school counselors*. Retrieved from http://www.schoolcounselor.org/school-counselors-members/legal-ethical/ethical-tips-for-school-counselors

American School Counselor Association. (2010). *Ethical standards for school counselors*. Alexandria, VA: Author.

Benjamin, G. A. H., Kent, L., & Sirikantraporn, S. (2009). A review of duty to protect statutes, cases, and procedures for positive practice. In J. L. Werth, E. R. Welfel, & G. A. H. Benjamin (Eds.), *The duty to protect: Ethical, legal, and professional responsibilities of mental health professionals* (pp. 9–28). Washington, DC: American Psychological Association.

Berg, R., Hendricks, B., & Bradley, L. (2009). Counseling suicidal adolescents within family systems: Ethical issues. *The Family Journal, 17,* 64–68.

Capuzzi, D. (2002). Legal and ethical challenges in counseling suicidal students. *Professional School Counseling, 6,* 36–45.

Center for Disease Control. (2014). *Lesbian, gay, bisexual and transgendered youth health*. Retrieved from http://www.cdc.gov/lgbthealth/youth.htm

Center for Effective Collaboration and Practice. (1999). *Early warning, timely Response: A guide to safe schools*. Retrieved from http://www.cecp.air.org/guide/guide.pdf

Corey, G., Corey, M. S., & Callanan, P. (2010). *Issues and ethics in the helping professions* (8th ed.). Pacific Grove, CA: Brooks/Cole.

Corr, C. A., & Balk, D. E. (2010). *Children's encounters with death, bereavement, and coping*. New York, NY: Springer.

Cottone, R. R. (2001). A social constructivism model of ethical decision making in counseling. *Journal of Counseling and Development, 79,* 39–45.

Cottone, R. R., & Tarvydas, V. M. (2007). *Counseling ethics and decision making* (3rd ed.). Upper Saddle River, NJ: Pearson.

Crespi, T. D. (2009). Group counseling in the schools: Legal, ethical, and treatment issues in school practice. *Psychology in the Schools, 46,* 273–280.

Dahir, C. A., & Stone, C. B. (2013). *The transformed school counselor* (2nd ed.). Boston: Lahaska Press.

Daniels, J. A. (2001). Managed care, ethics, and counseling. *Journal of Counseling and Development, 79,* 119–122.

Drogin, E. Y., Connell, M., Foote, W. E., & Sturm, C. A. (2010). The American psychological associations revised "record keeping guidelines": Implications for the practitioner. *Professional Psychology: Research and Practice, 41*(3), 236–243. doi:10.1037/a0019001

English, A., Bass, L., Boyle, A. D., & Eshragh, F. (2010) *State minor consent laws: A summary* (3rd ed.). Chapel Hill, NC: Center for Adolescent Health and the Law.

Family Educational Rights and Privacy Act of 1974 (FERPA or Buckley Amendment), 20 U.S.C. §1232g (2006).

Fischer, L., & Sorenson, G. P. (1996). *School law for counselors, psychologists, and social workers* (3rd ed.). White Plains, NY: Longman.

Foreman, T., & Bernet, W. (2000). A misunderstanding regarding duty to report suspected child abuse. *Child Maltreatment, 5*, 190–196.

Forester-Miller, H., & Davis T. E. (1995). *A practitioner's guide to ethical decision-making.* Alexandria, VA: American Counseling Association.

Francis, P. C., & Dugger, S. M. (2014). Professionalism, ethics, and value-based conflicts in counseling: An introduction to the special section. *Journal of Counseling and Development, 92*, 131–134.

Fundudis, T. (2003). Current issues in medico-legal procedures: How competent are children to make their own decisions?*Child and Adolescent Mental Health, 8*, 18–22.

Garcia, J. G., Cartwright, B., Winston, S. M., & Borzuchowska, B. (2003). A transcultural integrative model for ethical decision making in counseling. *Journal of Counseling and Development, 81*, 268–277.

Glosoff, H. L., Herlihy, B., & Spence, E. B. (2000). Privileged communication in the counselor-client relationship. *Journal of Counseling and Development, 78*, 454.

Glosoff, H. L., & Pate, R. H., Jr. (2002). Privacy and confidentiality in school counseling. *Professional School Counseling, 6*, 20–27.

Granello, D. H., & Granello, P. F. (2007). *Suicide: An essential guide for helping professionals and educators.* Boston, MA: Allyn and Bacon.

Green, J. P., Duncan, R. E., Barnes, G. L., & Oberklaid, F. (2003). Putting the informed into consent: A matter of plain language. *Journal of Pediatric Child Health, 39*, 700–703.

Guttmacher Institute. (August 2014). An overview of minor consent laws. Retrieved from www.guttmacher.org

Health Information Technology for Economic and Clinical Health (HITECH) Act, Title XIII of Division A and Title IV of Division B of the American Recovery and Reinvestment Act of 2009 (ARRA). Pub. L. No. 111-5 (2009).

Hendrix, D. H. (1991). Ethics and intrafamily confidentiality in counseling with children. *Journal of Mental Health Counseling, 13*, 323–358.

Herlihy, B., & Corey, G. (2015). *ACA ethical standards casebook* (7th ed.). Alexandria, VA: American Counseling Association.

Huey, W. C. (1996). Counseling minor clients. In B. Herlihy & G.Corey (Eds.), *ACA ethical standards casebook* (5th ed., pp. 241–245). Alexandria, VA: American Counseling Association.

Hussey, D. (2008). Understanding minor clients. In K. Strom-Gottfried (Ed.), *The ethics of practice with minors* (pp. 47–63). Chicago, IL: Lyceum Press.

Isaacs, M. L. (1997). The duty to warn and protect: *Tarasoff* and the elementary school counselor. *Elementary School Guidance and Counseling, 31*, 326–342.

James, R. K., & Gilliland, B. (2013). *Crisis intervention strategies* (7th ed.). Pacific Grove, CA: Thomson.

Jobes, D. A., & O'Connor, S. S. (2009). The duty to protect suicidal clients; Ethical, legal, and professional considerations. In J. L. Werth, E. R. Welfel, & G. A. H. Benjamin (Eds.), *The duty to protect: Ethical, legal, and professional responsibilities of mental health professionals* (pp. 163–180). Washington, DC: American Psychological Association.

Jungers, C. M., & Gregoire, J. (2013). Philosophy and counselor ethics. In C.M. Jungers & J. Gregoire (Eds.), *Counseling ethics: Philosophical and professional foundations* (pp. 3–24). New York, NY: Springer Publishing.

Kachgian, C., & Felthous, A. R. (2004). Court responses to *Tarasoff* statues. *Journal of the American Academy of Psychiatry and Law, 32*, 263–273.

Kaplan, D. (2006, January). The end of 'clear and imminent danger.'*Counseling Today, 10.*

Kitchener, K. S. (1984). Intuition, critical evaluation, and ethical principles: The foundation for ethical decision in counseling psychology. *Counseling Psychologist, 12*, 43–55.

Koocher, G. P. (2008). Ethical challenges in mental health services to children and families. *Journal of Clinical Psychology: In session, 64*, 601–612.

Lawrence, G., & Kurpius, S. E. R. (2000). Legal and ethical issues involved when counseling minors in non-school settings. *Journal of Counseling and Development, 78*, 130–136.

Maples, M. R., Packman, J., Abney, P., Daughtery, R. F., Casey, J. A., Pirtle, L. (2005). Suicide by teenagers in middle school: A postvention team approach. *Journal of Counseling & Development, 83*, 397–406.

McFarland, W. P., & Dupuis, M. (2001). The legal duty to protect gay and lesbian students from violence in the schools. *Professional School Counseling, 4*, 171–179.

Meara, N., Schmidt, L., & Day, J. (1996). Principles and virtues: A foundation for ethical decisions, policies, and character. *Counseling Psychologist, 24*(1), 4–77.

Mitchell, C. W., Disque, J. G., & Robertson, P. (2002). When parents want to know: Responding to parental demands for confidential information. *Professional School Counseling, 6*, 156–162.

Mitchell, C. W., & Rogers, R. E. (2003). Rape, statutory rape, and child abuse: Legal distinctions and counselor duties. *Professional School Counseling, 6*, 332–338.

Mitchell, R. (2007). *Documentation in Counseling Records*. Alexandria, VA: American Counseling Association.

National Association of Social Workers. (2008). *Code of ethics*. Retrieved from http://www.socialworkers.org/pubs/code/default.asp

National Board of Certified Counselors. (2012). *Code of ethics*. Retrieved from www.nbcc.org/ethics

National District Attorneys Association. (2013). *Minor consent to medical treatment laws*. Retrieved from www.ndaa.org

Nystul, M. S. (2010). *Introduction to counseling: An art and science perspective* (4th ed.). Boston: Allyn & Bacon.

Pope, K. S., & Vasquez, M. J. T. (2010). *Ethics in psychotherapy and counseling* (4th ed.). San Francisco: Jossey-Bass.

Prout, S. M., & Prout, H. T. (2007). Ethical and legal issues in psychological interventions with children and adolescents. In H. T. Prout & D. T. Brown (Eds.), *Counseling and psychotherapy with children and adolescents: Theory and practice for school and clinical settings* (4th ed., pp. 32–63). Hoboken, NJ: Wiley.

Rave, E. J., & Larsen, C. C. (Eds.). (1995). *Ethical decision making in therapy: Feminist perspectives*. New York: Guilford Press.

Remley, T. (1990). Counseling records: Legal and ethical issues. In B. Herlihy & L. Golden (Eds.), *Ethical standards casebook* (pp. 162–169). Alexandria, VA: American Association for Counseling and Development.

Remley, T. P., & Herlihy, B. (2014). *Ethical, legal, and professional issues in counseling* (4th ed.). Upper Saddle River, NJ: Merrill.

Rokop, J. J. (2003). The effects of CPS mandated reporting on the therapeutic relationship: The client's perspectives. *Dissertations Abstracts International, 64*(5-B), 135.

Sandhu, D. S. (2000). Special issue: School violence and counselors. *Professional School Counseling, 4*, iv–v.

Salo, M. (2015). Counseling minor clients. In B. Herlihy & G. Corey (Eds.), *ACA Ethical standards casebook* (7th ed., pp. 205–214). Alexandria, VA: American Counseling Association.

Salo, M., & Shumate, S. (1993). Counseling minor clients. In T. Remley, Jr. (Ed.), *The ACA Legal Series* (Vol. 4). Alexandria, VA: American Counseling Association.

Small, M. A., Lyons, P. M., Jr., & Guy, L. S. (2002). Liability issues in child abuse and neglect reporting statutes. *Professional Psychology: Research and Practice, 33*, 13–18.

Stadler, H. A. (1986). Making hard choices: Clarifying controversial ethical issues. *Counseling and Human Development, 19*, 1–10.

State Law Survey for Use in Applying the State Personal Representative for Minor Section of the HIPAA Privacy Rule, 45 CFR § 164.502 (g)(3) www.ermerlaw.com/PDFs/hipaa _state_law_survey_version_3_0.pdf

Stone, C. (2005). *Ethics and law: School counseling principles*. Alexandria, VA: American School Counselor Association.

Strom-Gottfried, K. (2008). *The ethics of practice with minors*. Chicago, IL: Lyceum Press.

Tarvydas, V. M. (1987). Decision-making models in ethics: Models for increasing clarity and wisdom. *Journal of Applied Rehabilitation Counseling, 22*, 11–18.

U.S. Department of Education. (n.d.). *Family educational rights and privacy act (FERPA)*. Retrieved from http://www2.ed.gov/policy/gen/guid/fpco/ferpa/index.html

Wagner, W. G. (2008). *Counseling, psychology, and children* (2nd ed.). Upper Saddle River, NJ: Pearson.

Weiner, N., & Robinson Kurpius, S. W. (1995). *Shattered innocence: A practical guide for counseling women survivors of childhood sexual abuse*. Washington, DC: Taylor & Francis.

Welfel, E. R. (2013). *Ethics in counseling & psychotherapy: Standards, research, & emerging issues* (5th ed.). Belmont, CA: Thomson.

Wheeler, A. M., & Bertram, B. (2014). *The counselor and the law: A guide to legal and ethical practice* (7th ed.). Alexandria, VA: American Counseling Association.

Younggren, J. N., & Harris, E. (2008). Can you keep a secret? Confidentiality in psychotherapy. *Journal of Clinical Psychology, 64*, 589–600.

Zingaro, J. C. (1983). Confidentiality: To tell or not to tell. *Elementary School Guidance and Counseling, 17*, 261–267.

PART II

COUNSELING THEORIES AND TECHNIQUES

Adaptations for Children

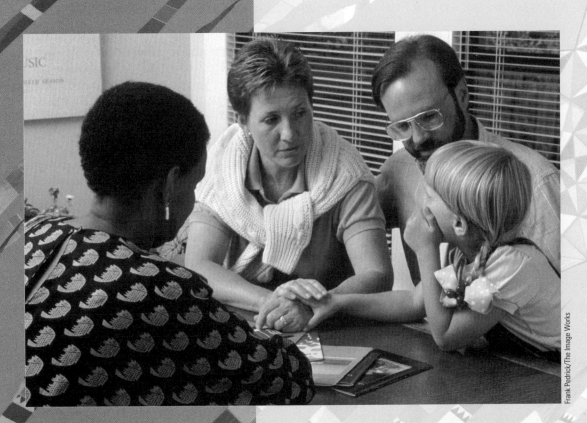

Frank Pedrick/The Image Works

CHAPTER 5

Psychoanalytic Counseling

A moment's insight is sometimes worth a life's experience.
—OLIVER WENDELL HOLMES

Psychoanalytic thought may be traced to Paul Dubois (1848–1918) whose treatment of people with psychosis involved talking to them reasonably. Dubois may have introduced a different way of working with people but indubitably the person whose name is most commonly associated with the origins of psychoanalysis is Sigmund Freud. Freud and his colleagues in the Wednesday Psychological Society met in the early part of the 19th century to discuss personality theory, therapy, and the analysis of the *psyche* (Merydith, 2007). From these beginnings, psychoanalysis has branched into a way to understand the human being as well as a system of treatment. As Luborsky, O'Reilly-Landry, and Arlow (2008) explain, "whether because it is rejected, adapted, or accepted, Freud's legacy is still with us" (p. 16). We will begin our discussions of counseling theories with psychoanalysis, the forerunner of all other types of therapy.

After reading this chapter, you should be able to:

- ▶ Outline the development of psychoanalysis and Sigmund Freud
- ▶ Explain the theory of psychoanalysis including its core concepts
- ▶ Discuss the counseling relationship and goals in psychoanalysis
- ▶ Describe assessment, process, and techniques in psychoanalysis
- ▶ Demonstrate some therapeutic techniques related to psychoanalytic therapy
- ▶ Clarify the effectiveness of psychoanalysis
- ▶ Discuss psychoanalytic play therapy

SIGMUND FREUD
(1856–1939)

Sigmund Freud was born in Freiberg, Moravia, in 1856 and died in London in 1939. However, he is considered to have belonged to Vienna, where he lived for nearly 80 years. Freud was the first of his mother's eight children; he also had two half brothers more than 20 years his elder.

Freud graduated from the gymnasium at age 17 and, in 1873, entered the medical school at the University of Vienna. He became deeply involved in neurological research and did not finish his M.D. degree for 8 years. Never intending to practice medicine because he wanted to be a scientist, Freud devoted his next 15 years to investigations of the nervous system (Hall, 1954). However, the salary of a scientific researcher was inadequate to support the wife and the six children he had at that time. In addition, the anti-Semitism prevalent in Vienna during this period prevented Freud from achieving university advancement. Consequently, Freud felt forced to take up the practice of medicine.

Freud decided to specialize in the treatment of nervous disorders; at the time, not much was known about this particular branch of medicine. First, he spent a year in France learning about Jean Charcot's use of hypnosis in the treatment of hysteria (Stone, 1971). Freud (1963) was dissatisfied with hypnosis because he thought its effects were only temporary and the treatment did not get at the center of the problem. Freud then studied with Joseph Breuer, learning the benefits of the catharsis (or "talking out your problems") form of therapy.

Noticing that his patients' physical symptoms seemed to have a mental base, Freud probed deeper and deeper into the minds of his patients. Hall (1954) notes, "His probing revealed dynamic forces at work which were responsible for creating the abnormal symptoms that he was called upon to treat. Gradually there began to take shape in Freud's mind the idea that most of these forces were unconscious" (p. 15). According to Stone (1971), this finding was probably the turning point in Freud's career. To substantiate some of his ideas, Freud decided to undertake an intensive analysis of his own unconscious forces in order to check on the material he had gathered from his patients. Hall further notes, "On the basis of the knowledge he gained from his patients and from himself he began to lay the foundations for a theory of personality" (p. 17).

Freud's early support of Charcot and his new and revolutionary ideas cost him the support of most scholars and doctors. Later in his lifetime, however, Freud was accepted as a genius in psychotherapy. Many influential scientists, including Carl Jung, Alfred Adler, Ernest Jones, and Wilhelm Stekel, recognized Freud's theory as a major breakthrough in the field of psychology; however, these scientists disagreed with some of Freud's ideas so adamantly that they broke with him early on.

Freud's penultimate recognition in academic psychology came in 1909, when he was invited by G. Stanley Hall to give a series of lectures at Clark University in Worcester, Massachusetts. According to Fancher (2000), Hall single-handedly made Freud's name a household word in the United States by ensuring full press coverage for all of Freud's lectures on psychoanalysis. It was Clark University's 20th anniversary, and Hall marked it by bringing Freud to the United States for his first and only trip. Freud's name began to appear in popular songs, and *Time* magazine featured him on the cover.

Freud's writing career spanned 63 years, during which he authored more than 600 publications. His collected works have been published in English in 24 volumes as *The Standard Edition of the Complete Psychological Works of Sigmund Freud* (Strachey, 1953–1964). Among Freud's most famous works are *The Interpretation of Dreams* (1900/1965a), *The Psychopathology of Everyday Life* (1901/1971), and *New Introductory Lectures in Psychoanalysis* (1933/1965b).

Freud never seemed to think his work was finished. "As new evidence came to him from his patients and his colleagues, he expanded and revised his basic theories" (Hall, 1954, p. 17). As an example of his flexibility and capability, at age 70, Freud completely altered a number of his fundamental views: He revamped motivation theory, reversed the theory of anxiety, and developed a new model of personality based on id, ego, and superego.

Freud developed his psychoanalytic model of people over five decades of observing and writing. The major principles were based on the clinical study of individual patients undergoing treatment for their problems. Free association, or saying whatever comes to mind, became Freud's preferred procedure after he discarded hypnosis.

Just as Sigmund Freud was the father of psychoanalysis, he was the grandfather of child psychoanalysis. His therapy with adults conducted at the Vienna Psychoanalytic Institute was continuous and lengthy, often requiring several years to complete. Yet his most famous case with a child was with Little Hans, a 5-year-old boy who was afraid of large animals. Freud met with Little Hans and his father only once and then began consulting with the father who followed Freud's advice for helping Hans. The treatment was based on Freud's theory of development. Psychoanalysis includes theories about the development and organization of the mind, the instinctual drives, the influences of the external environment, the importance of the family, and the attitudes of society. As useful as psychoanalysis is as a therapeutic tool, its impact and value reach far beyond medical applications. It is the only comprehensive theory of human psychology. Psychoanalytic theory has proved helpful to parents and teachers in the upbringing and education of children.

The psychodynamic approach to therapy includes theories based on the belief that human functioning is the result of the drives and forces within the person. Those drives and forces are often unconscious. Freud's psychoanalysis was the first psychodynamic theory and the focus of this chapter. Other psychodynamic approaches like those of Jung (1964) and Adler (1927) are based on Freud's ideas.

Although psychoanalytic theory has been modified in some areas, its basic concepts remain unchanged. The fact that almost all counseling theories include some of the basic premises from the psychoanalytic method shows the influence and durability of the theory.

THE NATURE OF PEOPLE

Freud believed that humans existed in perpetual turmoil. He considered innate drives, or instincts, as the determining factors in life. According to Freud, a person's behavior is organized in efforts to satisfy those drives—even the acts that seem random have a basis in fulfilling those instinctual needs. Thus mental processes are considered the causal factors of human behavior.

The concept of human nature in psychoanalytic theory assumes two hypotheses—psychic determinism and dynamic unconscious. Psychic determinism implies that mental life is a continuous manifestation of cause-related relationships, and that nothing happens by chance (Merydith, 2007). Dynamic unconscious implies that some basic needs, desires, and impulses are outside a person's awareness. Therefore, mental activity may be kept below the conscious level. The goal of psychoanalytic counseling involves helping a person fulfill their development by understanding human behavior through investigating that unconscious, inner experience. Counseling leading to catharsis then leads to confronting the unconscious mind in ways that promote learning, understanding, and growth in mental development and coping skills.

Freud viewed people as basically evil and victims of instincts that must be balanced or reconciled with social forces to provide a structure in which human beings can function. Freud wrote about two types of innate drives—sex and aggression. To achieve balance, people need a deep understanding of those forces that motivate them to action. According to Freud, people operate as energy systems, distributing psychic energy to the id, ego, and superego; human behavior is determined by this energy, by unconscious motives, and by instinctual and biological drives. Psychosexual events during the first 5 years of life are critical to adult personality development.

In summary, according to psychoanalytic theory, the basic concepts of human nature revolve around the notions of psychic determinism and dynamic unconscious mental processes. Psychic determinism simply implies that our mental life is a continuous logical manifestation of cause-and-effect relationships. Nothing is random; nothing happens by chance. Although mental events may appear unrelated, they are actually closely interwoven and depend on preceding mental signals. Closely related to psychic determinism are unconscious mental processes, which exist as fundamental factors in the nature of human behavior. In essence, much of what goes on in our minds, and hence in our bodies, is unknown, below the conscious level; thus, people often do not understand their own feelings or actions. The existence of unconscious mental processes is the basis for much of what is involved in psychoanalytic counseling.

Concepts

THE UNCONSCIOUS   As noted in Figures 5-1 and 5-2, the *unconscious* holds about 85 percent of the material in our minds. The concept of the *unconscious* is the foundation of psychoanalytic theory and practice. The *unconscious* is a part of the mind beyond our awareness: drives, desires, attitudes, motivations, and fantasies that exist and exert influence on how people think, feel, and behave in the conscious area of functioning. The *conscious* refers to the part of mental activity that we are aware of at any given time. As children grow, their conscious minds become more logical and realistic. The unconscious mind does not become more mature (Shapiro, Friedberg, & Bardenstein, 2006). The *preconscious* refers to thoughts and material that are not readily available to the conscious but can be retrieved with some effort. For example, students may struggle to find an answer to a test question lost in the preconscious. The *subconscious* refers to those involuntary bodily processes such as digestion and breathing that have been with the person since birth. Carl Jung added a concept of *collective unconscious*, which refers to the vast reservoir of inherited wisdom, memories, and insights that individuals share with all humankind (see Figure 5-2).

PERSONALITY

Freud's concepts of a three-part personality form the basis of a psychoanalytic counseling theory. The principal concepts in Freudian theory can be grouped under three topic headings: structural, dynamic, and developmental. The structural concepts are id, ego, and superego. The dynamic concepts are instinct, cathexis, anticathexis, and anxiety. The developmental concepts are defense mechanisms and psychosexual stages.

Structural Concepts

Freud believed human behavior resulted from the interaction of three important parts of the personality: id, ego, and superego.

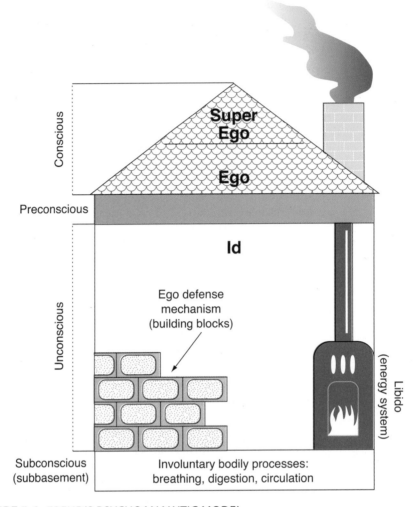

FIGURE 5-1 FREUD'S PSYCHOANALYTIC MODEL

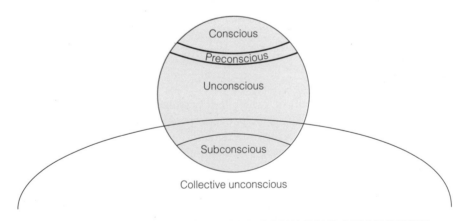

FIGURE 5-2 THE RELATIVE IMPORTANCE OF THE CONSCIOUS, PRECONSCIOUS, UNCONSCIOUS, SUBCONSCIOUS, AND COLLECTIVE UNCONSCIOUS

ID   The id, the basic unit in Freud's personality structure, contains the basic human instincts plus each person's genetic and constitutional inheritance. Thus the id contains our basic instincts or drives to satisfy basic needs, including thirst, hunger, sex, and aggression. These drives can be constructive or destructive. Constructive, pleasure-seeking (sexual) drives provide the basic energy of life (libido). In Freud's system, anything pleasurable is labeled sexual. Destructive, aggressive drives tend toward self-destruction and death. Life instincts (libido) are opposed by death instincts (Thanatos). Libido motivates someone toward survival and prosperity whereas Thanatos pushes toward chaos and destruction. The id, working on the pleasure principle, exists to provide immediate gratification of any instinctual need, regardless of the consequences. The id is incapable of thought, but can form, for example, mental pictures of hamburgers for a hungry person. The formation of such images and wishes is referred to as *fantasy* and *wish fulfillment* (the *primary process)*.

EGO   As a result of interacting with reality, the id developed a liaison between itself and the environment that Freud labeled the ego. Often called the "executive" of the personality, the ego strives to strike a balance between the needs of the id and the superego. The ego operates out of the reality of the external world and transforms the mental images formed by the id (the hamburgers, for example) into acceptable behavior (purchasing a hamburger). These reality-oriented, rational processes of the ego are referred to as the *secondary process*. The ego, operating under the *reality principle,* is left with the task of mediating a balance among the demands of the id, superego, and reality.

The ego's primary mission is self-preservation, which is accomplished by mediating the demands of the id (instinctual demands) with the realities of the environment. The well-functioning ego is able to achieve the right balance between seeking pleasure and avoiding the consequences of infringement on the societal rules and mores. The goal of all mental activity, as Freud explained, is to keep tension at a steady level.

As noted in Figure 5-3, children are generally dependent on their parents to a large extent during their first two decades of life. During this time, the ego develops a superego that continues the parents' influence over the remainder of the person's lifetime.

SUPEREGO   Composed of two parts—the *ego ideal* (developed from the child's idea of what parents and significant others thought was good) and the *conscience* (what parents and significant others thought was bad)—the superego is, in essence, a personal moral standard. It incorporates the standards that have been learned from parents and from society and internalized over time. The superego works to control the id by imposing ideals of right and wrong. Often thought of as the judicial branch of the personality, the superego can act to restrict, prohibit, and judge conscious actions.

Dynamic Concepts

Freud believed that energy could be directed into three parts of the personality: id, ego, and superego. This is the hydraulic element of personality, the stresses, conflicts, and dynamic interactions between drives and reality (Luborsky, O'Reilly-Landry, & Arlow, 2008). The more energy that goes into one part, the less energy is available for the other structures. So if strong energy is fed to the id, the person will have less

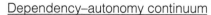

Dependency–autonomy continuum

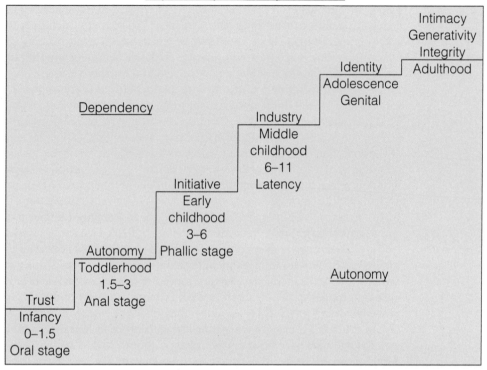

FIGURE 5-3 DEVELOPMENTAL STAGES AND THE DEPENDENCY–AUTONOMY CONTINUUM

power for the superego to prevent the impulsive action or for the ego to mediate and find a realistic way to satisfy the impulse. Shapiro, Friedberg, and Bardenstein (2006) explain that according to psychoanalytic thought, rather than a unified whole, the mind contains mental structures that have different aims, content, and operations.

INSTINCT   An instinct is an inborn psychological representation, referred to as a *wish* which stems from a physiological condition referred to as a *need*. For example, hunger is a need that leads to a wish for food. The wish becomes a motive for behavior. Life instincts serve to maintain the survival of the species. Hunger, thirst, and sex needs are served by life instincts. Freud believed that human behavior is motivated by basic instincts. *Libido* is the energy that permits life instincts to work.

CATHEXIS   Cathexis refers to directing one's libidinal energy toward an object, person, or idea that will satisfy a need.

ANTICATHEXIS   Anticathexis refers to the force the ego exerts to block or restrain the impulses of the id. The reality principle or superego directs this action of the ego against the pleasure principle emanating from the id.

ANXIETY   Anxiety refers to a conscious state in which a painful emotional experience is produced by external or internal stimulus; that is, a welling up of autonomic nervous energy. Closely akin to fear, but more encompassing, is the anxiety that originates from internal and external causes. Freud believed there were three types of anxiety: reality, neurotic, and moral. Reality anxiety results from real threats from the environment. Neurotic anxiety results from the fear that our instinctual impulses from the id will overpower our ego controls and get us into trouble. Moral anxiety results from the guilt a person feels when he or she fails to live up to his or her own standards.

Defense Mechanisms

The ego protects itself from heavy pressure and anxiety with defense mechanisms, which are patterns of thoughts or behaviors that protect someone from overwhelming anxiety. Safran and Kriss (2014) explain that defenses are the operations of the mind used to avoid emotional pain by pushing thoughts, wishes, feelings, or fantasies out of awareness (p. 21). The healthy, high-functioning ego attempts to cope with anxiety, depression, and stress with effective, reality-based, task-oriented, coping skills. When the load becomes too heavy, the ego may resort to defense-oriented coping methods that provide short-term relief but deny or distort reality and generally cause more problems in the long term.

People use *defense mechanisms* to respond to situations that cause them unconscious fears; this is called "psychic danger" (Luborsky, O'Reilly-Landry, & Arlow, 2008).

McWilliams (1994) explains that we rely on a particular defense mechanism based on our temperament, the stresses of our childhood, defenses that we saw caretakers use, and what has worked previously, therefore becoming automatic, habitual responses. Counselors are generally able to detect their clients' defense mechanisms. Seligman and Reichenberg (2014) listed some defense mechanisms that are healthy and common in the well-adjusted life.

Affiliation or turning to others when you need help and support yet continuing to recognize personal responsibility.

Altruism means receiving satisfaction in helping other people.

Anticipation involves thinking about the future and relieving anxiety by finding ways to address situations effectively.

Humor allows you to focus on the amusing parts of circumstances.

Sublimation refers to redirecting emotions or impulses that could be unhealthy into acceptable ones.

Suppression leads to intentionally ignoring nonproductive, troubling experiences, and emotions.

Other mechanisms may lead to maladaptive situations. Based on McWilliams's (1994) distinctions, defense mechanisms are listed as primary or high order. Both types function to protect the ego from anxiety. Young children, with their limited view of the world outside themselves, most often choose primary defenses that ignore the world or wish problems away, such as magical thinking, or believing they can wish for something and it will magically happen. Higher-order defenses are more sophisticated and may serve to distort reality or focus attention away from the unpleasant.

PRIMARY DEFENSES

Acting Out   Acting out means reducing the anxiety aroused by forbidden desires by expressing them. The behavior of a revenge-seeking child is one example. An underachieving student may engage in violence, vandalism, or theft to express forbidden hurt feelings.

Compensation   Compensation is covering up a weakness by emphasizing some desirable trait or reducing frustration in one area of life by over gratification in another area; for example, the class clown may compensate for poor academic performance by engaging in attention-getting behavior. An underachiever may be an attention-getting clown of the first order or may overachieve in another area (e.g., sports, hobbies, or gang activities) to compensate for low grades.

Denial   Denial is a refusal to face unpleasant aspects of reality or to perceive anxiety-provoking stimuli. Children may deny the possibility of falling while climbing high trees. An underachieving child may say, "Things are going fine; my grades will be much higher this time." Counselors need to remember that denial is common in young children when they use magical thinking, but it is maladaptive for adolescents.

Fantasy   Fantasy is a way of seeking gratification of needs and frustrated desires through the imagination. A fantasy or imagined world may be a more pleasant place than a child's real world. An underachieving child may say, "Just wait, one of these days I'll become a doctor and show that teacher. She'll be sorry she made fun of my bad test score."

Fixation   Fixation differs from regression in that the individual does not always regress to a more pleasant stage of development to avoid the pain or stress in a current developmental stage, but instead might decide to remain at the present level of development rather than move to the next stage, which poses more difficulties and problems to solve. The tendency is to stay with a situation that is pleasurable and comfortable and in which the person has been successful. Counselors often are confronted with dependent, underachieving students who have a difficult time, first, in developing alternative problem solutions and, second, in making commitments to try their new alternatives.

Identification   Identification is the development of role models that people identify with or imitate. They may choose to imitate either a few traits of the model or the total person. Identification often occurs with the same-sex parent and may be borne out of love or power; for example, "I love Dad so much I want to be just like him," or "If I can't beat him, I'll join him until I get big, too." Adolescents may be at the point where they are challenging all issues raised by their parents. The underachieving student might say, "I know a high school student who dropped out and is making a lot of money. He says school is a waste of time."

Projection   Projection is attributing one's own unacceptable characteristics to others or to things in the external world. For instance, a teacher may find it uncomfortable to admit he does not like the children in his class, so instead he says the children do not like him. In this way, he projects his dislike for his students onto the students. An underachieving child may say, "My teacher doesn't like me; he thinks I'm stupid."

Rationalization   Rationalization is an attempt to prove that one's behavior is justified and rational and is thus worthy of approval by oneself and others. When asked why they behaved in a certain manner, children may feel forced to think up logical excuses or reasons. An underachieving child may say, "I could finish my homework if my little brother would stop bothering me."

Undoing   Undoing is engaging in some form of atonement for immoral or bad behavior or for the desire to participate in such behavior; for instance, after breaking a lamp, a child may try to glue it back together. An underachieving child may say, "I get in a lot of arguments with my teacher, but I always try to do something to make up for it." Adolescents may become fixated on trying to repair a relationship that is beyond mending.

Withdrawal   Withdrawal means reducing ego involvement by becoming passive or learning to avoid being hurt; examples of withdrawn children include the shy child or school-phobic child. A withdrawn, underachieving child will probably not say much as he or she tries to avoid "risky" situations.

HIGHER-ORDER DEFENSES

Displacement   Displacement means redirecting energy from a primary object to a substitute when an instinct is blocked. For example, anger toward a parent may be directed toward a sibling or another object because of the fear of reprisal from the parent. The underachieving child might say, "The stuff we study is so boring I'll never make good grades." The child may be redirecting hostile feelings from the teacher to the subject matter.

Intellectualization   Intellectualization is the act of separating the normal affect, or feeling, from an unpleasant or hurtful situation; for example, a child whose dog has been hit by a car might soften his or her grief by saying, "Our dog is really better off dead; he was feeble and going blind." An underachieving child may say, "I learn best from doing things outside school," or "I don't learn from the boring things we do at school."

Reaction Formation   Reaction formation refers to the development of attitudes or character traits exactly opposite to ones that have been repressed. Anxiety-producing impulses are replaced in the conscious by their opposites; for example, "I would love to drink" is replaced by "Liquor should be declared illegal." An underachieving child may say, "I don't want to be a nerd; nerds suck up to the teacher just to make good grades."

Regression   Regression is a retreat to earlier developmental stages that are less demanding than those of the present level. An older child may revert to babyish behavior when a baby arrives in the family. An underachieving child may say, "All we do is work; recess and lunch should be longer."

Repression and Suppression   Repression forces a dangerous memory, conflict, idea, or perception out of the conscious into the unconscious and places a lid on it to prevent the repressed material from resurfacing. In repression, the person unconsciously bars a painful thought from memory. Suppression is a conscious effort to do the same thing. An underachieving child might have repressed painful memories about failure in a prior school experience.

Sublimation   Sublimation often has been referred to as the backbone of civilization. Through it, people redirect their libidinal desires and energy into productive and acceptable activities and outlets. Often the products of this redirected energy have resulted in significant advances in the arts, sciences, quality of life, and civilization in general. Parents and teachers would do well to help children find productive outlets for their great energy. Underachieving students do not need a lot of unstructured time to fill with negative addictions such as video games, gang activity, overeating, and drugs.

These examples of ways a child might express a preference or behave with patterns built around one, two, or a combination of defense mechanisms, may become automatic ways to avoid situations they do not think they can tolerate.

Psychosexual Stages and Erikson's Stages

Freud (1940/1949) viewed personality development as a succession of stages, each characterized by a dominant mode of achieving libidinal pleasure and by the pleasure-seeking drives related to specific tasks. How well one adjusts at each stage is the critical factor in development. Successful resolution of the psychosexual conflicts in each stage allows a child to develop and move on to the next stage. The key to successful adjustment in each stage is how well parents help their child adjust to that stage and make the transition to the next stage. The difficulty with Freud's system comes when counselors emphasize the extremes rather than the normal range of behaviors. The key seems to lie in maintaining a balance between extremes in Freud's five developmental stages which are oral, anal, phallic, latency, and genital.

Erikson's (1950, 1968) developmental theory expands psychoanalytic theory by emphasizing the psychosocial crises at each stage of life. According to Erikson, each person faces a crisis that must be resolved in order to achieve a new stage of social interaction. Unsuccessful resolution may hinder further development and can have a negative impact. Erikson places more emphasis on society and the demands of the world whereas Freud focuses on internal conflicts. Erikson's childhood and adolescent stages are trust versus mistrust, autonomy versus shame and doubt, initiative versus guilt, industry versus inferiority, and identity versus role confusion. The following section contains the similarities and differences in Freud's and Erikson's stages of development.

FREUD'S ORAL STAGE (BIRTH TO 2 YEARS OLD): ERIKSON'S TRUST VERSUS MISTRUST   The oral-erotic substage is characterized by the sucking reflex, which is necessary for survival. The child's main task in the oral-sadistic substage is to adjust to the weaning process and to learn to chew food. Pleasure comes when the tension is reduced by using the mouth. The mouth is characterized as an erogenous zone because one obtains pleasure from sucking, eating, and biting. Adult behaviors, such as smoking, eating, and drinking, and the personality traits of gullibility, dependency (oral-erotic), and sarcasm (oral-sadistic) originate in the oral period.

Winnicott (1971, 1977) and Piaget and Inhelder (1969) believe that children at 12 to 18 months old begin to form an identity based on their "me" and "not me" worlds during this oral or trust-building stage. Erikson explains the conflict as learning to trust or mistrust based on how well the child's basic needs are met. The process of developing an identity begins when infants see their image reflected in their mothers' expression as they look at their babies. Mothers who are depressed or under stress and have difficulty expressing their love by their looks and expressions send a disturbing message to their infants. The infant begins to sense, "If Mother seems not to love me or be pleased with what she sees, I may be unlovable." Children who fail to form a sense of trust may face a lifelong struggle with relationships.

FREUD'S ANAL STAGE (2 TO 3 YEARS OLD): ERIKSON'S AUTONOMY VERSUS SHAME AND DOUBT   During the anal stage, the membrane of the anal region presumably provides the major source of pleasurable stimulation. There are anal-expulsive and anal-retentive substages. The major hurdle is the regulation of a natural function (bowel control). Toilet training requires the child to learn how to postpone immediate gratification. Again, the manner in which the parents facilitate or impede the process forms the basis for a number of adult personality traits. Stubbornness, stinginess, and orderliness (anal-retentive) and generosity and messiness (anal-expulsive) are among the adult traits associated with the anal stage.

Erikson talks about the child separating personal identity at this stage and struggling to become more independent. The conflict resolves around shame and doubt versus autonomy. Again parents influence this stage of development as they help their child learn about controlling their bodily functions. Children who fail to develop a sense of autonomy may become dependent, unconfident adults.

FREUD'S PHALLIC STAGE (3 TO 6 YEARS OLD): ERIKSON'S INITIATIVE VERSUS GUILT   Self-manipulation of the genitals provides the major source of pleasurable sensation at this age. The Oedipus complex also occurs during this stage; the female version is sometimes referred to as the Electra complex. Sexual and aggressive feelings and fantasies are associated with the genitals. Boys have sexual desires for their mothers and aggressive feelings toward their fathers; girls develop hostility toward their mothers and become sexually attracted to their fathers. Attitudes toward people of the same sex and the opposite sex begin to take shape. The key question for healthy development, according to classical psychoanalysis, in the phallic stage is, "How does the child handle competition with the same-sex parent for the affection of the opposite-sex parent?" The answer lies within whether the child has chosen to identify with the same-sex parent as a power figure or love object. In other words, Dad has the power, so if you cannot beat him, join him; or, Dad is a great guy and I would like to be like him.

Erikson's explanation of the stage of initiative versus guilt focuses on the child's social involvement and relationships. Children who spend their time in play and other constructive activities develop initiative and competence. If children do not develop initiative, they may experience guilt and feelings of incompetence during their life.

FREUD'S LATENCY STAGE (6 TO 11 YEARS OLD): ERIKSON'S INDUSTRY VERSUS INFERIORITY   Sexual motivations presumably recede in importance during the latency period as the child becomes preoccupied with developmental skills and activities. Children generally concentrate on developing same-sex friendships. Sexual and aggressive impulses are relatively quiet during this phase.

The school years incorporate the conflict between industry and inferiority according to Erikson. During this time, children learn to be productive. They also develop their sense of gender during these years. This unresolved stage may lead to life span feelings of failure, inferiority, and inadequacy.

FREUD'S GENITAL STAGE (ADOLESCENCE): ERIKSON'S IDENTITY VERSUS ROLE CONFUSION   The final stage of Freud's developmental theory follows the latency stage and last through the rest of life. During this stage, personal identities, caring relationships, and loving, sexual relationships are formed. All those growth areas also involve the risk of rejection and fear of rejection that has a tremendous impact on future relationships.

Erikson captures the identity conflict of adolescence during this time of life. Teens confront the dimensions of life—career, social, sexual, and life meaning—and must determine their sense of self across those aspects. The experimentation and confusion of this time of life characterize this stage of development. Role confusion results if adolescents fail to navigate these struggles successfully.

Oral, anal, and phallic stages are classified as narcissistic because children derive pleasure from their own erogenous zones. During the genital stage, the focus of activity shifts to developing genuine relationships with others. The goal for the young person is to move from a pleasure-seeking, pain-avoiding, narcissistic child to a reality-oriented, socialized adult.

In summary, over gratification of the child's needs could result in the child's fixation at a particular stage; deprivation may result in regression to a more comfortable developmental stage. For example, a 3-year-old only child suddenly finding a rival for his parents' attention in the form of a new baby sister regresses to his pre-toilet-training period in an effort to compete. Too much frustration in coping with a particular developmental stage also could result in fixating the child at that stage. Freud believed that personality characteristics are fairly well established by the age of 6. Gratification of need during each stage is important if the individual is not to become stuck at that level of development because, according to Freud, the residue from regression and fixation may reappear in adult personality development.

Finding the healthy balance between unhealthy extremes is the key to mental health and a theme that runs throughout this book. Parents always have the difficult task of walking the thin line between too much and too little gratification of their child's needs. Perhaps the answer lies in the nurturing and preservation of the child's feelings of worth, confidence, and trust.

RELATIONSHIP

Freud was a physician; therefore, his approach to therapy incorporates the doctor–patient style. In psychoanalysis, the relationship is the agent of change. The counselor is an expert who interprets the client's drives and defenses. Clients are encouraged to talk about whatever comes to mind, a technique known as free association. By their passive, unobtrusive behaviors, psychoanalysts encourage clients to develop *transference*, reacting to the counselor as the client has responded to other people in the past. As therapy progresses, the counselor takes a more active role, interpreting what has been learned from free association and transference. Luborsky, O'Reilly-Landry, and Arlow (2008) explain that, as therapy proceeds, the counselor hears patterns in the client's stories and recurring troubles. The counselor listens for the inner conflicts that may be connected to the symptoms and problems. Therapy is long term, often lasting for several years.

Arlow (2005) noted three characteristics of a psychoanalyst. The first is the empathy to identify with the cognitive and emotional aspects of the client's experience and also to maintain separation from the client. A critical second characteristic is intuition in order to organize all the information a client gives into a meaningful configuration (Seligman & Reichenberg, 2014). Arlow noted the third capacity needed by a psychoanalyst is introspection, which allows the therapist to understand and interpret. Through the psychoanalytic process, the therapists serves as "a third ear attuned to underlying meanings, symbols, contradictions and important omissions that may point the way to unlocking the unconscious" (Seligman, 2006, p. 58).

Goals

The goal of psychoanalytic counseling is to help a person "achieve a more adaptive compromise between conflicting forces through understanding the nature of the conflicts and dealing with them in a more mature and rational manner" (Arlow, 2005, p. 35). The objectives include increasing self-understanding, improving acceptance of feelings and desires, replacing unconscious defense mechanisms with conscious coping tactics, and developing relationships.

Novie (2007) said goals of psychoanalysis are for clients' to (1) resolve their problems so they can improve their abilities to cope with changes, (2) work through unresolved developmental stages, and (3) cope more effectively with the demands of society. Those goals are reached by exploring unconscious material, especially as it relates to the relationship between client and therapist.

Luborsky, O'Reilly-Landry, and Arlow (2008) outlined the reasons for using psychoanalysis. One purpose is to reveal the inner problems that have been disguised as symptoms by reaching an "emotional understanding" of the meaning and the function of the symptom. Another intent is to become integrated by finding solutions that work for all parts of a person. A third target is to find the sources of past pain that are contributing to present distress, thus intermingling the past in the present. Finally, therapists help clients recognize what prevents their taking appropriate action.

Change occurs through a course of opening up to self-discovery, finding patterns that interfere in life, unraveling the influence of the past from the present and finding new coping skills. In the opening phase of counseling, free association helps in self-discovery. The second phase includes communicating, understanding, interpreting, and analyzing transference and countertransference. In this phase, the therapist and client begin to recognize patterns (Weiner & Bornstein, 2009). The third part of therapy allows the counselor and client to identify sources of pain in order to untangle the past from the present. In the final phase of counseling, therapeutic relationship becomes a place to develop new competence (Luborsky, O'Reilly-Landry, & Arlow, 2008).

COUNSELING METHODS

Merydith (2007) alerted therapists to be cautious in using psychoanalysis with children. First, he noted that children attribute their distress to external rather than internal causes, or they accept suffering as part of their lives. He questioned whether insight-oriented change is possible with children. Using only indirect interpretation through stories and metaphors are techniques that may lead to age-appropriate self-awareness. Sugarman (2008) announced that insight and consciousness in children and adults exist on a continuum rather than polarities. Furthermore, children are dependent on their parents, and that relationship will likely interfere with transference to the therapist, a critical part of psychoanalysis. He suggested play therapy as a primary method to access emotions and to analyze children's thinking. Fundamentally, the principles to keep in mind when analyzing children are the following:

- Develop a warm, friendly relationship
- Accept the child
- Create an atmosphere of permissiveness in the relationship
- Recognize the child's feelings and reflect them
- Respect the child's ability to solve problems
- Allow the child to lead and follow that lead
- Do not hurry
- Use only necessary limits (Merydith, 2007, p. 112)

Assessment

Freudian psychoanalysis includes little formal assessment. Free association is the mirror to the mind and therefore provides a look into unconscious material to be analyzed and connected to behavior. Dream interpretation could also be considered the assessment of symbolic events in the client's world. Some analysts may use projective assessment techniques such as the Rorschach inkblot test in which the client projects thoughts and feelings on pictures and the Thematic Apperception Test in which a person tells a story about pictures. Shapiro, Friedberg, and Bardenstein (2006) explain that projection involves people perceiving in the external environment the emotional qualities and meanings that are actually theirs internally. An example would be an angry adolescent who believes all adults are "out to get me." Goldman and Anderson (2007) recommended that therapists consider the security and quality of the client's relationships in order to build a strong alliance.

Freud believed unresolved conflict, repression, and free-floating anxiety often go together. Painful and stressful conflicts that cannot be resolved in the conscious may be buried and forgotten in the unconscious. Later on, a person may experience anxiety that cannot be readily traced to any ongoing situation in the person's life. Relief from such anxiety may come only from accessing the unconscious and uncovering and resolving the original conflict. Recall and integration of repressed memories into one's conscious functioning often provide symptom relief from free-floating anxiety.

Freud also was interested in how people handled the tension of being pulled in opposite directions by the polarities in life. He saw people as born with the pleasure principle, or the will to seek pleasure; however, people are confronted with an opposite force, the reality principle, which demands that the will to pleasure be bridled. The tension that results from being pulled in opposite directions by the pleasure principle and by the reality principle becomes the essential, motivating force in one's life. People can either find productive ways to reduce the tension or give in to the tension and be destroyed by it. The task of humankind is to find a way to integrate the polarities into choices that neither compromise nor deny the opposing sides. For example, taking your textbook to the beach on spring break may be an attempt to find a middle ground between doing what you want and what you should. A synergistic solution might be completing the work before leaving on the trip, which would probably result in higher-quality work and play. Living becomes a process of either mastering or succumbing to the tension resulting from life's polarities.

Process

Luborsky, O'Reilly-Landry, and Arlow (2008) outline the process of psychoanalysis focusing on discovery and recovery. The beginning or *opening phase* revolves around the reasons for seeking treatment at this time, triggers to current problems, and the degree of distress the client is demonstrating. The elements of treatment are building the therapeutic relationship and exploring the client's concerns. The middle phase of psychoanalysis is the *working through* part in which themes are revisited and explored. The therapist and client increase their understanding of the forces, past patterns, and inner conflicts that are causing the client's problems. The analysis of transference and examination of other relationships occurs in the working phase of treatment. In the final phase, the therapist and client agree that goals have been reached, transference is resolved, and separation is the next step.

Psychoanalytic counselors often search for repressed, traumatic events in the lives of their clients as possible causes for the symptoms and problems brought to counseling. Severe trauma is often associated with damaged egos, low self-esteem, and anxiety disorders; however, counselors can overlook the devastating effects on self-worth from the daily onslaught of negative criticism heaped on some children throughout their developing years. Most of that criticizing behavior falls short of legally being abuse and occurs in relatively small doses, so it often goes unnoticed and unchecked. Therefore, we are presenting a system for evaluating how well a child's self-esteem, mental health, and other personal needs are being supported by the family and, to a great extent, by the school.

COUNSELING AND DEVELOPMENT OF SELF

Neff and Vonk (2009) compare global self-esteem to self-compassion, positive self-regard that encompasses being kind to ourselves and seeing self as part of a larger, interconnected world. For children, the keys to mental health are their schoolwork and their relationships with family, peers, and other significant people. Children's realistic expectations for themselves and their growing positive impact on their worlds lead to healthy productive lives. Some conditions complement the productivity and relationship equation. These conditions are as follows:

Belonging: Children need to feel connected to their family or to a family of their own creation if the family of origin did not work out. As children grow older, they need to feel connected to a peer group.

Child advocacy: Children need at least one advocate who can be trusted to help them through crisis periods.

Risk management: Children need to take risks and master challenging tasks. The difficulty is finding tasks that are challenging yet not impossible. Children need to believe that they are successful if they have given a task their best effort and that it is all right to take risks and fail. Self-compassion incorporates not only forgiveness for not being the "star" but also the motivation to continue to try.

Empowerment: Children need to exercise developmentally appropriate amounts of control over their own lives. Opportunities to make choices and decisions contribute to their abilities to improve those skills.

Uniqueness: Children and adults need to feel they have a unique purpose and value.

Productivity: As children get things done, they feel better. Encouragement and reinforcement of productive activity can move children toward finding intrinsic rewards in accomplishment.

Counseling children through Freud's five stages of development often requires an assessment of how well their basic needs are being met. A rating scale of 0 to 10 (0 for unmet needs and 10 for fully met needs) can be used to assess the child's progress in each level of Maslow's (1970) hierarchy, including acceptance of self (Table 5-1).

Problems in adult development are often traced to childhood frustration from failure to meet basic human needs during the developmental years. Psychoanalytic counseling can focus on the child's level of human needs attainment in past years, as well as in the present. Questions of how children handle the pain of not getting what they want can be treated in psychoanalytic counseling. Are conflict and stress repressed in the unconscious or handled in the conscious area of functioning? Are depression and anxiety handled in task-oriented or defense-oriented ways? Both are good questions for psychoanalytic counselors to address.

Techniques

The primary goal of counseling within a psychoanalytic frame of reference is to make the unconscious conscious. All material in the unconscious was once in the conscious. Once brought to the conscious level, repressed material can be dealt with in rational ways by using any number of methods discussed in this book.

TABLE 5-1 CHILD'S NEEDS ASSESSMENT

Physiological needs			
Nutrition, sleep, exercise, general	0	5	10
Safety needs			
Safety within the family and peer group settings	0	5	10
Love and belonging needs			
Affection shown to the child	0	5	10
Promises made and kept to the child	0	5	10
Someone listens to the child	0	5	10
Family follows a dependable schedule	0	5	10
Child has own space, possessions, and a right to privacy	0	5	10
Someone is there when the child arrives home	0	5	10
Child is loved unconditionally	0	5	10
Child has a place and role in the family	0	5	10
Child has found acceptance and a place in his/her peer group	0	5	10
Self-esteem needs			
Someone affirms the child's worth	0	5	10
Child is given the opportunity to achieve and accomplish tasks	0	5	10
Child is given the opportunity to make choices	0	5	10
Self-actualization needs			
Child is not blocked by unmet needs in the previous four levels	0	5	10
Child is developing potential abilities, strengths, and skills	0	5	10
Problem-solving skills enable the child to engage in developmental rather than remedial activities	0	5	10

Several methods can be used to uncover the unconscious. Detailed counselors take detailed case histories, with special attention given to the handling of conflict areas. Hypnosis, although rejected by Freud, is still used to assist in plumbing the unconscious. Analyses of resistance, transference, and dreams are frequently used methods, as are catharsis, free association, interpretation, and play therapy. All these methods have the long-term goal of strengthening the ego. The principal counseling methods discussed in this chapter are catharsis, free association, interpretation, analysis of transference, analysis of resistance, analysis of incomplete sentences, bibliocounseling, storytelling, and play therapy.

Catharsis

Hirschmüller (1989) said that Freud collaborated with Breuer (1842–1925) in discovering the benefits of catharsis through hypnosis. Freud found that if, under hypnosis, hysterical patients were able to verbalize an early precipitating causal event, hysterical symptoms disappeared. Freud soon discarded hypnosis because he was unable to induce in every patient the deep hypnotic sleep that enabled the patient to regress to an early enough period to disclose the repressed event. Freud discovered that for many people the mere command to remember the origin of some hysterical symptom worked quite well. Unfortunately, many of his patients could not remember the origin of their symptoms even on command. Freud thus decided that all people were aware of the cause of their illness, but that for some reason certain people blocked this knowledge. Freud believed that unless this repressed traumatic infantile experience could be retrieved from the unconscious, verbalized, and relived emotionally, the patient would not recover. Because not everyone had the ability to find this unconscious material, the analyst had to use more indirect means to gain access to the unconscious mind. Freud developed free association and interpretation to bring everyone to the emotional state of catharsis he believed was necessary for cure.

Free Association

In traditional psychoanalysis, the client lies on a couch and the analyst sits at the head of the couch beyond the client's line of vision. The analyst then orders the client to say whatever comes to mind. Through this method, the unconscious thoughts and conflicts are given freedom to reach the conscious mind. A great struggle takes place within the client to keep from telling these innermost thoughts to the analyst. The analyst must constantly struggle against this resistance. The fundamental rule of psychoanalytic counseling requires clients to tell the counselor whatever thoughts and feelings come into their minds, regardless of how personal, painful, or seemingly irrelevant.

While the client is trying to associate freely, the counselor must remain patient and nonjudgmental and insist that the client continue. The counselor must also look for continuity of thoughts and feelings. Although the client may appear to be rambling idly, psychoanalytic counselors believe there is a rational pattern to this speech. To interpret what the client is saying, the counselor must pay attention to the affect, or feeling, behind the client's verbalization, noting the client's gestures, tone of voice, and general body language during free association.

Luborsky and Luborsky (2006) developed the *Core Conflictual Relationship Theme (CCRT) Model* as one way to understand the relationship patterns patients reveal in their stories. The pattern consists of three elements: (1) the wish (W), either stated or implied; (2) the response of others (RO), either real or expected; and (3) the response of self (RS). These authors explain that common wishes are to be loved, respected, and/or accepted. At this point, the counselor offers some interpretations of the patterns in the client's statements to try to open another door for free association.

Shapiro, Friedberg, and Bardenstein (2006) describe three other types of patterns: discrepancies, omissions, and excesses. Discrepancies happen when what is said and what is done are inconsistent. An example would be the child who insists she does not care that her friend has moved but has isolated herself since that event. Omissions involve what is not said, the absence of thoughts or feelings such as having been the victim of a trauma but never expressing anger. Finally, excesses are the extreme acts or expressions, or the overreacting to something. An example would be a school-age boy having a tantrum when he was told his session was finished. The emotion often is related to another source that seems more difficult to discuss.

Interpretation

Free association, in turn, leads to another important technique: interpretation. Three major areas of interpretation are dreams, parapraxia, and humor.

INTERPRETATION OF DREAMS   Freud (1901/1952, 1965a) believed dreams expressed wish fulfillment. To correctly interpret the power of the id, the analyst must learn about and interpret the client's dreams. There are three major types of dreams: those with meaningful, rational content (almost invariably found in children); those with material very different from waking events; and those with illogical, senseless episodes. All dreams center on a person's life and are under the person's psychic control. Every dream reveals an unfulfilled wish. In children's dreams, the wish is usually obvious. As the individual matures, the wish, as exposed in the dream, becomes more distorted and disguised. The ego fights the initial conscious wish, which thus is pushed back to the unconscious mind; it brings itself back into the conscious mind by means of a dream. The dream guards against pain. When people are sleeping, repressive defenses are weaker, and forbidden desires and feelings can find an outlet in dreams. Freud referred to dreams as the royal road to the unconscious. The counselor's role is to listen to the client's dream and help the client interpret the dream's symbolism.

Freud's method of dream interpretation was to allow the client to free-associate about the dream's content. Certain objects in dreams were universal symbols for Freud. For example, a car in someone's dreams usually represented analysis. Car dreams also may refer to one's direction in life or how one treats his or her body and takes care of his or her personal health. Dreams about falling are related to fears about falling from one's moral standards. Dreams about teeth were associated with lying, as in lying through your teeth. Dreams about a person may relate to positive or negative traits that person has that the dreamer may wish to emulate or discard. The same may be true for animal dreams that symbolize the dreamer's own negative traits or behaviors he or she should discard. House and building dreams may refer to specific concerns in one's life; for example, dreams in a kitchen may relate to one's eating habits. Dreams about children may indicate one's need for fun, happiness, spontaneity, and doing something new and different; in contrast, they may signify indulging in childish behavior. Clothing dreams could relate to changing one's mood or state of mind. Death dreams could refer to anxiety about significant changes in one's life.

The key for understanding one's dream is identifying the basic theme being communicated in the dream. This is done by stripping away such details as names, places, and things, leaving only the action. For example, a dream about someone drowning could be reduced to the theme that something bad is happening to a person the dreamer cares about and his or her help is needed. Next, match the bare-bones theme to an ongoing part of the dreamer's life and give full attention to the feelings and emotions that are generated. One's feelings are the best indicators of what needs attention in one's life or the unfinished business that needs to be completed according to psychoanalysis.

Freud (1952/1901) believed every dream to be a confession and a by-product of repressed, anxiety-producing thoughts. He thought that many dreams represented unfulfilled sexual desires and expressed the superego's guilt and self-punishment. Nightmares result from the desire for self-punishment. Because we are consciously and unconsciously aware of those things that we fear most, we put these things into our nightmares to punish ourselves.

PARAPRAXIA   Parapraxia, or "Freudian slips," are consciously excused as harmless mistakes, but through them the id pushes unconscious material through to the conscious. The counselor must be aware of any slips of the tongue while dealing with a client. The Freudians also believe there are no such things as "mistakes" or items that are "misplaced." According to psychoanalytic thinking, everything we do—for example, forgetting a person's name, cutting a finger while peeling potatoes—has unconscious motivation. The analyst must take all these unconscious mistakes and arrange them into a conscious pattern.

HUMOR   Jokes, puns, and satire are all acceptable means for unconscious urges to gain access to the conscious. The things we laugh about tell us something about our repressed thoughts. One of the fascinations of humor, according to psychoanalytic theory, is that it simultaneously disguises and reveals repressed thoughts. Repressed thoughts, released by humor, are usually generated from the id or superego. Because sexual thoughts are usually repressed, many jokes are sexually oriented; because aggressive thoughts are usually repressed, they are expressed in humor by way of satire and witticisms. Again, the counselor must watch for patterns and themes. What does the client think is funny? How does the client's sense of humor fit into a pattern from the unconscious?

Analysis of Transference

Transference occurs when the client views the counselor as someone else. Freud was genuinely surprised when his patients first regarded him as someone other than an analyst, helper, or adviser. During the course of psychoanalytic counseling, clients usually transfer their feelings about some significant individual from their past to the therapist. Transference generally is a product of unfinished business with a significant person from the client's childhood. Clients commonly transfer their feelings, thoughts, and expectations about the significant other to the counselor. Counseling provides a stage for reenacting unresolved conflicts with the counselor, who can help clients deal with them in more effective and functional ways. Transference relationships can become a real battleground when love feelings directed toward the counselor are rejected and the client, in turn, rejects the counselor by resisting the counselor's every effort to be helpful. Both transference and resistance can be analyzed for cause-and-effect implications for the client's life. Countertransference occurs when the counselor begins to view a client as someone other than a client.

Referral to another competent professional is recommended for a counselor who loses his or her balance on the objectivity–empathy continuum.

Analysis of Resistance

Freud also was surprised by the amount of resistance his patients mounted against his attempts to help them. Resistance took the form of erecting barriers to free association, thus breaking Freud's rule against censoring or holding back the material. Freud's patients were often unwilling or unable to talk about some of their thoughts during free association or descriptions of their dreams. Resistance prevents painful and irrational content from reaching the conscious, and it must be eliminated for the person to have the opportunity to face and react to these repressed conflicts in realistic and healthy ways. Therefore, the essential task of any counselor is building a trusting relationship with each client that undermines the client's need to resist the counselor's attempts to be helpful. Analysis of resistance can also provide valuable information regarding the client's need to withhold information from the counselor.

Analysis of Incomplete Sentences

Psychoanalytic counselors often use projective techniques such as the House-Tree-Person or Children's Apperception Test in an attempt to understand their clients' thoughts, behaviors, and feelings. Ecker and Hulley (1995) recommend asking children to complete stimulus statements about likes, dislikes, family, friends, goals, wishes, and things that make the child happy or sad to help counselors understand children and find problem areas. This procedure may be especially useful in acquainting counselors with children and in establishing better rapport with those who are anxious, fearful, or reluctant to talk.

Examples

The thing I like to do most is _____.

The person in my family who helps me most is _____.

My friends are _____.

I feel happiest (or saddest) when _____.

My greatest wish is _____.

The greatest thing that ever happened to me was _____.

I wish my parents would _____.

When I grow up, I want _____.

Brothers are _____.

Sisters are _____.

Dad is _____.

Mom is _____.

School is _____.

My teacher is _____.

Bibliocounseling

Bibliocounseling—that is, reading and discussing books about situations and children similar to themselves—can help clients in several ways. Children unable to verbalize their thoughts and feelings may find them expressed in books. From selected stories, children can learn alternative solutions to problems and new ways of behaving; by reading about children similar to themselves, clients may not feel so alone or different.

In an article citing the benefits of bibliocounseling for abused children, Watson (1980) suggests that children may become psychologically and emotionally involved with characters they have read about. Vicarious experiences through books can be similar to the child's own thoughts, feelings, attitudes, behavior, or environment. Directed reading can lead to expression of feelings or problem solving. Watson lists the goals of bibliotherapy as (1) teaching constructive and positive thinking, (2) encouraging free expression concerning problems, (3) helping clients analyze their attitudes and behaviors, (4) looking at alternative solutions, (5) encouraging the client to find a way to cope that is not in conflict with society, and (6) allowing clients to see the similarity of their problems with those of others. The proposed stages of bibliotherapy include identification, catharsis, and insight—goals closely aligned with psychoanalysis.

With bibliocounseling, discussion focused around characters' behaviors, feelings, thoughts, relationships, cause and effect, and consequences is more effective than just asking the child to retell the story. Discussion also clears up questions that arise from the reading. Counselors can guide children to see how the story applies to their own lives. Rapee, Abbott, and Lyneham (2006) used bibliotherapy for children with anxiety disorders. Paparoussi, Andreou, and Gkouni (2011) outline a classroom-based intervention using books to help children face their fears of death and of darkness. Davis, Thompson, May, and Whiting (2011) identified bibliotherapy as effective for treating anxiety and phobia in children and adolescents. Bibliocounseling is also a means of educating children about certain areas of concern such as sex, physical disabilities, divorce, and death. Pardeek (2014) and Shechtman (2009) have written excellent books about the use of bibliotherapy. Once children have enough information about a problem, their attitudes and behaviors tend to change.

Storytelling

Richard Gardner (1986) developed the mutual storytelling technique as a therapeutic means for working with children. It uses a familiar technique to help children understand their own thoughts and feelings and to communicate meaningful insights, values, and standards of behavior to children. The counselor sets the stage and asks the child to tell a story, which is recorded on tape. The counselor instructs the child that the story should have a beginning, a middle, and an ending, and that the child will be asked to tell the moral (lesson) of the story at the end. The counselor may need to clarify some points of the story after the child has finished. The counselor then prepares a story using a similar theme and setting and including the significant figures from the child's story. The counselor's story, however, provides the child with better alternatives or responses to the situation.

Platteuw (2011) identifies elements to create a therapeutic story. First the counselor identifies the child's issues and then creates a character, place, and situation as a metaphorical structure for the identified difficulty. The main character, who is also struggling with the issue, uses coping strategies similar to those used by the child client with the difficulties of those strategies coming to light. The counselor then describes a pathway out of the crisis to a solution, shifting to a positive outcome. This process is especially useful when a child is stuck during the therapy session.

We have found storytelling to be an excellent counseling technique to help children cope with feelings, thoughts, and behaviors they are not yet ready to discuss in a direct manner with the counselor. Storytelling also has been useful in helping children realize possible consequences of their behavior. (See the case study of Pete later in this chapter.)

Psychoanalytic Play Therapy

Psychoanalytic play therapy began with Anna Freud (1926) adapting the work of Sigmund Freud for the treatment of children by incorporating play activities into therapy. She used toys and games to put the child at ease, create an alliance with the child, and discover clues about the child's inner life. Other prominent figures in psychoanalytic play therapy include Hiam Ginott (1994), Melanie Klein (1984), and Otto Weininger (1984, 1989). These therapists recognize that play often expresses the emotional issues of the child.

Traditional psychoanalytic play therapists help children recognize and understand their unconscious motivations, bringing those driving forces into consciousness. They assume that two or more parts of the child's personality clash. Those battling aspects occur from the differences in the desire from the child's pleasure-seeking id colliding with the needs and direction of the moralistic superego. As explained in earlier sections of this chapter, the ego mediates those conflicts. When that intervention of the ego no longer works, problems emerge (Brems, 2008), symptoms develop, and defense mechanisms operate to allow the child to function.

The fundamental goal is the child's insight into self. More specific goals of psychoanalytic play therapy (Bromfield, 2003) involve decreasing suffering, recovering from trauma, adjusting to life, following a medical treatment plan, eliminating fears, advancing academically, managing anger, and accepting disabilities. Bromfield explains the aim as moving past the current pain in order to accept one's self and develop security, adaptability, and self-accepting ways.

From a Freudian view, play is used symbolically and equates to adult free association. Play offers the counselor opportunities to see the child's hidden internal conflicts. Interpretations of play are based on the counselor's understanding of that conflict. Play is also used as a means to build a counseling relationship and to establish a basis for interpretation, which is expected to resolve the conflict, reduce the symptoms, and make the defenses irrelevant. The therapist then is the interpreter, as Brems (2008) explains "the person solving the riddle behind the symptom and the person who explains the riddle to the child, which in turn relieves conflicts (p. 283)." Levy (2011) details the neurobiology of that process.

Lee (2009) emphasizes the nondirective process. The therapist invites the child to play and choose the toys, games, drawings, logs, or other material. The child creates the themes and sets the direction of the play. The therapist follows the child's lead and offers remarks to label, describe, or question the flow of play. The relationship between child and counselor allows transference, which then supports the therapist's theories about the conflict and is interpreted accordingly.

Weiner and Bornstein (2009) outlined three steps for interpretation: clarification, confrontation, and then interpretation, and Kernberg and Chazan (1991) translated those strategies for children. Therapists clarify by asking questions about what the child meant by words or actions. Examples would be "Talk to me about what that means" or "What happens when you…" Confrontation means drawing attention to something that is inconsistent. The formula suggested is to use some sentences like "On one hand, you say (or do)——but, on the other hand, you say (or do)——how do you put these things together?" This type of confrontation allows two discrepant elements to be noticed and unraveled. Interpretations are offered in tentative ways with phrases such as "I wonder if," "Could it be." More complete explanations of these strategies can be found in Shapiro, Friedberg, and Bardenstein (2006).

Some psychoanalytic play therapists provide a private toy box for each child and bring the container to each session. The toys include dolls, animals, blocks, balls, houses, fences, vehicles, pencils, crayons, and other materials that can be used in different ways. The toys become recipients of the child's thoughts and feelings. No other child is allowed to use these toys so the child's work is protected, safe from intrusion, and shared only between the child and the counselor (Klein, 1932, 1984; Weininger, 1989). Weininger highlights maintaining the same place, time, length of session, and therapy process when working with children to add to the security needed for a transference relationship to evolve.

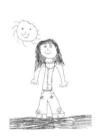

FIGURE 5-4
SELF-PORTRAIT
DRAWING BY A
10-YEAR-OLD
GIRL

(Reprinted with permission of Jessica Marie Martin.)

Toys symbolize important objects for the child. The child uses the playthings in ways she might want to use the original object. The counselor interprets to ease the child's anxiety about the conflict. In the safe place the counselor has created, a child can explore inner thoughts and feelings in order to acknowledge what is reality and what needs to be changed (Bromfield, 2003). Self-portrait drawings are good indicators of how children see their world. See Figure 5-4 for a drawing done by a 10-year-old girl who has love and support from her family, does well in school, makes friends easily, and excels in her sport of gymnastics. Contrast this drawing with Pete's drawing later in this chapter (see Figure 5-5).

Chethik (2000) outlines four concepts important to the psychodynamic play therapy process: therapeutic alliance, resistance, transference, and interventions. The therapeutic alliance involves the observing part of the process, in which the child works and shares treatment goals. Resistance is the deadlock that occurs when the child has no desire to change. Transference occurs when the child projects unconscious feelings and wishes on the counselor that the child feels toward an important adult in the child's life. Finally, interventions are used to help improve the problems. In psychoanalytic play therapy, confrontation, clarification, interpretation, and working through are used to help identify the phenomenon by defining it, analyzing it, and exploring it. In one case study of psychoanalytic play therapy, a South African game of masekitlana was used with those techniques to help a child who had seen relatives killed overcome his trauma (Kekae-Moletsane, 2008).

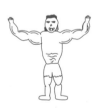

**FIGURE
5-5** PETE'S
DRAWING

Winnicott (1971, 1977) worked extensively with children from the 1920s through the early 1960s. He used a squiggle game play technique that combined drawing and storytelling to build rapport with children. He would draw a few neutral lines (a squiggle) on paper and say "I shut my eyes and go like this on the paper and you turn it into something, and then it is your turn and you do the same thing and I turn it into something" (p. 12). The counselor and child alternate drawing squiggles and turning them into meaningful pictures. Each time a drawing was finished, the "artist" made up a story about the completed pictures. Through the storytelling and conversation surrounding the squiggle game, children were able to express thoughts, feelings, and ideas from their unconscious that previously were not accessible to them (Wagner, 2008).

Leudar et al. (2008) examined four group psychotherapy sessions to document therapists' practices and the conversations that turned play into therapy. Therapists introduced therapeutic themes and reflected on children's ways of coping. These focused interactions allowed a single focus of attention that led to change. Sugarman (2008) talked about the use of play to promote children's insight of their suffering from cumulative trauma. Finally, a special issue of the *Journal of Infant, Child, and Adolescent Psychotherapy* (McCarthy & Conway, 2011) has been devoted to children with attention deficit hyperactivity disorder and the psychoanalytic process.

In psychoanalytic play therapy, the counselor's role is to interpret the child's symbolic play in words that are meaningful to the child. Chazan and Wolf (2002) detail the specifics of using a play therapy instrument to measure change in psychotherapy. Likewise Schneider, Midgley and Duncan (2010) suggest the use of the child psychotherapy Q-set as a measure of both process and outcome with children in psychotherapy. Both those instruments would be useful in measuring the impact of play therapy with the goal of successful play therapy resulting in higher levels of self-esteem, communication, trust, confidence, and problem-solving ability.

Object Relations Theory

As mentioned earlier, love and work are important concepts in Freud's system. He believed that a quick assessment of mental health could be based on how well people were managing their relationships and careers. Object relations theory assumes emotional life and relationships center on the unconscious images of our earliest and most intense relationships (Luborsky, O'Reilly-Landry, & Arlow, 2008). In other words, object relations theory focuses on how the early family relationships affect the type of relationships formed outside the family. For example, missing a solid father figure during her childhood years may motivate a woman to seek the love and attention she did not get from her father from older, fatherly types of men. Freud used the word *object* to refer to people or things used to satisfy sexual or aggressive drives, a means to an end. Object relations theorists stress the importance of the person's relationship to that object. To avoid loss and abandonment, humans will do whatever they can to maintain connections to love objects. This may be done by looking for others to have relationships that match the idealized earlier ones. Object relations theory helps therapists understand reasons people continue to have relationships that seem to be maladaptive, perhaps even self-destructive (Luborksy, O'Reilly-Landry, & Arlow, 2008).

Family relationships that model appropriate and healthy models for future relationship development are the best assistance children can have in learning to build relationships outside the family. Children who receive proper nurturing during their dependent years do not seek parent figures in their adult relationships. Parents who facilitate their children's movement through the developmental stages toward the achievement of independence and identity provide them with blueprints for fulfilling and healthy adult relationships. As children begin differentiating themselves from their families, they carry their internalized view of how relationships operate to their peer group and eventually to their adult world. For example, a woman might carry a repressed image of her father as a hostile and rejecting person who did not provide the love and nurturing she needed and project this image of her father on all men in general. Seeing this hostile father image in her husband, she reacts accordingly, causing him to act out the hostile role of her father.

Treatment for children educates parents to be better models of how to provide the right amount of love and nurturing. Treatment for adults accesses the unconscious to find the history of the unresolved conflicts with their parents and to find out how the repressed conflicts contribute to their difficulties in establishing and maintaining the relationships they would like to have.

As previously mentioned, Donald Woods Winnicott (1896–1971) was a British psychoanalyst who, through his clinical experience as a pediatrician and child psychiatrist, came to believe that the first few months of a child's life were critical to the development of good mental health and adjustment in the future life of the child. He strongly emphasized the mother's role in her child's development. Winnicott's view was that mothers did not have to be extraordinary in their duties, and that the "good enough mother" would be sufficient in facilitating the development of good mental health in her children. He believed that most mothers instinctively know how to meet their children's needs through providing the love, caring, and support needed to get their children started on the road to mature independence, providing they do not let themselves become misguided by child-rearing books. Winnicott (1971, 1977) recognized the importance of physical holding by the mother when the child is totally dependent and the "holding environment" mothers create through their empathy, which meets the child's physiological and emotional needs in reliable and consistent ways. He viewed holding as a form of ego support that is needed for children, adolescents, and adults when they are under stress. Well-cared-for infants do not experience the anxieties produced by environmental failure that some children experience during their stage of total dependence. These anxieties include feelings of falling, depersonalization, and generalized insecurity. To handle these intolerable feelings and anxieties, children create elaborate defenses such as repression to avoid having to face these difficulties on a day-to-day basis. Splitting themselves from reality (schizophrenia) would be an extremely costly, but not uncommon, measure for developing a position of invulnerability to defend against these anxieties. Winnicott believed that the analyst should "stand in" for the important people (objects) in a person's psychological history who literally let the person down. He used these transference relationships in treatment to help people relive and reevaluate their pasts. The analyst assumes the "holding" role the child never experienced, including the environmental support or holding that was lacking in the person's past. Such environmental support was the forerunner of case management, which includes helping people meet their basic survival needs so that they can benefit from counseling.

In summary, Freud (1930) viewed the personal unconscious as the repository of the primitive, the antisocial, and the evil within us. Repressed below the conscious area of functioning, these three forces tend to cause anxiety and tension through conflicts that affect our behavior in negative ways. The solution is to bring these forces into conscious awareness.

Psychoanalytic counselors are interested in accessing the personal unconscious to bring these repressed conflicts into conscious awareness, where they can be treated. As noted previously, the most common means of returning unconscious content to the conscious are dream interpretation, free association, analysis of resistance, analysis of transference, hypnosis, meditation, reflection, and analysis of slips of the tongue, selective remembering and forgetting, and accidents. Play therapy, in combination with the expressive arts, provides the preferred treatment modality for any theoretical orientation for younger children.

Case Studies

Identification of Problem I[1]

Dennis, age 9, was considered a disturbed, slow, resistant boy who had to be pushed into doing everything he was supposed to be doing. He rarely participated in any family activities and had no friends in the neighborhood. His school records listed such problems as regression, playing with much younger children, thumb sucking, daydreaming, soiling, bullying, and tardiness. An excerpt from the first counseling session begins with Dennis entering the playroom.

Transcript

DENNIS: Well, what are we going to do today?

COUNSELOR: Whatever you'd like. This is your time.

DENNIS: Let's talk.

COUNSELOR: All right.

DENNIS: Let's go back in history. We're studying about it in school. I'm going to be studying about Italy next week. I can't think of anything to talk about. I can't think of one thing to say. Can you?

COUNSELOR: I'd rather discuss something you suggest.

DENNIS: I can't think of a thing.

COUNSELOR: We can just sit here if you like.

DENNIS: Good. Do you want to read?

---

[1] The case of Dennis was contributed by Michael Gooch.

COUNSELOR:	Okay.
DENNIS:	You be the student, and I'll be the teacher. I'll read to you. Now you be ready to answer some questions. I don't like spelling. I like social studies, and I like history more than any other subject. I'd like being the teacher for a change. [Dennis asks the counselor questions from a reading text.]
COUNSELOR:	You like to ask questions you think I'll miss.
DENNIS:	That's right. I'm going to give you a test next week. A whole bunch of arithmetic problems, and social studies, and other questions.
COUNSELOR:	You like getting to be the teacher and getting to be the boss.
DENNIS:	Yeah, I never get to be the boss.
COUNSELOR:	You would like to have a chance to tell people what to do.
DENNIS:	Yeah, I hate getting bossed around all the time.
COUNSELOR:	It would be nice if you got to be your own boss sometimes and not have to take orders from your teacher and your parents.
DENNIS:	Right, I never get to do anything I want to do.
COUNSELOR:	It would be really nice if your teacher or parents would let you choose some things to do.
DENNIS:	Yeah, but they don't let me.
COUNSELOR:	It's hard for you to get your own way at school and home.
DENNIS:	Sometimes I do.
COUNSELOR:	How were you able to do that?
DENNIS:	I raised a fuss.
COUNSELOR:	You mean you got what you wanted by making a lot of noise.
DENNIS:	I cried, kicked, and screamed.
COUNSELOR:	So one time you got what you wanted.
DENNIS:	I got punished, too; I couldn't play video games for a week.
COUNSELOR:	So you need a better way to get to do something you want to do.
DENNIS:	I don't know what to do.
COUNSELOR:	Well, we can practice in here on how to get things you want.
DENNIS:	How?
COUNSELOR:	Kind of like you are doing now, when you are the teacher and I am the student.
DENNIS:	Okay. Now, I'm going to read like my friend does. [Dennis imitates his friend's reading style.] Notice how he reads?
COUNSELOR:	He seems to read fast without pausing.
DENNIS:	Yes.
COUNSELOR:	You'd like to be able to read like that.

DENNIS: Not much. Let's name the ships in the books. [Dennis names each type of boat.] I have so much fun making up those names. That's what we'll do next week. [Dennis begins reading again.] Stop me when I make a mistake or do something wrong.

COUNSELOR: I'd rather you stop yourself.

DENNIS: The teacher always stops me.

COUNSELOR: I'm a listener, not a teacher.

DENNIS: Be a teacher, all right? [Dennis begins reading again.] That reminds me, I have three darts at home. The set cost me three dollars. Two broke. [The session is about to end. The counselor examines some darts and a board.] Oh boy, darts. Maybe we can play with them next week.

COUNSELOR: You're making lots of plans for next time.

DENNIS: Yeah.

Several counseling sessions followed this one. Dennis showed marked improvement at school and at home. Dennis's mother and teacher spoke more positively of him. The counselor gave Dennis his complete, undivided attention, participating in his games, tasks, projects, and plans. The counselor was someone with whom Dennis could talk and share his interests and ideas at a time when no one else would understand and accept him. He needed someone who would let him lead the way and be important in making decisions and plans. Dennis played the role of the initiator, the director, the teacher. He needed to have someone else know how it felt to be the follower who is told what to do, ordered into activity, and made to meet expectations. He needed to gain respect, as well as confidence, in his ability to face tasks and problems and see them through successfully. In short, he used the therapy experience to improve his relationships and skills. He became a competent, self-dependent person by practicing behavior that gave him a sense of adequacy and self-fulfillment.

Identification of Problem II[2]

A family sought therapy for problems with Pete, their rebellious 12-year-old son. The boy and his younger sister had been adopted 5 years earlier after a series of foster care arrangements. The adopting couple had no children before the adoption.

A history-gathering first session with the adoptive parents revealed that Pete had been physically abused by his biological mother and by at least one subsequent foster mother. The parents described Pete as rebellious and disrespectful, especially toward his mother. During the second session, the counselor met separately with Pete to establish rapport and continue assessing the context of the presenting problem. Although the boy was 12 years old, his social and emotional development appeared to be more like that of a 6- or 7-year-old child. The counselor wanted to help Pete feel comfortable, as well as elicit more information about his inner thoughts. With these objectives in mind and in view of Pete's apparent developmental

---

[2] The case of Pete was contributed by Robert Lee Whitaker, Ph.D.

stage, the counselor asked him to draw a picture of a person. Pete drew a very muscular, threatening-looking young adult (Figure 5-5). Then the counselor asked Pete to make up a story about the picture. Pete then told the following story. Note how the story's themes metaphorically describe Pete's experiences and his frustrated efforts to cope with them.

Pete's Story

He was born in a hollow tree. His mom was a dog; his dad was a cat. He was green, and he was the strongest person who ever lived. People called him Starman. He could throw a car, and it wouldn't come down for a week.

Then one day he met a baby. The baby had a race with him in the Olympics and beat him. The baby asked if he thought he could beat him again. For 2 years, they competed, and the baby always won. So the guy trained for 2 more years to beat the baby, but by that time, the baby was so big his head went out of the earth. He could jump out the earth. The guy knew he couldn't do anything about it, so he retired and went off to be a wimp and was never seen again. There were stories that he was beat up, killed, shot. And that was the last they saw of him.

A week later, the counselor asked Pete to tell the story of Starman's early life.

He lived in a jungle and helped his dad fight off the beasts that tried to attack his family. He's been alive 300 billion years. He was a god and a very powerful prince of the world then. His dad was the king. The prince made up the rules for the kingdom (which was communist). People could only work when the prince wanted them to work, and no family could have over $700. If so, they had to see him, and they couldn't leave the country.

The queen was named Laura. She was as skinny as a toothpick, and she was so powerful she could make it rain or snow or any kind of weather when she wanted. She could make people feel like they were dying and could make them grow old real fast. She could make them have nine lives or make them look ugly. She could change their bodies into beasts. She was very wicked.

The prince didn't like her because she was trying to overrule him and get all the power he had. So, the prince got all the other gods in all the world or universe and his dad and formed all their powers together and killed her. When she died, she turned into a planet called Saturn (her remains). The queen is dead now.

The prince grew up, and his dad died because of Zeus. Zeus gave him poison, and the prince was in charge from then on, except for Zeus (the god over all). The prince enforced all the laws the same way the lady did, and Zeus threatened to kill him. The lady had enforced the laws because Zeus threatened to kill her. The prince killed her because he didn't like the rules and what she was doing to the people, but he didn't know Zeus was making her do it by threatening to kill her.

The prince went on doing things the way Zeus wanted until he died. Now he is just a strong person.

Interpreting the Story This story suggested to the counselor a need to explore issues of anger and powerlessness with Pete. "Starman," or "the prince," felt powerless against the exceptional power and influence of the queen and the baby. Queen "Laura" had absolute control over the environment and could make whatever kind of weather she wanted (usually bad), make people grow old quickly, make them experience a feeling of death, make them ugly, and even turn them into beasts. Leadership, no matter who was in power, was always threateningly authoritarian.

The prince's battle for power or control is described as a violent act against the leader, made possible by combining the power of all oppressed victims. The story appears to reflect the trauma of Pete's upbringing and the particularly negative feelings he has toward female individuals with power over him. Furthermore, the story seems to parallel closely his history of abuse and development into an aggressive person involved in a power struggle with his adoptive mother. The information elicited from the story alerted the counselor to Pete's experience of the reported historical events. It is unlikely that Pete could have conveyed the impact of his history and its present relevance to his life in a form more insightful and descriptively meaningful than the story he told.

Intervention From the initial assessment interview with Pete's parents and the issues identified within the story, the counselor chose the following initial interventions: First, he decided to continue combining direct assessment procedures with picture-drawing and storytelling strategies to identify additional problematic areas for Pete. Second, the counselor began formulating a story to be used later about an abused person or animal who learned to adapt to a new environment by gradually learning to trust. Third, he asked Pete's permission to share with Pete's parents the story and the counselor's impressions of it. He then used the story to show the parents the relationship between Pete's present behavior and the trauma of his early experiences. The parents appeared to expect Pete to behave like any normal 12-year-old boy and not manifest any significant behavioral deficits related to the care he received during the first 7 years of his life. The counselor suggested that Pete was attempting to cope with these early experiences and that his parents might be able to help him and themselves by reconsidering the long-range impact of such an experience, adjusting their expectations, mutually deciding on and concentrating on just a few rules, giving Pete choices within limits they could accept, and selecting the roles each of them wanted to serve in Pete's life in light of what the story might suggest. Finally, the counselor suggested they try an experiment to begin their exploration of the new roles they wished to assume in Pete's life by letting the mother have a vacation from her job as the primary disciplinarian.

Rationale The therapeutic intentions of this plan were (1) to reinforce consistency in the parents' rules and expectations; (2) to empower Pete with choices his parents could accept; (3) to empower Pete's mother by providing more involvement and support from his father in parenting; (4) to foster an expectation of trust rather than distrust ("I know he'll do the right thing," instead of "I know he'll do the wrong thing"); (5) to focus less on punishment and more on logical consequences for Pete's misbehavior; and (6) to do away with any "mystery" rules or consequences.

Outcome Pete and his family settled into a more trusting relationship as Pete continued to express his early trauma and other emotional distress throughout his 4 years of psychoanalytic therapy.

DIVERSITY APPLICATIONS OF PSYCHOANALYTIC COUNSELING

Foster (2010) and Haaken (2008) call for more attention to cultural diversity in psychoanalysis—a theory that values intellectualism, individuation, and individual achievement, goals that do not translate across theories. Long-term treatment focused on attainment of insight to bring more of the unconscious into conscious awareness does not hold much appeal for clients from cultures that have neither the resources, patience, nor desire for such treatment and outcomes. Traditional psychoanalysis conditions of therapist anonymity, self-satisfaction, and individual development do not mesh with cultures that value social involvement and dedication to the group. However, as the oldest treatment approach and having been developed in Austria, psychoanalysis has a classical acceptance worldwide that many counseling theories do not have. As psychoanalytic counselors move toward treating families, their acceptance of other cultures should increase. Likewise, moving from stressing the individual to focusing on the welfare of the family and community should appeal to those cultures where group needs are considered over individual needs. Kekae-Moletsane (2008) explored one cultural adaptation of psychotherapy by using a South African traditional game as a tool in therapy. Seligman and Reichenberg (2014) note that contemporary psychoanalysis has increased flexibility, more collaborative treatment alliance, and the acknowledgement of cultural backgrounds and thus may be more appropriate for a diverse population.

Novie (2007) talked about two techniques that are relevant. One is free association, which creates an environment of unfolding that is unique to each client. The second technique is countertransference or the reactions of the therapist toward the client. The in-depth consideration of the interaction between client and analyst helps the understanding of the age, gender, race, class, as well as other social and biological factors of the client.

EVALUATION OF PSYCHOANALYSIS

Mander (2000), in agreement with Alexander (2004), details the psychodynamic approach to brief therapy that can be adapted to working with children and adolescents within the school setting. Several other publications have appeared under the title "brief psychoanalytic counseling." Laor (2001) notes that brief psychoanalytic psychotherapy can be adapted to individual clients by varying the time limits, therapist's activity, and therapeutic focus. Midgley and Kennedy (2011) review psychoanalysis with children. This approach continues to grow.

Safran and Kriss (2014) argue that evidence of the effectiveness of psychodynamic psychotherapy exists. They cite two meta-analytic studies (Abbass, Hancock, Henderson, & Kisely, 2006; Leichsenring & Rabung, 2008), with not only strong effect size for symptom improvement but also follow-up of large and stable effects. Shedler (2010) asserts that psychodynamic psychotherapy has a wide range of effectiveness for a wide range of conditions. Weiner and Bornstein (2009) affirm that psychotherapy works with adolescents and adults, with severely disturbed psychotic clients, with people who have personality disorders, and with people with less severe disorders. Blatt and Zuroff (2005) found positive effects of psychotherapy in symptom reduction and increase in patient's adapting and coping. Furthermore, Mackrill (2008) described ways that clients' strategies for change affect the process and outcome of analysis. Likewise Cogan (2007) found that the goals of symptom reduction, being able to work and love and being content with life challenges differentiated those who benefited from those who did not.

Research on psychoanalysis with children and adolescents is also sparse. Muratori, Picchi, Bruni, Patarnello, and Romagnoli (2003) treated 58 young children with psychoanalysis for 11 sessions. The control group included children of the same age who had the same diagnosis of anxiety or depression but did not receive services. The results indicate support for psychoanalysis as a treatment for anxiety and depression in children (Shapiro, Friedberg, & Bardenstein, 2006).

Luborsky and Luborsky (2006) have developed the Core Conflictual Relationship Theme (CCRT) as an objective way to study and measure the therapeutic relationship. By rating client statements, the counselor identifies relationship patterns that can be interpreted to the client. This objective way to study the transference aspect of psychoanalysis has promising implications for more research. Additionally, the Symptom-Context Method tracks the connection of the symptom to its context.

SUMMARY

Some of the key assumptions of psychoanalysis are fundamental to understanding its process. The beliefs that behavior and feelings result from unconscious motives rooted in childhood experiences support the need the therapeutic need to uncover those repressed motives. Freud believed behavior is determined and always has a cause again based on those unconscious, instinctual drives. The three parts of the personality, the id, ego, and superego, form the unconscious mind. The id and superego conflict constantly with the ego. That creates anxiety which humans mediate with the use of defense mechanisms.

Freud (1918) identified the task of analysts as bringing to patients' knowledge of their unconscious, repressed material and uncovering the resistances that oppose this extension of their knowledge about themselves. He believed that frustration made his patients ill, and that their symptoms served them as substitute satisfactions. Freud clearly noted the harm that may come to patients who receive too much help and consolation from their therapists, but also pointed out that many patients lack the strength and general knowledge to handle their lives without some mentoring and instruction, in addition to analysis, from their therapists.

Freud considered his theory of repression to be the cornerstone of the entire structure of psychoanalysis. However, Grünbaum (1993) notes that more research is needed to validate the link between such things as repressed childhood molestation and adult neurosis. He points out that a first event followed by a second event does not prove causality between the events. The theories of dreams and parapraxia also suffer from lack of hard data to prove causality.

In Freud's defense, much of his data collecting was similar to what passes today for acceptable, phenomenological research. In fact, data collecting through free association has many similarities to the open-ended, phenomenological interviewing method in which participants are encouraged to free-associate about the topic under study. In addition, Morgan and Morgan (2001) make a strong case for using single-participant designs in counseling research. Freud used a single-participant design method in his case study research. Finally, much of what is being done in counseling today has its roots in Freud's many contributions to the current theory and practice of counseling.

WEB SITES FOR PSYCHOANALYTIC COUNSELING

Internet addresses frequently change. To find the sites listed here, visit www.cengage.com/counseling/henderson for an updated list of Internet addresses and direct links to relevant sites.

National Psychological Association for Psychoanalysis (NPAP)

International Psychoanalytical Association (IPA)

American Psychoanalytic Association (APsaA)

Sigmund Freud Museum, Vienna and London

New York Psychoanalytic Society and Institute

REFERENCES

Abbass, A. A., Hancock, J. T., Henderson, J., & Kisely, S. (2006). Short-term psychodynamic psychotherapies for common mental disorders. *The Cochrane Database of Systematic Reviews, 4*, CD004687.

Adler, A. (1927). *Understanding human nature.* New York: Greenburg.

Alexander, F. (2004). A classic in psychotherapy integration revisited: The dynamics of psychotherapy in light of learning theory. *Journal of Psychotherapy Integration, 14*, 347–359.

Arlow, J. A. (2005). Psychoanalysis. In R. J.Corsini & D.Wedding (Eds.), *Current psychotherapies* (7th ed., pp. 15–51). Pacific Grove, CA: Brooks/Cole.

Blatt, S. J., & Zuroff, D. C. (2005). Empirical evaluation of the assumptions underlying evidence-based treatments in mental health. *Clinical Psychology Review, 25*, 459–486.

Brems, C. (2008). *A comprehensive guide to child psychotherapy* (3rd ed.). Long Grove, IL:Waveland Press.

Bromfield, R. (2003). Psychoanalytic play therapy. In C.Schaefer (Ed.), *Foundations of play therapy* (pp. 1–13). New York: Wiley.

Chazan, S. E., & Wolf, J. (2002). Using the children's play therapy instrument to measure change in psychotherapy: The conflicted player. *Journal of Infant, Child, and Adolescent Psychotherapy, 2*, 73–102.

Chethik, M. (2000). *Techniques of child therapy.* New York: Guilford Press.

Cogan, R. (2007). Therapeutic aims and outcomes of psychoanalysis. *Psychoanalytic Psychology, 24*, 193–207.

Davis, T. E., Thompson E., May, A., & Whiting, S. E. (2011). Evidence-based treatment of anxiety and phobia in children and adolescents: Current status and effects on the emotional response. *Clinical Psychology Review, 31*(4), 592–602. doi: 10.1016/j. cpr.2011.01.001

Ecker, B., & Hulley, L. (1995). *Depth-oriented brief therapy*. New York: Jossey-Bass.

Erikson, E. (1950). *Childhood and society*. New York: Norton.

Erikson, E. (1968). *Identity: Youth and crisis*. New York: Norton.

Fancher, R. (2000). Snapshots of Freud in America. *American Psychologist, 55*, 1025–1028.

Foster, R. P. (2010). Considering a multicultural perspective for psychoanalysis. In A. Roland, B. Ulanov, & C. Barbre (Eds.), *Creative dissent: Psychoanalysis in evolution (pp. 173–185)*. Westport, CT: Praeger/Greenword Publishing Group.

Freud, S. (1918). *Lines of advance in psychoanalytic therapy*. Paper presented at the fifth International Psychoanalytic Congress, Budapest, Hungary.

Freud, A. (1926). *Psychoanalytic treatment of children*. London: Imago.

Freud, S. (1949). *An outline of psychoanalysis* (J.Strachey, Trans.). New York: Norton. (Original work published 1940.)

Freud, S. (1952). *On dreams* (J. Strachey, Trans.). New York: Norton. (Original work published 1901.)

Freud, S. (1963). *An autobiographical study* (J. Strachey, Trans.). New York: Norton. (Original work published 1925.)

Freud, S. (1965a). *The interpretation of dreams* (J.Strachey, Trans.). New York: Norton. (Original work published 1900.)

Freud, S. (1965b). *New introductory lectures in psychoanalysis* (J. Strachey, Ed. & Trans.). New York: Norton. (Original work published 1933.)

Freud, S. (1971). *The psychopathology of everyday life* (A.Tyson, Trans.). New York: Norton. (Original work published 1901.)

Gardner, R. (1986). *Therapeutic communication with children: The mutual storytelling technique* (Rev. ed.). Lanham, MD: Jason Aronson.

Ginott, H. (1994). *Group psychotherapy with children: The theory and practice of play-therapy*. Northvale, NJ: Aronson.

Goldman, G. A., & Anderson, T. (2007). Quality of object relations and security of attachment as predictors of early therapeutic alliance. *Journal of Counseling Psychology, 54*, 111–117.

Grünbaum, A. (1993). *Validation in clinical theory of psychoanalysis*. Madison, CT: International Universities Press.

Haaken, J. (2008). When white buffalo calf woman meets Oedipus on the road. *Theory and Psychology, 18*, 195–208. doi: 10.1177/0959354307087881

Hall, C. (1954). *A primer of Freudian psychology*. New York: Mentor.

Hirschmüller, A. (1989). *The life and work of Josef Breuer*. New York: New York University Press. (Original German edition 1978.)

Jung, C. G., et al. (1964). *Man and his symbols*. New York: Doubleday.

Kekae-Moletsane, M. (2008). Masekitlana: South African traditional play as a therapeutic tool in child psychotherapy. *South African Journal of Psychology, 38*, 367–375.

Kernberg, P. F., & Chazan, S. E. (1991). *Children with conduct disorders: A psychotherapy manual*. New York: Basic Books.

Klein, M. (1932). *The psychoanalysis of children*. London: Hogarth.

Klein, M. (1984). *Love, guilt, and reparation and other works, 1921–1945*. New York: Free Press.

Laor, I. (2001). Brief psychoanalytic psychotherapy: The impact of its fundamentals on the therapeutic process. *British Journal of Psychotherapy, 18*(2), 169–183.

Lee, A. C. (2009). Psychoanalytic play therapy. In K. J.O'Connor & L. D.Braverman (Eds.) *Play therapy theory and practice: Comparing theories and techniques* (2nd ed., pp. 25–82). Hoboken, NJ: Wiley.

Leichensenring, F., & Rabung, S. (2008). Effectiveness of long-term psychodynamic psychotherapy: A meta-analysis. *Journal of the American Medical Association, 300*, 1551–1565.

Leudar, I., Sharrock, W., Truckle, S., Colombino, T., Hayes, J., & Booth, K. (2008). Conversations on emotions: On turning play into psychoanalytic psychotherapy. In A. Peräkylä, C. Antaki, S. Vehviläinen, & I. Leudar (Eds.), *Conversation analysis and psychotherapy* (pp. 152–172). Cambridge, England: Cambridge University Press.

Levy, A. J. (2011). Neurobiology and the therapeutic action of psychoanalytic play therapy with children. *Clinical Social Work Journal, 39*(1), 50–60. doi: 10.1007/s10615-009-0229-x

Luborsky, L., & Luborsky, E. (2006). *Research and psychotherapy: The vital link*. Lanham, MD: Jason Aronson.

Luborsky, E. B., O'Reilly-Landry, M., & Arlow, J. A. (2008). Psychoanalysis. In R. J. Corsini & D. Wedding (Eds), *Current psychotherapies* (8th ed., pp. 15–62). Belmont, CA: Thomson.

Mackrill, T. (2008). Exploring psychotherapy clients' independent strategies for change while in therapy. *British Journal of Guidance and Counselling, 36*, 441–453.

Mander, G. (2000). *A psychodynamic approach to brief therapy*. London: Sage Publications.

Maslow, A. (1970). *Motivation and personality* (2nd ed.). New York: Harper & Row.

McCarthy, J., & Conway, F. (2011). Introduction: Attention deficit hyperactivity disorder in children and the psychoanalytic process. *Journal of Infant, Child, and Adolescent Psychotherapy, 10*, 1–4.

McWilliams, N. (1994). *Psychoanalytic diagnosis: Understanding personality structure in the clinical process*. New York: Guilford.

Merydith, S. P. (2007). Psychodynamic approaches. In H. T. Prout & D. T. Brown (Eds.) *Counseling and psychotherapy with children and adolescents: Theory and practice for school and clinical settings* (pp. 94–130). Hoboken, NJ: Wiley.

Midgley, N., & Kennedy, E. (2011). Psychodynamic psychotherapy for children and adolescents: a critical review of the evidence base. *Journal of Child Psychotherapy, 37*(3), 232–260. doi: 10.1080/0075417X.2011.614738

Morgan, D., & Morgan, R. (2001). Single-participant research design: Bringing science to managed care. *American Psychologist, 56*, 119–127.

Muratori, F., Picchi, L., Bruni, G., Patarnello, M., & Romagnoli, G. (2003). A two-year follow-up of psychodynamic psychotherapy for internalizing disorders in children. *Journal of the American Academy of Child and Adolescent Psychiatry, 42*, 331–339.

Neff, K. D., & Vonk, R. (2009). Self-compassion versus global self-esteem: Two different ways of relating to oneself. *Journal of Personality, 77*(1), 23–50. doi: 10.1111/j.1467-6494.2008.00537.x

Novie, G. J. (2007). Psychoanalytic theory. In D. Capuzzi & D. R. Gross (Eds.), *Counseling and psychotherapy: Theories and interventions* (4th ed.). Upper Saddle River, NJ: Merrill.

Paparoussi, M., Andreou, E., & Gkouni, V. (2011). Approaching children's fears through bibliotherapy: A classroom-based intervention. In J. Hagen & A. T. Kisubi (Eds.), *Best practices in human services: A global perspective*. Oshkosh, WI: Council for Standards in Human Services.

Pardeek, J. A. (2014). *Using books in clinical social work: A guide to bibliotherapy*. New York: Haworth.

Piaget, J., & Inhelder, B. (1969). *The psychology of the child*. New York: Basic Books.

Platteuw, C. (2011). Narrative play therapy with adopted children. In A. Taylor de Faoite (Ed.) *Narrative play therapy theory and practice* (pp. 214–229). London: Kingsley.

Rapee, R. M., Abbott, M. J., & Lyneham, H. J. (2006). Bibliotherapy for children with anxiety disorders using written materials for parents: A randomized controlled trial. *Journal of Consulting and Clinical Psychology, 74*, 436–444.

Safran, J. D., & Kriss, A. (2014). Psychoanalytic psychotherapies. In D. Wedding & R. J. Corsini (Eds.), *Current psychotherapies* (10th ed, pp. 19–54.). Belmont, CA: Cengage.

Schneider, C., Midgley, N., & Duncan, A. (2010). A "motion portrait" of a psychodynamic treatment of an 11-year-old girl: Exploring interrelations of psychotherapy process and outcome using the child psychotherapy Q-Set. *Journal of Infant, Child, and Adolescent Psychotherapy, 9*, 94–107.

Seligman, L. (2006). *Theories of counseling and psychotherapy: Systems, strategies, and skills* (2nd ed.). Upper Saddle River, NJ: Pearson.

Seligman, L., & Reichenberg, L. W. (2014). *Theories of counseling and psychotherapy: Systems, strategies and skills* (4th ed.). Upper Saddle River, NJ: Pearson.

Shapiro, J. P., Friedberg, R. D., & Bardenstein, K. K. (2006). *Child and adolescent therapy: Science and Art.* Hoboken, NJ: Wiley.

Shechtman, Z. (2009). *Treating child and adolescent aggression through bibliotherapy.* New York: Springer.

Shedler, J. (2010). The efficacy of psychodynamic psychotherapy. *American Psychologist, 65*, 98–109.

Stone, I. (1971). *The passions of the mind: A biographical novel of Sigmund Freud* (5th ed). New York: Doubleday.

Strachey, J. (Ed. & Trans.). (1953–1964). *Standard edition of the complete psychological works of Sigmund Freud.* London: Hogarth Press.

Sugarman, A. (2008). The use of play to promote insightfulness in the analysis of children suffering from cumulative trauma. *The Psychoanalytic Quarterly, 77*, 799–833.

Wagner, W. W. (2008). *Counseling, psychology and children* (2nd ed.). Upper Saddle River, NJ: Pearson.

Watson, J. (1980). Bibliotherapy for abused children. *School Counselor, 27*, 204–208.

Weiner, I. B., & Bornstein, R. F. (2009). *Principles of psychotherapy: Promoting evidence-based psychodynamic practice* (3rd ed.). Hoboken, NJ: Wiley.

Weininger, O. (1984). *The clinical psychology of Melanie Klein.* Springfield, IL: Charles C. Thomas.

Weininger, O. (1989). *Children's phantasies: The shaping of relationships.* London: Karnac.

Winnicott, D. W. (1971). *Playing and reality.* London: Tavistock.

Winnicott, D. W. (1977). *The piggle: An account of the psychoanalytic treatment of a little girl.* New York: International University Press.

CHAPTER 6

Person-Centered Counseling

I'm looking for the angel within.
—MICHELANGELO

Humanistic philosophy characterizes people as capable and autonomous beings who have the capacity to solve their own problems, work toward their full potential, and make positive changes in their lives. These positive beliefs undergird a counseling approach that focuses on the emotional experiences of the client and the conditions counselors demonstrate that allow people to discover their inherent strengths in their journey to self-actualization.

After reading this chapter, you should be able to:

- Outline the development of client-centered counseling and Carl Rogers
- Explain the theory of client-centered counseling, including its core concepts
- Discuss the counseling relationship and goals in client-centered treatment
- Describe assessment, process, and techniques in client-centered counseling
- Demonstrate some therapeutic techniques
- Clarify the effectiveness of client-centered counseling
- Discuss client-centered play therapy

CARL ROGERS
(1902–1987)

Carl Rogers was born in Oak Park, Illinois, the fourth of six children. His early home life was marked by close family ties, a strict religious and moral atmosphere, and an appreciation of the value of hard work (Rogers, 1961). During this period, Rogers's family did not mix socially but rather enjoyed their own company. His family moved to a farm when he was 12 so the children could resist the temptations of suburban life.

His father, a civil engineer, required the farm be run scientifically; thus from raising lambs, pigs, and calves, Rogers learned about matching experimental conditions with control conditions and about randomization procedures as well as respect for other scientific methods.

Rogers started college at the University of Wisconsin to study scientific agriculture. After 2 years, however, he switched his career goal to the ministry as a result of attending some emotionally charged religious conferences. In his junior year, he was chosen to go to China for 6 months for an international World Student Christian Federation conference. During this period, two things greatly influenced his life. First, at the expense of great pain and stress on his family, Rogers freed himself from the religious thinking of his parents and became an independent thinker, although he did not abandon religion entirely. He wrote, "From the date of this trip, my goals, values, aims, and philosophy have been my own" (Rogers, 1967, p. 351). Second, he fell in love with a woman he had known most of his life. He married her, with reluctant parental consent, as soon as he finished college so they could attend graduate school together.

Rogers chose to go to graduate school at Union Theological Seminary, where Goodwin Watson's and Marian Kenworthy's courses and lectures on psychology and psychiatry interested him. He took courses at Teachers College, Columbia University, across the street from Union and found himself drawn to child guidance while working at Union. Rogers obtained a fellowship at the Institute for Child Guidance, and he was on his way to a career in psychology.

At the end of his time at the Institute for Child Guidance, Rogers accepted a job in Rochester, New York, at the Society for the Prevention of Cruelty to Children. He completed his Ph.D. at Columbia Teachers College and spent the next 12 years in Rochester raising his son and daughter. Rogers once said that his children taught him far more about the development and relationships of individuals than he ever learned professionally.

Rogers spent 8 years in Rochester immersed in his work, conducting treatment interviews and trying to be effective with clients. He gradually began teaching in the sociology department at the University of Rochester. He was also involved in developing a guidance center and writing a book, *The Clinical Treatment of the Problem Child* (1939). At this time, Otto Rank's work influenced Rogers's belief in people's ability to solve their own problems, given the proper climate.

In 1940, Rogers accepted a full professorship at Ohio State University. Realizing he had developed a distinctive viewpoint, he wrote the then-controversial book *Counseling and Psychotherapy* (1942), in which he proposed a counseling relationship based on the warmth and responsiveness of the therapist. Rogers believed that in such a relationship clients would express their feelings and thoughts. This was a radical change in a field that had been dominated by psychoanalysis and directive counseling. He and his students at Ohio State University made detailed analyses of counseling sessions and began to publish cases in "client-centered therapy." The theory developed as Rogers and his colleagues began to test the hypotheses they formed from their case studies.

In 1945, Rogers moved on to the University of Chicago, where he organized the counseling center and spent the next 12 years doing research. While associated with the University of Chicago, he wrote his famous work, *Client-Centered Therapy*, which was published in 1951. Rogers described his years at Chicago as very satisfying, but he eventually accepted an opportunity at the University of Wisconsin, where he was able to work in both the departments of psychology and psychiatry. He had long wanted to work with psychotic individuals who had been hospitalized.

In 1966, Rogers moved to the Western Behavioral Science Institute in La Jolla, California. Two years later, he and several colleagues formed the Center for Studies of the Person. During the next 20 years, he wrote about using person-centered therapy with groups and the application of his theory to education, marriage, administration, and politics. He spoke in South Africa, Eastern Europe, the Soviet Union, Northern Ireland, and Central America (Fall et al., 2010). Kirschenbaum (2009) has released *The Life and Work of Carl Rogers*, a book that includes materials taken from Rogers's diaries and reveals the subtleties of this influential man.

Rogers's theory evolved through distinct phases. The first was the "nondirective" phase that focused on the differences between directive and nondirective approaches to counseling. In *Counseling and Psychotherapy* (1942), he argued that clinicians should not tell clients how to change but rather to help clients express, clarify, and gain insight into their emotions. The next phase shifted to the client's responsibility as well as the counselor's therapeutic stance. In his book *Client-Centered Therapy* (1951), Rogers explained that treatment could not be totally nondirective. He talked about the counselor's role as being more active. The counselor must communicate empathy, congruence, and acceptance to create a therapeutic alliance. In *On Becoming a Person* (1961), Rogers introduced his third phase by discussing healthy and fully functioning people as those who are open to experience and appreciative of themselves. The last part of his career centered on the expanded application of the therapy principles, the person-centered phase in which Rogers represented his concern with all of humanity. In his work, Rogers promoted the belief that people have within them resources for understanding themselves (Fall et al., 2010; Seligman & Reichenberg, 2014). Kirschenbaum (2009) noted that Rogers's theories reflect his personal development in that his ideas grew richer as Rogers's insight, personality, and compassion strengthened.

THE NATURE OF PEOPLE

Carl Rogers viewed people as rational, socialized, forward-moving, and realistic beings. He considered people as strong and capable, trusting their capacity for handling problem. He argued that negative, antisocial emotions are only a result of frustrated basic impulses; an idea related to Maslow's hierarchy of needs. For instance, extreme aggressive action toward other people results from a failure to meet the basic needs of love and belonging. Rogers believed that once people are free of their defensive behavior, their reactions are positive and progressive.

Rogers considered people at their most fundamental level to be essentially positive with a tendency to grow, to heal, and to move toward their fullest potential (Fall et al., 2010). People possess the capacity to experience—that is, to express rather than repress—their own maladjustment to life and move toward a more adjusted state of mind. Rogers believed that people move toward actualization as they move toward psychological adjustment. Because people possess the capacity to regulate and control their own behavior, the counseling relationship is merely a means of tapping personal resources and developing human potential. People learn from their external therapy experience how to internalize and provide their own psychotherapy.

In summary, a child-centered counselor believes that people:

- Have worth and dignity in their own right and therefore deserve respect
- Have the capacity and right to self-direction and, when given the opportunity, make wise judgments
- Can select their own values
- Can learn to make constructive use of responsibility
- Have the capacity to deal with their own feelings, thoughts, and behavior
- Have the potential for constructive change and personal development toward a full and satisfying life (self-actualization)

Rogers (1994) provided perhaps the best description of his view of human nature:

> One of the most satisfying experiences I know—is just fully to appreciate an individual in the same way that I appreciate a sunset. When I look at a sunset … I don't find myself saying, "Soften the orange a little on the right hand corner, and put a bit more purple along the base, and use a little more pink in the cloud color…." I don't try to control a sunset. I watch it with awe as it unfolds. (p. 189)

CORE CONCEPTS

Child-centered counselors focus on the ways children discover who they are capable of becoming. Counselors understand that development flows and the maturing process leads to a deepening sense of self. Three concepts apply to that understanding: the person, the world, and the self.

Person

The foundation of this approach to counseling is the idea of the sovereign human being (Raskin, Rogers, & Witty, 2014). The person includes all components of the human being—the thoughts, behaviors, feelings, and physical self—and that wholeness should not to be reduced to a diagnosis or a label. The person develops and "exists in a continually changing world of experience of which he is the center" (Rogers, 1951, p. 483). People are motivated by their inner-directed progress to become more fully functioning, improving, becoming more independent, and enhancing themselves. Landreth (2012) talks about this progression as a goal-directed activity toward satisfying personal needs in the child's unique world of experiences—the child's world.

World

World, another central concept of child-centered counseling, means everything the child experiences internally as well as externally. Rogers (1959) used the word *experience* as a noun to refer to everything that is taking place within the person at any given time. Those internal references contain the basis for looking at life. Whatever the child perceives to be happening makes up his reality. Counselors must understand the child's view of reality if they want to understand the child's behavior. Counselors "look through the child's eyes" (Sweeney & Landreth, 2009, p. 125), avoid evaluating any behaviors, and work hard to understand the child's frame of reference (world). The point of focus, therefore, becomes the child's reality, not some predetermined set of categories (Landreth, 2012). In other words, counselors need to know the unique "self" of the child.

Self

Parts of all of the child's experiences gradually form what the child considers self. Self is the person's private world that becomes recognized as "me" across interactions with others. The differentiation results in developing ideas about self, about the external world, and about oneself in the world. Rogers (1951) defines *self* as the totality of the perceptions of the child. He explains that even infants have times in which they recognize "I am hungry, and I don't like it," even though they have no words to match their experience. Thus begins the natural process of the child's appreciating things seen as self-enhancing and devaluing experiences that are threatening or negatively impact self. Rogers (1951) describes self-concept as:

> An organized configuration of perceptions of the self which are admissible to awareness. It is composed of such elements as the perceptions of one's characteristics and abilities; the percepts and concepts of the self in relation to others and to the environment; the value qualities which are perceived as associated with experiences and objects; and the goals and ideals which are perceived as having positive or negative valence. (p. 501)

As children develop, they realize that parents and others evaluate them. They believe that love and their sense of being lovable depends on their behavior. The child may become confused when actions that satisfy them (such as screaming when they are angry) are labeled as bad by their caretakers. The child has trouble integrating the satisfaction of expressing anger with the disapproval of parents.

As a person ages, relying only on evaluations from other people may lead to doubt, denial, or even disapproval of self. The person may eventually become psychologically maladjusted. In order to decrease the likelihood of those external evaluations replacing a healthy sense of self, the child-centered counselor acknowledges the person, world, and the self of the child, believing each person has the capacity to move steadily toward growth and health.

The need for positive regard accompanies the development of self-concept. Children want to be valued, accepted, and understood, the ingredients of unconditional positive regard. The child associates self with the degree of positive regard received or denied. If children receive conditions of worth such as evaluative and critical messages that they are only loveable if they think, feel, and act as others demand, their acceptance of themselves may be impaired. Children may internalize the criticisms and devalue the aspects of themselves they consider unworthy. This causes inner conflicts and incongruities and limits their natural tendency toward growth.

If children are given unconditional positive regard—messages that they are special just because of who they are—they are more likely to become fully functioning adults. That does not mean children's misbehavior is ignored or condoned, but rather that caretakers correct the behavior and still accept the child. For example, "I love you and I can tell that you are upset that I insisted you come to your grandparents, but your screaming at me must stop" (Fall et al., 2010; Seligman & Reichenberg, 2014).

When children doubt themselves, their perceptions and experiences, they may acquire "conditions of worth" and a self that is "incongruent" and stumble in their attempts to self-define and regulate (Raskin et al., 2014). Children develop positive self-concepts if what they value in themselves and what parents and significant others value match (Presbury, McKee, & Echterling, 2007). Child-centered counseling creates an atmosphere in which people can talk about preferences or feelings or opinions, a step in redefining and accepting self.

THEORY OF COUNSELING

Child-centered counselors create an environment in which a child can discover and explore self. Counselors focus on the relationship with the child, knowing that partnership is vital to the success or failure of counseling. Landreth (2012) explains that counselors concentrate:

- On the child rather than the problem
- The present rather than the past
- Feelings rather than thoughts and behaviors
- Understanding rather than explaining
- Accepting rather than correcting
- The child's wisdom and direction rather than the counselor's

The inner person of the child and what the child is and can become are the focal points.

Rogers (1992), in a reprint of his classic 1957 article about the necessary and sufficient conditions of therapeutic change, addressed the question, "Is it possible to state in clearly definable and measurable terms what is needed to bring about personality change?" Accepting the behaviorists' challenge, Rogers proceeded to answer in descriptive terms. The six *core* conditions for personality change have become the classic conditions for child-centered counseling, expressed by Rogers and explained by Presbury et al. (2007):

1. Two people are in psychological contact. A degree of caring and investment in the relationship exist.
2. The client is in a state of incongruence. The client may be vulnerable or anxious and thus motivated to change.
3. The therapist is congruent and involved in the relationship. The counselor, a genuine, trusted, and actualizing model, is crucial to the effectiveness of counseling.
4. The therapist offers unconditional positive regard for the client. The counselor has an unqualified faith in the worth and dignity of the person.
5. The therapist experiences empathetic understanding of the client's internal frame of reference. By expressing empathy and the implicit aspects of the person's experience, the counselor creates a place in which the client can increase self-awareness.
6. The communication of empathetic and positive regard is achieved. If clients feel valued by the counselor, they can value themselves more.

Rogers believed that each core condition is necessary to create optimal opportunity for personality change. The sixth condition, the basis for trust between counselor and client, is especially vital to the counseling process. We agree with Rogers that the six conditions, which need not be limited to the child-centered method of counseling, provide a sound foundation for most standard methods of counseling both children and adults.

As noted previously, Rogers first called his process *nondirective therapy* because of the therapist's encouraging and listening role. Later, he adopted the term *client-centered*, because of the complete responsibility given to clients for their own growth, and then *person-centered*, in hopes of further humanizing the counseling process. As this book focuses on counseling children, we will use the terminology *child-centered* for Rogers's counseling approach.

Relationship

Rogers (1967) was convinced that personality change does not happen except within a relationship. He explained that the counseling relationship was between two equal and capable people who work together in their alliance in which both grow and are enriched by their association. The counselor's job is to create a place to release the client's potential. The role of the client is to be who she is.

Child-centered counselors see people positively, accepting people as they are and assuming they can solve their own problems. Counselors focus on strengths and successes, and they encourage clients to move forward. Client-centered practitioners offer acceptance, respect, understanding, and valuing to promote clients' self-exploration.

Most importantly, child-centered counselors live the qualities of congruence, unconditional positive regard, and empathy, the core conditions of therapy. Congruence refers to the counselors' ability to be genuine and aware of themselves and the way others see them. Counselors are open and authentic, present and aware of the experience of interacting with the client (Rogers, 1959). Unconditional positive regard can be defined as caring about, respecting, liking, and accepting people without applying any conditions on them to act, feel, or think in certain ways (Kirschenbaum, 2009). Unconditional positive regard implies communicating warmth and acceptance what Rogers sometimes called *prizing*. Rogers (1980) defined empathy as "temporarily living in the other's life, moving about in it delicately without making judgments; it means sensing meanings of which he or she is scarcely aware, but not trying to uncover totally unconscious feelings, since this would be too threatening.... It means frequently checking with the person as to the accuracy of your sensings" (p. 142). Empathy then is the sense of what people are thinking, feeling, and experiencing, as well as the ability to communicate that understanding. Sensitive, accurate, and active listening expose counselors to the subjective world of the other person.

To maintain himself in the nondirective role of the child-centered counselor, Rogers refrained from giving advice, asking questions, and making interpretations of the client's message, thoughts, feelings, and behaviors. He believed all three of these counselor behaviors tend to shift the counseling process from a child-centered to a counselor-centered focus. When pressed for advice, a common Rogers's response would be, "I would like to know the advice you would like to hear from me."

Rogers believed that one way people get themselves into trouble is letting other people direct their lives and that a counselor who does likewise makes the client's problem situation worse. Therefore, Rogers believed he could facilitate his clients' progress if he put them in the position of charting the direction of their counseling interviews. He was successful in doing so by replacing advice, interpretations, and questions with the active listening process of limiting his responses to summaries and clarifications of the content, feelings, and expectations for counseling presented in his clients' interviews. Hence, the direction of child-centered interviews is left to the client. Visualize two people riding side by side in a horse-drawn carriage with the reins lying on the floor of the driver's seat. Each rider is waiting for the other to pick up the reins and drive the horse. Finally, out of clear frustration, if not fear, one of the riders picks up the reins and guides the horse. Rogers maintained the counselor should not be the one to pick up the reins unless possible bodily injury demanded it. Some scholars are not all that sure that he would have done it even then. Rogers believed that directing the counseling interview would be an important first step for clients to begin directing their lives outside the counseling interview.

In the child-centered counseling process, if the counselor creates a warm and accepting climate in interviews, children trust the counselor enough to risk sharing their ideas about their lives and the problems they face. During this sharing with a nonjudgmental counselor, children feel free to explore their feelings, thoughts, and behaviors as they relate to their personal growth, development, and adjustment. Such explorations should, in turn, lead to more effective decision making and to productive behavior. Rogers (1951) wrote that the counselor operates from the point of view that people have the capacity to work effectively with all aspects of their lives that come into conscious awareness. Expansion of this conscious awareness occurs when the counseling climate meets Rogers's core conditions and children realize that the counselor accepts them as competent to direct their own lives.

Child-centered counseling deals primarily with the organization and function of self. The counselor becomes an objective, unemotional "mirror" who reflects the person's inner world with warmth, acceptance, and trust. This mirroring allows people to judge their thoughts and feelings and to begin to explore the effects on their behavior. Thus, people are enabled to reorganize their thoughts, feelings, and behaviors and function in a more integrated fashion.

Hutchby (2005) talked about eliciting feelings-talk with children by active listening skills. Clients are the experts whose task is to teach the counselor about their life situation. Clients thereby learn more about themselves, because teaching also generally helps the teacher learn. The teaching factor may be the main reason that child-centered therapy helps many people. Child-centered counselors create an environment in which a person's natural tendency toward growth can flow. The counselor accomplishes this by cultivating and communicating the facilitative conditions.

Bratton, Ceballos, and Ferebee (2009) outline a group experience designed for preadolescents. They wanted to encourage the preteens to become more aware of their own resources in order to help them handle frustrations more effectively. Building on both positive desires and on negative impulses without being afraid of consequences, participants discovered an internal strength and more creative self-development.

Goals

In child-centered counseling, the child is to be understood instead of diagnosed, treated, or changed. The main goal of child-centered therapy is assisting people in becoming more autonomous, spontaneous, and confident (Rogers, 1983). As people become more aware of what is going on inside themselves, they can stop fearing and defending their inner feelings. They learn to accept their own values and trust their own judgment, rather than live by the values of others. The ultimate goal of child-centered therapy is for the client to be a fully functioning person who has learned to be free.

According to Rogers (1983), learning to be free is the essential goal of education. People who have learned to be free can confront life and face problems; they trust themselves to choose their own way and accept their own feelings without forcing them on others. Such individuals prize themselves and others as having dignity, worth, and value.

Some general expectations of child-centered therapy include a change from immature to mature behavior; fewer defensive behaviors; more tolerance for frustration; and improved functioning in life tasks. Sweeney and Landreth (2009) describe a child as being more open to a range of experiences and to other people. They explain that the child feels less helpless and less threatened and has more realistic, objective expectations. The child becomes more confident and more self-directed.

Central to child-centered counseling is helping children trust and be honest with themselves. Other goals include promoting awareness of self, optimism, responsibility, congruence, and autonomy. When these strengths are developed, people build an internal control and make better use of potential. This counseling approach does not focus on resolving a problem but on allowing people to lead more rewarding lives and to deal with the joys and challenges of life (Seligman & Reichenberg, 2014).

COUNSELING METHOD

As has already been mentioned, the counselor as a person is vital to child-centered counseling. The conditions the counselor models become the ultimate counseling goals for all clients, to be genuine, accepting, and independent. Effective child-centered counselors must possess openness, empathic understanding, spontaneity, acceptance, mutual respect, and intimacy. After clients move through the immediate counseling goals of self-exploration with auxiliary goals, such as improving a math grade or making a new friend, they begin to work toward achieving the ultimate counseling goals for the effective child-centered counselor: developing the same traits modeled by child-centered counselors. Counselors promote the person's self-awareness and personal growth.

Assessment

Child-centered counselors rarely use diagnostic and assessment tools, which are considered distracting from the counseling relationship. Rather than strategies or treatment, counselors use themselves and the core conditions to promote the relationship and enhance the client's self-awareness (Murdock, 2013).

People react to love that depends on conditions and then may become maladjusted. The core to this difficulty is the incongruence between the self-experience that pushes them toward growth and the experiences that occur as they try to please others. Children may deny parts of themselves that others do not value and come to view themselves as only the aspects of themselves prized by others. So if the child feels loved when making good grades but dismissed when playing the piano, he may begin to deny his pleasure in musical performance. The person becomes afraid of genuine feelings, and the conflict between the authentic self and the self that has become dependent on conditional acceptance escalates (Presbury et al., 2007). The distress that discrepancy causes can be expressed in a variety of symptoms. Since humans have an innate tendency to move toward inner consistency and harmony, the person will feel a need to resolve the tension of unsettled feelings. Therefore, the perception of inner turmoil motivates the client to change (Fall et al., 2010).

Process

The counseling process outlined by Rogers (1942) includes 12 steps.

1. The individual comes for help.
2. The helping situation is characterized as a chance to grow.
3. The counselor promotes free expression of feelings about the concerns.
4. The counselor accepts, recognizes, and clarifies these feelings.
5. When the person's negative feelings have been fully expressed, they are often followed by a tentative expression of positive drives toward growth.
6. The counselor accepts and recognizes the positive feelings, which gives the person a chance to understand himself as he is. Insight and self-understanding emerge.
7. This insight, the understanding and acceptance of self, provides a foundation from which the person can move to a new level of integration.
8. Mingled with the insight is an awakening to clarification of possible decisions and courses of action.
9. The beginning of small but significant positive actions begins.
10. Further insight occurs.
11. More integrated positive action, less fear, and more confidence follow.
12. The person feels less need for help and recognizes the relationship is near an end (Fall et al., 2010; Rogers, 1942).

The person-centered model for helping, as modified by Carkhuff (1973), involves three general stages through which the client proceeds. In the first phase, self-exploration, people examine exactly where they are in their lives, including a type of self-searching in which they question themselves concerning their status at the present moment. In the second phase, people begin to understand the relationship between where they are in life and where they would like to be. That is, they move from a type of discovery in self-exploration to an understanding. The third phase involves action. In this context, action is goal directed; people engage in some program or plan to reach the point where they want to be. The only exception to the logical order of these three stages might be in helping children; their movement through the process may be more meaningful if action is followed by understanding and then self-exploration. Children problem-solve better when they can move from concrete to abstract thinking. Self-exploration is the most abstract area of the process in Rogers's system.

Techniques

Perhaps the strongest techniques in the child-centered counselor's repertoire are attitudes toward people: *congruence* (genuine), *unconditional positive regard* (accepting), and *empathy* (understanding). Rogers (1957) said that a person who was given those 'core conditions' would naturally grow and move toward a more self-accepting position. Congruence reveals the trustworthy counselor who is not playing an artificial role. Wood, Linley, Maltby, Baliousis, and Joseph (2008) designed a scale of the authentic personality which may be helpful to estimate congruence.

Unconditional positive regard implies that the counselor accepts clients as people who have the potential to become good, rational, and free. All humans have self-worth, dignity, and unique traits as individuals, thus they require individualized counseling approaches. People direct their own counseling sessions. For the process to succeed, clients must believe they can reveal themselves to the counselor in an atmosphere of complete acceptance.

Empathy is the attitude that holds the counseling process together. By attempting to understand, the counselor helps convince people that they are worth hearing and understanding. Rogers (1995), in a reprint of a 1956 speech, identified six principles he believed helped him become more effective in understanding and showing empathy in counseling. He believed that acceptance and understanding of his clients kept him from trying to fix their problems. Once he came to believe that people have a basic positive direction, he wanted his clients to discover their own paths to resolving their problems as he explained in the six principles that follow:

First principle: "In my relationships with people I have found that it does not help, in the long run, to act as though I am something I am not." Rogers found it harmful to pretend to be feeling a certain way with a client if he actually felt differently. Constructive relationships cannot be built on pretense.

Second principle: "I have found it effective in my dealings with people to be accepting of myself." He learned to trust his reactions to clients, which he thought made his relationships with clients much more authentic. He believed that real relationships were always in the process of change and never static.

Third principle: "I have found it to be of enormous value when I can permit myself to understand another person." This principle became the cornerstone for his theory of child-centered counseling. He believed a therapist should be completely open to hearing exactly what the client is trying to relate. He believed that most people had an opinion formed before hearing what another person was trying to communicate. Consequently, Rogers thought the best thing that counselors could do was listen. He placed great value on learning from his students' reactions to each of his classes. Any success he enjoyed as a teacher was attributed to understanding each student's point of view.

Fourth principle: "I have found it to be of value to be open to the realities of life as they are revealed in me and in other people." He believed there was balance to life, the fragile as well as the tough.

Fifth principle: "The more I am able to understand myself and others, the more that I am open to the realities of life and the less I find myself wishing to rush in." That is, he was less likely to try to manipulate people into meeting certain goals or conforming to certain modes of living. Rogers did not believe clients should learn what a therapist thought they should learn, but he did hold that other people change as the therapist changes.

Sixth principle: "It has been my experience that people have a basically positive direction." He believed that the more individuals felt they were being understood and well received, the more they would drop false pretenses. Having seen the negative side of human behavior—immaturity, destructiveness, regression, and antisocial behavior—he still maintained that people in general were positive and constructive, moving forward toward self-actualization, and growing toward maturity. Most rewarding to Rogers were the times when his clients discovered their positive directions in life.

Therefore the child-centered counselor refrains from giving advice or solutions, diagnosing, interpreting, moralizing, and making judgments, which would defeat the plan for teaching clients how to counsel themselves and imply that the counselors know and understand their clients better than the clients know themselves—an assumption totally out of line with Rogers's view. Instead, child-centered counselors use the methods of (1) active and passive listening, (2) reflection of thoughts and feelings, (3) clarification, (4) summarization, (5) confrontation of contradictions, and (6) general or open leads that help client self-exploration. Many of those skills are outlined in Chapter 3; below we turn our attention to a model for listening.

The major technique for child-centered counseling is active listening, which lets the client know that the counselor is hearing and understanding correctly what the client is saying. Active listening is especially important for counseling children. If the counselor fails to receive the correct message, the child attempts to reteach it to the counselor. Once counselor and child agree that the counselor has the story straight and that the counseling service will be helpful, counseling can continue.

Carkhuff (1973, 1981) systematized Rogers's concept of active listening (reflection) into a highly understandable, usable model (Table 6-1). Carkhuff believes that counselors typically respond on any one of the five levels relating to the three phases of counseling: Phase I is where you are now in your life; Phase II is where you would like to be; and Phase III is planning how to get from Phase I to Phase II. He classified Levels 1 and 2 as harmful, Level 3 as break even, and Levels 4 and 5 as helpful. It is often assumed that the worst thing that can happen in counseling is that clients show no change. However, this is not true. The conditions of clients who receive a preponderance of Level 1 and 2 responses could grow worse as the result of counseling.

Level 1 and 2 responses in Carkhuff's model also appear in Gordon's (1974) "dirty dozen" list of responses that tend to close or inhibit further communication: (1) ordering, directing; (2) warning, threatening, stating consequences; (3) moralizing, shoulds, oughts; (4) advising, giving suggestions and solutions; (5) messages of logic, counterarguments; (6) judging, criticizing; (7) praising, buttering up; (8) name-calling, ridiculing; (9) psychoanalyzing; (10) reassuring, giving sympathy, consoling; (11) probing: "who, what, when, where, why?"; and (12) humor, distracting, withdrawing.

TABLE 6-1 FIVE LEVELS OF COMMUNICATION

Levels	Phase I	Phase II	Phase III
	Thoughts and feelings about where you are now	Thoughts and feelings about where you would like to be	Plans for getting from where you are to where you would like to be
1			
2			X
3	X		
4	X	X	
5	X	X	X

Note: The Xs indicate which phases of counseling are treated by each of the five levels of communication.

Level 1 responses tend to discount what a person is feeling and thinking with statements such as:

- "Oh, don't worry about that. Things will work out."
- "If you think you have a problem, listen to this."
- "You must have done something to make Mrs. Jones treat you that way."

Level 1 responses may also be indications that the counselor simply was not listening. As such, Level 1 responses do not help with any of the three counseling phases in Table 6-1.

Level 2 responses are messages that give advice and solutions to problems. These responses do not allow the counselor and the client to fully explore the problem situation so are not helpful. Ignoring the active listening process deprives clients of the opportunity to work out their own solutions to their problems. Level 2 responses keep clients dependent on the counselor's authority and prevent clients from learning to counsel themselves. Typical Level 2 responses include the following:

- "You need to study harder."
- "You should eat better."
- "You should be more assertive."
- "Why don't you make more friends?"
- "How would you like your brother to treat you the way you treat him?"

Even though the advice may be excellent, the client—child or adult—may not have the skills to do what you suggest. The advice clients seek may often be something they already know but wish they did not. Moreover, rebellious children and adolescents may work especially hard to show that your advice is ineffective, just to receive the satisfaction of knowing that an "expert" counselor is no more successful than they are in solving day-to-day problems. We do, however, want to distinguish between giving advice and giving information. Information could be news about a job opening. Advice, in contrast, could be, "I think you need to quit your job." In summary, Levels 1 and 2 are ill-advised attempts to disregard or fix the client's problem.

Level 3 responses are classified as break-even points in the counseling process; they are neither harmful nor helpful. However, these responses provide bridges to further conversation and exploration in the counseling process; they are the door openers and invitations to discuss concerns in more depth.

Level 3 responses reflect what the client is thinking and feeling about the present status of the problem; for example, "You are feeling discouraged because you haven't been able to make good grades in math." Such responses are checkpoints for counselors in determining whether they are hearing and understanding the client's problem. Either the client acknowledges that the counselor has understood the message correctly, or the client makes another attempt to relate the concern to the counselor. At this point in counseling, clients are teaching the counselors about their problems and are thereby learning more about their problems themselves.

According to Carkhuff's model, counselors make Level 3 responses when asking themselves whether the client is expressing pain or pleasure, then finding the correct feeling word to describe the pain or pleasure. Seven feeling words are listed in Figure 6-1. To build your counseling vocabulary, add three synonyms of your own under each word. In reflecting the client's feeling and thoughts, do not parrot the exact words of the client. An example of a level 3 response would be "You are sad because your grandparents are moving far away." Also counselors may find time used for a summary helpful and may begin with "Let's see if I understand what you have told me up to now."

Remember that the focus on feelings is to help clients to recognize and be aware of their feelings so they can use them as indicators of whether they are making good decisions and doing the behaviors they need to be doing. To ignore feelings is much like driving a car without paying attention to the red lights and gauges on the car's dashboard. Feelings are one of the best indicators that people have for helping them find direction in their lives. Children may prefer to discuss their feelings by selecting one of the faces on the feelings chart in Figure 6-1. In fact, they may prefer to draw a face that represents how they feel.

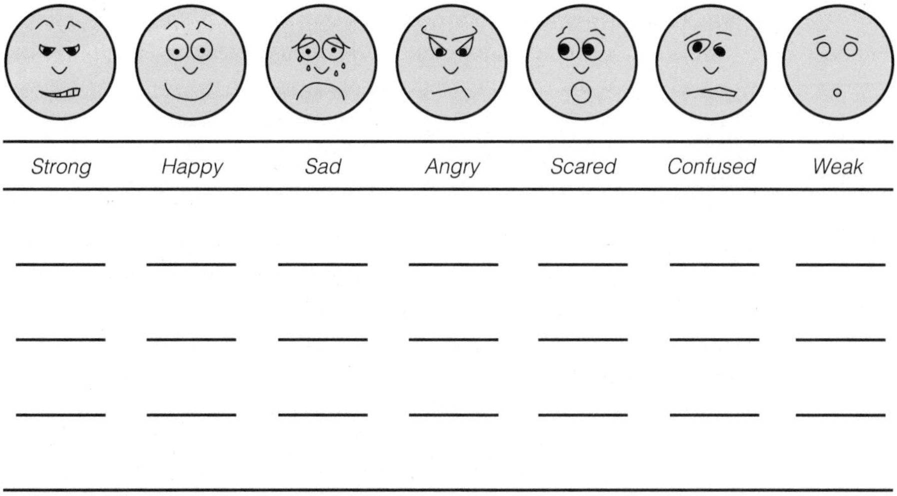

Strong	Happy	Sad	Angry	Scared	Confused	Weak
____	____	____	____	____	____	____
____	____	____	____	____	____	____
____	____	____	____	____	____	____

FIGURE 6-1 SYNONYMS FOR FEELING WORDS

Level 4 responses reflect an understanding of Phases I and II in Carkhuff's model; for example, "You are feeling discouraged because you haven't been able to make good grades in math, and you want to find a way to do better." Rephrase the responses in your own words as you summarize the client's thoughts and feelings.

Level 5 responses are appropriate when the client agrees that the counselor understands the problem or concern. Now it is time to assist the client in developing a plan of action. Reality therapy provides a good framework for planning after child-centered counseling has helped the client relate the concern to the counselor. Following is an example of a combined Level 5 response:

Child-centered therapy: You feel _____ because _____, and you want _____.

Reality therapy: Let's look at what you have been doing to solve your problem.

Combined child-centered and reality therapies: You feel discouraged because you haven't been able to make good grades in math, and you want to find a way to do better. Let's look at what you have been trying to do to make better grades in math.

The entire counseling interview cannot be accomplished in one response. Several sessions of Level 3 and 4 responses may be necessary before the problem is defined well enough to solve.

The success of the child-centered approach to counseling depends on the relationship between counselor and client. Counselors who do not trust or like children would be unable to create the curative conditions needed for this approach and would most likely be unsuccessful. Children, to a greater degree than adults, are sensitive to the real feelings and attitudes of others. They intuitively trust and open up to those who like and understand them. Phony expressions of understanding may not fool children, and certainly not adolescents, for very long. Virginia Axline's *Dibs: In Search of Self* (1964) presents a good example of a child-centered counseling method using play therapy.

Young children can distinguish between positive and negative behaviors and are able to choose the positive once the counselor has established an open dialogue in which feelings and emotions can be aired and conflicts resolved. Again, the counselor uses active listening to give children an opportunity to release emotions without feeling threatened by the counselor.

Listening carefully and observing the child increase the counselor's ability to understand what the child is trying to communicate. All clients convey both verbal and nonverbal messages, and the counselor needs to be alert to these messages. Nonverbal messages may be the most important clue to what the child is really feeling and trying to communicate. The focus on feeling is done to help clients learn how to recognize and use their feelings as indicators of whether they are making good choices and decisions in their lives. Lacking the verbal skills of most adults, children can benefit from bibliocounseling, storytelling, and play therapy (see Chapter 17) as aids to teaching about and communicating their problem situations.

Case Study[1]

Identification of the Problem

Ginger Wood, an 11-year-old girl in the sixth grade at Hill Middle School, was referred to the school counselor because her grades recently had fallen and she seemed depressed.

Individual and Background Information

Academic School records show that Ginger has been an A student for the past 3 years. On her last report card, however, her grades dropped to a C average.

Family Ginger is the elder of two children; her younger brother is 9. Her mother is an elementary school teacher, and her father is a computer systems analyst; they recently have separated.

Social Ginger is approximately 30 pounds overweight. She has a friendly personality, and teacher reports indicate that she has no problem relating to her peers.

Counseling Method

The counselor chose to use Rogers's (1965) child-centered counseling method. The counselor believes that Ginger's problem originates from emotional blocks. Her goal is to establish a warm relationship with Ginger, aid her in clarifying her thoughts and feelings, and enable her to solve her problems.

In this method, the counselor uses five basic techniques: (1) unconditional positive regard, (2) active listening, (3) reflection, (4) clarification, and (5) summarization.

Transcript

COUNSELOR: Hi, Ginger. I'm Susan Morgan. Your teacher, Ms. Lowe, told me that you might come to talk to me.

GINGER: Yeah, I decided to.

COUNSELOR: Do you know what a counselor's job is?

GINGER: Yeah, Ms. Lowe told me that you help people with their problems.

COUNSELOR: That's right. I try to teach people how to solve their own problems. Do you have something on your mind that you'd like to talk about?

GINGER: Well, I haven't been doing so well in school lately.

COUNSELOR: Yes, Ms. Lowe said you are normally an A student.

GINGER: I used to be, but not now. I made Cs on my last report card. My mom was really upset with me; she yelled at me and then grounded me.

COUNSELOR: It sounds as though she was angry with you because your grades went down.

GINGER: Well, not so much angry as unhappy. [Ginger looks ready to cry.]

---

[1]The case of Ginger was contributed by Anne Harvey.

COUNSELOR:	So she was disappointed that you weren't doing as well in school as you usually do, and this made you upset too.
GINGER:	I guess so. She maybe thought it was her fault too, and that could have made her feel worse.
COUNSELOR:	You mean that she felt responsible for your grades going down.
GINGER:	Well, maybe. Things aren't going so well at home. Mom and Dad aren't living together right now, and they may get a divorce. She hasn't had a lot of time for me and my brother lately. I guess she's really been scared about what is going to happen to us.
COUNSELOR:	The problem at home has made it tougher for you to do well at school because you're worried about what's happening.
GINGER:	Yeah, I think about it a lot. It's harder to study when I'm thinking about my mom and dad.
COUNSELOR:	It would be for me too. This must be a very hard situation for you to go through.
GINGER:	It sure is; everybody's mad. My little brother doesn't understand what's going on, and he cries a lot. Mom does too.
COUNSELOR:	So the whole family is hurting.
GINGER:	Well, I guess so. My dad doesn't seem to be, but why should he be? It's all his fault. He's getting what he wants.
COUNSELOR:	I guess he's the one who wants the divorce. It doesn't seem fair to the rest of you.
GINGER:	Yeah. He's got a girlfriend. My mom didn't even know anything about her until Daddy said he was leaving. I hate him! [Ginger starts to cry.] And that makes me feel even worse 'cause I know I shouldn't hate my father. I wish he were dead!
COUNSELOR:	[Handing her a tissue] So you're all torn up between the way you feel and the way you think you should feel.
GINGER:	Yeah, it's so hard to sort everything out. Do you think that makes me a bad person for me to hate my father?
COUNSELOR:	I think you are a good person who doesn't know what to do with all of her feelings right now. I'm wondering if you think you are a bad person.
GINGER:	Sometimes I do but then I think most of my friends would feel about the same way I do if they were in my shoes. In fact I know a girl who had the same thing happen last year and she was really unhappy all the time.
COUNSELOR:	Knowing your parents are fighting is a tough thing to handle.
GINGER:	Yes! That is exactly how it is. But I don't want to always be worrying and then making things worse because my grades are going down.
COUNSELOR:	You are concerned about things at home but want to concentrate on some school work too. How about if we think about ways you could start making better grades? Would you like to make another appointment to talk with me tomorrow to see what you have figured out by then?
GINGER:	Okay. Could I come back during lunch? Thanks, Ms. Morgan. I'm glad we talked about it. I feel a little better now.
COUNSELOR:	That will be fine.
GINGER:	Bye, Ms. Morgan, and thanks.
COUNSELOR:	You're welcome.

CHILD-CENTERED COUNSELING AND THE DEVELOPMENT OF SELF-ESTEEM[2]

A centerpiece of child-centered counseling, self-esteem can be increased by helping clients improve these two important areas in their lives. Radd (2014) developed a process to integrate self-esteem development into life skills education, a theme consistent with the application of child-centered theory to education. The process includes a series of activities that focus on teaching children about self-esteem and ways of applying that information to daily living.

Each of the activities has three steps. The counselor may choose to teach these statements in the first person or in the format given. The counselor begins by saying:

1. "All people are special and valuable because they are unique." This statement is discussed to teach the concept of unconditional valuing of people simply because they are people. For children in kindergarten through fourth grade, the words *special* and *different* are effective. "No matter what you do, you are still special because you are a person." For children in grades 5 through 8, variations of the words *unique* and *valuable* are effective. "If everyone were the same, it would be boring." "It is impossible for people to be better than other people because everyone is unique." In other words, "I'm the best me there is." The counselor continues with the second step.

2. "Because people are special and unique, they have a responsibility to *help* and *not hurt* themselves. People *show* they remember that they are important by the way they *choose* to act. If people choose to hurt themselves or others, they are forgetting that they are special. Likewise, if people choose to help themselves or others, they are remembering that they are special. What is special to you? How do you treat it? Do you help or hurt the things you think are special? Are your toys and computer games more important to you than people? Toys and games can be replaced, but people are different and irreplaceable. If you are remembering that you are as special as your toys, will you help or hurt yourself? When people help others, they are helping themselves. People hurt themselves when they hurt other people by forgetting that all people are special and unique. What people give is generally what they receive. The point we want to teach is that, if we like ourselves, we do not hurt ourselves or others." The counselor continues with the third step.

3. "People are responsible for 'watching' their actions to see if they are remembering the *truth* that they are special. People are 'with' themselves at all times and are accountable for remembering to treat themselves as important people. When people blame others for their actions, they are forgetting their responsibility to others. Who is with you all the time? Who will live with you forever? Who decides what happens to you? Who is the only one you can change?"

---

[2]Tommie R. Radd, Professor in the College of Education, University of Nebraska at Omaha, contributed this section.

Integrating Self-Esteem-Building Activities with the Child's Life

After the self-esteem activities are introduced into all environments children experience, the concepts are related to the children's daily life experiences and are associated with various situations, interactions, and other skills, such as decision making, self-control, and group cooperation.

The continuing process of relating self-esteem activities to a child's life is the *self-esteem series weave*. After this information is taught and processed, the children experience the integration of these concepts into their daily life experiences. The weaving process makes the concepts about self alive and relevant for children.

The self-esteem series weave process is implemented consistently, regardless of the counseling approach or setting. The self-esteem activities and weave can become the core of classroom group guidance, small-group counseling, individual counseling, and positive behavior management. The self-esteem activities are introduced and taught. Then, each subsequent session begins with a brief review of the self-esteem activities and a weave of the self-esteem activities into the process of the group or individual session.

An example of the self-esteem series weave process follows. Although it is part of the second individual counseling session with a third-grade student, the same process is used in classroom group guidance, in small-group counseling, and within the classroom behavior plan.

In the first session, the self-esteem activities were introduced and woven throughout the session. Bill was referred to counseling because of his problems with work completion. Following is an extract from Bill's counseling session:

BILL: I'm still in trouble with my teacher this week.

COUNSELOR: You are not feeling very good about this.

BILL: I think my teacher doesn't like me. She thinks I'm dumb.

COUNSELOR: Your bad feelings come from what your teacher thinks about you. I'm wondering how this fits in with what we talked about last week.

BILL: You said that I am special, no matter what I do, because no one else is like me anywhere in the world.

COUNSELOR: It seems this week you are feeling as though you're not special.

BILL: I don't know. My teacher doesn't think so.

COUNSELOR: So you think you are not important or special because you think your teacher does not think you are special.

BILL: Yeah. I know you think I'm special, but it is hard for me to think so when my teacher doesn't like me.

COUNSELOR: You may be showing that you forget you are special by the way you have been acting in your class. You and your teacher told me you have been deciding not to complete your work. I'm wondering if you have been hurting yourself with your choices.

BILL: I've been hurting myself because I'm not doing my work. But other people aren't doing their work and they don't get picked on.

COUNSELOR: It sounds as though you feel cheated because the teacher likes the other children better than you and does not treat you fairly. Let's see if we can figure this out with the ideas we learned last week.

BILL: Okay.

COUNSELOR: I wonder if you remember what we said about whom children hurt when they choose not to do their work.

BILL: I think they are hurting themselves.

COUNSELOR: So, we could take a look at what happens to you when you don't do your work.

BILL: I guess it hurts me.

COUNSELOR: If you want to, we can think of some ways to help you stop hurting yourself.

BILL: Okay. Maybe I can ask the teacher for help when I get lost on my work, or I can get a friend to help me. I can ask for help remembering the homework too.

COUNSELOR: These ideas might help you. We need to know which ones you want to try.

BILL: I guess I just need to do what it takes to turn in all my assignments.

COUNSELOR: Next week we can see if you've been remembering to do all those things you need to do to help yourself. Maybe you could show me the work you get done each day.

BILL: Okay.

The process of integrating self-esteem building with life skill development is most effective if it becomes the focus and foundation of group guidance, group counseling, behavior management, and individual counseling (Radd, 2014). The consistent exposure of children to self-concept activities related to life experiences clarifies and personalizes these difficult concepts so they become part of the children's knowledge base. Once again, however, self-esteem development is best served by helping children improve their academic performance and develop more friendships.

MOTIVATIONAL INTERVIEWING

Motivational interviewing is a person-centered but directive approach for increasing intrinsic motivation to change by investigating and confronting ambivalence (Miller & Rollnick, 2013). This method mixes person-centered fundamentals of warmth and empathy and techniques of questioning and reflective listening. Motivational interviewing also incorporates goals about change and provides specific interventions to encourage the client toward behavioral change (Miller & Rollnick, 1991; Moyers & Rollnick, 2002).

Motivational interviewing grew from Miller becoming frustrated with his research on treatment with problem drinkers. Treatment groups and control groups had comparable outcomes. As his investigations continued, Miller discovered therapist empathy predicted client success better than any specific treatment did. His conclusion was that empathy and reflective listening were critical parts of effective brief therapy. Motivational interviewing avoids assessment and any direct attempts to sway the client who is allowed to control the agenda. The counselor's role is that of a partner who aids in the exploration of attitudes about change. Resistance is considered ambivalence to change (Zinbarg & Griffith, 2008). The goal of motivational interviewing is to help someone move away from the uncertainty through self-talk and consideration of advantages and disadvantages of changing.

Miller and Rollnick (2013) have delineated four principles of motivational interviewing.

1. The counselor uses reflective listening to convey understanding of the message and caring for the person.
2. The counselor must develop the discrepancy between the person's stated values and his or her current behavior. The perceived discrepancy creates motivation for change. Clients talk themselves into change.
3. The counselor addresses resistance with reflection rather than confrontation. Resistance is seen as clients expressing the current side of ambivalence. The counselor should not argue for change, but he or she should know that client resistance signals using a different response. Resistance indicates energy that needs to be redirected.
4. The counselor supports the client's self-efficacy by giving the message that the client is capable of change. The counselor builds confidence that change can happen and provides brief interventions that allow change and reinforce optimism. The client is the resource for answers and solutions (Presbury et al., 2007; Prochaska & Norcross, 2007, p. 155).

Strait et al. (2012) tested the effectiveness of motivational interviewing with 103 middle school students. Some of the students participated in a single motivational interviewing session related to academic performance. The remaining students were in a waitlist control condition. The students who received the treatment showed improvements in class participation, positive academic behavior, and higher math scores. The researchers concluded a single motivational interviewing session can have beneficial effects on academic behavior and could be an effective approach for adolescents.

One of the techniques of motivational interviewing is developing a motivational discrepancy between the current behaviors (real self) and the desired goals (ideal self). That type of discrepancy motivates change. The following is an example based on Miller and Rollnick (2013).

CLIENT: Maybe I did pick on her more than I thought. I never counted how many times I called her a name before.

COUNSELOR: You're surprised.

CLIENT: Yes, I didn't think about how many bad things she hears from me. But everyone talks trash to other people.

COUNSELOR: You're confused. On one hand you see you've been saying lots of hurtful things but on the other hand you know other folks do the same thing.

Motivational interviewing can be used early, as a prelude to treatment, as a stand-alone brief intervention, or in combination with other treatments (Prochaska & Norcross, 2007). It has been used with different groups of clients and in situations in which resistance is a factor (Seligman & Reichenberg, 2014). A meta-analysis of research over the past 25 years indicates the intervention often empowers reluctant clients to change (Lundahl, Kunz, Brownell, Tollefson, & Burke, 2010).

CHILD-CENTERED PLAY THERAPY

Virginia Axline (1947) translated the nondirective counseling approach of Carl Rogers to work with children. Her book *Dibs: In Search of Self* (1964) describes this play therapy model. As discussed previously, the philosophy of child-centered therapy incorporates the belief that each child inherently strives for growth and has the capacity for self-direction. Axline believed that each child has an internal, powerful drive toward complete self-realization. She suggested that the evidence of this would be the move toward maturity, independence, and self-direction. Children need a fertile environment to develop a well-adjusted personality (Carmichael, 2006). Therefore, the child-centered counselor trusts the child and creates an environment in which the child's inner direction and self-healing strength will surface. As Axline explained, child-centered play therapy (CCPT) is a way of being with children instead of doing something to them.

Landreth (2002) provides further details on the child-centered approach to play therapy. His definition follows:

> Play therapy is defined as a dynamic interpersonal relationship between a child (or person of any age) and a therapist trained in play therapy procedures who provides selected play materials and facilitates the development of a safe relationship for the child (or person of any age) to fully express and explore self (feelings, thoughts, experiences, and behaviors) through play, the child's natural medium of communication, for optimal growth and development. (p. 16)

Landreth (2012) says that CCPT is an attitude, a philosophy, and a way of being. This model is based on beliefs in the child's innate tendency toward growth, maturity, and capacity for self-directed healing and self-direction. The focus is on the relationship, which is central to the success or failure of counseling. In child-centered play therapy, the child leads. The counselor focuses on the child's strengths, reflects the child's feelings, and recognizes the power of warmth, caring acceptance, and sensitive understanding in their relationship. The counselor must be attentive, caring, healing, serving, and patient throughout the process (Carmichael, 2006). Basic principles of the child-centered relationship are as follows:

1. The counselor has a genuine interest in the child and builds a warm, caring relationship.
2. The counselor accepts the child unconditionally, not wishing the child were different.
3. The counselor institutes a feeling of safety and permissiveness in the relationship, allowing the child freedom to explore and express himself or herself.
4. The counselor maintains sensitivity to the child's feelings and reflects them in a way that increases the child's self-understanding.
5. The counselor strongly believes in the child's capacity to act responsibly and solve personal problems, and allows the child to do so.
6. The counselor trusts the inner direction of the child, allowing the child to lead the relationship and refusing to override the child's direction.
7. The counselor does not hurry the therapeutic process.
8. The counselor uses only the limits necessary for helping the child accept personal and appropriate responsibility (Axline, 1947; Landreth, 2012).

The counselor who practices CCPT expresses an attitude of being completely with the child, an emotional and verbal participant. The process involves the counselor being open to the child's experience by living out these messages:

I am here (nothing will distract me).
I hear you (I am listening carefully).
I understand you.
I care about you (Landreth, 2002).

Play Therapy: The Art of the Relationship (Landreth, 2012) contains details about accomplishing these goals and about setting up a play area. Landreth suggests that toys in the playroom should capture the child's creative and emotional expressiveness. Counselors should choose toys that can be used in a number of ways, that are sturdy, and that provide ways to explore life, test limits, develop self, and provide chances to gain self-control. He talks about real-life toys, acting out toys, and creative expression toys.

Children become familiar with their inner value when the counselor accepts the child. Child-centered play therapists create a place where children can play without interference, suggestions, solutions, or interpretation. They do not direct in even subtle ways and seldom ask questions in order to avoid moving the relationship toward the counselor's interest and away from the child's play. The counselor does not interpret play, does not label any items, and does not ask the child to explain anything. Child-centered play therapists track the child's play with comments that reflect only what the child is doing such as "You are putting that right there." Evaluation is avoided even if requested by the child. The counselor might respond with what is seen such as "You used many colors and covered the entire sheet."

Throughout the play therapy the counselor appreciates the process of play and encourages free expression so that the child can discover inner motivation. Counselors do set boundaries for what is not acceptable. The only limits would include prohibiting any dangerous, disruptive behavior. Additionally, taking materials out of the playroom or destroying the room or materials in it would be discouraged as would inappropriate displays of affection. When limits are needed, the counselor would state in a matter-of-fact way what is inappropriate rather than commanding the child. Sweeney and Landreth (2009) summarize the necessity of attending to the child's desire to stretch the limit because the counselor deals with intrinsic factors such as motivation, perception of self, independence, acceptance, and relationships with other people. Most importantly, the counselor believes the child will cooperate when he or she feels accepted.

Landreth (2012) provided specific steps for play therapists to use in setting limits in his ACT model. These steps should help in communicating understanding and acceptance of the child's motives, making the limit clear, and offering alternatives. "You would like to take the doll home with you, but the doll stays in the playroom so that you will have it next week."

Step 1 is Acknowledging the child's feelings and wishes; Step 2 is Communicating the limit; and Step 3 is Targeting acceptable alternatives. The following is an example:

CHILD: "I'm going to paint your face now."

A and C steps:

COUNSELOR: "You want to share your paint with me, but I'm not for painting."

CHILD: "But I want to...."

T step:

COUNSELOR: "You really want to use your paint more. You could draw something on that clown over there."

CHILD: "Oh, okay."

Kottman (2009) described five distinct phases of CCPT.

1. Children use play to express a range of negative feelings.
2. Children use play to express ambivalent feelings, usually fear or anger.
3. Children use play to express negative feelings, but the focus has shifted to specific targets like parents or teachers or the counselor.
4. Ambivalent feelings, both positive and negative, come back but now are directed toward parents, siblings, or others.
5. Positive feelings prevail with the child expressing negative emotions appropriately (p. 136).

Moustakas (1997) explains relationship play therapy as the creation of play dramas. Within the relationship, the counselor demonstrates acceptance, receptiveness, and openness, together with the skills of "listening and hearing, teaching and learning, directing and receiving, participating actively and quietly observing, confronting and letting be" (p. 2). He discusses the use of play therapy as a prevention strategy in which parents and teachers participate. The brief therapy—one to four play sessions—is supportive. The relationship and counseling process encourage self-disclosure, expression of feelings, and limits.

CCPT has been supported as effective across a range of problems (Bratton, Ray, Rhine, & Jones, 2005; Carmichael, 2006; Ray & Bratton, 2010) with the exception of severe autism or active schizophrenia (Guerney, 2001). Bratton et al. (2005) conducted a review of play therapy research outcomes comparing studies to identify overall treatment effects. VanFleet, Sywulak, and Sniscak (2010) summarized those findings as "play therapy is effective, nondirective play therapy is very effective and the inclusion of parents is highly effective" (p. 213). Some examples of that effectiveness follow.

Bratton et al. (2013) studied CCPT with low income preschool children who had disruptive behaviors such as aggression, destroying property, and attention problems. One group of children received therapy and the other group had reading mentors. Counselors used a CCPT protocol for a total of 17 to 21 sessions. Results based on teacher ratings indicated a significant decrease in disruptive behavior problems for the children who participated in CCPT. The authors noted this promising finding indicated child-centered play therapy as a responsive early mental health intervention for preschool children. Other studies have supported CCPT as an effective treatment for behavior problems in elementary children (Cochran,

Cochran, Nordling, McAdam, & Miller, 2010; Garza & Bratton, 2005; Ray, Blanco, Sullivan, & Holliman, 2009; Ray, Schottelkorb, & Tsai, 2007; Schottelkorb & Ray, 2009; Schumann, 2010).

Additionally, Baggerly and Jenkins (2009) investigated the effectiveness of CCPT and children who were homeless. Their results indicated improvement in self-limiting and positive trends in development with the 36 elementary children who participated.

Johnson, McLeod, and Fall (1997) studied CCPT with children who had special needs. Six children were identified in two rural Midwestern elementary schools. Six weekly 30-minute play therapy sessions were held. The transcripts and videotapes of the sessions were analyzed for expression of feelings and of control. These authors concluded that nondirective child-centered play therapy was effective in allowing the children chances to express feelings, experience control, and develop coping skills. They also noted that therapists' perceptions were altered more favorably toward the children. Griffith (1997) discusses a client-centered empowerment model of play therapy for working with children who have been sexually abused. Her report also documents the effectiveness of CCPT.

DIVERSITY APPLICATIONS OF CHILD-CENTERED COUNSELING

Cornelius-White (2005, 2007) stated that person-centered counselor facilitates learning regardless of age, race, ethnicity, or geographic location. As a result of this approach incorporating a respectful, accepting attitudes as well as an emphasis on understanding the person from that person's frame of reference, people from diverse background are likely to respond well.

Cardemil and Battle (2003) recommend suspending preconceptions about a client's race/ethnicity and suggest that counselors should engage clients in an open dialogue on these facts. Moodley, Lago, and Talahite (2004) agree that child-centered counseling is based on understanding the uniqueness of the individual through empathic understanding, genuineness, and unconditional positive regard by the therapist. Just as clients experience their environment in their own unique way, the child-centered counselor's role is to perceive the client unlike any client seen before.

Person-centered counseling has been effective not only in the United States but also in African, African American, Puerto Rican, Japanese, Chinese, Canadian, Egyptian, white and black South Africans, and Austrian cultures. Several researchers (Abdel-Tawab & Roter, 2002; Follensbee, Draguns, & Danish, 1986; Hayashi, Kuno, Osawa, Shimizu, & Suetake, 1998; Hill-Hain & Rogers, 1988; Jenni, 1999; Spangenberg, 2003; Stipsits & Hutterer, 1989; Waxer, 1989) have provided information relative to child-centered counseling in their cultures. The effectiveness of child-centered play therapy has been documented with African American boys (Baggerly & Parker, 2005), Chinese children (Shen, 2002, 2010), Latino children (Garza, 2010; Garza & Bratton, 2005), and Japanese children (Ogawa, 2007).

Approximately 200 organizations and training centers located around the world are dedicated to the research and application of principles developed by Rogers (Kirschenbaum & Jourdan, 2005). Landreth (2009) suggested the child-centered approach may be uniquely suited for children from different economic and ethnic backgrounds because the counselor's philosophy remains constant. Counselors offer acceptance and understanding, regardless of a person's ethnicity, circumstance, or concern. They posit that the child is free to communicate through play in a way that is comfortable and typical for the child, including any cultural variations in play or expression.

Fall et al. (2010) and Sue and Sue (2008) point out that child-centered counseling can be problematic for clients from cultures that expect their "counselors" to be experts who will advise and guide them regarding decisions to be made and problems to be solved. In other words, when expectations are not met, clients are likely to become frustrated with the child-centered process and drop out of counseling. Additionally some groups do not value insight and may find self-actualization a goal not suited to their ideals and goals. The expression of emotions may be difficult for some and indeed some cultures encourage the suppression of feelings. Those clients may be uncomfortable with empathic responses so that counselors need to adapt to the person's needs.

Cain (2010) advised that person-centered counseling has strengths that are relevant to people from diverse backgrounds. Seligman and Reichenberg (2014) agree that person-centered theory reflects American ideals and many aspects of the approach are relevant across diverse societies. Those relevant aspects include the following:

- Emphasis on a people's rights to their own feelings and thoughts
- Significance of respect, genuineness, acceptance, and empathy
- Focus on the person's own experience and viewpoint
- Attention to personal growth and development
- Interest in relationships and similarities among people
- Attention to awareness of the present time (p. 164)

Sweeney and Landreth (2009) and Fall et al. (2010) suggested that counselors explain their approach to therapy and discuss how that approach fits with the client's expectations. People in action-oriented cultures who are frustrated with the child-centered process will need to be told that child-centered counseling is designed to solve immediate problems by teaching clients how to be their own counselors. However, this theory may be inherently incompatible with cultures that value collective wisdom rather than inner wisdom.

Finally Raskin et al. (2014) conclude that person-centered counselors who stay true to core conditions for all clients and maintain their openness, appreciation, and respect for all kinds of differences will build an effective therapeutic relationship.

EVALUATION OF PERSON-CENTERED COUNSELING

Carl Rogers has had profound impact on the practice of counseling. He was the first person to study counseling effectiveness (Hergenhahn & Alson, 2007) opening the field to investigations that continue today. He systematically used transcripts from recorded session to study the process of counseling and worked with his associates at the University of Chicago Counseling Center to test locus of evaluation, counseling process, and core conditions of counseling (Murdock, 2013). Across all his work

Rogers maintained an unfaltering emphasis on the importance of person-centered relationships everywhere.

Seligman and Reichenberg (2014) noted that Rogers's explanations of the counseling relationship has influenced all theories and listed these as notable contributions:

- His development of a comprehensive theory of *self*.
- His beliefs in the dignity and worth of each person and in the innate progression toward actualization and growth
- A theory that is appropriate and relevant over 70 years after its inception
- A solid foundation on which other theories can build
- An optimistic, affirming, and positive view of human beings
- Outcome research that supports the major tenets of person-centered counseling
- A theory that can easily be integrated into other treatment approaches

Rogers initiated investigations into *process research*, research that focuses on the interactions between client and counselor. Most of that line of research has focused on empathy, genuineness, and positive regard that Rogers (1957) considered facilitative interpersonal condition "necessary and sufficient conditions of therapeutic personality change." Researchers have demonstrated those conditions contribute to positive outcomes but are neither necessary nor sufficient (Kirschenbaum & Jourdan, 2005; Prochaska & Norcross, 2014). Client perception of the counselor's empathy is a strong indicator of successful therapy (Elliott, Bohart, Watson, & Greenberg, 2011) and the facilitative conditions are the common factors across many forms of counseling (see Chapter 3). Raskin et al. (2014) echo the strong support researchers have found for empathic understanding and positive regard.

Outcome research tracks the effectiveness of therapy. Reviews of person-centered therapy indicate it is more effective than no treatment and to a placebo treatment (Prochaska & Norcross, 2014). In a meta-analysis on the treatment of mild to moderate depression, nondirective therapies such as person-centered worked just about as well as any other treatment (Cuijpers et al., 2012). In a large study of people who were suffering from anxiety and depression, all patients treated with person-centered, cognitive-behavioral, and psychodynamic therapies had equivalent outcomes (Stiles, Barkham, Mellor-Clark, & Connell, 2008).

In an expanded study of humanistic therapies that assessed almost 180 outcome studies, Elliott and Freire (2010) found that those who participated in person-centered counseling changed more than untreated clients, with large pre-post change in clients and with therapeutic gains that were maintained over time. They concluded the studies show strong support for person-centered counseling. In a more recent analysis Elliott, Greenberg, Watson, Timulak, and Freire (2013) stated that person-centered therapy "appeared to be consistently, statistically and practically equivalent in effectiveness to cognitive-behavioral therapy" (p. 502). Those authors also reviewed studies for specific client problems and determined strong support for humanistic therapies in treating depression, relationship problems, coping with chronic health problems, and psychosis.

However the effectiveness of person-centered counseling with children and adolescents has less robust results. Weiss and Weisz (1995, 2004) found the effectiveness of child-centered therapy as better than no treatment but lower than behavioral, cognitive, and parent-training interventions. Yet Raskin and Rogers (2005) identified positive changes in self-acceptance and internal evaluations in short-term child-centered counseling. Others have also reported progress with children in only a few sessions (Barlow, Strother, & Landreth, 1985; Ray, Schottelkorb, & Tsai, 2007; Shen, 2002). Additionally, the reported outcomes of child-centered play therapy discussed earlier indicate that earlier analysis by Weiss and Weisz have been questioned (Shirk & Russell, 1992; Wampold, 2001) with the conclusion that research evaluations of child therapy underrepresent the actual practice of therapy and in research studies (Prochaska & Norcross, 2014).

Presbury et al. (2007) reported that the efficacy of the child-centered approach occurs in the counseling relationship, the use of the core conditions and attitudes, and the flexibility and openness of the counselor. Prochaska and Norcross (2003) noted that the combination of humanistic and cognitive approaches was the second-most utilized combination of theory, and the blend of behavioral and humanistic was the fourth. Cepeda and Davenport (2006) provided an example of this combination with their integration of person-centered therapy with solution-focused counseling.

These studies confirm the potential for client-centered counseling. Those practitioners who use this approach may wish to assess their progress with the child clients. Landreth (2012) suggested these guidelines to determine if someone is benefiting from therapy:

1. Is this person becoming less defensive, more open to his or her experiences?
2. Is this person more able to take responsibility for his or her feelings and actions?
3. Is this person becoming less rigid, more tolerant or accepting of self, others, and the world?
4. Is this person becoming more independent, more self-directing?
5. Is the person becoming more objective, more rational?
6. Is the person more able to live in and enjoy the present?
7. Is the person less anxious, less fearful, less unhappy than when he or she entered therapy?

Two examples of the results of person-centered therapy follow.

Myers (2000) has found that clients in her phenomenological study on the experience of being heard put high values on their therapists' active listening, feedback, and expressions of empathy. They reported that these methods gave them room for self-exploration, the opportunity to move further and deeper into their own experience, and the feelings of safety, trust, and being understood, all of which were reported as being necessary to give them the freedom to examine their personal experiences.

In a similar vein, Siebert (2000) studied the efficacy of empathy on the "recovery" of an 18-year-old woman who had been diagnosed as an "acute paranoid schizophrenic" on her commitment to a hospital by her parents. She was telling her parents that God told her she was to have his baby. Her physician and the hospital staff thought she should be committed to the state psychiatric hospital, where they predicted she would spend the rest of her life. Siebert viewed this as an opportunity to try something different in his interview with her, because she was headed to what he termed "the snake pit" anyway. It was definitely a "What have you got to lose?" situation for him. Before his interview with the patient, he developed a game plan of four questions for himself. What would happen if:

- I just listened to her and did not allow my mind to put any psychiatric labels on her?
- I talked to her believing that she could turn out to be my best friend?
- I accepted everything she reports about herself as being the truth?
- I questioned her to find out whether there is a link between her self-esteem, the workings of her mind, and the way others have been treating her?

Siebert, following the child-centered counseling model he designed for himself, brought about dramatic improvement in his patient, and she was not committed to the state hospital. Several days after that first session, she mentioned to Siebert that she had been doing a lot of thinking about what they had talked about. She asked, "I've been wondering, do you think I imagined God's voice to make myself feel better?" This case led Siebert to do a lot of thinking also.

SUMMARY

Child-centered counselors are optimistic. They value the dignity and inherent worth of each person and they trust that all people know what they need to grow toward their best selves. People get in trouble when their need for the love of others is based on external conditions of worth such as "being a good boy" or "making perfect grades." When a child internalizes those conditions as standards that define him, that opposes his own regard for self and the discrepancy promotes uncertainty of his worth. Child-centered counselors create an atmosphere through their congruence, empathy, and unconditional positive regard. They focus on the present rather than the past or future and allow the child to lead the way from the state of incongruence to a more fully functioning being. Rogers established the collaborative alliance as the most important strategy for change and those core conditions of empathy, congruence, and unconditional positive regard are considered necessary for building and maintaining a therapeutic relationship, regardless of theoretical approach (Seligman & Reichenberg, 2014).

Kirschenbaum and Jourdan (2005) and Kirschenbaum (2009), reviewing the history and current status of child-centered counseling, noted that Rogers was the first to tape record and transcribe entire sessions of therapy for research and teaching. He was the first psychotherapist to receive both the APA's Distinguished Scientific Contribution Award and its Distinguished Professional Contribution Award. Currently, numerous books, book chapters, and journal articles have been published about Rogers's work, many since his death in 2004.

Rogers (2007) gave a simple explanation of why the person-centered attitude is effective in therapy. In his words:

> As the therapist listens to the client, the client comes more to listen to himself or herself; as the therapist cares with a more unconditional caring for the client, the client's self-worth begins to develop. As the client responds in herself in both those ways then the client is becoming more real, more congruent, more expressing of what is actually going on inside. (p. 4)

INTRODUCTION TO CHILD-CENTERED COUNSELING VIDEO

To gain a more in-depth understanding of the concepts in this chapter, visit www .cengage.com/counseling/henderson to view a short clip of an actual therapist–client session demonstrating child-centered counseling.

WEB SITES FOR CHILD-CENTERED COUNSELING

Internet addresses frequently change. To find the sites listed here, visit www.cengage .com/counseling/henderson for an updated list of Internet addresses and direct links to relevant sites.

Center for Studies of the Person

Association for the Development of the Person-Centered Approach (ADPCA)

Association for Humanistic Psychology (AHP)

Association for Play Therapy (APT)

Carl Rogers

Natalie Rogers

Motivational Interviewing

Roots of Empathy

REFERENCES

Abdel-Tawab, N., & Roter, D. (2002). The relevance of client-centered communication to family planning settings in developing countries: Lessons from the Egyptian experience. *Social Science and Medicine, 54,* 1357–1368.

Axline, V. (1947). *Play therapy: The inner dynamics of childhood.* Boston: Houghton Mifflin.

Axline, V. (1964). *Dibs: In search of self.* Boston: Houghton Mifflin.

Baggerly, J., & Jenkins, W. W. (2009). The effectiveness of child-centered play therapy on developmental and diagnostic factors in children who are homeless. *International Journal of Play Therapy, 18*(1), 45–55. doi:10.1037/a0013878

Baggerly, J., & Parker, M. (2005). Child-centered group play therapy with African American boys at the elementary school level. *Journal of Counseling & Development, 83,* 387–396.

Barlow, K., Strother, J., & Landreth, G. (1985). Child-centered play therapy: Nancy from baldness to curls. *School Counselor, 32,* 347–356.

Bratton, S. C., Ceballos, P. L., & Ferebee, K. W. (2009). Integration of structured expressive activities within a humanistic group play therapy format for preadolescents. *The Journal for Specialists in Group Work, 34,* 251–275 doi:10.1080/0193920903033487

Bratton, S. C., Ceballos, P. L., Sheely-Moore, A. I., Meany-Walen, K., & Pronchenko, Y., & Jones, L. D. (2013). Head start early mental health intervention: Effects of child-centered play therapy on disruptive behaviors. *International Journal of Play Therapy, 22,* 28–42. doi:10.1037/a0030318

Bratton, S. C., Ray, D., Rhine, T., & Jones, L. (2005). The efficacy of play therapy with children: A meta-analytic review of treatment outcomes. *Professional Psychology: Research and Practice, 36*(4), 376–390.

Cain, D. J. (2010). *Person-centered psychotherapies*. Washington, DC: American Psychological Association.

Cardemil, E., & Battle, C. (2003). Guess who's coming to therapy? Getting comfortable with conversations about race and ethnicity in psychotherapy. *Professional Psychology: Research and Practice, 34*, 278–286.

Carkhuff, R. (1973, March). Human achievement, educational achievement, career achievement: Essential ingredients of elementary school guidance. Paper presented at the National Elementary School Guidance conference, Louisville, KY.

Carkhuff, R. (1981, April). Creating and researching community based helping programs. Paper presented at the American Personnel and Guidance Association convention, St. Louis, MO.

Carmichael, K. D. (2006). *Play therapy: An introduction*. Upper Saddle River, NJ: Prentice Hall.

Cepeda, L. M., & Davenport, D. S. (2006). Person-centered therapy and solution-focused brief therapy: An integration of present and future awareness. *Psychotherapy: Theory, Research, Practice, Training, 43*, 1–12.

Cochran, J. L., Cochran, N. H., Nordling, W. J., McAdam, A., & Miller, D. T. (2010). Two case studies of child-centered play therapy for children referred with highly disruptive behavior. *International Journal of Play Therapy, 19*, 130–143. doi: 10.1037/a0019119

Cornelius-White, J. H. D. (2005). Teaching person-centered multicultural counseling. *The Journal of Humanistic Counseling, Education, and Development, 44*, 225–239.

Cornelius-White, J. H. D. (2007). Learner-centered teacher-student relationships are effective: A meta-analysis. *Review of Educational Research, 77*, 113–143.

Cuijpers, P., Driessen, E., Hollon, S. D., et al. (2012). The efficacy of non-directive supportive therapy for adult depression: A Meta-analysis. *Clinical Psychology Review, 32*, 280–291.

Elliot, R., Bohart, A. C., Watson, J. C., & Greenberg, L. S. (2011). Empathy. In J. C. Norcross (Ed.), *Psychotherapy relationships that work* (2nd ed., pp. 132–151). New York: Oxford University Press.

Elliott, R. & Freire, E. (2010). The effectiveness of person-centered and experiential therapies: A review of the meta-analyses. In M. Cooper, J. C. Watson, & D. Hölldampf (Eds.), *Person-centered and experiential therapies work: A review of the research on counseling, psychotherapy, and related practices* (pp. 1–15). Ross-on-Wye, UK: PCCS Books.

Elliott, R., Greenberg, L. S., Watson, J., Timulak, L., & Freire, E. (2013). Research on humanistic-experiential psychotherapies. In M. J. Lambert (Ed.), *Bergin and Garfield's Handbook of Psychotherapy and Behavior Change* (6th ed.). Hoboken, NJ: John Wiley & Sons.

Fall, K. A., Holden, J. M., & Marquis, A. (2010). *Theoretical models of counseling and psychotherapy* (2nd ed.). New York: Brunner Routledge.

Follensbee, R. W. Jr., Draguns, J. G., & Danish, S. J. (1986). Impact of two types of counselor intervention on Black American, Puerto Rican, and Anglo-American analogue clients. *Journal of Counseling Psychology, 33*, 446–453.

Garza, Y. (2010). School-based child-centered play therapy with Hispanic children. In J. N. Baggerly, D. C. Ray, & S. C. Bratton (Eds.), *Child-centered play therapy research: The evidence base for effective practice* (pp. 177–192). Hoboken, NJ: John Wiley & Sons.

Garza, Y., & Bratton, S. (2005). School-based child-centered play therapy with Hispanic children: Outcomes and cultural consideration. *International Journal of Play Therapy, 14*, 51–80.

Gordon, T. (1974). *Teacher effectiveness training*. New York: Wyden.

Griffith, M. (1997). Empowering techniques of play therapy: A method for working with sexually abused children. *Journal of Mental Health Counseling, 19*, 130–143.

Guerney, L. F. (2001). Child-centered play therapy. *International Journal of Play Therapy, 10*, 13–31.

Hayashi, S., Kuno, T., Osawa, M., Shimizu, M., & Suetake, Y. (1998). Client-centered therapy in Japan: Fujio Tomoda and Taoism. *Journal of Humanistic Psychology, 38*, 103–124.

Hergenhahn, B. R., & Olson, M. H. (2007). *An introduction to the theories of personality* (7th ed.). Upper Saddle River, NJ: Pearson Prentice Hall.

Hill-Hain, A., & Rogers, C. (1988). A dialogue with Carl Rogers: Cross-cultural challenges of facilitating child-centered groups in South Africa. *Journal for Specialists in Group Work*, *13*, 62–69.

Hutchby, I. (2005). "Active Listening": Formulations and the elicitation of feelings-talk in child counseling. *Research on Language and Social Interaction*, *38*, 303–329.

Jenni, C. (1999). Psychologists in China: National transformation and humanistic psychology. *Journal of Humanistic Psychology*, *39*, 26–47.

Johnson, L., McLeod, E. H., & Fall, M. (1997). Play therapy with labeled children in the schools. *Professional School Counseling*, *1*, 31–34.

Kirschenbaum, H. (2009). *The life and work of Carl Rogers*. Alexandria, VA: American Counseling Association.

Kirschenbaum, H., & Jourdan, A. (2005). The current status of Carl Rogers and the child-centered approach. *Psychotherapy: Theory, Research, Practice, Training*, *42*, 37–51.

Kottman, T. (2009). Play therapy. In A.Vernon (Ed.), *Counseling children & adolescents* (4th ed., pp. 123–146). Denver, CO: Love Publishing.

Landreth, G. (2002). *Play therapy: The art of relationship* (2nd ed.). New York: Routledge.

Landreth, G. (2009). Child Parent Relationship Therapy (CPRT). New York: Routledge.

Landreth, G. (2012). *Play therapy: The art of relationship* (3rd ed.). New York: Routledge.

Lundahl, B., Limz. C., Brownell, C., Tollefson, D., & Burke, B. I. (2010). A meta-analysis of motivational interviewing: Twenty-five years of empirical studies. *Research on Social Work Practice*, *22*, 137–160.

Miller, W. R., & Rollnick, S. (1991). *Motivational interviewing: Preparing people for change*. New York: Guilford.

Miller, W. R., & Rollnick, S. (2013). *Motivational interviewing: Preparing people for change* (3rd ed.). New York: Guilford Press.

Moodley, R., Lago, C., & Talahite, A. (2004). *Carl Rogers counsels a black client: Race and culture in child-centered counseling*. Ross-on-Wye, UK: PCCS Books Ltd.

Moustakas, C. (1997). *Relationship play therapy*. Northvale, NJ: Jason Aronson, Inc.

Moyers, T. B., & Rollnick, S. (2002). A motivational interviewing perspective on resistance in psychotherapy. *Journal of Clinical Psychology: In Session*, *58*, 185–194.

Murdock, N. L. (2013). *Theories of counseling and psychotherapy: A case approach* (3rd ed.). Upper Saddle River, NJ: Pearson.

Myers, S. (2000). Empathic listening: Reports on the experience of being heard. *Journal of Humanistic Psychology*, *40*, 147–173.

Ogawa, Y. (2007). Effectiveness of child-centered play therapy with Japanese children in the United States. *Dissertation Abstracts International*, *68*, 884.

Presbury, J. H., McKee, J. E., & Echterling, L. G. (2007). Person-centered approaches. In H. T. Prout & D. T. Brown (Eds.), *Counseling and psychotherapy with children and adolescents: Theory and practice for school and clinical settings* (4th ed., pp. 180–240). Hoboken, NJ: Wiley.

Prochaska, J. O., & Norcross, J. C. (2003). *Systems of psychotherapy: A transtheoretical analysis* (5th ed.). Pacific Grove, CA: Brooks/Cole.

Prochaska, J. O., & Norcross, J. C. (2014). *Systems of psychotherapy: A transtheoretical analysis* (8th ed.). Pacific Grove, CA: Brooks/Cole.

Radd, T. R. (2014). *Teaching and counseling for today's world: Pre-K-12 and beyond* (2nd ed.). Omaha, NE: Grow with Guidance.

Raskin, N., & Rogers, C. (2005). Person-centered therapy. In R.Corsini & D.Wedding (Eds.), *Current Psychotherapies* (7th ed., pp. 130–165). Belmont, CA: Brooks/Cole.

Raskin, N., Rogers, C., & Witty, M. C. (2014). Client-centered therapy. In R. J.Corsini & D.Wedding (Eds.), *Current psychotherapies* (10th ed., pp. 95–150). Belmont, CA: Brooks/Cole.

Ray, D. C., Blanco, P. J., Sullivan, J. M., & Holliman, R. (2009). An exploratory study of child-centered play therapy with aggressive children. *International Journal of Play Therapy, 18*, 162–175. doi:10.1037/a0014742

Ray, D. C., & Bratton, S. C. (2010). What the research shows about play therapy: Twenty-first century update. In J. N. Baggerly, D. C. Ray, & S. C. Bratton (Eds.), *Child-centered play therapy research: The evidence base for effective practice* (pp. 3–33). Hoboken, NJ: Wiley.

Ray, D., Schottelkorb, A., & Tsai, M. (2007). Play therapy with children exhibiting symptoms of attention deficit hyperactivity disorder. *International Journal of Play Therapy, 11*, 43–63.

Rogers, C. R. (1939). *The clinical treatment of the problem child*. Boston: Houghton Mifflin.

Rogers, C. R. (1942). *Counseling and psychotherapy*. Boston: Houghton Mifflin.

Rogers, C. R. (1951). *Client-centered therapy*. Boston: Houghton Mifflin.

Rogers, C. R. (1957). The necessary and sufficient conditions of therapeutic personality change. *Journal of Consulting Psychology, 21*, 95–103.

Rogers, C.R. (1959). A theory of therapy, personality, and interpersonal relationship, as developed in the client-centered framework. In S. Koch (Ed.), *Psychology: A study of a science: Formulations of the person and the social context* (Vol. 111, pp. 184–256). New York: McGraw Hill.

Rogers, C. R. (1961). *On becoming a person*. Boston: Houghton Mifflin.

Rogers, C. R. (1967). The conditions of change from a client-centered viewpoint. In B.Berenson & R.Carkhuff (Eds.), *Sources of gain in counseling and psychotherapy*. New York: Holt, Rinehart, & Winston.

Rogers, C. R. (1977). *Carl Rogers on personal power: Inner strength and its revolutionary impact*. New York: Delacorte.

Rogers, C. R (1980). *A way of being*. Boston: Houghton Mifflin.

Rogers, C. R. (1983). *Freedom to learn for the 80's*. Columbus, OH: Merrill.

Rogers, C. R. (1992). The necessary and sufficient conditions of therapeutic personality change. *Journal of Consulting and Clinical Psychology, 60*, 827–832.

Rogers, C. R. (1994). Rogers's quote. *Journal of Humanistic Education and Development, 32*, 189.

Rogers, C. R. (1995). What understanding and acceptance mean to me. Illinois Personnel and Guidance Association Meeting (1956, Urbana, Illinois). *Journal of Humanistic Psychology, 35*, 7–22.

Rogers, C. R., (2007). *Counseling and psychotherapy: Newer concepts in practice*. Boston: Houghton Mifflin.

Schottelkorb, A. A., & Ray, D. C. (2009). ADHD symptom reduction in elementary students: A single-case effectiveness design. *Professional School Counseling, 13*, 11–22. doi: 10.5330/PSC.n.2010-13.11

Schumann, B. (2010). Effectiveness of child centered play therapy for children referred for aggression. In J. N. Baggerly, D. C. Ray, & S. C. Bratton (Eds.), *Child-centered play therapy research: The evidence base for effective practice* (pp. 193–208).

Seligman, L., & Reichenberg, L. W. (2014). *Theories of counseling and psychotherapy: Systems, strategies and skills* (4th ed.). Upper Saddle River, NJ: Pearson.

Shen, Y. (2002). Short-term group play therapy with Chinese earthquake victims: Effects on anxiety, depression and adjustment. *International Journal of Play Therapy, 11*, 43–63.

Shen, Y. (2010). Effects of post-earthquake group play therapy with Chinese children. In J. N. Baggerly, D. C.Ray, & S. C.Bratton (Eds.), *Child-centered play therapy research: The evidence base for effective practice* (pp. 85–104). Hoboken, NJ: John Wiley & Sons.

Siebert, A. (2000). How non-diagnostic listening led to a rapid "recovery" from paranoid schizophrenia: What is wrong with psychiatry? *Journal of Humanistic Psychology, 40,* 34–58.

Spangenberg, J. (2003). The cross-cultural relevance of child-centered counseling in post-apartheid South Africa. *Journal of Counseling & Development, 81,* 48–54.

Stiles, W. B., Barkham, M., Mellor-Clark, J., & Connell, J. (2008). Effectiveness of cognitive-behavioural, person-centred, and psychodynamic therapies in UK primary-care routine practice: Replication in a larger sample. *Psychological Medicine, 38,* 677–688.

Stipsits, R., & Hutterer, R. (1989). The child-centered approach in Austria. *Child-centered Review, 4,* 475–487.

Strait, G. G., Smith, B. H., McQuillin, S., Terry, J., Swan, S., & Malone, P. S. (2012). A randomized trial of motivational interviewing to improve middle school students' academic performance. *Journal of Community Psychology, 40*(8), 1032–1039. doi:10.1002/jcop.21511

Sweeney, D. S., & Landreth, G. L. (2009). Child-centered play therapy. In K. J. O'Connor & L. D. Braverman (Eds.), *Play therapy theory and practice: Comparing theories and techniques* (pp. 123–162). Hoboken, NJ: Wiley.

VanFleet, R., Sywulak, A. E., & Sniscak, C. C. (2010). *Child-centered play therapy.* New York: The Guilford Press.

Wampold, B. E. (2001). *The great psychotherapy debate: Models, methods, and findings.* Mahwah, NJ: Erlbaum.

Waxer, P. H. (1989). Cantonese versus Canadian evaluation of directive and non-directive therapy. *Canadian Journal of Counseling, 23,* 263–271.

Weiss, B., & Weisz, J. R. (1995). Relative effectiveness of behavioral versus non-behavioral child psychotherapy. *Journal of Consulting and Clinical Psychology, 63,* 317–320.

Weisz, J. R., Hawley, K. M., & Doss, A. J. (2004). Empirically tested psychotherapies for youth internalizing and externalizing problems and disorders. *Child & Adolescent Psychiatric Clinics of North America, 13,* 729–815.

Wood, A. M., Linley, P. A., Maltby, J., Baliousis, M., & Joseph, S. (2008). The authentic personality: A theoretical and empirical conceptualization and the development of the authenticity scale. *Journal of Counseling Psychology, 55,* 385–399.

Zinbarg, R. E., & Griffith, J. W. (2008). Behavior therapy. In J. L. Lebow (Ed.), *Twenty-first century psychotherapies: Contemporary approaches to theory and practice* (pp. 8–42). Hoboken, NJ: John Wiley & Sons.

CHAPTER 7

Gestalt Therapy

Be who you are and say what you feel because those who mind don't matter and those who matter don't mind.

—DR. SEUSS

Rather than emphasize the unconscious, some counselors focus on consciousness—those parts of experience that are more readily accessible. Gestalt counselors want to build the client's abilities to fully experience their emotions. No theory builds the capacity of clients to become more aware of themselves and the things around them than Gestalt therapy. The German word *Gestalt* defines the unique way parts are integrated into a whole and Gestalt therapy transfers that integration into a directive, holistic treatment.

After reading this chapter, you should be able to:

▸ Outline the development of Gestalt therapy and Fritz Perls
▸ Explain the theory of Gestalt therapy including its core concepts
▸ Discuss the counseling relationship and goals in Gestalt therapy
▸ Describe assessment, process, and techniques in Gestalt therapy
▸ Demonstrate some therapeutic techniques
▸ Clarify the effectiveness of Gestalt therapy
▸ Discuss Gestalt play therapy

FRITZ PERLS
(1893–1970)

Fritz Perls's estranged wife, Laura, once referred to him as half prophet and half bum. In his autobiography, *In and Out the Garbage Pail* (1969b), Perls wrote that, at the age of 75, he liked his reputation of being both a dirty old man and a guru. Unfortunately, he continued, the first reputation was on the wane and the second ascending.

Born in a Jewish ghetto on the outskirts of Berlin on July 8, 1893, Friedrich Salomon Perls was the third child of Amelia Rund and Nathan Perls. From his late teens through his university schooling, Perls studied and acted with the Reinhard School of Drama, earning money to pay for most of his education. Clarkson and Mackewn (1993) suggest Perls's emphasis on nonverbal behavior began with his theater work. He earned his M.D. degree from the Friedrich Wilhelm University in 1921. He was in psychoanalysis with Karen Horney, Clara Happel, and Wilhelm Reich and studied with Helene Deutsch at the Psychoanalytic Institute in Vienna.

Perls was a medic in World War I and worked at the Goldstein Institute for Brain-Damaged Soldiers. Those experiences initiated his appreciation of perception. During that time he also met Laura Posner whom he married in 1930 (Fall, Holden, & Marquis, 2010).

After some hard times in Europe, Perls found success as a training analyst in Johannesburg, South Africa. In 1934, he founded the South African Institute for Psychoanalysis in Johannesburg. In 1936, Perls flew to Czechoslovakia to deliver a paper to the Psychoanalytic Congress. He met with his hero, Sigmund Freud, but was given only a cool reception—a brief 4-minute audience while he stood in Freud's doorway. Perls experienced another disappointment when most of the other analysts gave his paper an icy reception. From then on, Perls challenged the assumptions and directions of Freud and the psychoanalysts. It would not be until his final years that people would begin to listen to his theories, though he never would get the opportunity to show Freud his mistakes in ignoring Perls.

Perls spent 12 years in South Africa, during which he formulated all the basic ideas underlying what he would later call Gestalt therapy. At 53, he moved his family to New York, where the "formal birth" of Gestalt therapy took place. The people involved debated what to call the new theory. Perls held out for *Gestalt*, a German term that cannot be translated exactly into English, but the meaning of the concept can be explained as:

> A form, a configuration or a totality that has, as a unified whole, properties which cannot be derived by summation from the parts and their relationships. It may refer to physical structures, to physiological and psychological functions, or to symbolic units. (English & English, 1958, p. 225)

Carroll (2009) explains Gestalt as a neurological operation in which unfinished forms are completed and meaning is created. Laura Perls (1992) provided this definition of Gestalt: "a structured entity that is more than and different from its parts. It is the foreground figure that stands out from its ground, it 'exists'" (p. 52).

In late 1951, *Gestalt Therapy: Excitement and Growth in the Human Personality* was published. Perls is listed as one of the authors, although Ralph Hefferline wrote nearly all of the first half of the book and Paul Goodman the second. The book contains a comprehensive explanation of the theory and practice of the Gestalt approach to therapy. Perls's other writings include *Ego, Hunger, and Aggression: The Beginnings of Gestalt Therapy* (1947), *Gestalt Therapy Verbatim* (1969a), *The Gestalt Approach and Eye Witness to Therapy* (1973), *Gestalt Is: A Collection of Articles about Gestalt Therapy and Living* (1975), and, with Patricia Baumgardner, *Gifts from Lake Cowichan and Legacy from Fritz* (1975).

At first, the new therapy had almost no impact. Perls began traveling to major U.S. cities to run groups for professionals and laypeople interested in the new idea. As he traveled, he discovered that he was received far better on the road than he was in New York, prompting Perls to leave the city— and his wife—for the warmth of Miami. Although he and Laura worked together in the development of Gestalt therapy, Perls came to realize that the roles of husband and father gave him little satisfaction.

Miami was important to Perls because there he met "the most significant woman in [his] life," Marty Fromm. In Florida, he also found LSD and became involved in the drug subculture. He moved to California in 1964 and became widely known at the Esalen Institute in Big Sur, where he had to compete with people such as Rollo May, Abraham Maslow, Virginia Satir, Bernard Gunther, and Will Schutz (Clarkson & Mackewn, 1993). Perls contended that the techniques Gunther and Schutz employed used other people's ideas and offered "instant joy." Perls, who opposed quick cures and respected only originality, next moved to Canada and established his own Gestalt Institute of Canada at Cowichan Lake, Vancouver Island, British Columbia, in 1969.

Nine months after beginning work at the center in Canada, Fritz Perls died of advanced pancreatic cancer. He died as he had lived. On the last evening of his life, March 14, 1970, Perls sat on the edge of his bed in the intensive care unit ready to light a cigarette. His nurse rushed in, took his cigarettes and lighter, and said, "Dr. Perls, you can't smoke in here." Perls glared at her, said "Nobody tells Fritz Perls what to do," fell back on his bed, and died.

Perls viewed Gestalt theory as being in progress at the time of his death. He thought that theory development, like human development, was a process of becoming. Thus he revised the theory to fit his observations of human behavior across his lifetime. Over the course of his life, his philosophy evolved from conservative psychoanalysis to a theory rejecting traditional norms and promoting freedom and "do your own thing" (Murdock, 2013). Former students of Gestalt therapy such as Erving Polster, Miriam Polster, and Isadore From continue to advance a more moderate version of this approach which continues to be defined by the ways it is practiced—spontaneous, creative, and authentic.

THE NATURE OF PEOPLE

The Gestalt view of human nature is positive: People are capable of becoming self-regulating beings who can achieve a sense of unity and integration in their lives. Human beings have the ability to cope with their lives successfully, but sometimes may need help. Yontef and Jacobs (2014) explained that in Gestalt thought there is no meaningful way to understand a person if that human is considered apart from the person's interactions with environment or interpersonal relations. Consequently, people have psychological problems because they have become separated from important parts of themselves such as their emotions, bodies, or contacts with others. Helping individuals become aware of those neglected parts and restore, integrate, and balance themselves is the purpose of gestalt therapy (Seligman & Reichenberg, 2014).

Gestalt therapy helps individuals know themselves, their strengths, and self-sufficiency (Seligman & Reichenberg, 2014). According to Gestalt theory, the most important areas of concern are the thoughts and feelings people are experiencing at the moment. Additionally, the meaning that comes from the person's interpretation of the immediate experience is critical (Fall et al., 2010).

The interconnected general principles for healthy functioning in Gestalt perspective are these:

1. Valuing the here and now in order to experience each minute fully
2. Embracing self-awareness and experience, understanding, and accepting all parts of self
3. Prizing wholeness or responsibility and understanding life is a process; as people mature they move past old ways and become more self-sufficient, self-observing, and self-understanding (Fall et al., 2010).

Unhealthy functioning happens when people restrict their awareness and develop patterns that do not fulfill their needs. Many people fragment their lives, distributing their concentration and attention among several variables and events at one time—multitasking. The results of such fragmentation can be seen in an ineffective living style, with outcomes ranging from low productivity to serious accidents.

Perls (1969a) saw the person as a total organism—not just as the brain. His saying that people would be better off losing their minds and coming to their senses meant that our bodies and feelings are better indicators of the truth than our words, which we use to hide the truth from ourselves. Body signs such as headaches, rashes, neck strain, and stomach pains may indicate that we need to change something in our lives. Perls believed that awareness alone can be curative. With full awareness, a state of organismic self-regulation develops, and the total person takes control. Harmony with environment, maturity, or actualization comes from embracing what is good and rejecting what is bad for the person (Greenberg, Rice, & Elliott, 1993).

CORE CONCEPTS

Awareness

For Gestalt therapists, awareness signifies emotional health. Perls (1969a) explained, "Because with full awareness you become aware of this organismic self-regulation, you can let the organism take over without interfering, without interrupting; we can rely on the wisdom of the organism" (p. 17). Seligman and Reichenberg (2014) stated that awareness is both the hallmark of wellness and the goal of counseling.

Self-regulation requires awareness of one's inner self and of the external environment. Conscious awareness or focused attention involves full use of all the senses: touching, hearing, seeing, tasting, and smelling. Mentally healthy people can maintain their awareness without being distracted by the various environmental stimuli that constantly vie for their attention. Such people can fully and clearly experience their own needs and the environmental alternatives for meeting them. Healthy people still experience their share of inner conflicts and frustrations, but, with their higher levels of concentration and awareness, they can solve their problems without complicating them with fantasy elaborations. They likewise resolve conflicts with others when it is possible; otherwise, they dismiss the conflicts. People with high levels of awareness of their needs and their environment know which problems and conflicts are resolvable and which are not. In Perls's theory, the key to successful adjustment is the development of personal responsibility—responsibility for one's life and responsibility to one's environment. Much of the Perls's doctrine is summarized in his famous Gestalt Prayer:

> I do my thing and you do your thing.
>
> I am not in this world to live up to your expectations,
>
> And you are not in this world to live up to mine.
>
> You are you and I am I.
>
> And if by chance we find each other, it's beautiful.
>
> If not, it can't be helped. (Perls, 1969b, p. 4)

The healthy person focuses sharply on one need (the figure) at a time, thereby relegating other needs to the background. When the need is met—or the Gestalt is closed or completed—it is relegated to the background and a new need comes into focus (becomes the figure). The smoothly functioning figure—ground relationship characterizes the healthy personality. The dominant need of the organism at any time becomes the foreground figure and the other needs recede, at least temporarily, into the background. The foreground figure is the need that presses most sharply for satisfaction, whether the need is to preserve life or is related to less physically or psychologically vital areas. For individuals to be able to satisfy their needs, close the Gestalt, and move on to other things, they must be able to determine what they need, and they must know how to manipulate themselves and their environment to get it. Even purely physiological needs can be satisfied only through the interaction of the organism and the environment (Perls, 1975).

Gestalt counselors enhance a person's awareness through experiment, a here-and-now focus and process statements. Gestalt practitioners avoid reflective listening, believing that talking leads to overthinking rather than to awareness. These counselors instead focus on body movements and other nonverbal to understand a person (Seligman & Reichenberg, 2014).

Contact

The interaction of the person with the environment is called *contact*, the central feature of life. In Gestalt therapy, contact means recognizing what is occurring here and now, moment to moment (Yontef & Jacobs, 2014). Contact is the process of knowing about a need and trying to fulfill that need by engaging with the environment. Contact occurs through the functions of looking, listening, touching, talking, moving, smelling, and tasting (Polster & Polster, 1973).

Carroll (2009) explains that children use aggression to interact with the world, to ask for what's needed, and to organize their excitement or energy. Aggression then is essential for children to express their needs; their means of contact.

Humans interact with their environment at the *contact boundaries* of the person. The psychological contact boundaries are the exchange between the person and resources within the environment. Polster and Polster (1973) explained the point at which one faces the "me" in relation to that which is "not me" is the contact boundary. As the distinction of me–not me happens, a sense of self develops.

Self

In Gestalt thought, the self is always in the process of becoming. As stated above, self emerges as the person has experiences and develops the sense of "who I am and who I am not" or "me." A nurturing environment is necessary for the child to develop this sense of self. Rejection or lack of support leads to a diminished ability to self-regulate and interact with the environment. Carroll (2009) explains that all our interactions involve adjusting to the contact between what is me and what is not me. In a healthy person, self is always changing, transforming by taking in what nourishes and rejecting what obstructs growth.

Integration

Therefore, healthy functioning equates with integration; all parts of the person work in a well-coordinated, wholesome manner. Perls defined neurotic people or those with "growth disorders" (1969b, p. 30) as those who try to attend to too many needs at one time and, as a result, fail to satisfy any one need fully. People with growth disorders deny or reject parts of themselves and their world, do not live in the present, and do not make healthy contact with others. They feel guilty and resentful, use the past to blame others for their problems, and are trapped in this unhealthy state. They may have a great deal of unfinished business that overwhelms them (Seligman & Reichenberg, 2014).

Neurotic people also use their potential to manipulate others to do for them what they have not done for themselves. Rather than running their own lives, they turn them over to others who will take care of their needs. In summary, people cause themselves additional problems by not handling their lives appropriately in the following six categories:

1. *Lacking contact with the environment:* People may become so rigid that they cut themselves off from others or from resources in the environment.
2. *Confluence:* People may incorporate too much of themselves into others or incorporate so much of the environment into themselves that they lose touch with who and where they are. Then the environment takes control.
3. *Unfinished business:* People may have unfulfilled needs, unexpressed feelings, or unfinished situations that clamor for their attention. (This situation may manifest itself in dreams.)
4. *Fragmentation:* People may try to discover or deny a need such as to show aggression. The inability to find and obtain what one needs may be the result of fragmenting one's life.
5. *Top dog/underdog:* People may experience a split in their personalities between what they think they "should" do (top dog) and what they "want" to do (underdog).
6. *Polarities (dichotomies):* People tend to flounder at times between existing, natural dichotomies in their lives, such as body–mind, self–external world, fantasy–reality, infantile–mature, biological–cultural, poetry–prose, spontaneous–deliberate, personal–social, think–feeling, and unconscious–conscious. Much of everyday living seems to be involved in resolving conflicts posed by these competing polarities.

THEORY OF COUNSELING

"Gestalt therapy is an exploration rather than a direct attempt to change behavior" (Yontef & Jacobs, 2014, p. 317). The client and counselor collaborate to increase understanding toward the goal of growth through increased consciousness.

Gestalt therapists emphasize direct experiences. They focus on achieving awareness of the here and now. Gestalt counselors block the client in any attempt to break out of this present awareness by talking about the past or future. As an experiential approach, Gestalt therapy is not concerned with symptoms and analysis, but rather with total existence and integration. Integration and maturation, according to Perls (1969a), are never-ending processes directly related to a person's awareness of the here and now. A "Gestalt" is formed in a person as a new need arises. If a need is satisfied, the destruction of that particular Gestalt is achieved, and new Gestalts can be formed. This concept is basic in Gestalt therapy. Incomplete Gestalts are referred to as "unfinished business."

Perls, Hefferline, and Goodman (1951) outlined four main emphases in Gestalt work as the following:

- Pay attention to experience, become aware of, and concentrate on the present
- Maintain and promote connections of social, cultural, historical, physical, emotional, and other factors
- Experiment
- Encourage creativity

Relationship

In Gestalt therapy, counselors are considered tools of change (Fall et al., 2010). With respect, compassion, and commitment to the person's perception of the world, Gestalt counselors focus totally on the client's immediate experiences (Yontef & Jacobs, 2014). Awareness is the capacity to focus, to attend, and to be in touch with the present. The function of the Gestalt counselor is to facilitate the client's awareness in the "now." The Gestalt counselor is both supportive and confrontational, an aggressive therapist who frustrates the learner's attempts to break out of the awareness of here and now. The counselor stops client's attempts to retreat into the past or jump into the future by relating the content to the immediate present. That does not mean the past or future is not part of therapy, but those are examined as being experienced in the present (Parlett & Hemming, 1996).

Miller (1989) points out that Perls often used sarcasm, humor, drama, and shock to rouse people from neurosis. For Perls, Gestalt therapy was a search for a workable solution in the present. The counselor's job is to assist the client in experimenting with authentic new behaviors, rather than to explain and maintain the unhelpful or harmful behaviors of the past. Clients are discouraged from talking about something. Clients are asked to experience and act (Murdock, 2013). Perls (1970a) said, "Lose your mind and come to your senses" (p. 38).

The Gestalt counselor works to create an authentic relationship with the client that Yontef and Jacobs (2014) refer to as a fluid back-and-forth attention to counseling process and to relationship. Haley (2010) said counselors build a client's awareness and growth by the following activities: identifying themes central to the client; thinking about client concerns that will guide the sequence, timing, and methods of counseling; establishing and maintaining a safe environment; and creating an atmosphere of contact.

Goals

Perls (1969a) wrote that the aim of his therapy was to help people themselves to grow up—to mature, take charge of their lives, and become responsible for themselves. The central goal in Gestalt therapy is deeper awareness, which promotes a sense of living fully in the here and now. Two kinds of awareness involve awareness of the moment, process, or content and awareness of the awareness process, knowing about choices (Mann, 2010). When that goal is achieved, people have the ability to track what is happening as well as the responsibility for interacting with the world differently (Fall et al., 2010).

Integration is also promoted in Gestalt counseling. The aim of integration is to help people become systematic, whole persons whose inner state and behavior match so completely that little energy is wasted. Such integration allows people to give their full attention and energy to meeting their needs appropriately. The ultimate measure of success in Gestalt therapy is the extent to which clients grow in awareness, take responsibility for their actions, and move from environmental support to self-support.

Seligman and Reichenberg (2014) highlighted these as the most important goals of Gestalt therapy: promoting attention, clarity, and awareness; helping people live in the here and now; and encouraging people's wholeness, integration, and balance (p. 209). Gestalt counselors also want to help people find closure for their unfinished business and access their own resources. Promoting self-sufficiency, actualization, and meaningful contact and developing skills to manage life are also included in successful therapy outcomes. Perls (1969a) stated that the essential difference between Gestalt therapy and other types of psychotherapy is that Gestalt practitioners do not analyze, they integrate. Awareness is the vehicle of change.

COUNSELING METHOD

After viewing the Gloria interviews with Rogers, Perls, and Ellis in *Three Approaches to Psychotherapy* (Shostrom, 1965), it is obvious that Perls is the only one of the three therapists who challenges Gloria on her core issue of trying to please others by being the person she thinks others want her to be. Her lifestyle was an excellent example of a phony layer of neuroses. Perls, confronting Gloria with the inconsistencies in her verbal and nonverbal behavior, penetrated her well-defended lifestyle of playing roles she thought others would prefer to the actual person she was trying to conceal. Basically, the point of Gestalt therapy is to treat the client's lifestyle, rather than treat the fragments of the client's life. To Perls, spending time talking with Gloria about her daughter, father, ex-husband, boyfriends, and transference issues would be like trying to put a jigsaw puzzle together, one piece at a time, without looking at the picture of the completed puzzle before starting. Perls wanted to work with the whole person, not fragments of the person's life.

The general reaction students have to watching Perls working with Gloria is, first, they cannot visualize themselves counseling a client in the same confrontational manner. Second, they do not see a counseling framework or guideline, such as those provided in reality therapy, solution-focused brief counseling, cognitive-behavioral therapy, and rational-emotive behavior therapy. However, they do become interested in various Gestalt methods that help clients work through impasses in their personal development. Certainly the film illustrated the power of Fritz Perls—who in person or on film—never left anyone feeling neutral; he made everyone think and react.

Gestalt counseling has three critical elements: the authentic relationship between counselor and client, exploration of awareness and experiments in awareness (Clarkson, 2013). In order to create a therapeutic environment to lead to greater awareness of one's real self, how one interacts with others and how one functions in the here and now, clients are encouraged to follow these guidelines (Fall et al., 2010):

1. Be aware of a continuum of awareness: notice everything
2. Commit to the here and now: speak in present and then discuss how experiences impact the present moment
3. Own everything: take responsibility for all thoughts, actions, feelings, and sensations
4. Commit to meaningful discussion: communicate in a clear, responsible way and be willing to listen to feedback
5. Avoid questions: change questions to statements
6. Take risks: face fears and risk being rejected to gain awareness of true self and explore
7. Accept personal responsibility: clients have the power to change and the responsibility to decide when and how to do so

Finally unlike other counseling theories, the emphasis in Gestalt therapy is on physical or body sensations as important parts of lives (Murdoch, 2013) as well as clues to fuller awareness.

Process

As stated earlier Gestalt therapy is exploring rather than attempting to change behavior. It is a therapy of process, the counselor is always emphasizing the what and how of behavior rather than the why (Yontef & Jacobs, 2014). The goal is growth and autonomy accomplished by increasing consciousness. Gestalt therapists focus on the awareness process, the range of a person's experiences. The patterned processes of a person's awareness are the foci of counseling. Knowing those patterns allows the person to clarify thoughts, feelings, and decisions in the current experience and to realize the ways those cognitions, emotions, and choices happen. What does not come to awareness is sometimes also highlighted (Yontef & Jacobs, 2014).

Gestalt counseling emphasizes the immediate interaction between practitioner and client. Those interactions proceed through building a relationship, determining and investigating the problem, experimenting with change, and ending. In the early part of treatment, the client learns about the here-and-now focus rather than the there-and-then approach. Reflection and encouragement are used to move the client to the second stage of exploring the problem. Some Gestalt experiments, such as the ones described below, may be used during this portion of therapy. As the awareness grows, the client begins to experiment and work toward integration of self and elimination of blocks to contact and awareness. At the ending stage, counselors continue to support change (Fall et al., 2010).

While Gestalt counselors consider the person as always becoming, Perls (1969a) presented a somewhat structured model of five layers used to depict how people fragment their lives and prevent themselves from succeeding and maturing. The five layers form a series of counseling stages, or benchmarks, for the counseling process; in fact, they could be considered as five steps to a better Gestalt way of life. These five layers as described by Perls and Fall et al. (2010) are as follows:

1. *The phony layer:* Many people are trapped in trying to be what they are not. The phony layer is characterized by unresolved conflicts and failure to find integration of competing polarities. People have social masks to hide themselves.

2. *The phobic layer:* As people become aware of their phony games, they also become aware of their fears that maintain the games. This experience is often frightening and may scare people back into the phony layer.

3. *The impasse layer:* This is the layer people reach when they shed the environmental support of their games and find they do not know a better way to cope with their fears and dislikes. People at this point of paralysis face the terror of moving from external support to relying on self. People often become stuck here and refuse to move on because they believe that a life of limited awareness is better than the pain and fear of change.

4. *The implosive layer:* People become aware of how they limit themselves, and they begin to experiment with new behaviors within the safe confines of the counseling setting. The exploration may be awkward and scary as old ways are discarded.

5. *The explosive layer:* If experiments with new behaviors are successful outside the counseling setting, people can reach the explosive layer, where they find much unused energy that had been tied up in maintaining a phony existence.

Perls (1969a) believed that progress through the five layers of neuroses is best achieved by observing how psychological defenses might be associated with muscular position, or what he called *body armor*. He believed the client's body language would be a better indicator of the truth than the client's words, and that awareness of hidden material could be facilitated by acting out feelings. Perls asked people to project their thoughts and feelings on empty chairs representing significant people in their lives. People were often asked to play several roles in attempting to identify sources of personal conflict. Perls expanded on Rogers' idea of feedback as a therapeutic agent by including body posture, voice tone, eye movements, feelings, and gestures.

In many ways, Gestalt interventions are breakthrough mechanisms that help clients reframe their problems into manageable projects, resolve decision-making conflicts, and find a reasonable balance between taking too much or too little responsibility in their lives.

Techniques

Several language, game, and fantasy methods may be used to maintain the present-time orientation of the counseling interview. We have used some of the following techniques with 5- to 12-year-old children, as well as with adolescents and adults.

Language

Use of language is an important part of Gestalt therapy. The careful use of words helps counselors create a place that encourages change. The following are some of the word structures important to Gestalt therapy.

"I" LANGUAGE   Counselors encourage use of the word *I* when the client uses a generalized *you* when talking; for example, "*You* know how it is when *you* can't understand math and the teacher gets on *your* back." When *I* is substituted for *you*, the message becomes, "*I* know how it is when *I* can't understand math and the teacher gets on *my* back." The client tries on such substitutions of "I" for "you" like a pair of shoes to see how they fit. "I" language helps children take responsibility for their feelings, thoughts, and behaviors.

SUBSTITUTING *WON'T* FOR *CAN'T*   Again, the client tries on the "shoes" for comfort, substituting "I *won't* pass math" for "I *can't* pass math." How much of the responsibility the child will own is the question to be answered.

SUBSTITUTING *WHAT* AND *HOW* FOR *WHY*   The counselor asks the client to substitute *what* and *how* for *why* in this technique; for example, "*How* do you feel about what you are doing?" "*What* are you doing with your foot as we talk about your behavior?"

PRESENT TENSE   When clients discuss past events, counselors encourage a focus on the present, in the here and now. So rather than discussing how a mother's scolding ruined a relationship, the client would be asked to describe how those rebukes affect feelings and thoughts in the counseling relationship right now.

NO GOSSIPING   If the client must talk about someone who is not present in the room, let the talk, all in the present tense, be directed to an empty chair. For example, a student might say, "I think you treat me unfairly, Ms. Clark. I wish you would be as nice to me as you are to the other kids." The student can then move to the other chair and answer for Ms. Clark, "Joan, I would find it easier to like you if you would be more helpful to me during the day." The dialogue between Joan and Ms. Clark would continue until the child finished her complaint and the anticipated responses from her teacher. Person-to-person dialogues not only update the material into the present but also increase Joan's awareness of the problem. Side benefits include a better picture of the situation for the counselor and rehearsal time for Joan, who may wish to discuss the problem later with her teacher. Some empathy on Joan's part for the teacher's side of the conflict may also emerge from the dialogue.

CHANGING QUESTIONS INTO STATEMENTS   The method of changing questions into statements has the effect of helping children to be more authentic and direct in expressing their thoughts and feelings. For example, rather than asking, "Don't you think I should stop hanging around those guys?" the child should say, "I think I should stop hanging around those guys" or "I think you want me to stop hanging around those guys." Perls believed that most questions are phony in that they are really disguised statements.

TAKING RESPONSIBILITY   Clients are asked to fill in sentence blanks as another way of examining personal responsibility for the way they manage their lives. For example, "Right now I'm feeling _____, and I take _____ percent responsibility for how I feel." The exercise is quite an eye opener for those clients who tend to view outside sources as the total cause of their good and bad feelings.

INCOMPLETE SENTENCES Incomplete sentence exercises, like the exercise on taking responsibility, help clients become aware of how they help and hurt themselves. For example, "I help myself when I _____," or "I block or hurt myself when I _____."

Experiments

Gestalt therapy defines experimentation as the act of trying something different to increase awareness. That testing may enhance emotions or may bring a recognition that something has been kept from awareness. Experimentation is an alternative to the verbal means of psychoanalysis and the control of behaviorism (Yontef & Jacobs, 2014). Experiments should not be threatening or negative but should promote growth. Experiments are suggestions for focusing the awareness that clients can use to increase their intensity, power, flexibility, and creativity (Haley, 2010). When counselors suggest possible experiments, they should be timely, inviting, and respectful (Seligman & Reichenberg, 2014). Polster and Polster (1973) list enactments, role-plays, homework, or other activities as experiments for clients to complete between sessions.

THE EMPTY CHAIR TECHNIQUE The Gestalt technique of the empty chair often is used to resolve a conflict between people or within a person (Greenberg & Malcolm, 2003; Stumpfel & Goldman, 2002). Barnard and Curry (2012) suggested the empty chair technique may help people become aware of their self-judgments and their responses to those judgments as well as develop some compassions for themselves. The child can sit in one chair, playing his or her own part; then the child can sit in the other chair, playing out a projection of what the other person is saying or doing in response. Similarly, a child may sit in one chair to discuss the pros of making a decision, and then argue the cons of the decision while sitting in the opposite chair.

For example, Sharon was having trouble deciding whether to tell of her friend's involvement in destruction of property. She thought her friend had behaved wrongly and should not let other children take the blame for the incident, yet she was reluctant to tattle on the friend and get her in trouble. The counselor suggested that Sharon sits in one chair and talk about what would happen if she did tell on her friend, and then move to the other chair to describe what would happen if she did not. The technique helped Sharon to look at the consequences of both acts and make her decision. In this instance, Sharon decided to talk with her friend to give her the opportunity to confess and make amends for the damaged property.

The empty chair technique is a powerful intervention for working with clients of all ages who are in conflict with a third party who is not present in the session. For example, the conflict might be with a spouse, sibling, teacher, parent, friend, or boss. Rather than having clients talk on and on about how awful this other person is, the client is asked to speak directly to the offending person as if she or he were sitting in the empty chair. Then, because the client knows this person well, the client is asked to sit in the empty chair and reply the way the offending person would respond. The back-and-forth dialogue continues until clients finish expressing all of their thoughts and feelings on the subject.

Three productive things happen with this version of the empty chair technique. First, the counselor gets a better, firsthand account of the dynamics of the relationship. Second, the client may develop some empathy for the offending party's position. Third the client receives some rehearsal practice for confronting the absent person. The counselor might even model some possible methods of confronting the third party by taking the client's role and having the client play the part of the other person. Then, the client can practice confronting the offending third person, with the counselor taking the role of that person. This method has been particularly useful in helping students protest effectively to their teachers when they have questions about their grades.

The empty chair method also has been useful with clients who have "unfinished business." Stumpfel and Goldman (2002) explained that unmet needs equate to unclosed gestalts that have not moved from awareness. The dialogue in the empty chair can address those unclosed gestalts. For example, people who have lost a loved one have continuing regrets about the relationship. In the empty chair they talk to their lost loved one as though that person were sitting in the chair and, in many cases, sit in the empty chair and reply as they "know" this person would reply. For example, a son might say to his deceased father, "Dad, I always wanted to tell you how much I loved you, and I was never able to do this." Speaking for his father from the other chair, the reply is almost always, "Son, you didn't have to say it. I knew all along that you loved me." Counselors have only to witness such an event one time to "see" the heavy burden of guilt lift from the shoulders of their client.

In a variation of the empty chair method, a problem can be explored in an individual or group situation by introducing the empty chair as a hypothetical person with behaviors and characteristics similar to those of the child and his or her particular problem. It is sometimes easier for children to discuss a hypothetical child and how this child feels or could change than to discuss their own feelings and behaviors. While discussing an imagined person, children learn about themselves.

The empty chair method is useful for angry children, who can talk to the angry self in another chair and find out why they are so upset. It can also serve as projection for the child who is afraid of an ugly monster. The child can become the monster and allow that creature to explain its motives for scaring children. Retroflection also may be used to help students express difficult or frightening thoughts and feelings. Retroflection is giving voice to that part of the body that is exhibiting muscular tension. The counselor may ask a child who tightens up his or her mouth to say what the mouth would like to say.

Engle and Holliman (2002) write that the expression of emotional experiences allows for the formation of a new Gestalt when people are in conflict over opposing values or over what they should do versus what they want to do. Experiments such as the empty chair dialogue are useful in developing new schematic structures for bringing the conflict into focus so that it can be integrated into a workable solution. Greenberg and Malcolm (2003) present a method for using the empty chair. The intervention begins with clients addressing an individual with whom they have unfinished business, followed by clients responding as they believe the other person would respond. The dialogue continues until clients reach a point of resolution in completing the unfinished business, which, in effect, moves the issue of "unfinished" business from figure to ground in the client's field of awareness.

Wagner Moore (2004) points out that the two-chair method has been shown to be superior to person-centered, empathic responding in resolving inner conflicts. Kellogg (2004) presents an update on the various Gestalt methods involving "chair-work" in saying "good-bye" when a client is holding on to a relationship that no longer exists, in working with dreams, and in finding integrations of bipolar opposites in a person's life. Greenberg (2011) has further details related to testing the empty chair dialogue and other expressive techniques.

REVERSAL   Many people act as though they have only one side of a trait whether it's the "good" side or the "bad" side. In the reversal experiment, the client speaks the opposite of any thought, feeling, or action to bring into awareness the other end of the continuum.

BIPOLARITIES   Perls applies the term *differential thinking* to the concept of thinking in terms of opposites. Much of everyday life appears to be spent resolving conflicts posed by competing polarities, such as "I should" versus "I want" when one is confronted with a difficult decision. This dialogue experiment can be used with empty chairs in the following ways.

TOP DOG VERSUS UNDERDOG   One of the most common bipolarities is what Perls (1969a) labeled *top dog* and *underdog*. The top dog is righteous, authoritarian, and knows best. The top dog is a bully and works with "you should" and "you should not." The underdog manipulates by being defensive or apologetic, wheedling, and playing crybaby. The underdog works with "I want" and makes excuses such as "I try hard" and "I have good intentions." The underdog is cunning and usually gets the better of the top dog because the underdog position appeals to the pleasure-seeking side of our personality.

Two chairs can be used to help clients resolve "I want" versus "I should" debates. Label one chair top dog (I should) and the other chair underdog (I want). Clients are asked to present their best "I should" argument while sitting in the top dog chair and facing the empty underdog chair. On completion of the first "I should" point, the client moves to the underdog chair to counter with an "I want" argument. The debate continues back and forth until the client completes all arguments from both points of view. Talking about the activity often reveals in which chair (or on which side of the argument) the client feels and thinks the greatest integration of shoulds and wants occurs, thus allowing the client to have the best of both sides.

The top dog–underdog technique works for individuals and groups. To use the technique in a group, the counselor can divide the clients into two subgroups, the top dogs and the underdogs. The top dog group members list reasons they *should* do a certain thing, whereas the underdog group members think of reasons they *want* to do something. The lists generally lead to much discussion. Children and adolescents respond well to this activity.

The best outcomes from the top dog–underdog debate occur when clients can identify areas in their lives where the shoulds and wants agree; for example, "I love to read, and I should read." These synergistic solutions help children and adolescents integrate the polarities in their lives.

MY GREATEST WEAKNESS   In another exercise, clients are asked to name their greatest weakness and write a short paragraph on how this weakness is really their greatest strength; for example, "My greatest weakness is procrastination, but I'll never give it up because by putting things off I create the motivation I need for completing unpleasant tasks." Once clients realize that their greatest weakness may, in fact, be the greatest strength they have going for them, they begin to realize that they control the weakness rather than vice versa. Clients also realize that the counselor who uses this technique is not pushing them to fix their "weakness." Maybe all that is needed is to just manage the weakness more efficiently such as by not procrastinating too long.

RESENT, DEMAND, AND APPRECIATE: THE INTEGRATION OF OPPOSING THOUGHTS, FEELINGS, AND BELIEFS   Clients list the three people to whom they are closest and, for each of them, write one thing they resent about the person, one thing they demand from the person, and one thing they appreciate in the person. Such an exercise helps clients become more aware of the mixed feelings they have about others, how it is possible to resent and appreciate a person at the same time, and how opposing thoughts and feelings can be integrated.

The purpose of working with these bipolarities, or splits in the personality, is to bring each side into awareness so reorganization that does not exclude either side can take place. Gestalt therapy is directed toward making life easier by integrating the splits in existence; each side is necessary and has its place in the well-integrated personality.

Name	Something You Resent	Something You Demand	Something You Appreciate
John	I resent that you don't spend enough time with me.	I demand more time.	I appreciate your company and friendship.
Mary			
Sue			

FANTASY GAMES FOR CREATING AWARENESS   Fantasy games can be great fun for children while enabling them to become aware of their present feelings. As a group activity, the children choose an animal they would like to be, and then move around as they think this animal would. The children sit down in pairs and discuss what they would feel if they were this particular animal. As a culmination of the activity, they write stories about how they would feel, think, and behave if they were actually the animal. By the end of the exercise, children should have a real awareness of how they feel and think, and they should be able to discuss this with their counselor, teacher, or parents.

Fantasy games can be devised from almost any object or situation. The rosebush and wise-person fantasies are two favorites. In the first fantasy, the client pretends to be a rosebush and then considers the following points:

1. Type of bush—strong or weak?
2. Root system—deep or shallow?
3. Number of roses—too many or too few?
4. Number of thorns—too many or too few?
5. Environment—bad or good for growing?
6. Does your rosebush stand out?
7. Does it have enough room?
8. How does it get along with the other plants?
9. Does it have a good future?

The wise-person fantasy involves asking a fantasized source of wisdom one question, which the wise person ponders for a few minutes before answering—speaking through the client, of course. Both question and answer should add some awareness and understanding to the client's life. For example, a client may ask, "What should I do with my life?" Then he or she answers, as the wise person, "Develop all your talents and skills as much as you can."

Clients are asked to discuss their fantasies in depth with the counselor in individual sessions and with groups of two to four if a group is meeting. A good follow-up procedure for clients is to complete the statement "I learned that _____" after each exercise is completed.

During fantasy activities such as the rosebush or wise-person fantasies, children may need help as they reacclimate to their environment. Counselors may ask these children to count backward slowly from ten or to touch something solid or to move their bodies to reconnect with their location. Directing clients in a group setting to look slowly around the area and become reacquainted with their environment also is effective.

DREAMWORK Dreaming is a way of becoming aware of the world in the here and now. Awareness is the dominant theme of Gestalt, so dreaming and Gestalt seem to work well together. Perls saw dreams as a road to integration (Seligman & Reichenberg, 2014). He believed the parts of a dream represented aspects of the dreamer. Dreaming is a guardian of one's existence because the content of dreams always relates to one's survival, well-being, and growth; therefore, Gestalt therapists have helped clients overcome impasses in their lives through serious consideration of dreams. The Gestalt approach to dreams is helpful not only to people experiencing dilemmas in their lives but also to the average "healthy" person who may spend many of their waking hours out of touch with the here and now because they are worrying compulsively about the future or doting on memories of failure or past pleasures.

Spontaneity is an important feature of Gestalt therapy, and according to Perls, dreams are the most spontaneous expression of the existence of the human being. The Gestalt approach is concerned with integration rather than analysis of dreams. Such integration involves consciously reliving a dream, taking responsibility for being the objects and people in the dream, and becoming aware of the messages the dream holds. According to Perls, all parts of the dream are fragments of the dreamer's personality that must be pieced together to form a whole. These projected fragments must be reowned; thus, hidden potential that appears in the dream also is to be reowned. As clients play the parts of all the objects and persons in the dream, they may become more aware of the message the dream holds. They may act out the dream until two conflicting roles emerge—for instance, the top dog and the underdog. This want–should conflict is essentially the conflict from which the dreamer suffers. Gestalt counselors believe that dreams have hidden existential messages that, once discovered, can fill the voids in people's personalities, help with solving problems and developing self-awareness.

Basically, the Gestalt method for working with dreams requires clients to describe the dream and then list all the parts of the dream, including people, objects, animals, buildings, rooms, and trees. Each of these is fully described so the client paints a verbal picture of the dream. Clients are asked what, if anything, the dream might mean to them. Interpretation is left to the client, based on the philosophy that to interpret the client's dream for the client would suggest that the counselor would know the client better than the client knows himself or herself. Next, the client is asked to speak or give voice to each part of the dream, much like an animated movie in which trees and animals talk.

Each object in the dream offers clients the opportunity to project parts of their personality onto that object. For example, a client may say, "I am the bedroom in Harriet's house and I like being her bedroom. She is very particular about keeping me clean, neat, and orderly." These projections are done for all of the objects and people in the client's dream. The counselor may suggest that Harriet's bedroom have a conversation with Harriet's house and ask the client to role-play the dialogue for such a conversation. Following the talking exercise for each object in the dream, the client is again asked for an interpretation of the dream. It may come in the form of a best guess. Regardless of the interpretation or best guess about the dream's meaning, the client is not likely to have this dream again. This method has a way of finishing up unfinished business that retires the dream to the background of the client's experience.

Joyce and Sills (2010) expanded this play-the-part dream work. They described other useful approaches as using the present tense to tell the dream, creating different endings, using movement rather than words to tell the story, and including dialogues between the elements.

Seligman and Reichenberg (2014) emphasize that the Gestalt approach to therapy puts the clients in charge of interpreting dreams. It also helps dreamers take responsibility for their dreams and to see dreams as part of themselves. Integrating the dreams into their lives and acknowledging thoughts and emotions reflected in the dream that might otherwise be ignored leads to greater awareness, what Perls (1970b) called "the royal road to integration" (p. 204).

Using the Body to Build Awareness

As noted earlier, Gestalt therapy goals include people growing by becoming more aware of their thoughts, feelings, and physical self. Because some individuals deny their body sensations, Gestalt counselors pay attention to the message of the body.

Seligman and Reichenberg (2014) explained that counselors may use these strategies to accomplish this awareness.

IDENTIFICATION   If counselors notice a person showing reactions in a part of their body, they may call attention to it. For example, if a person starts tapping her fingers on the desk, the counselor may say something like "I see your fingers drumming on the table. What are your fingers saying?" or "Become your fingers and tell me what they feel."

LOCATING EMOTIONS IN THE BODY   Counselors may help people locate their emotions in order to feel more fully. An example would be a statement such as "You are talking about your anger at your classmate. Show me where that madness is in your body." When the client explains the rage is in his neck, the counselor explores that physical sensation with him.

REPETITION AND EXAGGERATION   When they see a client's body movements, clinicians may encourage clients to repeat and exaggerate those actions, focusing attention on the energy. A counselor may say "I see your leg swinging. Try exaggerating that, swing it as strongly as you can, and let's talk about what feelings come up."

These body awareness activities as well as the modifications in language and other experiments such as the empty chair are techniques Gestalt clinicians employ to increase clients' awareness of thoughts, feelings, and the world.

Gestalt Play Therapy

Violet Oaklander (1978, 1988) translated Gestalt theories to play therapy in her book *Windows to Our Children* and expanded her thoughts in her recent book *Hidden Treasure* (2006). Her definition of play therapy is an improvisational drama in which children experiment with the world. She talks about play being serious, full of purpose, and essential to mental, physical, and social growth. Oaklander contends that awareness of self and of one's existence is the overarching goal of Gestalt play therapy.

Oaklander (2011) explains that Gestalt therapy is a process-oriented approach focused on the healthy, integrated person—senses, body, emotions, and intellect. The concern of the therapy is the functioning of all aspects of the person so that senses, body, emotions, and intellect are well coordinated in a creative adjustment. According to Oaklander, children who constrict or immobilize their emotions display symptoms as they attempt to find a balance that integrates all aspects of their beings. She states that the child's capacity to represent experiences in symbolic fashion allows a self-reflective manner that helps the child develop a greater sense of self. Oaklander describes the process of Gestalt play therapy as being like a dance that sometimes the counselor leads and other times the child leads. Oaklander directs the counselor to meet the child where she or he is and suggest, but not push.

Oaklander (2001) says that play gives children chances to learn and to take safe risks. Through fantasy, children can test possibilities of doing something different to resolve fears, confusions, and conflicts. She also explains the important concept of *contact* in Gestalt play therapy. Contact is having the ability to be completely present in a situation by using one's senses that connect with the environment such as looking, listening, and smelling. Being aware of feelings and using the intellect are also part of making contact. Recognizing what is being done and how it is being done is the contacting process. When children are anxious or troubled, they do not use their senses fully. They block emotions and inhibit contact. Oaklander (2011) notes that children deserve "small segments" of therapy and larger segments of play. She recommends honoring a child's resistance, explaining that reluctance grows from the child not having the support to go further. Her discussions on the timing of work with children emphasize the slower, more careful pace counselors take with children.

Gestalt play therapy includes exercises and experiences that involve the senses and the expression of feelings. Oaklander's book *Windows to Our Children: A Gestalt Therapy with Children and Adolescents* (1988) contains examples of these exercises in which she uses various creative activities and explains how they work. Enhancing the self increases a person's ability to be in contact. Experiencing the contacting process leads to integration, choice, and change.

Oaklander (1978, 1993, 2006) also adapted several Gestalt techniques for children. She recommends projection through art and storytelling as a way of increasing the child's self-awareness and cites fantasy and imagery such as the wise-person fantasy, as good ways to tap intuitive thought in children and adults. Oaklander has also frequently used the empty chair method as a helpful way to handle unfinished business, frustration, and anger. Carmichael (2006) provided some examples of activities a Gestalt play therapist might try.

- Ask children to draw how they feel.
- Ask children to draw how they would like to be.
- Have children look at an object and draw how it made them feel. Children could also draw their emotional response to a story, dream, fantasy, poem, or music.
- Draw or use clay to illustrate opposites such as happy/sad, angry/calm, love/hate.
- Have children create a road map of their lives, showing bumps, slips, and so on.

When the child completes the drawing, sand tray, clay figure, or whatever media has been used, the counselor asks "Tell me about this" and continues to ask about all aspects of the creation.

Wheeler and McConville (2002), in agreement with Oaklander, point out that Gestalt techniques in working with children are focused on the development of inner strength and confidence in the child through opportunities to make choices, achieve mastery, own their projections, participate in imaginative play, and expel aggressive energy appropriately.

CONFIDENCE COURSES FOR PLAY THERAPY This gentle form of obstacle course, designed to build confidence, uses combinations of pit jumps, incline balances, boxes, barrels, ladder climbs, rope slides, and other similar objects. (Children also can be involved in constructing such a course.) As children attain better motor coordination and balance, they form a better self-image, a feeling of mastery, and an

"I can do it" attitude about themselves. They begin to feel they can solve problems and deal with their world competently. The same holds true for adolescents who negotiate tougher ropes or challenge courses.

Case Study

Many short-term counseling sessions with children can be conducted using the empty chair technique. For example, consider the following method for working with anger:

CHILD: I hate my dad. He's mean. I hate his guts.

COUNSELOR: Let's pretend your dad is sitting in that empty chair. What do you want to say to him? You can walk over there and say whatever you want.

CHILD: Get off my back! Leave me alone! I cleaned my room just as good as I could.

COUNSELOR: Now sit in the other chair. Pretend to be your dad.

CHILD: I've told you and told you that this room looks like a pigpen.

COUNSELOR: Now be yourself again.

CHILD: I cleaned my room good, Dad! Then you came in and said it still isn't good enough. Nothing was left out in the room but my toys!

COUNSELOR: Now be your dad.

CHILD: This is the last time I'm telling you, Son. The room better be finished when I get back. That means toys too.

COUNSELOR: Now be you.

CHILD: You don't care about me! You don't care about how I feel. You just worry about the house being messed up. You get mad when I get out my toys. Kids are supposed to have toys! It's MY ROOM! Quit it! Stop complaining about what I do. [This outburst is accompanied by much nonverbal expression of anger, as well as the overt angry verbal content and eventually tears.]

The child has expressed his strong thoughts that his room should be his territory, that it should be all right to have his toys out. A global "hatred" for the father has been reduced to anger about a specific recurring problem (the differing standards for the room held by the parent and the child). After release of the built-up anger, some problem solving could achieve a compromise about the room situation.

Another sample counseling session involves the top dog–underdog debate, using an empty chair for each "dog." This technique is useful when the child has a decision-making problem. Most decision-making problems involve a debate between the inner voice of "I should do …" (top dog) versus "Yes, but I want to do …" (underdog). An empty chair is assigned to each point of view.

Identification of the Problem

Susan is experiencing a conflict whether to live with her mother or her father when their divorce is final.

Individual and Background Information

Susan Adams is a 10-year-old girl in the fourth grade. Her mother and father are getting a divorce, and she has a role in deciding whether to live with her mother or her father. Susan is the second of three children. This was the second marriage for Susan's mother and the first marriage for Susan's father. Her elder brother is not her father's biological son. Both parents work in factory jobs, but their income seems to be limited by the fact that Susan's father spends most of his paycheck on alcohol. Susan is an average student in school; she is quiet and has never had behavioral problems. She gets along well with her peers at school. Susan's physical health is good, but she has a vision problem that requires a new pair of glasses, which her parents claim they do not have the money to buy.

Transcript

COUNSELOR: Susan, we have the next 30 minutes for our talk. Where would you like to start?

SUSAN: Well, you know my problem about having to decide whether to live with Mom or Daddy after their divorce is final. I just don't know what I'm going to do.

COUNSELOR: I know that when we talked about this the other day, you were feeling really upset about this situation of having to choose between your mom and dad. I can tell you still feel this way.

SUSAN: Yes, I do. I did all the things we talked about—like talking to both of them. That made it even harder to decide because they both want me to live with them. I still don't know what to do. I wish they would stop the divorce.

COUNSELOR: Well, it's a good feeling to know that they both want you, but a bad feeling to know you have to choose. You would really like to have them stay together.

SUSAN: Yes, I really would, but that's impossible! I've tried every way I can to keep them together.

COUNSELOR: Susan, would you try an experiment with me that might help clarify your thinking about this decision?

SUSAN: I'll try anything to help.

COUNSELOR: [explains and demonstrates the top dog—underdog technique] So, when you are in the top dog chair, you say, "I should …," and when you are in the underdog chair, you say, "I want …" Okay?

SUSAN: Okay. [goes to the top dog chair first]

TOP DOG: I should go with Daddy because he'll be all alone.

UNDERDOG: Yes, but I want to stay with Mom because I hate to give up my room, and I want to stay with my sister.

TOP DOG: What is Daddy going to do without anyone to cook for him and clean house?

UNDERDOG: Why can't he hire a maid, and I can visit him a lot too?

TOP DOG: If I don't live with Daddy, he won't have anybody, because he doesn't want Jake, and Sally is too young to move away from Mom.

UNDERDOG: Well, Daddy goes out and drinks a lot with his friends, and sometimes he gets sick and is not nice to be around when he gets drunk.

TOP DOG:	I think I should take care of him when he gets sick.
UNDERDOG:	I think it is better not to be near him when he drinks. I would like to visit him when he is not drinking.
TOP DOG:	How can I live with Mom and help Daddy too?
UNDERDOG:	I just know things will be better if I live with Mom in my room and see Daddy as often as I can.
COUNSELOR:	Do you think you've finished with this argument, Susan?
SUSAN:	Yes, I've said all I can think of.
COUNSELOR:	I'm wondering what you learned from doing this exercise.
SUSAN:	Well, I think things will be better if I stay where I am with Mom. But I'll need to see a lot of Daddy—as much as I can. I love them both so much. [starts to cry]
COUNSELOR:	I know this has to be a sad and rough time for you. It really hurts, doesn't it?
SUSAN:	It sure does. I need to be brave about this and not let it make me so sad.
COUNSELOR:	It's okay to feel sad about this. You can always come in here to talk to me when you want to. [Counselor terminates the interview and schedules another session for the next day.]

DIVERSITY APPLICATIONS OF GESTALT THERAPY

Gestalt therapy has certain aspects that appeal to some cultures and others that the same cultures might find offensive. Gestalt counselors attempt to understand each person's perspective of the world and thereby respect the individuality of humans (Fall et al., 2010). Gestalt therapy is directed more toward total lifestyle change than to individual problems that are mere fragments of a person's life and style of interacting with the environment. Most people from all cultures coming to counseling for the purpose of getting help for specific problems are frustrated when they find the Gestalt counselor taking a global focus of examining the total picture rather than the pieces of the presenting problem. In summary, Gestalt counselors believe that teaching clients how to behave in an authentic, honest, and open manner will be sufficient for handling any problem that might arise.

Gestalt therapy is the most present-oriented therapy discussed in this book; however, old, unfinished business can be updated to the present by having clients confront their "problem" people in the empty chair. Even unfinished business with deceased people can be addressed with the empty chair method. Techniques such as the empty chair may present problems for clients from cultures where verbal, emotional, and behavioral expressiveness contradict cultural norms (Duran, 2006).

Saner (1989) has voiced concerns about possible cultural bias in U. S. Gestalt therapy methods. He suggests several ways to make Gestalt therapy valid across cultures: He proposes dropping the ethnocentric emphasis on the individual in favor of stressing reciprocal interaction by all participants in a social setting, using psychodrama in group therapy rather than the hot-seat method of individual therapy, and incorporating contributions from other disciplines in Gestalt theory and practice. Jacobs (2005) and Lee (2004) assert that Gestalt therapists have an increased appreciation for interdependence and a better understanding of shame and cultural values. In the end, it is the counselor's responsibility to be aware of possible difficulties clients from other cultures may have with the interventions and theories the counselor practices.

EVALUATION OF GESTALT THERAPY

Wolfe (2012) wrote about his "two-chair dialogue" between his "practitioner head" and his "researcher head," capturing the problems of the art of therapy juxtaposed with the science. Ironically, he chooses to deliberate his dilemma using these well-known techniques from Gestalt therapy.

As noted earlier rather than examining each individual piece in a person's jigsaw puzzle, the Gestalt therapist prefers to work with the total person. This means that Gestalt counselors would replace discussions of getting a job or making better grades with the counselor with the goal of teaching the client to interact with people in an open, authentic manner. Counselors would also work to help people discard phony behavior and relate to others in an open, honest manner. Clients would be encouraged to invest the energy, formerly used to play phony roles, into more productive activities such as getting and maintaining employment and earning better grades.

In addition, the Gestalt counselor trains clients to trust the feelings their brains are sending to their bodies. In other words, people need to give their attention to those feelings that are indicators they are about to do the right or wrong thing, make the right or wrong decision, stay in the right or wrong job, or stay in the right or wrong relationship. Gestalt techniques facilitate discovery, confrontation, and resolution of the client's major conflict, often in a dramatically short time. The inexperienced therapist, observer, or client might assume that Gestalt therapy offers an "instant cure." Even experienced counselors are tempted to push the client to a stance of self-support too fast, too soon.

Strümpfel (2006) reviewed 74 studies of Gestalt therapy and concluded evidence for the effectiveness of this approach was significantly positive for a range of clients. Treatment effects were stable in follow-up. Clients evaluated the therapy favorably and nursing staff reported improvements in clients. Effects were greatest for clients with symptoms of depression, anxiety, and phobias as well as for school children with achievement difficulties. Brownell (2008) also synthesizes the growing body of research on the effectiveness of the Gestalt approach.

Gestalt therapy contributed the concepts of field theory, immediacy and wholeness, and mind–body integration to counseling. Similarly innovative strategies such as the empty chair, emphasis on nonverbal messages, dream processing, and "I" statements have had significant impact on the practice of counseling. Perhaps most significantly the Gestalt emphasis on the relationships between the counselor and the client provides the clearest support for the Gestalt approach to counseling.

Seligman and Reichenberg (2014) suggest that Gestalt therapy is particularly appropriate for individuals who feel they are not living fully. They may be detached and uninvolved, or they may be so involved in the pressures of life that they have no sense of joy. Gestalt therapy is also effective with people who have channeled their emotional problems into physical reactions such as illness or pain.

Brief Gestalt therapy (BGT) was created to adapt the practice of Gestalt therapy to managed care restrictions (Houston, 2003). There are some significant differences between BGT and brief therapy (BT). BGT counselors adapt the counseling process to fit the individual needs of clients and their presenting problems. There is greater emphasis on developing a working relationship between the counselor and client. Methods and assumptions from other systems of counseling are used. Solution-focused methods of expanding the positive aspects of one's life and scaling progress toward goals are two examples. Homework assignments or between-session experiments are used as they are in reality therapy and rational-emotive behavior therapy. Burley and Freier (2004), in a related article, point out that people get into difficulty when there are interruptions of the process of Gestalt formation and resolution, which may have developed in the early childhood years. They refer to this as a procedural memory problem that prevents people from retaining learned connections between stimuli and response (habits). It may not be long until we find behavioral methods finding their way into BGT.

SUMMARY

We urge caution regarding the misuse of popular Gestalt techniques with fragile children, adolescents, and adults who cannot handle the emotional intensity some of the methods generate. Additional caution, patience, and sensitivity also are recommended regarding Gestalt counseling with severely disturbed or psychotic clients. Therapeutic activity should be limited to procedures that strengthen clients' contact with reality, their self-confidence, and their trust in the counselor and the counseling process. With trust established between the counselor and the client, Gestalt counseling can be directed toward working with the painful, unfinished business of past and current conflicts.

Greenberg (2011) echoes similar concerns about using traditional Gestalt therapy with people who have borderline personality disorder, recommending interactive group therapy over talking to a dead parent in an empty chair and hot-seat confrontations. Therefore, the question of who should receive Gestalt therapy is as important as the skills, training, experience, and judgment of the therapist. A counselor who uses this approach must be neither afraid nor inept in allowing the client to follow through and finish the experience of grief, rage, fear, or joy. Without such skill, the counselor may leave the client vulnerable.

Gestalt therapy focuses on the here-and-now experience and on personal responsibility. As well as lessening worrisome symptoms, Gestalt counselors and clients work so that clients become more alive, creative, and free from unfinished business that has affected life satisfaction, fulfillment, and growth. Gestalt counselors focus on the present and on living. They believe that everything in life connects, a web of relationships meshes everything. Therefore, one can only know their self as existing in relation to other things. Gestalt therapy goals include helping people live in the present, use their resources, bring closure to unfinished business and achieve integration and wholeness.

INTRODUCTION TO GESTALT THERAPY VIDEO

To gain a more in-depth understanding of the concepts in this chapter, visit www .cengage.com/counseling/henderson to view a short clip of an actual therapist–client session demonstrating Gestalt therapy.

WEB SITES FOR GESTALT THERAPY

Internet addresses frequently change. To find the sites listed here, visit www .cengage. com/counseling/henderson for an updated list of Internet addresses and direct links to relevant sites.

Association for the Advancement of Gestalt Therapy (AAGT)

Center for Gestalt Development

Gestalt Therapy Page

Society for Gestalt Theory and Its Applications (GTA)

The Gestalt Therapy Network

REFERENCES

Barnard, L. K., & Curry, J. F. (2012). Self-compassion: Conceptualizations, correlates, & interventions. *Review of General Psychology, 15,* 289–303.

Baumgardner, P., & Perls, F. (1975). *Gifts from Lake Cowichan and legacy from Fritz.* Palo Alto, CA: Science and Behavior Books.

Brownell, P. (Ed.). (2008). *Handbook for theory, research, and practice in Gestalt therapy.* Newcastle, UK: Cambridge Scholars.

Burley, T., & Freier, M. (2004). Character structure: A gestalt-cognitive theory. *Psychotherapy: Theory, Research, Practice, Training, 41,* 321–331.

Carmichael, K. D. (2006). *Play therapy: An introduction.* Upper Saddle River, NJ: Pearson.

Carroll, F. (2009). Gestalt play therapy. In K. J. O'Connor & L. D. Braverman (Eds.), *Play therapy theory and practice: Comparing theories and techniques* (2nd ed., pp. 283–314). New York: Wiley.

Clarkson, P. (2013). *Gestalt counselling in action* (4th ed.). London: Sage.

Clarkson, P., & Mackewn, J. (1993). *Fritz Perls.* Thousand Oaks, CA: Sage.

Duran, E. (2006). *Healing the soul wound.* New York: Teachers College Press.

Engle, D., & Holliman, M. (2002). A Gestalt-experiential perspective on resistance. *Journal of Clinical Psychology, 58,* 175–183.

English, H., & English, A. (1958). *A comprehensive dictionary of psychological terms.* New York: Longmans, Green.

Fall, K. A., Holden, J. M., & Marquis, A. (2010). *Theoretical models of counseling and psychotherapy* (2nd ed.). New York: Brunner Routledge.

Greenberg, L. S. (2011). *Emotion-focused therapy.* Washington, DC: American Psychological Association.

Greenberg, L. S., & Malcolm, W. (2003). Resolving unfinished business: Relating process to outcome. *Journal of Consulting and Clinical Psychology, 70*, 406–416.

Greenberg, L. S., Rice, L., & Elliott, R. (1993). *Facilitating emotional change: The moment-by-moment process.* New York: Guilford Press.

Haley, M. (2010). Gestalt therapy. In D. Capuzzi & D. R. Gross (Eds.), *Counseling and psychotherapy: Theories and interventions* (5th ed., pp. 167–192). Upper Saddle River, NJ: Pearson.

Houston, G. (2003). *Brief Gestalt therapy.* Thousand Oaks, CA: Sage.

Jacobs, L. (2005). The inevitable intersubjectivity of selfhood. *International Gestalt Journal, 28,* 43–70.

Joyce, P., & Sills, C. (2010). *Skills in gestalt counseling and psychotherapy* (2nd ed.). Thousand Oaks, CA: Sage.

Lee, R. G. (Ed.). (2004). *The value of connection; A relational approach to ethics.* Cambridge, MA: Gestalt Press/Analytic Press.

Kellogg, S. (2004). Dialogical encounters: Contemporary perspectives on "chairwork" in psychotherapy. *Psychotherapy: Theory, Research, Practice, Training, 41,* 310–320.

Mann, D. (2010). *Gestalt therapy: 100 key points and techniques.* New York: Routledge.

Miller, M. (1989). Introduction to Gestalt therapy verbatim. *Gestalt Journal, 7,* 5–24.

Murdock, N. L. (2013). *Theories of counseling and psychotherapy: A case approach* (3rd ed.). Upper Saddle River, NJ: Pearson.

Oaklander, V. (1978). *Windows to our children.* Moab, UT: Real People Press.

Oaklander, V. (1988). *Windows to our children: A Gestalt therapy approach to children and adolescents.* Highland: Center for Gestalt Development.

Oaklander, V. (1993). From meek to bold: A case study of Gestalt therapy. In T. Kottman & C. Schaefer (Eds.), *Play therapy in action: A casebook for practitioners* (pp. 281–300). Northvale, NJ: Aronson.

Oaklander, V. (2001). Gestalt play therapy. *International Journal of Play Therapy, 10,* 45–55.

Oaklander, V. (2006). *Hidden treasure: A map to the child's inner self.* London: Karmac Books.

Oaklander, V (2011). Gestalt play therapy. In C. E. Schaefer (Ed.), *Foundations of play therapy* (pp. 171–186). Retrieved from http://www.eblib.com

Parlett, M., & Hemming, J. (1996). Gestalt therapy. In W. Dryden (Ed.), *Handbook of individual therapy* (pp. 194–218). Thousand Oaks, CA: Sage.

Perls, F. (1969a). *Gestalt therapy verbatim.* Moab, UT: Real People Press.

Perls, F. (1969b). *In and out the garbage pail.* New York: Bantam.

Perls, F. (1970a). Four lectures. In J. Fagan & I. L. Shepherd (Eds.), *Gestalt therapy now* (pp. 14–38). New York: Harper & Row.

Perls, F. (1970b). Dream seminars. In J. Fagan & I. L. Shepherd (Eds.), *Gestalt therapy now* (pp. 204–233). New York: Harper & Row.

Perls, F. (1975). *Gestalt is: A collection of articles about Gestalt therapy and living.* Moab, UT: Real People Press.

Perls, F., Hefferline, R., & Goodman, P. (1951). *Gestalt therapy: Excitement and growth in the human personality.* New York: Julian Press.

Perls, L. (1992). Concepts and misconceptions of Gestalt therapy. *Journal of Humanistic Psychology, 32,* 50–56.

Polster, W., & Polster, M. (1973). *Gestalt therapy integrated.* New York: Brunner/Mazel.

Saner, R. (1989). Culture bias of gestalt therapy: Made-in-U.S.A. *Gestalt Journal, 12,* 57–71.

Seligman, L., & Reichenberg, L. W. (2014). *Theories of counseling and psychotherapy: Systems, strategies, and skills* (4th ed.). Upper Saddle River, NJ: Pearson.

Shostrom, E. (Producer). (1965). *Three approaches to psychotherapy* [Film]. Orange, CA: Psychological Films.

Strümpfel, U. (2006). *Research on Gestalt therapy.* Retrieved from http://www.therapie-der-gefuehle.de/

Stumpfel, U., & Goldman, R. (2002). Contacting Gestalt therapy. In D. J. Cain & J. Seeman (Eds.), *Humanistic psychotherapies: Handbook of research and practice* (pp. 189–219). Washington, DC: American Psychological Association.

Wagner Moore, L. E. (2004). Gestalt therapy: Past, present, theory and research. *Psychotherapy: Theory, Research, Practice, Training, 41*(2), 180–189. doi:10.1037/0033-3204.41.2.180

Wheeler, G., & McConville, M. (2002). *The heart of development: Gestalt approaches to working with children, adolescents, and their worlds*. Hillsdale, NJ: Gestalt Press.

Wolfe, B. E. (2012). Healing the research-practice split: Let's start with me. *Psychotherapy, 49*(2), 101–108.

Yontef, G., & Jacobs, L. (2014). Gestalt therapy. In R. J. Corsini & D. Wedding (Eds.), *Current psychotherapies* (10th ed., pp. 299–335). Belmont, CA: Thomson.

CHAPTER 8

Behavioral Counseling

When all else fails, I become a behaviorist.
—HOWARD GARDNER

We are known by what we do. Human behavior shapes our lives and impacts those close to us. Our actions can be observed, whereas emotions, thoughts, and our past cannot be seen. Consequently, some scientists have focused on the study of human behavior, research that has provided the roots for what has become behavioral counseling, some forms of counseling that involve perspectives on the ways humans learn. In the early 20th century, John Watson conducted studies of classical conditioning with children. In 1913, he admonished professionals to focus on the objective study of observable behaviors. He talked about a "purely objective experimental branch of natural science" with the goal of "prediction and control of behavior" (Watson, 1913, p. 158). Watson became known as the father of behaviorism, a form of counseling that has evolved since about 1900.

After reading this chapter, you should be able to:

▶ Outline the development of behavioral theory
▶ Explain the theory of behavioral counseling, including its core concepts
▶ Discuss the counseling relationship and goals in behavioral counseling
▶ Describe assessment, process, and techniques in behavioral counseling
▶ Demonstrate some therapeutic techniques
▶ Clarify the effectiveness of behavioral counseling

EARLY BEHAVIORISM

The field of behavioral psychology has had numerous contributors over the years. The 1920s marked the time when the basic concepts of behavioral therapy were first used. It was not until the 1950s and 1960s, though, that systematic and comprehensive forms of behavioral therapy emerged. Primary contributors were Joseph Wolpe in South Africa, M. B. Shapiro and Hans Eysenck in Britain, and

John Watson and B. F. Skinner in the United States. During the first half of the 20th century, the roots of early behavioral counseling began with the work of a Russian physiologist, Ivan Pavlov. He identified a learning process called classical conditioning.

IVAN PAVLOV
(1849–1936)

Born in 1849, Pavlov began his education in a seminary school but abandoned his pursuit of the priesthood for his fascination with science. He received his M.D. in 1883 from the University of St. Petersburg and was made director of several research facilities, including the Imperial Institute of Experimental Medicines (Windholtz, 1997). Pavlov was awarded the Nobel Prize in 1904 for his book *Lectures on the Work of the Digestive Glands.*

Reminded that he had studied all the digestive juices of the body with the exception of saliva, Pavlov came out of retirement to research how saliva contributed to the digestive process, if at all. In collecting saliva from dogs, he made several observations. He noted that dogs salivated when they were fed and when they heard any noise that accompanied it, such as the click of opening the dog pen gate. This observation led to further experiments with Pavlov's classical, or respondent, conditioning model and to more efficient methods for collecting saliva for his research.

Wolpe and Plaud (1997) provide an overview of the development of behavior therapy, which features the contributions of Pavlov through his work on animal conditioning. Pavlov and his students discovered experimental neurosis, which could be produced and eliminated in animals through conditioning and counterconditioning. Many of his counterconditioning techniques are in use today to treat neurotic and anxiety reactions. Pavlov found he could eliminate undesirable conditioned responses and reduce associated anxieties by manipulating conditioned stimuli. The portion of his work that has withstood the test of time is his classical conditioning method first used to collect saliva from dogs.

John B. Watson, an experimental psychologist, used Pavlov's ideas in his work. Watson advocated studying observable variables that could be collected, counted, and analyzed in discrete parts. He rejected psychoanalytic introspection and, as stated earlier, became known as the father of behaviorism. His best-known experiment involved the application of classical conditioning to a child's phobia. Watson paired an unconditional stimulus (a loud sound) with a conditioned stimulus (a rat) to induce a fear response in the child, little Albert. Watson's student treated the child using behavioral techniques. Other practitioners used the principles of classical conditioning to problems of phobias, bedwetting, and tension. Joseph Wolpe developed a procedure known as systematic desensitization to treat fear and anxiety (Spiegler & Guevremont, 2009).

B. F. SKINNER
(1904–1990)

Just as behavioral therapy is rooted in Ivan Pavlov's experiments of respondent or classical conditioning, behavior modification stems from B. F. Skinner's work on instrumental or operant conditioning. Both scholars shared a common interest in using experimental methods to research abnormal behavioral patterns. Although he did not develop new principles of behaviorism, Skinner did the most to translate the theories and ideas of other behaviorists into the methods currently used by counselors and therapists around the world. He is also the person most associated with traditional behavioral counseling in the United States.

Burrhus Frederic Skinner was born and lived until he was 18 in Susquehanna, Pennsylvania. He had a younger brother, an attorney father, and a musical mother. He majored in literature at Hamilton College in Clinton, New York, with the goal of becoming a writer. After a few years with little success, Skinner regarded himself a failure as a writer. Reflecting later on this time in his life, Skinner commented that he failed because he had nothing to say.

Skinner then entered Harvard University to study psychology. The behavior of humans and animals was of special interest to him. He received a master's degree in 1930 and a Ph.D. in experimental psychology in 1931. After graduation, Skinner began his productive career as a teacher and researcher, first at Harvard and then at the University of Minnesota in 1936. While in Minnesota, he married Yvonne Blue. They had two daughters, the younger of which became famous for being reared in Skinner's air crib, a combination playpen and crib with a plastic mattress cover, glass sides, and air conditioning. In short, it resembled an aquarium for babies. His invention never caught on with crib-buying shoppers.

He was appointed chairman of the Psychology Department at Indiana University in 1945. He later returned to Harvard in 1948 to accept a professorship, which he held until his death. As he began to generate things to say in the field of behaviorism, Skinner's flair for writing returned. His numerous books include *The Behavior of Organisms* (1938), *Walden Two* (1948), The *Technology of Teaching* (1968), *Beyond Freedom and Dignity* (1971), *A Matter of Consequences: Part III of an Autobiography* (1983), and *Upon Further Reflection* (1987). R. Epstein also edited the book *Skinner for the Classroom* (1980).

Skinner's contribution to knowledge is not strictly confined to the laboratory. He made considerable contributions to solving educational problems. He developed and advanced the concepts of programmed instruction, operant conditioning in classroom management, and the teaching machine (first developed by Sidney Pressey in 1923). Perhaps the most controversial of Skinner's works is *Beyond Freedom and Dignity* (1971), which pictures a society where behavior is shaped and controlled by a planned system of rewards. His most helpful contributions to classroom management are found in *The Technology of Teaching* and *Skinner for the Classroom*.

Skinner (1990a), in an article he completed the evening before his death, attacked those who would use introspection or brain analysis as methods for analyzing behavior. He asserted that behavior is the product of three types of variation and selection: natural selection, operant conditioning, and modeling. Skinner had little use for cognitive psychology because he contended that it had not contributed, as behavior analysis, to the design of better environments for solving existing problems and preventing future problems. Summing up his 60 years in the profession, Skinner (1990b) said that the point he tried to make is that it can be demonstrated that people choose behavior based on anticipated consequences. According to Skinner, this selection by consequences has negative implications for the world and its future unless some vital changes are made. He concluded by saying that he would like to be remembered as fostering the needed changes.

Skinner's death in 1990 ended six decades of significant contributions to behavioral psychology that began with the publication of his first article in 1930. During his career, citations of Skinner's name in the literature exceeded those of the previous leader, Sigmund Freud (Banks & Thompson, 1995).

This first wave of behavior therapy focused on treating problem behaviors. By the 1960s behaviorists had amassed research that supported the efficacy, effectiveness and efficiency of behavior therapy which became a major force in psychology (Spiegler & Guevremont, 2009). The following sections of the chapter summarized that approach.

THE NATURE OF PEOPLE

A broad statement of the behaviorist view of the nature of people is Skinner's (1971) belief that children change because of the experiences they have. Behaviorists view human beings as neither good nor bad but merely products of their environment. People are essentially born neutral (the blank slate or tabula rasa idea), with equal potential for good or evil and for rationality or irrationality.

In this approach to counseling, behavior is defined as actions performed as a response to stimuli (Austad, 2009). Fall, Holden, and Marquis (2010) explain the philosophical foundations of behavioral counseling as *evolutionary continuity, reductionism, determinism,* and *empiricism. Evolutionary continuity* captures the view that animal behavior and human behavior are identical. Therefore, inferences about human behavior can be made based on experiments with animals. Behaviorists acknowledge the complexity of human behavior but argue that watching animals allows some generalizations to humans. *Reductionism* refers to considering behavior as components. Behavioral counselors believe that in order to find what is essential, each part of the whole must be considered. Personality then becomes the collection of discrete behaviors. Problems are addressed through the components of the behavior so that a shy child who wants more friends would learn ways to greet a peer, ask a question, take turns in a conversation, and smile, for example. *Determinism* implies that all behavior has cause and is never unpredictable or random. Reinforcement contingencies, or what happens before or after a behavior, determine actions. Finally, *empiricism* stresses the observable, testable, and measurable. These underpinnings of continuity, reductionism, determinism, and empiricism form the philosophical base of behaviorism.

Behaviorists contend that people are responders who act based on what they have learned. People make those reactions when the stimulus conditions are appropriate. Behavioral counselors, therefore, view individuals as products of their conditioning. The stimulus–response paradigm is the basic pattern of all human learning, according to behavioral theory. People react in predictable ways to any given stimulus according to what they have learned through experience. Humans react to stimuli much as animals do, except that human responses are more complex and organized on a higher plane. Personality is the total integration of behaviors a person has at any given time, a behavioral repertoire (Fall et al., 2010).

Skinner particularly regarded the human being as an organism who learns patterns of behavior, catalogs them within a repertoire, and repeats them at a later date. More specifically, the person learns a specific response when a satisfying condition follows an action. The number of these responses mounts as time passes and satisfying conditions are repeated. The behaviorist's interest is in the science of behavior as it relates to biology. Skinner believed:

> A person is a member of a species shaped by evolutionary contingencies of survival, displaying behavioral processes which bring him under the control of the environment in which he lives, and largely under the control of a social environment which he and millions of others like him have constructed and maintained during the evolution of a culture. The direction of the controlling relation is reversed: a person does not act upon the world, the world acts upon him. (1971, p. 211)

THEORY OF COUNSELING

Behavioral counseling is an action therapy in much the same way that reality therapy, solution-focused brief counseling, and cognitive-behavioral therapy are. Clients do something about their behavior rather than trying to understand it by talking about it. They may control, reduce, or eliminate troubling aspects of their behavior. They may also learn to increase behavior, such as exercising, as well as form new or better developed skills. Clients learn to monitor their behavior, practice skills, and complete therapeutic homework assignments to help them reach their goals.

Counselors help clients develop plans to reinforce adaptive or helpful behavior and extinguish maladaptive or unhelpful behavior. The counselor's role is, through reinforcement principles, to help clients achieve the goals they have set for themselves. Learning is structured and involves clients doing something, like practicing an action, recording behaviors, or confronting a situation with new skills.

This type of learning is considered to be a relatively enduring, observable change in behavior that comes after experience or practice. An ABC model outlines the sequence of action according to operant conditioning outlined by Skinner (1953). People tend to repeat the behavior when the same environmental conditions occur, the *antecedent (A)* to the behavior. Observable change means the person is doing something that is visible and measurable, the *behavior (B)* part of the equation. Finally, the phrase "experience or practice" refers to something that preceded or followed the action and that also caused the repetition of the behavior, or *consequence (C)*. Based on the premise that human behavior is learned, any or all behavior can be unlearned and new behavior learned in its place by attending to the antecedent and consequences of the behavior. Thus, the behaviorist is concerned with observable events that can be unlearned or enhanced by attending to the sequence of behavior. Antony and Roemer (2011) and Wilson (2008) listed the following as assumptions in this action-focused counseling:

- Individual differences emerge mostly from different experiences.
- Behavior, normal and abnormal, is learned and acquired primarily through modeling, conditioning, and reinforcement.
- Behavior has purpose.
- Behavioral counselors focus on understanding and changing behavior. Specificity is the foundation of behavioral assessment and treatment; a person is understood and described by what a person does in a particular situation.
- The focus of counseling is present functioning. Even if the child has a long-standing behavior, it is maintained by current reinforcers.
- Behaviors can only be understood by viewing the context in which they occur.
- A child's environment can be modified to increase appropriate behaviors and decrease harmful actions.
- Treatment begins with an analysis of the problem into components and continues by the formation of plans targeted to modify the subparts of the behavior.
- Treatment strategies are tailored to different problems in different individuals.
- Knowing the origins of psychological problems is not necessary for change. Rather than mental illness, behaviorists refer to "problems in living."
- Behavioral counselors commit to the scientific method. They have a testable framework, use treatment and techniques with measurable outcomes that can be replicated, evaluate methods and concepts, and emphasize research strategies that produce specific methods applied to particular problems. Counseling goals are stated in behavioral, specific, and measurable terms. Progress is assessed regularly.

Therefore, counselors who practice behavioral therapy focus on a person's current behavior to identify ways to modify the client's responses. That modification plan incorporates concepts related to principles of learning, consequences, schedules of reinforcement, chaining, and shaping.

CONCEPTS

Principles of Learning

Behavioral counseling includes several techniques based on principles of learning used to manage maladaptive behavior. Currently, behavioral counseling is used with covert processes (cognitions, emotions, and obsessive ideation), as well as with traditional overt behavior problems. The strength, presence, absence, and frequency of behavior are all considered the result of the reinforcement the person receives.

Behavioral counseling involves two types of behavior: operant and respondent. The assumption of operant conditioning is that when a person acts, if the behavior is promptly followed by some form of reinforcement, the person will likely make the same response in the same or similar environmental conditions. In operant conditioning, *operant behavior* refers to behavior that operates on and changes the environment in some manner. It is also referred to as *instrumental behavior* because it is instrumental in goal achievement. Respondent behavior will be discussed in the following sections on classical conditioning.

Consequences

Consequences have powerful control over behavior and can be divided into the two primary types: reinforcers and punishers. Reinforcers are consequences that are likely to increase the occurrence of the behavior. Someone who uses operant conditioning waits until the desired behavior or an approximation of the desired behavior occurs, and then reinforces it with a rewarding stimulus known as *positive reinforcement* or rewards (e.g., praise, money, candy, free time, and attention; something the person finds desirable). Therefore, positive reinforcers add something. *Negative reinforcement* (different from punishment) occurs when the operant behavior is reinforced by its capacity to stop an aversive stimulus, something the person wants to avoid. For example, rats learn to press a bar to shut off an electric shock, and children take their seats at school to shut off the aversive sound of their teacher's scolding. Therefore, negative reinforcers take something away to increase the desired behavior. If consequences increase or strengthen the behavior, they are defined as reinforcers which can be either positive or negative.

Punishers are consequences that weaken behavior and decrease the likelihood it will reoccur (Fink & Lotspeich, 2004). *Extinction* is the process of eliminating a behavior by ignoring the behavior or by not reinforcing it by withholding attention and other rewards. Fall et al. (2010) state that there is a sequence to the way a person may respond to extinction. The person may respond with denial she is being ignored, for example, and continue the behavior, then become angry, bargain to try to regain the reinforcement, and then accept that the reward will not be repeated. Therefore, using extinction requires consistency to maintain the

	Present	Withhold
Positive stimuli: Praise Tangible rewards	Positive reinforcement	Extinction

Negative stimuli:
Criticism
Unpleasant
  consequences
  and tasks
	Punishment	Negative
		reinforcement

FIGURE 8-1   EXAMPLES OF OPERANT CONDITIONING

elimination of the targeted behavior. *Punishment*, an aversive event, occurs after the behavior occurs. Punishment tends to decrease the occurrence of the behavior. Spanking, yelling, and sending children to time-out rooms are examples of widely used punishment. Spiegler and Guevremont (2009) explain that the child experiencing punishment, especially physical pain, may quickly stop the behavior but may also be anxious and avoid the person who inflicted the pain. Additionally the child may imitate the aversive behavior to others. Therefore, punishment should be the last strategy to use in order to avoid the harmful side effects it generates.

Figure 8-1 compares positive reinforcement, negative reinforcement, punishment, and extinction. A related behavioral concept is prompting, teaching someone a desirable response which can then be reinforced. The following would be choices of responding to a child who fights with her little sister over toys: yelling at her and telling her no one will ever like her (punishment); ignoring her (extinction); telling her you will stop saying "supercalifragilisticexpialidocious" when she stops grabbing the toy (negative reinforcement); or explaining to her that sharing is important and that when you get impatient waiting for your turn, you take a deep breath and smile till your teeth show (prompting) and that if she can do that for the next hour, she will earn 10 extra minutes of outside play time (positive reinforcement). The timing or schedule of responses to behavior also impacts the change.

Schedules of Reinforcement

Changing the balance of positive and negative consequences requires selecting an appropriate schedule of reinforcement for shaping behavior. There are two schedules of reinforcement for the acquisition and establishment of a new behavior: continuous and intermittent.

Continuous reinforcement happens each time the person has a particular response. Intermittent reinforcement happens only some of the time the response occurs. *Continuous reinforcement*, the reinforcement of each successful response, is best when the new behavior is first being learned. Once the new behavior has been learned, continuous reinforcement has the effect of extinguishing the behavior by satiating the learner. Reinforcement should be switched to *intermittent* reinforcement that occurs only some of the time the behavior occurs.

FIXED INTERVAL SCHEDULE   Reinforcement is provided on the first response after a fixed time has elapsed. The interval could be set, for example, at 30 seconds. Hourly wages paid weekly and tests given in a class each Friday are other examples of fixed interval schedules. Reinforced targeted behavior increases before the reinforcement and decreases dramatically after the reinforcement. For instance, study behavior increases before the test and decreases after the test.

VARIABLE INTERVAL SCHEDULE   Reinforcement is provided on the first response after some average time period. For instance, intervals could range from 15 to 45 seconds, averaging 30 seconds over several successful responses. Unannounced pop quizzes given in class are excellent examples of an application of the variable interval schedule. Study behavior is highest for classes where pop quizzes are given, but the teacher's popularity may suffer. Study behavior increases as the time between quizzes increases.

FIXED RATIO SCHEDULE   The participant is reinforced for every five, ten, or twenty correct responses made. The reinforcement rate is fixed at the same rate (e.g., every fifth correct response is reinforced). Piecework in a factory where people are paid according to the number of products produced is a good example of a fixed ratio schedule.

VARIABLE RATIO SCHEDULE   Participants are reinforced on an irregular intermittent schedule. That type of reinforcement results in the most frequent, long-lasting pattern of response. Playing slot machines is a good example of both how variable ratio reinforcement is applied and how strongly this method maintains the gambling addictions people have. Fishing is another good example of variable ratio reinforcement. An occasional bite will keep a fisherman "hooked" for hours.

However, reinforcement methods may serve to extinguish desired behavior when the reward or token replaces any intrinsic reward a person might receive from engaging in the desired behavior. For example, if parents reward or reinforce a child's piano practice or good grades, the message to the child may be that piano playing or being successful in school may not be worth doing without pay, and therefore is not worthwhile in and of itself.

Chaining and Shaping

Most behaviors are complex and require a combination of simpler behaviors. A behavioral chain is the arrangement of individual responses in a particular sequence (Kazdin, 2012). An example of a behavioral chain is answering the telephone. Some components of that chain such as hearing the ring, finding the telephone, picking up the phone, activating the answer mode, and speaking into the phone are all links in that chain. The links in behavior may be overlooked in planning interventions which should be developed by analyzing complex behavior and gauging the antecedents and consequences of each link in the chain (Wagner, 2008).

Shaping involves children learning complex behavior by mastering successive approximations, or small steps, toward the final behavior. Reading skills are examples of shaping behavior as are walking, tying shoes, and other tasks. Counselors help children learn new skills by breaking behavior into these manageable steps. The counselor and the child will need to be clear about the desired end sequence—what follow what or chaining. The combination of shaping and chaining often leads to improved behaviors (Gladding, 2005).

Classical Conditioning

Every person has many involuntary responses to some environmental conditions. Classical, or respondent, conditioning is the way in which a person learns to emit the involuntary response to new conditions rather than to only the condition that innately elicits that response. This form of learning that occurs when a neutral stimulus (the conditioned or learned stimulus) comes to elicit a response after multiple pairings with another stimulus (the unconditioned or unlearned stimulus). In the case of Pavlov's dogs, for example, Pavlov paired the unconditioned stimulus of food with the neutral stimulus of a bell. The response to the unconditioned stimulus was salivating—when the dogs smelled food, they salivated. After the bell rang at the same time food appeared for several times, the neutral stimulus (the bell) became the conditioned stimulus, and the response to the conditioned stimulus became the conditioned response (salivating). A relevant example for those working with children would be the child who is bullied at school (unconditioned stimulus) reacts with fear and distress. Later even if the bullying is eliminated, that child may be afraid and anxious (conditioned response) at school (conditioned stimulus).

Wilson (2008) explained that currently classical conditioning analysis incorporates more than only stimulus–response bonds. Analysis includes correlations or contingent relationships between the conditioned and unconditioned response rather than a simple pairing of a single conditioned stimulus with one unconditioned stimulus.

RELATIONSHIP

Behavioral counselors believe in establishing a positive, collaborative relationship by communicating empathy and positive regard for the client. Clients are expected to set goals, try new behaviors, work between sessions, and monitor themselves. Behavioral counseling is shared problem solving between counselor and client. Counselors use positive reinforcement such as paying attention, noting the child's strengths, recognizing progress, and being pleasant and patient. Emmelkamp, Vedel, and Kamphuis (2007) identified general features of a behavioral counseling relationship:

- Counselors treat clients as competent people who will learn about factors that reinforce the problem and will help design ways to change.
- Counselors and clients work together to decide the therapeutic objectives.
- The counselor pays attention to increasing motivation, explaining counseling, and introducing therapeutic and homework assignments.

In short, behavioral counselors help clients determine ways to modify problems in living. Wilson (2008) suggests the counselor consider these points: "What is causing this person to behave in this way right now and what can we do right now to change that behavior?" (p. 229). The focus is on the present and the future. Complaints are translated into goals of observable behavioral changes. Behavior is broken into its parts and treatment tailored to the problem of this individual. Counselors do a detailed analysis of the target behaviors—antecedent, behavior, consequences (ABC)—and then use operant conditioning principles to develop a plan for change. The counselor is active and directive in this type of counseling approach. Wilson explained that the behavioral counselor is instructive and compassionate, someone who helps solve problems and serves as a model of coping.

COUNSELING GOALS

As with most counseling, the ultimate goal of behavioral counseling is teaching children and adolescents to become their own counselors by changing their behavior to better meet their needs. Behavioral counselors assume that most abnormal behavior is learned and maintained in the same way normal behavior is acquired. All behavior change, internal and external, can be attempted through behavioral counseling. The change process involves the environment that controls the person's behaviors. Clients of behavioral counselors will be considering whether their current behavior produces too little reinforcement or too much punishment. Baldwin and Baldwin (2001) explained two foci of behavioral counseling: helping people learn how to decrease their excesses and/or learn skills to overcome deficits.

The goals of counseling are determined by the client and counselor. The counselor acts as collaborator who will outline the steps to be followed to reach goals and the client will report about behavior changes at each step. The process of change is modified and refined as needed.

Behavioral counseling differs from other approaches to counseling principally in terms of specificity. The behavioral counselor prefers to state goals as observable changes in behavior rather than hypothetical constructs. The focus is on a narrow definition of the problem in terms of the behavior to be changed and the basic counseling function involved is to help the client to learn to respond differently to situations (individuals, groups, institutions, and environmental settings). In behavioral counseling, the continuing assessment of the effects on outcomes of each counseling intervention determines if the procedure was effective or not. Antony (2014) provides a useful overview of all aspects of behavioral counseling.

After the problem has been identified and the desired behavior change agreed on by the counselor and the client, the behavioral counselor may use a variety of counseling procedures to help the client acquire the behaviors necessary to solve the problem. Specific techniques reduce and eliminate anxiety, phobias, and obsessive thoughts, as well as reduce inappropriate, observable behaviors. Other techniques may increase the occurrence of desired behaviors such as exercising, reading, or smiling. The ultimate outcome of behavioral counseling is to teach people to become their own behavior-modification experts—that is, to program their own reinforcement schedules (self-management).

Encouraging people to move from extrinsic to intrinsic reinforcement—to please themselves with their behavior rather than constantly seeking the approval .

of others—is even more desirable. The ultimate success of behavioral counseling lies in the client's success in transferring from an extrinsic reward system to an intrinsic reward system for maintaining the target behavior. For example, a child who receives extra privileges at home for completing homework assignments reaches the intrinsic level when she realizes that her life is better when she does well at school and then continues the target behavior, reinforced only by the realization that her life is more pleasant. As her grades improve, she finds her parents more cooperative and nicer to be around, and she finds her teachers praising her efforts rather than nagging her about the missed homework assignments.

COUNSELING METHODS

When using behavioral counseling methods with children, the counselor needs to match reinforcement to the child's developmental level and reward preferences. Social development is one good predicator of effective reinforcers. Young children in the preoperational stage of development probably do not find sharing toys with siblings or friends to be an attractive reward. Preoperational-stage children find playing alone with favorite toys or playing a game in which they can make up all the rules much more reinforcing. Adolescents, in contrast, find the social contact involved in sharing and team activities reinforcing.

Assessment

Behavioral counselors consider assessment as a sample of behavior under certain conditions or context. Behavior counselors begin by identifying and understanding the client's problem by getting details about it. Questions usually begin with how, when, where, and what (Wilson, 2008). Practitioners may find instruments such as the *Achenbach Child Behavior Checklist* (CBCL; Achenbach, 1991), *the Behavior Assessment System for Children* (BASC; Reynolds & Kamphaus, 2002) and *Behavioral Objective Sequence* (Braaten, 1998) help with identifying the specifics of behavior. The *Conners's Teacher Rating Scale* (Conners, 1997) is designed for teachers to provide information about children's behaviors. More information about the process of assessment in behavioral counseling follows in the following section on counseling process.

Process

Seligman and Reichenberg (2014) outlined the procedure of behavior counseling in eight steps. The following is modified from their work.

1. Describe the targeted behavior
   a. Review the nature and history of the concern
   b. Consider the context of the behavior
2. Determine a baseline, the current frequency, duration, and severity of the targeted behavior
3. Establish goals
   a. Goals should be realistic, clear, specific, and measurable
   b. Check that goals are meaningful to the client
   c. State goals positively such as "compliment your brother's achievements" rather than "stop making fun of your brother"

4. Plan strategies for change
    a. Change antecedent conditions
    b. Teach skills and provide information for desired change
    c. Enhance impulse-control
    d. Use modeling, rehearsal, and other techniques
    e. Put together reinforcement contingencies
    f. Plan implementation of change process, monitoring, and recording outcomes
    g. Write out commitment and plan
5. Implement the plan
6. Measure progress
    a. Review the results of the plan
    b. Emphasize successes
    c. Find and address any obstacles
    d. Revise, if necessary
7. Reinforce success
8. Continue by planning for maintenance of gains

More information relative to the behavioral counseling process follows.

Describe the Behavior

A reiteration of assumptions begins the analysis of a behavior, beginning with the components:

- *Antecedents:* the stimuli or cues that occur before behavior that leads to its occurrence
- *Behavior:* what the person says or does (or does not do)
- *Consequences:* what the person perceives happens to him or her (positive, neutral, negative) as a result of his or her behavior

Accordingly behavioral problems are usually rooted in antecedents or consequences. Additionally people usually prefer behavior for which the consequences are known over behavior for which the consequences are uncertain. Fink and Lotspeich (2004) explained that the first step in behavioral counseling is specifying the target behavior by determining a precise, objective definition. Some specification may involve determining chains of behavior, the small links that connect the activities of the target behavior. Next, the counselor and client measure the behavior to establish its frequency, duration, and strength, a baseline against which the success of change will be gauged. The final part of beginning assessment is identifying the antecedents and consequences that are related to the behavior. Behaviors are not considered maladaptive unless they are causing the child or family difficulties.

Assessment happens throughout treatment in the cycle of assessing, treating, and evaluating the target behavior. A behavioral observation system involves identifying the target behavior and defining it specifically so that "behaving in class" would become "seated in desk," "facing the teacher," "raising hand to answer," and "speaking only with permission." The specificity in observable behaviors aids counselor and child in developing goals to change behavior.

Beveridge and Berg (2007), for example, provided a method to understand parent–adolescent interactions that may help caregivers describe young people's behavior. Children may self-monitor by using recording charts. Behavioral counselors are experts in observing, recording, and defining behaviors.

Behavioral counselors utilize many methods in assessment because a person's behavior varies across situations. Thus interviews, observation, self-report forms, checklist, and symptom measures completed by several people may be used.

Behavioral assessment aims to identify the behavior to be changed (*target behavior*), to assess the best course of treatment, to monitor the impact of treatment over time, and at the conclusion of counseling. Counselors use a *functional analysis* to find the variables that maintain the target behavior. Haynes, O'Brien, and Kaholokula (2011) give detailed information on functional analysis in their book on behavioral assessment. People other than the client who may be part of the assessment would be family, teachers, and friends. The child's behavior would be considered across settings such as home, school, play, and the counselor's office.

Some methods used to describe behavior include behavioral interviews, observations, monitoring forms, self-report scales, outcome samples, and physiological assessments. During behavioral interviews the counselor solicits a detailed description of the target behavior, including information about the frequency, duration, and intensity of the action. Generally the history of the problem is also discussed. Behavioral observations may be in the child's natural environment, such as a playground or other less-direct methods such as audio or video recordings or tracking the incidents of the behavior. Behavioral counselors often suggest clients' complete monitoring forms or diaries to measure where they started on their goal and where they are now. Self-report scales may be paper-pencil or computer based. Those scales are more general than the other descriptive methods but may require less time. Finally physiological assessments such as biofeedback apparatus may provide information relative to the objective, physical implications of behavior such as increased blood pressure readings during anxious periods. Therefore many methods may be used to aid in the process of describing behavior.

Then the counselor and client collaborate in determining ways to manipulate the antecedents and/or consequences and to identify the variables impact on the target behavior. For example, if a child refused to eat a meal, the counselor may suggest parents ignore the refusal to discover if the parents' attention was the consequence maintaining the behavior.

The crux of the assessment and the success of the treatment revolves around the counselor and child working toward a collaborative understanding of the problem whether it be a deficit such as limited anger control or excess such as overeating. A behavior analysis designed to determine causes of and solutions to performance problems requires four steps:

1. Identify the problem category. Is it a problem of *performing a task*, or is it a problem of *dealing with people*?
2. Identify the problem type. Is the person *unable* to do the task, or is the person *unwilling* to do the task? The acid test is whether the person could do the task if his or her life depended on it (not that a counselor would be that extreme).
3. Determine the problem cause if the person is unable to do the task. Is it due to a *lack of knowledge* about what, when, and how the task should be done, or is there an *obstacle* in the environment that is preventing accomplishment of

TABLE 8-1 DETERMINING CAUSES OF AND SOLUTIONS TO PERFORMANCE PROBLEMS

What category of problem?	Is it a problem of:	Is it due to:	Approach it by:
Performing a task / Dealing with people	Being unable*	Lack of knowledge about what, when, how	Providing training
		Obstacle in the environment	Removing the obstacle
	Being unwilling*	Lack of knowledge about why something needs to be done	Providing information/ feedback
		Simple refusal	Changing the balance of positive and negative consequences

* Could he or she do it if his or her life depended on it? No = unable; yes = unwilling.

the task? If the person is *unwilling* to do the task, is it because there is a *lack of knowledge* about why something needs to be done, or is it simple *refusal*? Behavioral methods often fail because of their tendency to assume that all problems with people are rooted in someone's refusal to do certain things.

4. Select a problem solution that is appropriate for the problem at hand. If the person is *unable* to perform the task and needs to know how to do it, *provide training*. If there is an *obstacle in the environment* (e.g., the student cannot see the whiteboard), fix the problem (e.g., move the student closer to the board) or *remove the obstacle*. If a person is refusing to do a task (e.g., showing up late every day), the counselor needs to determine what is reinforcing the *undesired* behavior and what is deterring the *desired* behavior. Then, the counselor must find a way to *decrease* or *eliminate* both of the things that maintain the undesired behavior and find a way to reinforce the desired behavior (showing up on time). Note that punishment of the undesired behavior is a last-resort option because it carries a possible side effect of damaging the relationship you are trying to build with your client. The behavior analysis process is outlined in Table 8-1 and Figure 8-2.

DETERMINING BASELINE

Common by-products of the accurate description of the target behavior include the clear definition of the problem in specific behavioral terms and the determination of the frequency, severity, and duration of the behavior. An example of that specificity would be changing *overeating after school* to how many candy bars were eaten and how often that happened—thus the baseline might be two candy bars, three times a week when getting home from school. Doing more school assignment might be defined as the number of incomplete math assignments and the dates completed work was submitted compared to the due date—so the baseline would be six incomplete

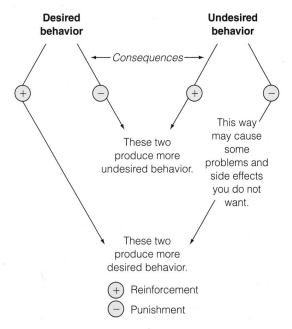

FIGURE 8-2 BALANCING CONSEQUENCES

daily math assignments out of ten; all incomplete turned in by Friday—two, three, or four days late. Next counselors and clients agree on a way to record such as in a diary, chart, checklist mentioned earlier.

ESTABLISHING GOALS

Goals emerge from the definition of the problem and the information revealed from describing the target behavior and determining the baseline. Goals establish the desired outcome of the counseling sessions. Goals should be tied to identified behaviors or outcomes with timelines for achieving the goals explicit. The useful acronym, SMART, allows a counselor to help children create understandable and manageable goals. Goals should be specific, measurable, attainable, relevant, and timely. Specific goals are clear, concise, and tangible; the goals identify what, where, and how. Measurable refers to goals that have a clear definition of way(s) or specific evidence to determine when the goal will be achieved and answer how much or how many. Measurable goals may state moving from something to more or less of the same thing (e.g., from 6 assignments to 12 assignments). Attainable means to be cautious that the goal is within reach. Attainable refers to something that can be achieved and answers the question about whether this is a realistic goal. Relevant goals relate to deciding if the goal ties to the desired accomplishment and answer the question about whether this is an important undertaking. Finally, timely denotes the amount of time to devote to accomplishing the goal.

Bovend'Eerdt, Botell, and Wade (2009) suggest building goals in four parts: the target activity, the support needed, quantification of performance, and time period for achievement. These authors tie the identified goals to a monitoring procedure, goal attainment scaling, a process we outlined in Chapter 3.

Treatment planning follows all the previous steps: description, baseline, and goals. The results of the behavioral assessment allow the functional analysis of the target behavior, the identification of the variables maintaining the behavior—treatment planning emerges as decisions about ways to change those variables. Another determination about how to proceed in counseling would be to match the treatment strategies to the client's diagnosis. Behavioral counselors may use standardized protocols from a treatment manual to choose the ways to proceed. Whether relying on the behavioral assessment or a treatment manual, counselors may choose from a variety of techniques for change, some of which are discussed in the following sections.

TREATMENT: STRATEGIES AND IMPLEMENTATION

Techniques for Change

Various treatment techniques may be employed to change the problem behavior. After the detailed behavioral assessment of the problem occurs, interventions begin quickly. Seligman and Reichenberg (2014) offered categories of strategies for behavioral counselors. Skill development and education include interventions such as training and practice of assertiveness, communication skills, time management, and parenting skills. Impulse control strategies involve learning and practicing relaxation, distraction, and avoiding triggers. Those techniques would be used after the assessment of the problem behavior is complete. Generally, the counselor works within the counseling session to help children acquire new behavioral responses. Children then practice those new behaviors within and outside the counseling session and monitor their move to mastery. Reinforcements or rewards motivate people to reach their goals, help them feel successful, and encourage them to undertake more. The length of therapy depends on the progress being made and the agreements between the counselor and the client. The following describe strategies for helping children increase desirable behaviors as well as decreasing unwanted behavior.

Modeling

Social learning theories have been influenced by the work of Albert Bandura. He combines the principles of both classical and operant conditioning and determines that as well as direct experience, learning occurs vicariously with the observation of other people's behavior (Bandura 1969, 1977, 1986). Modeling can be a treatment strategy for building complex skills such as sustaining a conversation, nurturing social skills, and building relationships or other situations in which a person would like to improve.

Bandura (1969) states people respond more positively to models similar to them in things like gender, age, race, and beliefs; as attractive and admirable in realistic ways; and as competent and warm. Counselors may use modeling in several ways:

- Counselors may be the models to demonstrate certain behaviors to the child such as ways to greet an adult. The child would then imitate the behavior.
- Child clients can observe their peers or other people who are performing the desired behavior such as finding a seat in the cafeteria. Children can watch

someone and identify the things that person is doing to make behavior successful. They can then report their observations to the counselor and practice what they have seen.

- Counselors can create situation for the child to imagine possible responses such as a young girl saying "I don't care" to someone who is calling her fat.
- Counselors may also use books, television, and other media that exhibit behaviors to be replicated by the child.
- Finally, children can use self-modeling by making audio or video recordings of their desired behaviors (Bandura, 1969).

If the model's behavior is only a step or two above the child's current level of competence, the behavior may be learned quickly. If the behavior is several steps beyond, the child may need more practice, reinforcement, and feedback before mastery. Behavioral counselors often use modeling to help children learn social skills.

For example, Charlene mentioned a friend, Patty, a number of times during the counseling sessions. She indicated that she admired Patty because Patty had a lot of friends, made good grades, and got along well with her parents and teachers. The counselor asked Charlene to observe Patty's behaviors closely for 1 week and to write on an index card those behaviors she particularly liked and wanted to imitate. The next week, Charlene brought back her list of six behaviors. The counselor and Charlene selected the most important one for Charlene (giving compliments) and began to work on that behavior. Role-playing and behavior rehearsal were included in the counseling to help Charlene learn the new behaviors. The observed behaviors were practiced and modified until they were appropriate for Charlene. As counseling progressed, Charlene continued to observe her model and to practice new behaviors until she became more like her ideal self.

Contingency Contracts

Contracts are effective for children if they have a part in writing the terms. Contract language must be simplified for understanding, and the goals should be quite clear, with as few steps as possible to meet the goals. Reinforcement should be immediate when the target behavior is being established. Readily available, cost-free, and developmentally appropriate rewards are preferable—being first in line, doing a favorite classroom job, being a student helper, running errands, tutoring a classmate—if they are reinforcing to the child. Counselors help by asking the child what a reward would be for them. Learning-enrichment activities are reinforcing for older students.

The contingency contracting process can be broken down into six steps:

1. The counselor and the student identify the problem to be solved.
2. The counselor collects data to verify the baseline frequency rate for the undesired behavior.
3. The counselor and the student set mutually acceptable goals.
4. The counselor develops a contingency plan that identifies the target behaviors and the number of times the target behavior has to be performed to earn the reward for the client. For example, completion of one homework paper per day in math earns 20 minutes of playing a favorite video game at home. The counselor selects interventions for attaining the goals.

5. The counselor evaluates the plan for observable and measurable change in the target behavior.

6. If the plan is not effective, the counselor repeats Step 4. If the techniques prove effective, the counselor develops a maintenance plan to maintain the new behavior and move the client from extrinsic rewards to the intrinsic reward of learning that life is better when math assignments are completed.

EXAMPLE 1   Jamal has been late for school so many times he is in danger of failing. He is referred to the counselor.

Step 1. The counselor talks with Jamal about the problem. Jamal is not happy with his tardiness but still has trouble getting out of bed because he has a job at night and both parents leave for work early in the morning so no one wakes him. He would like to do better but cannot figure out a way to improve.

Step 2. During the last month Jamal has been late 10 days by an average of 30 minutes.

Step 3. Jamal and the counselor discuss various ways he could get out of bed earlier and decide he will find two backups to his wake-up alarm system and try that strategy for the next two days. They will check after that time and then complete the contingency contract. After that evaluation, Jamal agreed to the next part of the contract.

Step 4. For each day he gets to school on time, Jamal will receive 20 points to be applied toward a total of 100 points, which can be exchanged for some gas money that his dad will contribute.

Step 5. Evaluation of the contingency contract indicates that Jamal got to school on time 4 days the first week, earning 80 points so received no money. The second week he arrived on time every day, for a total of 100 points. He then received $10 for gas. The following week, he earned 100 points and received the money again.

Step 6. The counselor, Jamal, and his father agree that continuing with the point system is not necessary. Jamal's attendance and grades are improving, and everyone seems happier—school officials, Jamal, and his parents. As a maintenance procedure, Jerry agrees to check in with the counselor each Friday afternoon for reports on his attendance.

EXAMPLE 2   Jason, a ninth grade student, was referred to the counselor for not completing assignments in his five classes. He was taking an advanced placement curriculum that required completion of daily school and homework assignments. Jason's prior work in middle school and his test scores were indicated he was capable of this level of work. His parents were punishing him for his inattention to school work by taking away privileges with his computer games. Baseline data collected over the past 2 weeks indicated that Jason was completing work in only one class, and that was done only on 4 of 10 school days. Individual counseling appeared to be somewhat effective during the first week it occurred; but at the conclusion of the second week, Jason's performance had nearly retreated to its baseline rate.

The counselor met with Jason and his parents for the purpose of designing a contract where he could be in charge of time for his computer games. An illustration of the plan and its progress can be found in Figure 8-3. Contingency contracts have

JASON'S CONTINGENCY CONTRACT RECORD

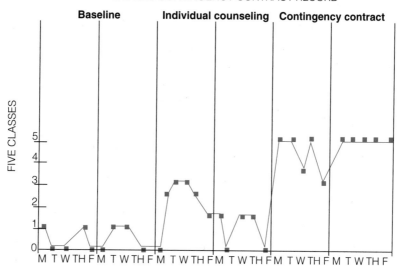

FIGURE 8-3   JASON'S CONTINGENCY CONTRACT RECORD

a "Let's make a deal" focus. The "deal" was that for each day of completed work in all five of his classes, Jason would earn 1 hour of game time that could be shared with his friends.

For a perfect week of completed work, he would earn a bonus of 3 hours. Jason's performance was a dramatic improvement over his baseline and counseling intervention record. He had 3 days with all work completed during the first week and a perfect week during the second week, in which he earned 8 hours of game time. After the behavior has been established, the goal would be to help Jason move from a dependence on extrinsic reinforcement to intrinsic reinforcement, where Jason would realize that life is better for him when he completes his work. His grades are going up. His parents and teachers are no longer nagging, and he controls the time he gets to spend on computer games. Eventually, the record-keeping and reinforcement schedule can be dropped, and as long as his grades remain high, Jason can monitor his free-time activities.

However, it is important to have a maintenance plan in place. One such plan would have Jason check in with his counselor at the end of the school day on each Friday with an index card, checked and signed by his teachers, indicating the days when all work was completed. The counselor would reinforce and encourage Jason to keep up his good work and place his card in a card file under his name.

Self-Management

An adaptation of the six-step contingency contract method, the self-management plan, is for people who can take more responsibility for their behavior. These plans also follow a step-by-step process: defining a problem in behavioral terms, collecting data on the problem, introducing a treatment program based on behavioral principles, evaluating the effectiveness of the program, and appropriately changing the program if the plan is not working. The major difference between self-management and other procedures is that clients assume the major responsibility for carrying out their programs, including arranging their own contingencies or reinforcement when they have the skills to do so.

Steps in developing a self-management plan are as follows:

1. Choose an observable and measurable behavior you wish to change, for example, completing daily home assignments.
2. Record the following for at least 1 week: (a) your target behavior, (b) the setting in which it occurs, (c) the antecedent events leading to the behavior, and (d) the consequences resulting from the behavior.
3. Set a goal you can achieve.
4. Change the setting and the antecedent events preventing the target behavior from occurring.
5. Change the consequences that reinforce the target behavior.
6. Keep accurate records of your target behavior—your successes and failures.
7. Develop a plan for rewarding yourself when you meet your daily goal and a plan to punish or levy a fine on yourself when you fail to meet your daily goal.
8. Arrange a plan to maintain the goals you have reached.

Self-management contracts are generally not effective for younger children unless the plan is managed by both the child and an older person. Self-tracking and self-rewarding usually are difficult for children younger than 11. Children can set goals and choose consequences, but they need an adult to monitor for tracking and reinforcing behavior. Training in self-management skills has been one of the best applications of behavioral principles to counseling children and adolescents.

Shaping

The basic operant technique of shaping is a general procedure designed to learn new behaviors by reinforcing behaviors that come close to or approximate the desired behavior. The behavior is changed using a series of steps from the original to a more complex level. Each successive approximation of the behavior is reinforced until the desired behavior is obtained. To administer the technique, the counselor must know how to skillfully use (1) looking, (2) waiting, and (3) reinforcing. The counselor looks for the desired behavior, waits until it occurs, and reinforces it when it does occur. In essence, the counselor is catching the child in good behavior—a much more difficult task than catching the child in bad behavior.

Adults who notice and reinforce successful approximations of the target behavior positively influence the child learning the desired behavior. Small correct steps need to be reinforced immediately each time they occur and poor approximations are ignored. Shaping offers a method for teaching complex behaviors to children because mediating steps are identified and rewarded. Extrinsic reinforcers are more likely to be effective with children. Sugar-free candy, stickers, trinkets, and "good behavior" ink stamps on the hand all work well. Pairing intrinsic rewards with extrinsic rewards is always good practice to help children move away from the need for extrinsic rewards.

Prompting

If a behavior is not occurring, the action can be prompted. Prompts can be visual, verbal, or physical stimuli such as notes, hints, or assistance with a task. Learning from prompting happens in three steps: prompting, reinforcing, and fading. Prompting is the stimuli that initiate the behavior such as a note reminding a child to take her lunchbox or a verbal explanation of a desired response such as "you may find you gloves by looking in your coat pocket." A valued consequence such as a gold star is provided as a reinforcer. Prompted behavior that is reinforced will be learned more quickly (Baldwin & Baldwin, 2001). Fading, the final step, involves gradually withdrawing the prompts until the desired behavior occurs without them.

Chaining

Chaining is the series of behaviors that lead to reinforcement. The smaller behaviors that are linked become the chain toward the complex behavior. Chaining involves strengthening all the parts of the chain that lead to the final behavior. Forward chaining involves starting at the beginning of the sequence, prompting and reinforcing each step until the segment is mastered, and then moving through the other steps (Fink & Lotspeich, 2004). Backward chaining involves starting with the last step and working backward to the first step. Each step receives prompting and reinforcing.

Behavioral Momentum

Behavioral momentum operates on much the same principle of Newton's law of motion, which states that a body in motion tends to remain in motion. Behavioral momentum has been used mostly to reduce noncompliant behavior in children and adults. Momentum is established by making three to five short, easy requests with a high probability of compliance to a person just before making a request having a low probability of compliance. Each high-probability request is reinforced by verbal praise on compliance. The theory is that the reinforcement gained from doing the easy tasks builds momentum that carries over to completion of the more difficult or low-compliance task. Romano and Roll (2000) have researched the level of compliance needed on the easy tasks to carry over for completion of the difficult task. High-probability tasks are generally defined as those having an 80 percent compliance rate. Romano and Roll have investigated the momentum effect that requests with medium levels of compliance probability might have. Medium levels of compliance probability were set at 50 to 70 percent of the time. The researchers found that both high and medium levels of compliance probability were effective in increasing compliance to low-probability requests.

Ray, Skinner, and Watson (1999), in a related study on behavioral momentum, found that momentum could be established by having parents of an autistic child administer the easy tasks, followed by the teacher administering the difficult task. Before the intervention, the student had consistently displayed noncompliant behavior toward the teacher. In this case, stimulus control did transfer from the parents to the teacher.

Biofeedback

In biofeedback, a machine accomplishes the three behaviors of looking, waiting, and reinforcing. Brain waves, muscle tension, body temperature, heart rate, and blood pressure can be monitored for small changes and fed back to the client by auditory and visual means. Biofeedback methods have been successful in, for example, teaching hyperactive children to relax. The more the child relaxes the slower and lower is the beeping sound on the monitor. The equipment may provide feedback with electric trains and recorded music. Both stop when the child stops relaxing and restart when the child takes the first small step toward relaxing again. An understanding of cause and effect by the children enhances biofeedback methods, but it is not a necessity.

Token Economies

Token economies are used on a group basis, as in a school classroom. The children earn tokens or points for certain target behaviors. These behaviors are classified as either on-task or socially appropriate. Children also lose tokens or points for off-task and socially inappropriate behaviors or alternatively earn points for on-tasks and appropriate behaviors. Children may periodically cash in tokens or points earned for rewards such as learning-enrichment activities, game time, trinkets, and sugarless candy.

Some teachers use token economies for their classroom groups. An empty jar sits on the teacher's desk. Every time something good happens in the classroom, the teacher drops some marbles in the jar. The marble noise becomes an auditory reinforcement to go with the visual image of the jar filling up. A full jar means all students get free popcorn during the lunch period. The Case Study describing Sue that appears later in this chapter is an example of how to use a token economy contract.

We have a caution with token economies and other types of group contingencies. Children prefer independent group contingencies over interdependent and dependent group contingencies. Independent group contingencies require the same response of all individuals in the group, but access to reinforcement is based only on each individual's response (e.g., everyone scoring 90 percent gets a reward). Interdependent contingencies depend on the collective performance of the group (e.g., the entire group receives a reward if the group mean equals 90 percent or better). Dependent group contingencies are based on the performance of a selected member or selected members of the group (e.g., if a paper drawn at random from a box containing all group members' test papers has a score of 90 percent or better, everyone receives a reward). Considerable evidence exists in the literature to support behavioral methods that use self-control, self-determination, and personal responsibility as motivators and reinforcers.

Behavior-Practice Groups

Behavior-practice groups have some advantages in counseling children. They provide a relatively safe setting for the child to practice new behaviors before trying them out in real-life situations. These groups are also useful in supporting and reinforcing children as they attempt new behaviors and reach goals. Behavior-practice groups may focus on any of several behavior changes, including the following:

- Weight loss
- Study habits
- Assertiveness training
- Communication skills
- Negative addictions such as drugs, alcohol, and smoking

In working with behavior-practice groups, the counselor needs to develop a lesson plan with behavioral objectives, instructional methods and activities, reinforcement, and evaluation. A good lesson plan maintains a balance among three teaching strategies: (1) tell me, (2) show me, and (3) let me try it. For example, a lesson plan in effective communication might have the following objectives: After six weekly group meetings, each child in the group will have demonstrated in at least three real-life settings the ability to do the following: (1) give positive feedback, (2) make a reasonable request, and (3) say no to an unreasonable request. The counselor would then identify the knowledge and actions needed for each objective, model the action, allow the participants to practice, and then reinforce the successful enactment of the task. The evaluation of the effectiveness of the group may be the number of times the participants perform the behavior outside the group setting.

Role-playing

Role-playing is a counseling technique that is not restricted to any one theory. Many counseling professionals use it. Behavioral rehearsal or role-play occurs when a client practices a new behavior in the counseling session and then tries the behavior in other places. The counselor and child enact a situation, the counselor uses prompting to help refine the behavior, and the child rehearses a newly learned or more appropriate behavior. Behavioral counselors often find that role-playing facilitates their clients' progress in self-management programs; for example, it can help clients see their behaviors as others see them and obtain feedback about these behaviors. Role-playing also can provide practice for decision making and exploring consequences. Negative role-playing or rehearsal can be helpful in identifying what *not* to do. Role-playing negative behaviors and their consequences may help children evaluate objectively what is happening and the consequences of their behavior.

Role-playing can help children learn about cause and effect and experience the consequences of their behavior in a relatively safe setting. Role-playing is useful to children who are working toward developing a sense of empathy and beginning to modify their egocentric views of the world.

Role-playing to Define a Problem

Children often have trouble describing exactly what occurred in a particular situation, especially one involving interpersonal problems with parents, teachers, or peers. Moreover, they may be unable to see clearly how certain behaviors have evoked an unwanted response or consequence. They may, however, be able to "put on a play" about the troubling situation to show the counselor the child's perspective. For example, suppose Nikita tells the counselor that he and his mother are in constant conflict. She is unfair and never allows him to do *anything* he asks. Role-playing could provide some insight into what occurs when Nikita asks for permission.

COUNSELOR: I'll be your mother, and you show me exactly how you ask her to allow you, for instance, to have a birthday party. Talk to me exactly as you would to your mother if you were to ask her for the party.

JASON: Mom, you never let me do anything! You always say no to anything I want. I want a birthday party, and you'll be mean if you don't let me have one this year!

The counselor can now readily see that if a conflict already exists between mother and child, this demand will increase the conflict and is unlikely to get Nikita his birthday party.

Children having trouble with peers might be asked to describe what happened, and then to role-play one or more persons in the incident. Verbal and nonverbal behaviors not adequately described in relating the incident often become more apparent when they are demonstrated through role-playing.

Role Reversal

When conflicts occur between children, adults frequently ask one child, "How would you feel if he hit you like that [said that to you, bit you, and so on]?" The purpose of this admonition is to have the child empathize with the other. However, many cognitive theorists, especially Piaget, emphasize that young children up through the preoperational stage (2–7 years old) lack the cognitive development to be able to put themselves in another person's place. Because children better understand what they see, hear, or experience directly, role-playing other children's positions could promote a better understanding than a verbal admonition.

COUNSELOR: Barbara, I understand from your sister that you hit her on the head quite often. Would you agree that this is what happens?

BARBARA: Yeah, I can really make her move if I threaten to hit her on the head!

COUNSELOR: Would the two of you describe to me what happened the last time you hit Judy? [The girls describe the incident.] Now, Barbara, I wonder if you would mind playing Judy and saying and doing exactly what Judy did. I would like Judy to say and do exactly what you did. [Remind the girls that hitting hard is not allowed during role-playing because people are not for hitting.]

The purpose of this role reversal is to help Barbara experience Judy's feelings when Barbara hit her, with the hope that Barbara will then want to explore better methods of relating to Judy.

Role reversal can be effective when communication breaks down between parents and children, between teachers and children, between peers, or between counselors and their clients. Each player can gain increased knowledge of the other's point of view.

Role-playing Used as Behavior Rehearsal

To refine a speech and ensure a smooth delivery, most adults rehearse a speech before presenting it to an audience. Children also may feel more comfortable about trying a new behavior if they can practice it before actually facing the real world.

Dave is a shy child who has no friends. In an effort to help Dave make friends, the counselor may want to help him decide exactly how to approach another child and what to say to the child after the opening "Hello." To build confidence, the counselor could first role-play another child and allow Dave to practice his new behaviors in a safe atmosphere. When Dave feels secure in role-playing with the counselor, another child can be involved in the role-playing to help Dave gain more realistic experiences in meeting other children. Dave can monitor his growing abilities to greet someone and begin to self-manage other behaviors he would like to develop.

Counseling Homework Assignments

Homework assignments may be given to children in counseling for a variety of reasons. Homework can build continuity between sessions and facilitate counseling by encouraging "work" on the child's problems between sessions. A homework assignment could be a commitment by the child to keep a record of some particular feeling or behavior, to reduce or stop a present behavior, or to try a new behavior. Homework assignments provide the child with an opportunity to try out new or different behaviors and discuss the consequences with the counselor. For example, after Dave (see preceding example) has rehearsed approaching a new person within the counseling session, the counselor might ask him to approach one new person during the coming week and try out this new behavior. Dave could evaluate whether the new behavior was effective for him and discuss the results with the counselor; if it was not effective, they could explore other methods.

CLASSICAL CONDITIONING METHODS

Systematic Desensitization

Systematic desensitization, developed by Wolpe (1958, 1969) from earlier work by Jacobsen (1938), is a procedure used to eliminate anxiety and fear. A response incompatible with anxiety, such as relaxation, is paired with weak and then progressively stronger anxiety-provoking stimuli. The approach is based on the principles of counterconditioning; that is, if all skeletal muscles are deeply relaxed, one cannot experience anxiety at the same time. Relaxation training may encompass a variety of exercises that range from deep, slow breathing to more complicated sequence procedures.

A student may be experiencing anxiety related to specific stimulus situations such as taking tests, performing in front of a group, being in high places, or seeing some animal. The first step for the treatment plan is to develop a hierarchy of scenes related to the fear or phobia, with mildly aversive scenes at the bottom and progressively more aversive scenes at the top. The counselor then teaches the student the process of deep muscle relaxation and asks the relaxed child to visualize the various scenes in the hierarchy.

One set of relaxation exercises involves successively tensing and relaxing 19 different muscle groups at 6-second intervals until a high level of relaxation is achieved. The process usually is performed with the student in a recliner chair or stretched out on a soft rug. The student is asked to go as high as possible on the hierarchy without feeling anxiety. When the student feels anxiety, he or she signals the counselor by raising one finger, and the counselor reverts to a less anxiety-provoking scene. Behavior practice facilitates the process. A student may successively practice giving a short speech in front of a mirror, with an audio tape recorder, with a video recorder, in front of a best friend, in front of a small group, and so on, until the student can give the speech in front of 25 classmates. The student's stimulus hierarchy might look like this:

0. Lying in bed in your room just before going to sleep—describe your room
1. Thinking about the speech alone in your room 1 week before you give it
2. Discussing the upcoming speech in class 1 week before it is due
3. Sitting in class while another student gives a speech 1 week before your speech
4. Writing your speech at home
5. Practicing your speech alone in your room or in front of your friend
6. Getting dressed in the morning of the speech
7. Eating breakfast and thinking about the speech before going to school
8. Walking to school on the day of your speech
9. Entering the classroom on the day of the speech
10. Waiting while another student gives a speech on the day of your presentation
11. Standing in front of your classmates and looking at their faces
12. Presenting your speech before the class

The technique consists of asking the student to relax, imagine, relax, stop imagining, relax, and so on, until, after repeated practice, the student learns to relax while visualizing each stage of the stimulus hierarchy.

Several relaxation exercises can be used with clients. Following are two types of exercises frequently used.

1. Tighten, then consciously "let go" of the various muscle groups, starting with your feet and moving to your legs, stomach, arms, neck, and head as you make yourself as comfortable as you can in a chair or lying down.
   a. Stop frowning; let your forehead relax.
   b. Let your hands, arms, and so on relax.
   c. Tighten 6 seconds, relax; tighten again 6 seconds, relax.
2. Form mental pictures.
   a. Picture yourself stretched out on a soft bed. Your legs are like concrete, sinking down in the mattress from their weight. Picture a friend coming into the room and trying to lift your concrete legs, but they are too heavy and your friend cannot do it. Repeat with arms, neck, and so on.
   b. Picture your body as a big puppet. Your hands are tied loosely to your wrists by strings. Your forearm is connected loosely by a string to your shoulder. Your feet and legs are also connected with a string. Your chin has dropped loosely against your chest. All strings are loose; your body is limp and sprawled across the bed.
   c. Picture your body as consisting of a bunch of rubber balloons. Two air holes open in your feet, and the air begins to escape from your legs. Your legs begin to collapse until they are flat rubber tubes. Next, a hole is opened in your chest, and the air begins to escape until your entire body is lying flat on the bed. Continue with your head, arms, neck, and so on.

d. Imagine the most relaxing, pleasant scene you can remember—a time when you felt really good and peaceful. If you remember fishing in a mountain stream, pay attention to the little things, such as quiet ripples on the water and leaves on the trees. What sounds were present? Did you hear the quiet rustling of the leaves? Is your relaxing place before an open fireplace with logs crackling, or is it the beach, with a warm sun and breezes?

Continued practice facilitates achievement of these mental pictures and relaxation levels.

Systematic desensitization, a classical conditioning technique, could be too complex for younger children, who are not always capable of handling sequential behaviors. Conscious relaxation and visualization may also be difficult for younger children, who benefit more by actual practice of the steps in the stimulus hierarchy. For example, the following systematic desensitization program could be used to help a 6-year-old child who is experiencing school phobia: The child indicates that he would like to work toward getting a favorite computer game. A chart is drawn up with spaces to star each day he followed the program and earned a dollar toward the purchase price of his game. Steps in the hierarchy were small enough not to overwhelm the child. Each session lasted 30 minutes.

Step 1. Child and his mother working together alone in the schoolroom, the child reading or talking to his mother

Step 2. Child, mother, and friend of the child in the schoolroom, with the child talking to his friend

Step 3. Child, mother, friend, and familiar adult (not on the school staff) together in the schoolroom, with child talking while playing

Step 4. Child, mother, friend, and teacher in the schoolroom, the child talking with the teacher; mother leaves them; friend leaves

Step 5. Child and teacher together in the schoolroom, talking to each other

Step 6. Child and teacher move to the classroom and talk to each other

Step 7. Child joins the classroom for half a day

Step 8. Child spends an entire day in the classroom

Classical conditioning and operant conditioning usually occur at the same time. A student is given after-school detention for disrupting her class. Detention has the operant effect of preventing the child's disruptive behavior; however, detention may also cause a classical conditioned response of hating school because more school is used as punishment. School time becomes associated with punishment. Associating being in school with a privilege would be much better. When the student misbehaves, she loses the privilege of being in class and has to spend her class time working in a time-out area or in the in-school suspension room. Additional school time (detention) would not be used as a punishment or consequence.

In summary, the technique of desensitization is based on a principle of learning referred to as *reciprocal inhibition*—that is, an organism cannot make two contradictory responses at the same time. If we assume that all responses are learned, relearning or reconditioning can extinguish them. Therefore, relaxation, being more rewarding than anxiety, can gradually replace anxiety as the response to the anxiety-evoking situation.

Wolpe (1989), attacking those who practiced cognitive therapy, makes the point that if a habit has been acquired by learning, the logical approach is to treat it by a method based on learning principles. He writes that the real difference between true behavioral therapy and cognitive therapy is those practitioners denying the possibility that some fears may be immediately triggered by a particular stimulus without the mediation of an idea of danger. Wolpe also criticizes cognitive therapists for dispensing with the behavior analysis required for successful treatment of neurotic suffering.

Flooding

Flooding, the opposite of desensitization, begins with the most feared stimulus in the stimulus hierarchy rather than the weakest or least feared. It is diving into cold water rather than getting used to it gradually. The clients are exposed to their strongest fears by putting themselves into the situation repeatedly over a short period of time. The continuous presentation of the anxiety-evoking situation leads to fatigue and eventual unlearning of the undesirable response. For example, a client might make several public speeches over a period of 2 weeks. The constant, concentrated approach has the effect of literally wearing out the stimulus. When a parent told you to get back on your bike after a crash, you were exposed to the flooding technique, also referred to as *reactive* or *internal inhibition*.

Counterconditioning

In counterconditioning, a stronger pleasant stimulus is paired with a weaker aversive stimulus as a procedure for overcoming the anxiety the aversive stimulus evokes. For example, a child may be given his or her favorite candy while sitting in a feared classroom. If the candy is sufficiently rewarding to the child, the anxiety evoked by the classroom should be diminished.

Aversive Conditioning

Aversive conditioning is the application of an aversive or noxious stimulus, such as a rubber-band snap on the wrist, when a maladaptive response or behavior occurs. For example, children could wear rubber bands around their wrists and snap them each time they found themselves daydreaming instead of listening to the teacher. Opportunity for helpful behavior to occur and be reinforced is recommended with this technique. Fall et al. (2010) noted that aversion therapy is used only when other change interventions have failed.

The following statements summarize each of the four classical conditioning methods presented earlier ($\oplus$ = pleasant stimulus; $\ominus$ = aversive stimulus):

1. Desensitization—where $\ominus$ is giving a speech. The aversive stimulus is handled in small steps by visualization or relaxation and by practice until increasingly larger steps can be handled.
2. Flooding (internal inhibition)—where $\ominus$ is getting back on the bike after falling off. The aversive stimulus is continually repeated until the fear response wears itself out.

3. Counterconditioning—where ⊕ is a candy bar and ⊖ is going to school. The larger pleasant stimulus overcomes the anxiety or fear evoked by the smaller aversive stimulus.
4. Aversive conditioning—where ⊖ is a snap of a rubber band on the wrist and ⊕ is daydreaming during class. The more painful stimulus overcomes the smaller reward gained from daydreaming in class.

Behavioral counselors have many strategies for helping children learn new behaviors or reduce the incidence of unwanted actions. Modeling, contingency contracts, self-management, shaping, prompting, chaining, and many other techniques are treatment options for the counseling using behavioral procedures. Additionally systematic desensitization, flooding, and counterconditioning may be useful. Aversive conditioning is used only when other methods have failed.

Measuring Progress

Counselors measure the progress of behavioral counseling by monitoring the treatment plans formed around specific, measurable goals that have generally been implemented during the first session. Plans are individual specific; therefore, they are closely tied to the problem resolution. Treatment periods are relatively brief, and client progress can be tracked on a daily or weekly basis. Costs for behavioral counseling treatments are relatively inexpensive, and client satisfaction with behavioral methods is generally high. Behavioral counseling, with accurate recording of baseline and post-treatment data, is well documented as an effective way to achieve rather impressive outcomes.

Lambert and Hawkins (2004) recommend the following instruments for validating the counseling outcomes: *Behavior and Symptom Identification Scale, Brief Symptom Inventory*, and *Outcome Questionnaire*. Each instrument is brief, easy to administer, and easy to score. Weaknesses include validity issues and weakness in constructs. Goal-attainment scales individualized for each client are excellent means for measuring progress in counseling.

Success

Children who have achieved some gains in their plans to change behaviors can learn to reward themselves and create their own self-management contingencies. Counselors can emphasize the children's efforts and growth, reinforcing the child's positive momentum. Counselors can also help children identify the people and things that reinforced changes, thereby encouraging children to acknowledge the environmental rewards that supported their work. Most importantly behavioral counselors can assist children by helping them determine the ways they encouraged themselves as they alter their responses.

Seligman and Reichenberg (2014) outlined three directions the last stage a behavioral change plan might include:

1. If the clients did not meet goals, the goals and strategies could be revised.
2. If clients met goals but want to continue changing behaviors, the counselor and client could agree to build on the success and work toward new goals.
3. If clients are pleased with their achievements, they develop plans to maintain the gains such as peer support groups, self-monitoring or periodic follow-up sessions.

The extended discussion of a general treatment plan to change behavior provides counselors with a roadmap that can be adapted to each person or problem. The steps detail ways to plan and assess change that is a collaborative effort of child and counselor.

Case Study

Identification of the Problem

Sasha is a 9-year-old girl in the fourth grade. She has exhibited some behavior problems in her classroom. She does not complete her classroom assignments, tells lies about her work and about things she does at home and at school, and is reported to be constantly out of her seat.

Individual and Background Information

Academic Sasha has been a successful student with above-average abilities. She is an excellent reader and has the ability to do any fourth-grade assignment.

Family Sasha is an only child. Her parents are in their 30s. She comes from an upper-middle-class family; her father and mother manage their own successful business.

Social Sasha seems to get along relatively well with the other children but has only one close friend, Marie. Sasha has been caught telling lies by the other children who tell her they do not like her lies. She brings money and trinkets to share with Marie and will give Maria clothes Sasha has discarded. Sasha plays only with Maria and is mostly around adults who let her have her own way, often ignoring her.

Counseling Method

The counselor in this case used a behavioral counseling technique to help Sasha evaluate her behavior. The criteria for determining when to use behavioral counseling are based on the frequency of the maladaptive behavior and the degree to which it hinders the child's healthy development and that of other children in the class.
In this case, the counselor used the following steps:

1. Establish a warm, talking relationship (therapeutic alliance) with the child.
2. List the problem behaviors on paper.
3. Identify one or two behaviors Sasha would like to change by eliminating or increasing the identified target.
4. Break the identified behaviors into ABC—antecedent, behavior, consequence.
5. Have Sasha spend a day recording how often the identified behaviors occur and how long those actions last as well as the strength of the reactions to the behaviors.
6. Work with Sasha to form a plan of action that would be most likely to help using the information from the baseline assessment and her preferences.
7. Develop a contingency contract with positive reinforcement in the form of a social reward (praise) for desirable behavior and token reinforcement (points to exchange for

learning-enrichment activities). Positive reinforcers are withdrawn (by loss of points) when undesirable behavior occurs.

8. These plans are discussed with, agreed on, and signed by the client, counselor, teacher, and parents to cover both school and home.

Transcript

COUNSELOR: Sasha, your teacher sent you to me because you seem to be having some problems in class. Would you like to tell me what kind of problems you are having? I'll write them down in a list so we can see what could be done to help you here and at home.

SASHA: People say I'm lying all the time and they don't want me on their teams. And my teacher yells at me because I just can't seem to get my work done or turned in on time. My mom and dad took me out of dance class because they said they didn't have time to take me to practice.

COUNSELOR: Sounds like lots of things not going your way right now. Let's start by looking at one thing you'd like to change and later we can go back to some of the other things that you don't like. What would you choose?

SASHA: I need to get the teacher to stop yelling at me but I just can't sit in my seat long enough to finish those math problems, and then time is always up before I'm done.

COUNSELOR: Who else is affected by your getting out of your seat?

SASHA: I guess I'm keeping the others from working when I go to their seats, and it bothers my teacher because she stops what she is doing and tells me to sit down and get busy.

COUNSELOR: What happens when you don't finish your work?

SASHA: Well, nothing really happens, except I try to get out of being fussed at and being kept in during play period for not doing my work.

COUNSELOR: What do you mean, Sasha?

SASHA: I make up stories about why I can't find my paper or somebody took it when I really hadn't even started it, or I hide what I have started in my desk or notebook and take it home and do it and then turn it in the next day and say I found it.

COUNSELOR: What do you tell your mom and dad about your work for the day when they ask you?

SASHA: Well, I tell a story to them too. I tell them I did all my work, and usually the same things I tell the teacher.

COUNSELOR: How do you feel about telling untrue stories?

SASHA: I don't really feel good about it, but I want Mom and Dad to be proud of me and I really do want to do my work, but I just can't seem to do it, so I just tell a story so people will stop bothering me.

COUNSELOR: Okay, Sasha, you say you want to change this, so let's look at the list of things you want to change and see what you and I can work out together.

SASHA: Okay, I'd like that. Could we talk about getting my work done so I won't have to tell stories about than anymore?

COUNSELOR: Okay, what kind of things could you do to stay in your seat and complete the math assignment? (After discussion about possibilities with Sasha a plan is developed for her to stay in her seat for 10 minutes, her estimate of the time needed to complete the math assignment. At school she receives tokens for her positive behaviors and earns privileges. At home for each week she completes her math assignments, one of her parents will spend at least10 minutes with her with no distractions.)

Let me read what we decided so you can see if you agree. If we need to change things, we will change it until we get it the way we think will help you the most. This contract tells you what will happen when you are able to finish your work and earn your tokens. If you do this for a week, your parents will spend time with you. Your teacher, your mom and dad, you, and I will all sign it to show you we are all willing to help you live up to the terms. Will you go over it with your mother and father and see if there is anything that needs to be changed?

SASHA: I think it's okay just the way it is.

COUNSELOR: Okay, you and I will sign first, and I will send copies to your teacher and your parents to sign. We will try this for a week, and then you and I will meet at the same time next week to see how you are doing and if any changes need to be made.

SASHA: Okay.

Contract for Behavior and Learning

Positive Behaviors	Tokens
1. Bringing needed materials to class	5
2. Working on class or home assignment until finished	5
3. Staying in seat	5
4. Extra credit (reading assignments or time on computer)	1,2,3,4,5

You may exchange tokens earned for positive behavior for time to do learning-enrichment activities.

Learning-Enrichment Activities	Tokens
1. Writing on the small chalkboards	15
2. Playing phonic rummy	15
3. Playing with the tray puzzles	15
4. Getting to be the library aide for a day	15
5. Getting to use the computer	15
6. Playing Old Maids with classmates	10
7. Using the iPad to hear and see a story	15
8. Using clay, finger paints, and other art supplies	10

I, _____, agree to abide by the terms set forth in this contract. It is my understanding that tokens earned will depend on my classroom work and behavior.

Signature

We, your teacher, your parents, and your counselor, agree to abide by the conditions specified in the contract. It is our understanding that we will assist you in any way we can with your work and problems.

Teacher

Parents

Counselor

Behavioral counseling helps individuals look at what they are doing and what happens when they do it. The contract helps children try different behaviors to see which ones work for them. It encourages parents to adhere to the terms of the contract and positively reinforce all desirable behaviors at home. If the child continues to receive positive reinforcement for socially desirable and classroom-adaptive behavior, the counselor gradually implements a self-reinforcement system and maintenance plan to help the child develop a sense of intrinsic reinforcement where he or she realizes that life is better at school and home when he or she makes good decisions about his or her school work and general behavior.

APPLICATIONS OF BEHAVIORAL COUNSELING

Behavioral counselors have more supporting research data available than counselors practicing other counseling approaches (Spiegler & Guevremont, 2009). As noted previously, behavioral counselors must collect accurate data if their procedures are to operate with maximum efficiency. Therefore, they have done a thorough job of validating their successful outcomes with the clients with whom they work. The research in behavioral counseling involves mostly single-case analysis so some of the methods of comparing applications, such as meta-analysis, cannot be completed.

The purpose of behavioral counseling is to change the client's overt and covert responses (cognitions, emotions, physiological states). Bandura (1974) reacted to the oft-repeated dictum, "Change contingencies and you change behavior," by adding the reciprocal side: "Change behavior and you change the contingencies ... since in everyday life this two-way control operates concurrently" (p. 866). Behavioral counselors work with behavior that is objective and measurable. Behavioral counseling methods, not confined to one stimulus–response theory of learning, are derived from a variety of learning principles.

Two particularly helpful aspects of behavioral counseling with children are specificity and small steps. Counselors who help children define abstract concepts in concrete, observable terms create understanding in young people of both the complexity of concepts as well as a way to manage the idea. As an example many children talk about not knowing how to be a friend. The child and counselor may discuss several ways of being a friend like saying hello, sharing toys, asking someone to eat lunch, or be on your team and other "friendly" behaviors. Thus the relationship problem becomes a possibility for doing something rather than a mysterious phenomenon. Another helpful strategy involves defining change in small steps rather than overwhelming differences. Counselors would encourage something like 20 minutes of movement rather than losing 10 pounds—the movement would probably eventually lead to weight loss but monitoring time each day is more realistic than waiting for many pounds to disappear.

The distinguishing features of behavioral counseling include the functional analysis of behavior (Fisher, Piazza, & Roane, 2011) and the development of the necessary technology to bring about change. Wilhite, Braaten, Frey, and Wilder (2007) explain an instrument for teachers working with students who are struggling with problem behaviors. The Behavioral Objective Sequence can be an assessment used in responding to the behaviors, developing instructional plans, and ensuring accountability. This translation of behavioral interventions can be readily applied in classroom settings. Thus, behavioral counseling is the application of specified procedures derived from experimental research to benefit individuals, groups, and organizations.

DIVERSITY APPLICATIONS OF BEHAVIORAL COUNSELING

Many aspects of behavioral counseling may be appealing to people from diverse backgrounds. People who prefer behavioral interventions over working with the cognitive and affective parts of the problems brought to counseling will appreciate the focus of behavioral approach. Behavioral counseling has a structure readily understood, focuses on present behavior and on achieving short-term behavioral changes leading to the attainment of specific, measurable goals. The behavioral counselor functions more as a directive, expert consultant than as a nondirective, active listener and facilitator for personal reflection. Additionally the interventions chosen in behavioral counseling are specific to the problem and the person and therefore can be sensitive to the client's background and current circumstances.

However, Diller (2004) and Ivey, D'Andrea, and Ivey (2012) point out that counseling approaches, such as behavioral counseling, often put a major focus on individual responsibility for changing one's life, neglecting cultural influences favoring an external locus of control in how people run their lives. These authors believe that directive approaches can still be effective if they are tailored to fit the cultural expectations of the clients.

Kauffman, Conroy, Gardner, and Oswald (2008) investigated cultural sensitivity in behavioral principles in education. They found no research suggesting that behavioral interventions work differently in children who have different ethnicity, gender, or religion. Those authors stated that cultural sensitivity requires respecting the individual student. They recommended that intervention choice is based on the science of behavior and the measuring of outcomes. Objectives of treatment should be discussed with parents and children to determine if the objectives are meaningful and worthwhile. The treatment procedures should be discussed in terms that parent and child can understand and those procedures must be acceptable to them. Behavioral counselors would do well to practice with those guidelines in mind.

Spiegler and Guevremont (2009) observed that behaviorists have not paid sufficient attention to matters of race, gender, ethnicity, and sexual orientation and challenge behavioral counselors to develop more clinical skills in diversity.

EVALUATION OF BEHAVIORAL COUNSELING

The research literature on the effectiveness of behavioral counseling abounds (Antony & Roemer, 2011) who suggest that there are few problems that behavioral therapies have not been found to bring some relief (p. 107). Some examples include anxiety disorders (Antony & Stein, 2009), substance use disorders (Hallgren, Greenfield, Ladd, Glynn, & McCrady, 2012; Vedel & Emmelkamp, 2012) and eating disorders (Touyz, Polivy, & Hay, 2008). Clients with obsessive-compulsive disorders improved after behavioral treatment (Barlow, 2004) as have those with post-traumatic stress disorder (PTSD). Foa et al. (2005) studied cognitive and behavioral techniques to treat PTSD and found the strongest evidence supporting exposure therapy in which a person develops a hierarchy of feared situations and learns to confront those conditions. Behavioral counseling has been successful in treating depression (Cuijpers et al., 2012; Dimidjian et al., 2006; Lewinsohn, Clarke, Hops, & Andrews, 1990), academic problems (O'Leary, 1980), and children's fears about surgery (Melamed & Siegel, 1980).

Wilson (2008) reported on the evaluations of clinical disorders treatment by the National Institute for Clinical Excellence (NICE) in the United Kingdom. Treatment guidelines are graded from **A**, meaning strong empirical support based on randomized controlled trials, to **C**, based on expert opinion with strong empirical data. Behavior therapy is typically rated as A and is the treatment of choice for specific mood and anxiety disorders, as well as eating disorders (Wilson & Shafran, 2005).

According to Kazdin (1991) and Weisz, Doss, and Hawley (2005) almost two-thirds of the outcome studies about treatment with children and adolescents have been behavioral treatments. Across many measures of treatment outcome, the young people in therapy improved more than those who received no treatment. The largest effects were found with using multiple behavioral methods, modeling, and desensitization/relaxation.

Zlomke and Davis (2008) reviewed the literature on one-session treatment (OST) for specific phobias. In these 3-hour sessions, clients create a hierarchy of fear. Counselor and client use these steps to create counselor-directed behavior experiments to overcome the fear. Two treatments for spider phobia in children indicated the OST was effective in reducing behavioral avoidance and subjective fear. One study included parents in the treatment and reported improvement at the end of the treatment as well as 1 year later. These authors concluded the application of OST for specific phobias in children leads to significant positive changes.

SUMMARY

Behavioral counselors operationalize terms referring to subjective states listed under such diagnostic categories as depression, anxiety, paranoia, shyness, obsession, and compulsion by describing these conditions as specific patterns of observable actions. For example, depression might be defined as loss of adequate reinforcement. Behavioral counselors are committed to defining problems precisely by breaking them down into observable and countable components of behavior. Behavioral goals are set in advance and systematically evaluated throughout the treatment process and follow-up period. Behavioral counselors view their work as re-educative rather than healing and reject diagnostic labels for behavior analysis. Often, behavioral counseling begins with a written contract outlining what the client is going to do and what outcomes are to be expected. Counseling begins with the behavior that is easiest to change, with accurate records maintained throughout the counseling experience. Behavioral counselors follow the scientific method in discarding ineffective interventions in favor of new intervention plans based on data collection and analysis.

Behavioral therapy has contributed to counseling by emphasizing the importance of research on treatment efficacy. Goal setting, accountability, specificity, and counseling outcomes have increasing importance in a world that demands efficiency and effectiveness. Antony and Roemer (2011) stated the essential goal of behavior therapy is helping clients establish a behavioral tools they need, not only to deal with their current concerns but also by developing skills they can use in other troubling situations. Most importantly the evidence indicates the positive outcomes often endure and generalize to other positive changes for the clients (Seligman & Reichenberg, 2014).

INTRODUCTION TO BEHAVIORAL COUNSELING

To gain a more in-depth understanding of the concepts in this chapter, visit www.cengage.com/counseling/henderson to view a short clip of an actual therapist–client session demonstrating behavioral counseling.

WEB SITES FOR BEHAVIORAL COUNSELING

Internet addresses frequently change. To find the sites listed here, visit www.cengage.com/counseling/henderson for an updated list of Internet addresses and direct links to relevant sites.

Association for Behavior Analysis

Association for Behavioral and Cognitive Therapies (ABCT)

Behavior OnLine: The Mental Health and Behavioral Science Meeting Place

B. F. Skinner Foundation

REFERENCES

Achenbach, T. H. (1991). *Manual for the child behavior checklist.* Burlington: University of Vermont, Department of Psychiatry.

Antony, M. M. (2014). Behavior therapy. In D. Wedding & R. J. Corsini (Eds.), *Current psychotherapies* (10th ed., pp. 193–228). Belmont, CA: Brooks/Cole.

Antony, M. M., & Roemer, L. (2011). *Behavior therapy.* Washington, DC: American Psychological Association.

Antony, M. M., & Stein, M. M. (Eds.) (2009). *Oxford handbook of anxiety and related disorders.* New York: Oxford University Press.

Austad, C. S. (2009). *Counseling and psychotherapy today: Theory, practice and research.* Boston: McGraw Hill.

Baldwin, J. D., & Baldwin, J. I. (2001). *Behavior principles in everyday life* (4th ed.). Upper Saddle River, NJ: Prentice Hall.

Bandura, A. (1969). *Principles of behavior modification.* New York: Holt, Rinehart, & Winston.

Bandura, A. (1974). Behavior therapy and the models of man. *American Psychologist, 29,* 859–869.

Bandura, A. (1977). *Social learning theory.* Upper Saddle River, NJ: Prentice Hall.

Bandura, A. (1986). *Social foundations of thought and action: A social cognitive theory.* Upper Saddle River, NJ: Prentice Hall.

Banks, S., & Thompson, C. (1995). *Educational psychology: For teachers in training.* St. Paul, MN: West.

Barlow, D. H. (2004). *Anxiety and its disorders* (2nd ed.). New York: Guilford Press.

Beveridge, R. M., & Berg, C. A. (2007). Parent-adolescent collaboration: An interpersonal model for understanding optimal interactions. *Clinical Child and Family Psychology Review, 10,* 25–52.

Bovend'Eerdt, J. H., Botell, R. E., & Wade, D. T. (2009). Writing SMART rehabilitation goals and achieving goal attainment scaling: a practical guide. *Clinical Rehabilitation, 23,* 352–361.

Braaten, S. (1998). *Behavioral objective sequence.* Champaign, IL: Research Press.

Conners, C. K. (1997). *Conners' Rating Scale – Revised manual.* North Tonawanda, NY: Mental Health Systems.

Cuijpers, P., van Straten, A. E., Driessen, D., van Oppen, P., Bockting, C., & Andersson, G. (2012). Depression and dysthymic disorder. In P. Sturmey & M. Hersen (Eds.), *Handbook of evidence-based practice in clinical psychology: Vol. II. Adult disorders* (pp. 243–284). Hoboken, NJ: John Wiley & Sons.

Diller, J. (2004). *Cultural diversity: A primer for the human services.* Belmont, CA: Brooks/Cole.

Dimidjian, S., Hollon, S. D., Dobson, K. S., Schmaling, K. B., Kohlenberg, R. J., et al. (2006). Behavioral activation, cognitive therapy and anti-depressant medication in the acute treatment of major depression. *Journal of Consulting and Clinical Psychology, 74,* 658–670.

Emmelkamp, P. M. G., Vedel, E., & Kamphuis, J. H. (2007). Behaviour therapy. In C. Freeman & M. Power (Eds.), *Handbook of evidence-based psychotherapies: A guide for research and practice* (pp. 61–81). West Sussex, England: Wiley.

Epstein, R. (Ed.). (1980). *Skinner for the classroom.* Champaign, IL: Research Press.

Fall, K. A., Holden, J. M., & Marquis, A. (2010). *Theoretical models of counseling and psychotherapy* (2nd ed.) New York: Routledge.

Fink, B. C., & Lotspeich, L. (2004). Behavior analysis and child and adolescent treatments. In H. Steiner (Ed.), *Handbook of mental health interventions in children and adolescents: An integrated developmental approach* (pp. 498–524). San Francisco, CA: Jossey-Bass.

Fisher, W. W., Piazza, C. C., & Roane, H. S. (Eds.) (2011). *Handbook of applied behavior analysis*. New York: Guilford Press.

Foa, E. B., Hembree, E. A., Cahill, S. P., Rauch, S. A. M., & Riggs, D. S., et al. (2005). Randomized trial of prolonged exposure for posttraumatic stress disorder with and without cognitive restructuring: Outcome at academic and community clinics. *Journal of Consulting and Clinical Psychology, 73*, 953–964.

Gladding S. T. (2005). *Counseling theories: Essential concepts and applications*. Upper Saddle River, NJ: Pearson.

Hallgren, K. A., Greenfield, B. L., Ladd, B., Glynn, L. H., & McCrady, B. S. (2012). Alcohol use disorders. In P. Sturmey & M. Hersen (Eds.), *Handbook of evidence-based practice in clinical psychology: Vol. II-Adult disorders* (pp. 133–165). Hoboken, NJ: John Wiley & Sons.

Haynes, S. N., O'Brien, W. H., & Kaholokula, J. K. (2011). *Behavioral assessment and case formulation*. Hoboken, NJ: John Wiley & Sons.

Ivey, A., D'Andrea, M. J., & Ivey, M. (2012). *Theories of counseling and psychotherapy: A multicultural perspective* (7th ed.). Thousand Oaks, CA: Sage.

Jacobsen, E. (1938). *Progressive relaxation*. Chicago: University of Chicago Press.

Kauffman, J. M., Conroy, M., Gardner, R., III, & Oswald, D. (2008). Cultural sensitivity in the application of behavior principles to education. *Education and Treatment of Children, 31*, 239–262.

Kazdin, A. E. (1991). Effectiveness of psychotherapy with children and adolescents. *Journal of Consulting and Clinical Psychology, 39*, 785–798.

Kazdin, A. E. (2012). *Behavior modification in applied settings* (7th ed.). Pacific Grove, CA: Brooks/Cole.

Lambert, M., & Hawkins, E. (2004). Measuring outcome in professional practice: Considerations in selecting and using brief outcome instruments. *Professional Psychology, Research, and Practice, 35*, 492–499.

Lewinsohn, P. M., Clarke, G. N., Hops, H., & Andrews, J. (1990). Cognitive-behavioral treatment for depressed adolescents. *Behavior Therapy, 21*, 385–401.

Melamed, B., & Siegel, L. (1980). *Behavioral medicine*. New York: Springer.

O'Leary, K. D. (1980). Pills or skills for hyperactive children? *Journal of Applied Behavior Analysis, 13*, 191–204.

Ray, K., Skinner, C., & Watson, T. (1999). Transferring stimulus control via momentum to increase compliance in student with autism: A demonstration of collaborative consultation. *School Psychology Review, 28*, 622–628.

Reynolds, C. R., & Kamphaus, R. W. (2002). *Behavior assessment system for children*. Circle Pines, MN: American Guidance Service.

Romano, J., & Roll, D. (2000). Expanding the utility of behavioral momentum for youth with developmental disabilities. *Behavioral Interventions, 15*, 99–111.

Seligman, L. & Reichenberg, L. W. (2014). *Theories of counseling and psychotherapy: Systems, strategies, and skills* (4th ed.). Upper Saddle River, NJ: Pearson.

Skinner, B. F. (1938). *The behavior of organisms*. New York: Appleton-Century-Crofts.

Skinner, B. F. (1948). *Walden two*. New York: Macmillan.

Skinner, B.F. (1953). *Science and human behavior*. Toronto, Canada: Free Press.

Skinner, B. F. (1968). *The technology of teaching*. Englewood Cliffs, NJ: Prentice Hall.

Skinner, B. F. (1971). *Beyond freedom and dignity*. New York: Knopf.

Skinner, B. F. (1983). *A matter of consequences: Part III of an autobiography*. New York: Knopf.

Skinner, B. F. (1987). *Upon further reflection*. Englewood Cliffs, NJ: Prentice Hall.

Skinner, B. F. (1990a). Can psychology be a science of mind? *American Psychologist, 45*, 1206–1210.

Skinner, B. F. (1990b, August). *Cognitive science: The creationism of psychology*. Keynote address presented at the meeting of the American Psychological Association, Boston.

Spiegler, M. D., & Guevremont, D. C. (2009). *Contemporary behavior therapy* (5th ed.). Belmont, CA: Wadsworth.

Touyz, S. R., Polivy, J., & Hay, P. (2008). *Eating disorders*. Göttingen, Germany: Hogrefe.

Vedel, E., & Emmelkamp, P. M. G. (2012). Illicit substance-related disorders. In P. Sturmey & M. Hersen (Eds.), *Handbook of evidence-based practice in clinical psychology: Vol. II – Adult disorders* (pp. 197–220). Hoboken, NJ: John Wiley & Sons.

Wagner, W. G. (2008). *Counseling, psychology, and children* (2nd ed.). Upper Saddle River, NJ: Pearson.

Watson, J. B. (1913). Psychology as the behaviorist views it. *Psychological Review, 20*, 158–177.

Weisz, J. R., Doss, A. J., & Hawley, K. M. (2005). Youth psychotherapy outcome research: A review and critique of the evidence base. *Annual Review of Psychology, 56*, 337–363.

Wilhite, K., Braaten, S., Frey, L., & Wilder, L. K. (2007). Using the behavioral objective sequence in the classroom. *Intervention in School and Clinic, 42*, 212–218.

Wilson, G. T. (2008). Behavior therapy. In D. Wedding & R.J. Corsini (Eds.), *Current psychotherapies* (8th ed., pp. 223–261). Belmont, CA: Thomson.

Wilson, G. T., & Shafran, R. (2005). Eating disorders guidelines from NICE. *The Lancet, 365*, 79–81.

Windholtz, G. (1997). Ivan P. Pavlov: An overview of his life and psychological work. *American Psychologist, 52*, 941–945.

Wolpe, J. (1958). *Psychotherapy by reciprocal inhibition*. Stanford, CA: Stanford University Press.

Wolpe, J. (1969). *The practice of behavior therapy*. New York: Pergamon.

Wolpe, J. (1989). The derailment of behavior therapy: A tale of conceptual misdirection. *Journal of Behavior Therapy and Experimental Psychiatry, 20*, 3–15.

Wolpe, J., & Plaud, J. (1997). Pavlov's contributions to behavior therapy: The obvious and the not so obvious. *American Psychologist, 52*, 966–972.

Zlomke, K., & Davis, T. E., III. (2008). One-session treatment of specific phobias: A detailed description and review of treatment efficacy. *Behavior Therapy, 39*, 207–233.

CHAPTER 9

Reality Therapy: Counseling with Choice Theory

Nothing strengthens the judgment and quickens the conscience like individual responsibility.
—ELIZABETH CADY STANTON

By the 1950s, therapists were becoming convinced that human experiences cannot be reduced to the past or the subconscious. Rather than using the deterministic point of view, counselors began considering ideas about the inner drive and the control people have over their lives. Counselors also began to explore the client's perceptions of the world, free will, and the present. From these changes in therapeutic focus arose the theory of reality therapy, a no-excuse, future-oriented approach that teaches self-determination and a process of change in behavior. This chapter focuses on this action-oriented theory.

After reading this chapter, you should be able to:

▶ Outline the development of reality therapy and William Glasser's involvement
▶ Explain the theory of reality therapy and choice theory including its core concepts
▶ Discuss the counseling relationship and goals in reality therapy
▶ Describe assessment, process, and techniques in reality therapy
▶ Demonstrate some therapeutic techniques
▶ Clarify the effectiveness of reality therapy

WILLIAM GLASSER (1925–2013)

Fritz William Glasser grew up in Cleveland, Ohio. Glasser (1998) described his mother as controlling and his father as the master of choice theory, a Russian Jewish immigrant who never tried to control anyone. His experiences with his parents led Glasser to a theory that covers a range of behaviors from external controls (his mother) to self-control (his father).

Glasser graduated from Case Institute of Technology as a chemical engineer in 1944, at the age of 19. At Case Western Reserve University, he earned a master's degree in clinical psychology at 23 and a medical degree at 28. While serving his last year of residency at the University of California at Los Angeles School of Psychiatry and in a Veterans Administration hospital, Glasser discovered that traditional psychotherapy was not for him. Glasser voiced reservations about psychoanalysis to his supervisor, G. Harrington, who reputedly agreed; however, such an attitude was not popular among his other colleagues. Glasser was denied a promised teaching position because of his rebellion against Freudian concepts. In an interview with Wubbolding (2000), Glasser recounted the encounter in which he began working differently. He was meeting with a client who had been in therapy for 4 years. She began by yet another iteration about her problems with her grandfather. Glasser's respond captures his stance:

> I can tell you that if you want to see me, I don't have any interest in your grandfather. There is nothing I can do about what went on with him, nothing you can do about what went on with him. He's dead. Rest in peace. But if that's what you want, then you'll have to say that you want another psychiatrist because I think you have some problems, but you have been avoiding them for a number of years by talking about your grandfather, and I want to talk about what is going on in your life right now. I have no interest in what was wrong yesterday (Wubbolding, 2000, p. 49).

In 1956, Glasser became head psychiatrist at the Ventura School for Girls, an institution operated by the State of California to treat seriously delinquent adolescent girls. For 12 years, Glasser conducted a successful program at the Ventura School; the theory and concepts of reality therapy evolved from this program. Glasser realized that the school was like a prison with strict guidelines, harsh punishment, and little sense of community. He thought that because the girls were treated as "losers," they believed they were. His program allowed each girl chances to make decisions and to assume personal responsibility. He treated each young woman with kindness, respect, and praise (Berges, 1976). The effectiveness of the school improved. Glasser outlined his methods in his first book, *Mental Health or Mental Illness?* (1961).

Glasser used the term *reality therapy* for the first time in April 1964 in a manuscript, "Reality Therapy: A Realistic Approach to the Young Offender." His widely read book *Reality Therapy* was published in 1965. In 1966, Glasser began consulting in California public schools for the purpose of applying reality therapy in education. These new ideas for applying reality therapy to teaching later became his third book, *Schools without Failure* (1969).

In 1968, Glasser founded the Institute for Reality Therapy in Los Angeles. It offers training courses for physicians, probation officers, police officers, nurses, lawyers, judges, teachers, and counselors. Introductory and advanced courses and programs are offered on a regular and continuing basis. The Educator Training Center, a special division of the Institute for Reality Therapy, was established after the publication of *Schools without Failure* (1969). In 1970, the William Glasser La Verne College Center was established at the University of La Verne in southern California to provide teachers with an off-campus opportunity to gain graduate and in-service credits while working within their own schools to provide an exciting educational environment for children. Currently the William Glasser Institute (http://www.wglasser.com/) offers trainings on choice theory across the world.

Control Theory

In 1977, Glasser incorporated the ideas of Powers' (1973) *Behavior: The Control of Perception* into a theoretical underpinning for reality therapy. The basis was the belief that people's choices result from trying to control their perceptions of their needs being met (Fall, Holden, & Marquis, 2010). Glasser then began to use control theory to identify his approach, explaining that when there is a difference between what a person wants (internal) and what the person perceives in the world (external), the mismatch leads to dissatisfaction. For example, troubled children may want love and attention but often have chosen irresponsible behavior to try to meet their needs (Fuller, 2007). The inner world of wants is like a picture album (Glasser, 1984) to be explored by the child and counselor. In control theory, the brain is considered the system that seeks to control, maneuver, and mold the world to satisfy internal needs (Wubbolding, 2011b).

Choice Theory

In the 1990s, Glasser moved to choice theory as a reflection of his ideas of self-control and the power of choice. Reality therapy is the delivery system and choice theory, the rationale. Choice theory explains human behavior by looking at motivation and communication (Wubbolding & Brickell, 2007). The idea behind choice theory is that people's problems are the results of unsatisfying relationships. To progress, people have to eliminate the external control psychology from relationship (Wubbolding, 2000). External control psychology uses things like blaming, nagging, criticizing, complaining, and punishing to get other people to comply. People need to replace that type of psychology with strategies to strengthen and support relationships such as love, support, negotiation, and trust. The following are ten axioms of choice theory which will be discussed in later parts in this chapter:

- The only person whose behavior we can control is our own.
- All we can give or get from other people is information.
- All long-lasting psychological problems are relationship problems.
- The problem relationship is always part of our present lives.
- What happened in the past that was painful has a great deal to do with what we are today, but revising this painful past can contribute little or nothing to what we need to do now—improve an important, present relationship.
- We are driven by five genetic needs: survival, love and belonging, power, freedom, and fun.
- We can satisfy these needs only by satisfying a picture or pictures in our quality worlds.
- All we can do from birth to death is behave. All behavior is total behavior and is made up of four inseparable components: acting, thinking, feeling, and physiology.
- All total behavior is designated by verbs and named by the component that is most recognizable.
- All total behavior is chosen, but we have direct control over only the acting and thinking components. We can, however, control our feelings and physiology indirectly through how we choose to act and think (Glasser, 1998, pp. 332–335).

Fuller (2007) explained that choice theory requires a counselor to connect to the client's inner quality world and to establish a trusting relationship. That inner quality world includes what the child would like to be.

Glasser's other books include *The Identity Society* (1972), *Positive Addiction* (1976), *Stations of the Mind* (1981), *Control Theory in the Classroom* (1986), *The Quality School: Managing Students without Coercion* (1990), *The Quality School Teacher* (1993), *Staying Together* (1995), *Choice Theory: A New Psychology of*

Personal Freedom (1998), *Getting Together and Staying Together* (2000b), *Reality Therapy in Action* (2000c), *Every Student Can Succeed* (2000a), *Unhappy Teenagers: A Way for Parents and Teachers to Reach Them* (2002), *Warning: Psychiatry Can Be Dangerous to Your Health* (2004), and *Treating Mental Health as a Public Health Problem: A New Leadership Role for the Helping Professions* (2005).

Another spokesman for reality therapy, Robert Wubbolding, worked with Glasser at the institute for several years. Wubbolding now heads the Center for Reality Therapy (http://www.realitytherapywub.com/) and is a faculty member at Xavier University in Cincinnati. His recent book *Reality Therapy* (2011) includes the most current overview of choice theory, and his other writings combine case studies and treatment protocols that clarify the practice of reality therapy.

THE NATURE OF PEOPLE

Choice theorists believe the essential nature of people is positive (Glasser & Wubbolding, 1995) but also acknowledge humans may be loving and productive as well as bedeviled, selfish, and self-absorbed. In this theory Glasser acknowledged a world that is defined differently due to the variation in values and needs among people.

Reality therapy focuses on the present. The focus of counseling is supporting people in their thoughts and actions so they can live more fulfilling lives. This therapy emphasizes self-determination, as Glasser (1998) explained, "We choose everything we do, including the misery we feel" (p. 3). Fuller (2007) explained that the driving force for all behavior is the goal of each person to have a distinct identity. Getting and keeping this sense of self, whether it is centered on either success or failure, is a critical component of living. Children who have a failure identity believe "I can't; I'm no good; I'm worthless." Children with success identity believe they are competent and worthwhile.

The basic human motivation is to increase pleasure and decrease pain (Glasser, 2011), feelings that occur based on the satisfaction (or lack) of basic needs. Those needs are survival, love and belonging, power, freedom, and fun (Glasser, 2004). Trying to narrow the gap between what a person wants and what a person has motivates behavior (Wubbolding et al., 2004). Choice theory incorporates all these ideas with assumptions about the ways people decide what to do.

As noted previously choice theory is based on the proposition that the only behavior we can control is our own. Glasser (1998) pointed out that people get into trouble when they try to control other people. He believed that the practice of control psychology is responsible for the widespread belief that people and their behaviors can be controlled. Consequently, people waste considerable energy and time trying to get other people to do things the others do not want to do. Equal amounts of time and energy are expended on resisting the efforts of others to get you to do things you do not want to do. Glasser saw these efforts as responsible for the breakdown of good relationships. In fact, Glasser believed that all long-lasting psychological problems brought to counseling are relationship problems resulting from these attempts to control others. According to Glasser, the remedy for fixing the damage done by the practice of control psychology is to teach choice theory to as many people as possible.

Glasser reminded us that having healthy relationships aids in positive development. Wubbolding (2011a) explained that interpersonal quality time builds relationships. Quality time requires effort and energy, an awareness of each other, and regular meetings. The time together is free of criticism and complaint and fills needs for all. The amount of time needed varies, and the activities involved are determined by the interests and ages of the people involved. Counselors want quality time with the children they see and use choice theory to build a quality relationship by attending to the child's needs, reality, and responsibility.

Concepts

The five basic *needs* of survival, love and belonging, power, fun, and freedom are innate and universal (Wubbolding, 2011a). Each person has the genetic motivation to fulfill those needs in order to avoid the pain that occurs when the needs are unfulfilled. The strength of each need varies among people. Although each need is distinct, needs can interact and overlap in a situation. Needs are translated and revised during the life span into *wants* which are defined as the specific people, things, or circumstances that the person desires because they meet his or her needs.

The five basic needs identified by Glasser sometimes conflict when a person tries to find a balance fulfilling the needs. The *survival* need is the biological drive to survive and to procreate, to have the essentials of life such as good health, food, air, shelter, safety, and security. The behaviors that support survival are eating, exercising, having shelter, and sexual behavior. *Love and belonging* are the needs of social creatures who want to get together, have friends, and be intimate with other people. Wubbolding (2000) surmised that when survival needs are largely met, the need for love and belonging will be the primary client concern. Glasser (2000c) agreed and said that having relationships with other people and meeting the need for love and belonging is a gauge of healthy or unhealthy living. He remarked, "To satisfy every other need, we must have relationships with other people" (p. 23) or we will be unable to satisfy the other four needs. Glasser suggests wanting power for power's sake is uniquely human. That need can be satisfied in malevolent ways by getting our way, bossing others, being right, getting more, and punishing others. However, doing things for the good of others is a better way of satisfying power needs. The need for *power* can be satisfied by a sense of accomplishment, doing a job well, working hard, and being recognized. Wubbolding (2011a) broadened the definition of the power needs to include inner control, achievement, self-esteem, and recognition. The need for *fun* is the pursuit of enjoyment, a feeling of invigorating playfulness and deep connection; the ability to laugh, play, and appreciate are components of this need for pleasure which can be satisfied in many ways (Wubbolding, 2011a). The need for *fun* also relates to the capacity to learn as Glasser (2004) wrote "Having fun, which produces a very good feeling, is our genetic reward for learning" (p. 20). The need for *freedom* is defined as the human desire for autonomy, to be able to choose with no excessive or unnecessary restrictions. This need reflects the innate human desire to expand options and to look for circumstances in which one can fulfill each need without impeding the fulfillment of others. Glasser believed all five needs have to be satisfied. While the needs are universal, the specific ways people choose to meet those needs are unique to the individual.

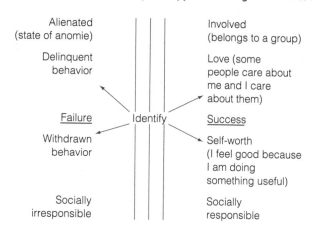

FIGURE 9-1 FAILURE AND SUCCESS IDENTITIES

Similar to Maslow's hierarchy of human needs, Glasser focused his early treatment plans on teaching people to love and be loved and to feel valued by themselves and others through success in their careers. Successful attainment of these two needs leads to a success identity (Figure 9-1). In fact, success in these two important areas can be a quick index for evaluating one's mental health. Both are keys to a healthy sense of self. Building a network of friends and supportive people puts children and adolescents on the road to achieving a healthy sense of self-esteem, a journey to be completed through success in the classroom.

Glasser believed that, despite varying manifestations, psychological problems are the result of one factor: the inability to fulfill one's basic needs. Throughout his career, he criticized the mental health community that understand mental illness as biological and often stated that psychotropic medications have great potential for harm, particularly the sense that there is nothing a person can do to help himself or herself (Glasser, 2004). Rather, he sees a correlation between people's lack of success in meeting their needs and the degree of their distress and unhappiness. His interest focuses on the symptoms people choose to ease the pain of not getting what they want. He maintained that psychological problems can result from people's denial of the reality of the world around them. *Denial of reality* in the reality therapy system refers to the tendency of people to try to avoid the unpleasant natural and logical consequences of their irresponsible behavior. In Glasser's system, *irresponsible behavior* is defined as attempts by people to satisfy their own basic needs in ways that infringe on the rights of others to meet their needs. For Glasser, feelings are the indicators that our behavior is on the right track; that is, if people feel good about their behavior and if others also feel good about it, chances are they are doing the right thing. In his incorporation of choice theory into reality therapy, Glasser (1998) stated that all problems brought to counseling have a relationship component and behavior in opposition to reality and responsibility is likely to lead to an abundance of relationship problems, especially as people try to meet their needs. The most important need, therefore, is love and belonging (Glasser, 2011).

Quality World

The quality world, or the world of wants, refers to the set of mental images that represent need-fulfilling things or people (Wubbolding, 2011a). Choice theory practitioners teach their clients that they can control only their own behavior and that they have the freedom to make choices that lead to better quality lives. Glasser (1998) held that each person maintains mental images of what and whom we would like to have in our quality world. Also called the inner picture album, the quality world consists of the perceptions of everything that has met—and we believe can continue to meet—one or more basic needs. According to Glasser, the components of our quality world represent three categories: people we want to be with, things we want to possess or experience, and beliefs that guide our behavior. The best way to bring reality to our quality world image is to make the changes in our lives that help us find better ways to meet our needs. Failure to satisfy a particular need often results in choosing a symptom behavior such as depression. These needs are satisfied only by fulfilling an image or picture we have included in our quality world. Hence, we see the importance of being able to visualize ourselves achieving the important and realistic goals we have set for ourselves. The amount of freedom we have in our lives is directly proportional to our success in satisfying the pictures and images in our quality worlds. We give up freedom when we put pictures in our quality worlds that we cannot satisfy. When we try to fill our album by controlling people, Glasser predicted other problems would occur.

Glasser believed that all we can give or get from other people is information. What we do with that information is our choice, as is the type and amount of information we give to others. Glasser stated that people have more control over thinking and doing than on feeling and physiology. He said it is easier to adjust one's thinking about a situation; so that rather than dwelling on the problems, one should start considering possible solutions. He reflected that people have inborn potential to control thoughts and actions directly. People control feelings and physiology only indirectly by changing their thinking and doing. The implications for counseling and change are that to have the highest chance of success, a person would focus on thoughts and actions. People are responsible only for what they choose to do with their behavior. Relationships become progressively better as people focus on changing their own behavior, as opposed to trying to get other people to change their ways.

Glasser (1998, 2011) pointed out that relationship problems are the causes of many other problems, such as pain, fatigue, weakness, and some chronic diseases commonly referred to as autoimmune diseases. He believed that people choose misery and depression rather than facing the problem of what they are doing to destroy an important relationship that is not working the way they want. Consistent with choice philosophy, Glasser (1998) stated that problem relationships are part of a person's present life. Although past painful events and relationships have significant influence on a person's present life, Glasser believed that to revisit the past is not nearly as productive as focusing on what needs to be done to improve a current important relationship.

Glasser has been influenced by W. Edwards Deming's (1966) philosophy that high-quality work is dependent on eliminating the fear that prevents people from getting along with each other. People do not perform well when there is an adversarial relationship between management and labor, teachers and students, and counselors and clients. To be successful, managers, teachers, and counselors must become a part of the quality worlds of the people with whom they work. Glasser believes that the practice of control psychology—that is, punishing wrong behavior and rewarding right behavior—is responsible for most of the human misery and adversarial relationships that exist worldwide. The problem is compounded by the fact that those who have power—government agencies, parents, teachers, business managers, and religious leaders who define right and wrong—totally support the practice of control psychology.

Glasser explained his educational model in four books: *The Quality School: Managing Students without Coercion* (1990), *The Quality School Teacher* (1993), *Every Student Can Succeed* (2000a), and *Unhappy Teenagers: A Way for Parents and Teachers to Reach Them* (2002). These books emphasize the business metaphor derived from Deming's work with Japanese factories. The message is that managers and teachers have a lot in common in that the results depend on how people are treated. The book presents two managerial models: the boss manager and the lead manager. Boss managers motivate by punishment rather than encouragement and reinforcement, tell rather than show, overpower rather than empower, and rule rather than cooperate. Lead managers do the reverse. In short, Glasser makes a case for cooperative teachers rather than controlling ones. Glasser (2002, 2005) believes that teachers can connect with their students if they give up the seven deadly habits that destroy all relationships: criticizing, blaming, complaining, nagging, threatening, punishing, and rewarding in order to control. The model works equally well in personal relationships, homes, schools, businesses, community agencies, and government because, regardless of setting, we are all in the business of managing people. The seven deadly habits should be replaced by the seven caring habits of encouraging, listening, negotiating, supporting, trusting, accepting, and respecting.

Theory of Counseling

The only assessment necessary in reality therapy counseling involves determining what relationships are problems (Murdock, 2013). According to choice theory, healthy functioning equates to responsible behavior, meeting one's own needs without preventing others from meeting theirs. Healthy people build, develop, and maintain relationships to fulfill their needs. The need for love and belonging is primary, but one must pay attention to all needs to accomplish a sense of well-being. Emotionally healthy people live by choosing thoughts, feelings, and behaviors responsibly. They improve their lives and try to make the world a better place (Wubbolding, 1991). Wubbolding (2000) called this "effective life direction."

Unhealthy functioning, according to reality therapy, is really people's breakdown in meeting their needs in responsible and effective ways. Glasser (1965) stated that people showing signs of maladjustment are not crazy and should not be labeled mentally ill. He argues that people are always responsible for their own behavior. Furthermore, he said that a range of behaviors called *abnormal* are really actions people choose when they are unable to satisfy their basic needs. The root of almost all maladjustment lies in the lack of a satisfying relationship (Glasser, 2000c). Maladjustment, then, is the result of a lack of connection between a person and other people. Glasser explained that what others say is mental illness is actually the way people choose to deal with the pain of loneliness or disconnection—choosing one form of pain to forestall an even greater pain. That means that the person who is functioning in an unhealthy way is having problems in choices, need satisfaction, and responsibility. Symptoms can be tied to needs in these ways. People may choose the emotional difficulty of loneliness instead of belonging; loss of control rather than feeling powerful; boredom and depression instead of fun; frustration or inhibition instead of freedom; and illness or deprivation rather than safety and security (Seligman & Reichenberg, 2014).

Glasser (2000c) said people create and endure misery for the following reasons. Choosing symptoms like depression and anxiety helps keep angering under control; choosing instead to depress has less painful potential consequences than jail or injury. Another reason is that choosing intense symptoms leads other people to comfort and care for the depressing person. Glasser suggested that if the person were not pampered when displaying symptoms, the behavior would disappear. Also, choosing intense symptoms allows people to avoid doing what they are afraid of doing. Therefore, by choosing their symptoms, people prevent the possibility of having satisfying relationships. People persist in their symptoms because it is the best way they know to meet their needs.

Counseling Relationship

Reality therapy counselors are verbally active (Fuller, 2007). Throughout the process, the counselor focuses on the person's real life, what the person is doing and plans to do. The relationship is built on a caring involvement of the counselor with the client. The counselor is encouraging, optimistic, concrete, and focused. The counselor builds an environment in which the client has enough security to evaluate current choices. Maintaining this safety is a critical part of the success of counseling. Fuller stated that the role of the counselor is to provide a partnership in which the child avoids excuses and accepts responsibility, emphasizes strengths, and learns and practices new behaviors.

Wubbolding (2007) listed skills to build a relationship with a client. His admonitions are "always be courteous, determined, enthusiastic, firm and genuine" (p. 298). He reminded counselors to suspend judgment by remembering that people are giving their best efforts to fulfill their needs. He suggested that counselors use humor and listen for the client's metaphors and themes. Counselors use reality therapy to establish rapport and trust in a brief, efficient way.

The counselor must build a choice theory relationship with clients. When experiencing a fulfilling relationship, clients can learn about handling the worrisome relationship that brought them into counseling. The client–counselor relationship becomes a bond in which clients learn how to build relationships based on choice theory. Glasser (2000c) explained that if the counselor does not connect to the client, change will not happen. The early stage of "making friends" is based on respect, boundaries, and choices. Some of the characteristics of the effective counselor who uses reality therapy have been outlined by Wubbolding (2007) and Wubbolding and Brickell (2008) and discussed earlier. These authors explained the ABCDEFG approach. The AB stands for *always be*, and the other letters denote ways to be with the client: *courteous, determined, enthusiastic, firm*, and *genuine*.

Wubbolding (2007) also talks about some things counselors should not do. Counselors do not accept excuses. Reality therapists are not concerned with the reasons behind a person's behaviors. The why's of behavior are considered unproductive and may distract from the healing power of making responsible choices. Counselors do not argue or criticize but instead accept the clients' ineffective choices and respect their freedom to choose. Finally, counselors do not give up but stay with the person past the time he or she expects to be abandoned. Counselors maintain an empathic and challenging attitude with continuing hope for the client's ability to change.

Reality therapy counselors use action verbs (depressing and angering) to help people take responsibility for their emotions and actions. They use first person pronouns (I and we) to emphasize the partnership of the counselor and client in the treatment process. They ask questions that use *what* rather than *why*. Finally, counselors use caring confrontation by asking thought-provoking questions.

The client in reality therapy must be willing to focus on behavior and must be ready to change. Reality therapists do not spend time looking at a client's past but instead concentrate on what is occurring now and on educating the client about choice theory. Clients must be open to having a relationship with the counselor and to being challenged about their choices.

Goals

The primary goal in using reality therapy is to help people have greater control over their lives by making better choices to fulfill their needs and do not interfere with or hurt others (Glasser, 2000c). Decisions, not circumstances, shape a person's behavior. Wise choices help people meet their innate needs and specific wants. Wise choices are responsible, respecting the rights of other people, and wise choices are realistic. Some appropriate goals are helping people form and sustain positive relationships, develop success identities, and have options of healthy actions that boost their total behavior. Reality therapy counselors help clients think clearly, experience happiness and other positive emotions, and take steps to remain physically healthy (Seligman & Reichenberg, 2014).

The biggest challenge counselors face in the practice of reality therapy based on choice theory is to teach their clients that control psychology will not work for them any better than it has worked for the rest of the world. Glasser (1998, 2000c), as we have mentioned earlier, believes that our attempts to control others are largely responsible for the misery in so many people's lives. Humankind, unfortunately, has a long history of turning to coercion and control to get others to follow our wishes.

The primary focus of choice theory in reality therapy is to prevent problems before they happen. Regardless of the skill of the counselor, it is often impossible to rescue failing students who have never been willing to put school and teachers in their quality world vision. People do not admit those who try to control them to their quality world. Glasser (1998, 2000a) believes then that a good way to learn choice theory is to treat others in your life like you treat your best friend, your boss, and most strangers. You rarely try to force these people to do anything. People, however, tend to believe that they own their spouses, children, students, and employees and so try to control them. For example, I have a right to control the people I own, and when they do not do what I want, I have a right to force them to do it. Consequently, we often have better relationships with those not so close to us because we do not try to own them and force them to do things. Glasser (1998, 2002) recommends that parents treat their children like the grandparents do, but he recognizes that there must be limits; natural or logical consequences should result when limits are breached.

Counseling Method

To reality therapists, change is a series of choices. In order to change, people have to be willing to assume responsibility for their decisions and for the direction of their lives. Primarily this means choosing new behavior. For the change process to work well, a person must realize the many options available in any situation. Glasser (1992) said that people change when they realize that what they are doing is not getting them what they want and that another behavior has a greater potential. Taking an active and responsible part in choices allows a person to assess the effectiveness of their behavior. Choice and assessment is the central process in reality therapy. Therefore, reality therapy based on choice theory includes an examination of the client's belief system. Clients will be challenged to explain the rationality of what they believe, as well as the utility of what they do when they act on their beliefs.

People may attempt control to build their quality world. The closer a person's reality world approaches his or her quality world, the happier he or she will be. The farther apart a person's reality and quality worlds are, the more pain the person experiences from not getting what he or she wants. Reality therapy counseling treatment plans are directed toward helping people handle the pain from not getting what they want. Treatment often involves changing strategies to help people get what they want and/or reviewing the pictures in their quality world. In all cases, counseling is focused on changing the client rather than how the client should try to change others. However, it must be noted that change in the client's behavior often influences change in others. The idea is to place one's quality world totally in one's hands and not have quality world objectives under the control of others.

Reality therapy counseling focuses on improving present relationships through personal change while learning from past relationships. As Wubbolding and Brickell (2007) explained, "Emphasizing the present without diminishing the importance of past experiences sends a subtle message ... that there is hope, and that life can be better" (p. 48). The success of the counseling process depends on creating a good relationship between the client and the counselor. The trust level between client and counselor needs to be high enough to handle confrontations, such as the following example:

COUNSELOR: What do you think caused the problem?

CLIENT: It's hard to say. It's really hard to say.

COUNSELOR: [In a friendly tone of voice] Well, try to say it anyway. This is the place to say hard-to-say things.

Clients sometimes choose to depress themselves when they do not get what they want. When this happens, counselors should confront them with the following four choices:

1. Continue to depress yourself.
2. Change what you are doing to get what you want.
3. Change what you want.
4. Both (2) and (3).

Glasser contends that choosing to depress, no matter how strongly or how long the duration, is not a mental illness. Like all behavior, it is a choice. He tested this premise in his work at a psychiatric hospital.

Process

The original practice of reality therapy followed eight steps which we still find helpful. Fuller (2007, pp. 341–348) provides summaries of the approach.

Step 1 is building good relationships with clients. Glasser calls this first step becoming involved, although *involvement* may not be the best word to describe this stage of counseling because it implies entangled or complex rather than positive, honest, and unencumbered relationships. All approaches to counseling include building a trusting climate in which clients feel free to express their innermost fears.

In Step 2, children focus on their present behavior. Glasser says he starts by saying to clients "Tell me the story" (Onedera & Greenwalt, 2007, p. 82), and that unhappiness is very often their story. The counselor and client describe what is the child doing now.

In Step 3, value judgment occurs. Children evaluate what is going on in their lives and how they are helping themselves. In other words, is their behavior helping them get what they want from life? If not, the counselor asks, "Do you want to change what is going on?" However, people do not change old behaviors until they are convinced that they are either not helping themselves or are actually harming themselves. In fact, people are more likely to change their behavior if they are thoroughly disgusted with their current behavior. Therefore, if in Step 3, clients do not give counselors negative evaluations about their current behaviors, counseling is not likely to generate any behavioral changes. Some helpful evaluation questions to ask in Step 3 include:

- How does this behavior help you?
- How does this behavior hurt you?
- How does this behavior help you learn math?
- How does this behavior improve your grade?
- Is your behavior getting you what you want?

Glasser (1998) believes that the only way for a person who feels bad to feel better is to make a positive change in behavior (see Figure 3-2). Reality therapy focuses on working with observable content, including behavior, plans, and goals.

Sometimes in a counseling relationship, counselors call attention to discrepancies in what the child says and what the child does. The careful use of confrontation provides a way to discuss those inconsistencies. Confrontations typically include three parts. The first part includes an introduction to the client's statement, action, or thought that prompts the statement. ["Several weeks ago you said you wanted to get along better with the boy who lives down the street."] The second part points out respectfully and tentatively the discrepancy. ["Today you talked about making fun of his new haircut."] The third part of a caring confrontation invites the client to respond by asking "What do you think about that?" or "Would you like to explore that with me?" Therapists use this type of confrontation to reflect and self-evaluate (Seligman & Reichenberg, 2014).

In Step 4, children plan responsible behavior in reasonable, specific, and positive terms. The counselor and child begin by looking at possible alternatives for getting what the child wants in life. A brainstorming format can be used in which the child looks at better ways of meeting his or her needs. If the child has difficulty selecting new things to try, he or she might focus on stopping something that is not working. However, the counselor will want to have clients plan for what they will be doing to fill the free time resulting from stopping ineffective behaviors. Counselors can also draw five idea circles, filling two with suggestions and leaving the rest empty for the child to fill. Children, preferring not to leave the circles empty, generally fill them. Counselors can ask children who their best friends are and what they might tell them to do.

In Step 5, children select alternatives for reaching their goals and commit to trying them. A key process in counseling children is helping them make commitments. When they are able to fulfill their commitments, they can build on these successes to achieve bigger goals.

In Step 6, counselors accept no excuses. The counselor and client examine the results of the commitment made in previous sessions. Children returning for a second interview often say, "Well, I made a commitment to turn in one homework paper a day, and I did not do that," and then begin to list all the reasons why they failed. Reality therapists do not dwell on rationalizing "why." No faultfinding or blaming is allowed (Murdock, 2013). At this point, the counselor and child discuss writing a new contract the child can handle; maybe one homework paper per day is too much for now and a less demanding contract is needed. Counselors do not accept excuses if children do not meet the commitments they made. Excuses are designed to avoid punishment, and when children learn they will not be punished for not meeting a commitment, they have no need for excuses.

In Step 7 counselors do not punish or manage reinforcement for the child client. Counselors do not interfere with the logical consequences of the child's poor choice—for example, a lower grade for failing to turn in a homework paper. Additional penalties that are not logical or natural consequences of failing to turn in the paper, such as paddling, are considered neither effective nor humane; however, logical and natural consequences are not removed.

In Step 8, never give up—perseverance is required. How long should counselors stick with children who seem stuck in their unhappiness? Glasser recommends working with such children three or four times longer than they expect. "Never give up" does not mean a lifelong commitment but rather building on whatever relationship that has been established in Step 1 and continuing to build this relationship through the entire eight-step process.

The key terms of *reality* and *responsibility* need further definition in different age groups. Developmental psychology provides understanding of ways the ideas change as people grow. Piaget (1973) described three stages of moral development, which match his stages of cognitive development:

1. Preconventional (preoperational stage, ages 2–7)
2. Conventional (concrete stage, ages 7–11)
3. Postconventional (formal stage, ages 11 to adulthood)

Kohlberg (1981) expands Piaget's three stages to six by defining two substages within each of Piaget's stages. The questions on which people make their moral judgments, choices, and decisions are listed for each substage.

Preconventional Morality

Stage 1: Will I get caught?

Stage 2: What is in it for me?

Conventional Morality

Stage 3: What will the neighbors think?

Stage 4: What is the rule or law?

Postconventional Morality

Stage 5: What is best for society?

Stage 6: What is best for humankind? Is human life at risk?

A strong case can be made that most problems brought to counseling are actually disorders of responsibility. Neurotic individuals assume too much responsibility; people with character disorders assume too little. Most people find themselves, at times, doing a little of both, depending on the situation. Sometimes knowing how much responsibility to take is difficult. We might assume Glasser would answer to consult your brain first; then, evaluate the feelings you have as indicators of whether you are expressing the right behavior which would be doing something you would like done to or for you.

Techniques

Reality therapy counseling combines challenge and encouragement to help children make new and better choices. Wubbolding (2007) talked about a **WDEP** system as a way to outline the system of reality therapy, which he described as a web of skills and techniques focused on helping the child choose more effective, healthy, responsible behavior. **W** (wants) is the stage in which the counselor learns about the client's wants, needs, and perceptions. Counselors help identify the core components of the person's quality world. Questions such as "What do you want?", "What are you not getting that you would like to get?", and "What is stopping you from getting what you want?" can be used to understand a person's wants. Change occurs only with client commitment, so counselors ask, "How hard do you want to work at changing your situation?" (p. 303) to determine the effort a person is ready to expend. The following client comments illustrate five increasing levels of commitment:

1. I don't want to be here.
2. I want the outcome but not the effort.
3. I'll try; I might.
4. I will do my best.
5. I will do whatever it takes (Wubbolding, 2007, p. 303).

D stands for direction and doing, exploring the current life situation with questions like "What are you doing?" and thereby asking for specifics that are currently happening. The question focuses on the client and behavior, opening the possibility of educating the client about how choice theory works. E involves evaluating what the person wants and what the person is doing to help determine whether or not the chosen behavior is effective. P refers to the state in which the person determines what action is needed and makes a commitment to change. Plans should meet these criteria:

- Simple—straightforward and easy for everyone to understand
- Attainable—realistic and within reach
- Measurable—for outcomes and timing, specifics need to be detailed and concrete
- Immediate—implemented as soon as possible
- Involves counselor—as a support and for objective feedback
- Controlled by the client—for personal accountability
- Commitment—"I will" statements
- Consistent—with the behavior hopefully becoming a healthy pattern

Clients may recycle through the WDEP process and may address multiple issues in this manner (Wubbolding, 2007).

As noted previously, Glasser provides specifics for the reality therapy counseling method. The following dialogue is an example:

COUNSELOR: Mary, can you tell me a little bit about your life right now here at school?

MARY: What do you mean?

COUNSELOR: Well, Mary, it seems as though you get sent to the office a lot to talk to me about problems you're having with your teachers. Tell me what you're doing and let's talk about it.

MARY: Well, I guess I talk out of turn in class too much sometimes. But my classes are so boring.

COUNSELOR: Okay, so you talk a lot in class and the teachers don't like what you're doing. Do you do anything else that seems to get you in trouble with Mr. Thompson and Mrs. Rudolph?

MARY: No, I don't think so.

COUNSELOR: Are you happy with what happens to you when you do these things?

MARY: I do the same old things that keep getting me in trouble, but I feel good for the moment.

COUNSELOR: I know you do feel better for a while. Are the good feelings worth the price you have to pay for them?

MARY: I guess not, because I'm sure tired of spending so much time in the office.

COUNSELOR: Would you like to work on a better plan?

MARY: Okay. Why not?

COUNSELOR: Let's start by thinking of some things you could do to get along better in your classes and some ways to make them less boring as well.

MARY: Well, I could stop talking out of turn! I know the teachers would like that.

COUNSELOR: Stopping unhelpful things is usually a good way to start. What about some things you could begin doing in class?

MARY: Doing more assignments would please the teachers, but I don't like all the work.

COUNSELOR: Your two suggestions will probably help you with the teachers, but they won't do much to make the class more enjoyable for you. Can you think of something to help you like school more?

MARY: Some of the kids get free time or get to go to the library when they turn in their work. Could I do this, too?

COUNSELOR: We can ask your teachers about that today. That might be a way to please both you and the teachers. Can you think of other ideas to try?

MARY: I guess that's about all for now.

COUNSELOR: Okay, Mary, how many of these ideas do you want to try?

MARY: I think I can do all of them if I can get free time too.

COUNSELOR: When do you want to start?

MARY: Today, if I can.

COUNSELOR: We can try. Can you go over these with me one time before we leave?

MARY: I think so. No more talking out of turn, and do enough work to earn some free time.

COUNSELOR: That sounds good to me. Do you want to shake hands and make this an agreement between you and me?

MARY: Okay.

COUNSELOR: Good. I'd like to talk with you a little each day to see how your plan is working. If it doesn't work, we'll have to make another plan. See you tomorrow?

MARY: Okay, see you tomorrow.

This is a typical reality therapy interview. Identifying and evaluating present behavior are followed by making a plan and building a commitment to follow through on it. Each step in the reality therapy process is supported by a relationship of trust, caring, and friendship between the counselor and the child.

As mentioned in an earlier chapter, the counseling process works better when the counselor uses statements rather than questions. Questioning moves the interview from a dialogue toward a teacher–student question-and-answer session that develops the counselor's plan rather than one for which the child feels ownership. More important, statements by the counselor allow the client more options in shaping the direction of the interview. As Carl Rogers noted, given the opportunity to take charge of the counseling interview, clients may gradually begin to take charge of their lives outside the counseling session as well. Following are examples of questions changed to reality therapy statements:

1. What are you doing to solve the problem? *Changed to statement:* If you are ready to do this, we can begin by looking at what you have been doing to solve the problem.
2. How is what you have been doing helping? Is your behavior getting you what you want? *Changed to statement:* It might be helpful to think about your behavior to see how each method is working for you if you feel ready to move to the next step.
3. If what you have been trying is not working, what are some things you could do that would help? *Changed to statement:* We could look at some new ideas to try when you are more comfortable about moving toward a plan.
4. Which of these new alternatives would you like to try? *Changed to statement:* You have several possibilities listed. Tell me what you think about trying any of them.
5. When can we meet again to find out how well your plan worked out? *Changed to statement:* It might be helpful to schedule a time for a follow-up of your plan. (Shake hands and sign a written plan if necessary.)

A second transcript from a case brought to a counselor follows as a way of demonstrating how reality therapy can be put into practice.

Case Study

Identification of the Problem*
Serena is a 10-year-old girl in the fourth grade at Anderson Elementary School. She was referred to the counselor because of an ongoing conflict she was having with another girl in her class.

Individual and Background Information

Academic Anderson's records indicate that Serena is a good student, receiving mostly "A" and "B" grades on her school work. Her teachers report that she typically has an excellent attitude in class and works hard on her assignments. Recently, she has been more disruptive in class than usual and will occasionally talk out of turn. Her grades have also been dropping somewhat on her recent schoolwork.

Family Serena has a supportive family. She lives with both of her biological parents. Teachers say that her parents have always been very kind and seem invested in the well-being of their only child.

---

*The case of Serena was contributed by David Naff.

Social According to her current teacher's reports, Serena is very friendly with her fellow classmates. This year, Serena has developed a close friendship with a girl named Destiny in her class who few other students have befriended due to her abrasive behavior. Serena and Destiny have a tumultuous relationship and go back and forth from being very close to very angry with each other.

Counseling Method

The counselor uses the reality therapy method of counseling to help Serena evaluate her behavior and identify what it is that she wants as a result of her behavior. This will allow her to investigate whether or not her behavior is leading to the results that she desires.

The five basic steps followed by the counselor in this case are (1) establishment of a relationship with the student, (2) identification of present behaviors (What is being done or has been done?), (3) evaluation of present behavior (Is it leading to the student's desired outcomes?), (4) development of plans that will help, and (5) commitment from the client to attempt at least one of these plans.

Transcript

COUNSELOR: Serena, I hear you have been having some trouble with your friend, Destiny. Tell me a little about that.

SERENA: Well ….

COUNSELOR: Let me tell you what I've heard and you tell me what's right and what's not. You two have gotten pretty close this year, but sometimes you disagree and get upset with each other.

SERENA: Yes that's it exactly. Sometimes she is my best friend and sometimes she is really mean to me.

COUNSELOR: Tell me about a time that has happened.

SERENA: Yesterday on the playground we were on the monkey bars and she pushed me off because she thought it was funny. But I did not think it was very funny.

COUNSELOR: What did you do when she pushed you off of the monkey bars?

SERENA: I yelled at her and told her that she was stupid.

COUNSELOR: How did that work?

SERENA: I got in trouble with the teacher and had to be in time-out for the rest of recess.

COUNSELOR: How did that help?

SERENA: It didn't! I got punished when Destiny started it all.

COUNSELOR: What else could you have done?

SERENA: Well, I could try to just walk away from Destiny when she does mean things to me. Or I guess I could just laugh at her, or I could tell a teacher what she's doing

COUNSELOR: What else could you do so that you are not kept from all of your friends during recess?

SERENA: Maybe I could try to play with some other people in my class more than Destiny. I get in trouble sometimes when I play with her.

COUNSELOR: You have talked about lots of thing you might do differently. Which of these would you like to try this week?

SERENA: I'm going to try to walk away when Destiny does something mean.

COUNSELOR: Okay. You have decided to walk away when Destiny hurts your feelings. Let's see how that works today and may you can come back tomorrow morning to talk about how well your plan worked.

SERENA: Okay. I'd like that.

As pointed out in earlier chapters, counselors must adapt their counseling style and language to their clients' developmental levels. A suggested reality therapy format for counseling younger children is as follows:

1. Tell me what happened. What did you do when that was going on?
2. How did that work for you? For everyone else?
3. What else could you do?
4. What would you like to try to do next time?
5. Do you want to write your plan for next time, or do you want me to write it?
6. Let's check tomorrow to see if your new plan is working. (Shake hands and sign names.)

Following is an outline of basic reality therapy for older children and teenagers who are capable of formal reasoning and abstract thinking.

1. Let's begin by talking about what you have been doing to solve the problem.
2. It would be helpful if you could give me an idea of how what you have been doing has been helping you in the situation. We may want to consider some questions: Is your behavior in touch with *reality* (as in the situation would be explained the same way by anyone who was present)? Is your behavior the *responsible* thing to do (as in does it hurt someone else or you)? Is your behavior the *right* thing to do (or would you want someone to do it to or for you)? [These questions would be addressed one at a time.]
3. If your behavior is not getting you what you want, what would you like to do differently?
4. What plan would you like to develop?
5. When can we follow up on your plan?

In summary, reality therapy is such a straightforward approach to counseling that some of our students question its utility for counseling difficult cases. Glasser's *Reality Therapy in Action* (2000c) is a strong answer to those who believe that, although reality therapy may be the treatment of choice for regular problems of adjustment, it is not sufficient for treating people with major disturbances in their lives. In *Reality Therapy in Action*, Glasser presents 18 of his most challenging cases from his 50-year career as a psychiatrist. These cases range from chronic depression to an extreme obsessive-compulsive disorder. Regardless of the various symptoms presented by these clients, they all had some things in common. Each of the clients had problems with establishing and maintaining relationships. All of them also lacked meaning in their careers or in their lives. As noted previously, Glasser believed that when people have difficulty meeting their basic needs of survival, freedom, power, fun, and love and belonging, they often choose a symptom as a way of compensating for failure to meet one or more of these basic needs. Choosing a symptom has the reinforcing effect of excusing the person for living an unproductive or even irresponsible life. After all, what can be expected from a person who has problems or who is "mentally ill"? If the symptom is sufficiently severe, further reinforcement for keeping the symptom is provided if the person receives total care for the disability. The road back to living a responsible life begins with a reality therapy type of plan to commit to doing those tasks or homework assignments the client can do and gradually increasing the tasks until the client decides, "I do not need my symptom anymore, and there are better ways to meet my basic needs." Therefore, treatment, via choice theory reality therapy, is geared toward taking the steps needed to put clients on track to finding better ways to meet their needs. The core of life is building loving relationships and a solid career or other meaningful activities that contribute to society. For students, academic progress is their career. Likewise, the foundation of choice theory reality therapy is building and maintaining relationships and improving academic or career performance to meet one's basic needs. Glasser presented a blueprint for how to use reality therapy to treat the most difficult cases you will ever face in your counseling career, and yes, it is the same basic choice theory reality therapy that you use with children and adolescents who are not completing their math assignments.

THE TEN-STEP REALITY THERAPY CONSULTATION MODEL

The ten-step reality therapy consultation model is an effective tool for counselors to use with teachers and parents who seek the counselor's assistance with their children's behavioral and motivation problems. Before deciding to use this model, counselors should assess whether the child's problems result from other people trying to control the child in coercive ways too often found in schools. We believe our current model, which has been adapted to be more consistent with Glasser's choice theory model, provides a step-by-step de-escalation for adults to help children control themselves.

The ten steps are divided into three phases, each with a special objective. Phase I, consisting of three steps, is designed to assist a teacher or parent in building a better relationship with the child.

Step 1. List what you have already tried that does not help. Stopping these ineffective interventions often stimulates a positive change in the child's behavior.

Step 2. If Step 1 is unsuccessful, make a list of change-of-pace interventions to disrupt the expected interactions between the adult and the child. For example, catch the child behaving appropriately, act surprised when the child repeats the same old aggravating behavior, ask yourself what the child expects you to do, and then do *not* do it.

Step 3. If Step 3 is necessary, make a list of things you could and would do to help the child have a better day tomorrow. For example, give the child at least three 20-second periods of your undivided positive attention, ask the child to run an errand for you, give the child some choices in how to complete a task or an assignment, ask the child's opinion about something relevant to both of you, give the child an important classroom or household chore, or negotiate a few rules (three to five) that you and the child think are fair to both of you.

Phase II, consisting of three steps, is devoted to counseling the child. In most cases, we find that successful interventions happen in the first phase. When this does not occur, we ask the adult to move to Step 4.

Step 4. Try one-line counseling approaches such as the following:

- Ask the child to stop the undesirable behavior. Use as few words as possible, relying instead on nonverbal gestures. Do not use threats. For example "Please put away your cell phone."
- Try the "Could it be?" questions recommended by the practitioners of individual psychology (see Chapter 11). Could it be the child wants your attention? Could it be the child wants revenge or control? Or could it be the child feels inadequate and wants to be left alone?
- Acknowledge the child's cooperative efforts, but do not thank the child for behaving responsibly as if this behavior is a favor to you. You might say something like "You were very careful with her crayons."

Step 5. Use reality therapy questions that emphasize the rules on which agreement was reached in a previous negotiation. For example:

- What did you do?
- What is our rule about this?
- What were you supposed to do?
- What else will you choose to do?

Step 6. Use the standard reality therapy questions that end with a written contract or a handshake. For example:

- What did you do?
- How did it help you?
- What could you do that would help you?
- What will you do?

Have the child dictate or write and sign a contract; have a follow-up meeting. If the contract is broken, have the child write or dictate a contract that he or she can meet. Eliminate punishment in favor of letting the child experience the logical consequences of appropriate and inappropriate behavior.

Phase III, consisting of four steps, is designed for children whose behavior makes teaching and learning difficult for everyone else in the classroom. In the home setting, Phase III is used when the child's behavior infringes on the rights of other family members. The hope is to solve the consultant problems in the six steps before Phase III, in which the primary intervention is isolation.

Step 7. In-class time-out is recommended. A quiet corner, study carrel, or private work area may be used. Time-out should not be in a punishment area or a "dunce's corner." The child has two choices: be with the group and behave, or be outside the group and sit in an isolated area. When the misbehavior occurs, send the child to the quiet area firmly with no discussion. The rest of the group does not have to be aware of the intervention. Have the child make a plan before returning to the group. The child's room may be used for time-out at home.

Step 8. Some children may require a time-out outside the classroom. The procedure is basically the same one described in Step 7. Some schools use a time-out room; others use an in-school suspension room. Contracts or plans for making a successful return to the classroom group can follow the questions used in the reality therapy method.

Step 9. Some children have difficulty getting through the entire school day without disrupting the class. Individual educational plans (IEPs) for these students may list four or five expectations or rules that the school has for all students. If the child does not meet one of these rules, have the child's parents remove the child from school for the remainder of the day. Allow the child to return the next day and remain as long as he or she follows the rules. Community agencies have been used when home isolation was not possible. Once again, no punishment needs to be administered in addition to the logical consequence of isolation. Such IEPs require the input of teachers, parents, administrators, the child, and the counselor.

Step 10. Step 10 often involves taking the child on a field trip to juvenile court to observe the probable consequences of continuing his or her present behavioral patterns. Interviews with the judge, other court officials, counselors, teachers, and inmates increase the child's awareness of logical consequences existing outside the home and school settings. Failure to meet consultation goals with a child who has not reacted positively to the ten-step method may mean that the child should be referred to a community agency better equipped to solve the child's problems.

The basic consultation model can be adapted to any situation in which the counselor is consulting with a client about how to work with a third person or is working directly with a client.

Yarbrough and Thompson (2002), using Step 6 in the ten-step consultation model with an underachieving student, were able to help the student significantly increase the number of school assignments completed from nearly 0 to 100 percent in five counseling sessions. (See Chapter 16 for more information about consultation.)

Donato (2004) recommends a maintenance program for students identified as proceeding through a school's discipline program too quickly. The program is for homeroom teachers to help these students meet their needs by connecting students with peers or groups (belonging), providing opportunities for students to make choices (freedom), giving students jobs and leadership roles to perform (power), and incorporating enjoyable activities into the day (fun).

Burns, Vance, Szadokierski, and Stockwell (2006) developed a scale, the Student Needs Survey, which included items for each of the five basic needs and tested the reliability and validity of the instrument. They determined the scale had the psychometric strength to be useful in applying and researching choice theory in schools.

Fox and Delgado (2008) discussed the use of choice theory in an after-school program for at-risk students. Meeting weekly, the students learned to accomplish missions related to responsibility. The authors noted that participation in the fun yet structured program allowed the elementary students to commit to projects that improved their world. Likewise Hakak (2013) provided group reality therapy and found increases in participant students' happiness scales. All these studies indicate the variety of applications and the successful outcomes of reality therapy.

DIVERSITY APPLICATIONS OF REALITY THERAPY

Glasser (1965) surmised that all humans have the same basic needs; these needs do not vary with age, sex, or race. Wubbolding (2007) agrees, saying, "Reality therapy is an eminently cross-cultural method" (p. 306). Reality therapists want to know people and understand their view of the world and their quality world. Wubbolding and Brickell (2007) noted that using reality therapy takes into account the worldview of the client by opening realistic choices that exist in the client's world.

Reality therapy was designed to help all types of people meet two basic needs: the need to love and be loved, and the need to feel worthwhile to ourselves and others. Glasser (1998, 2000c, 2005) has revised his list of human needs to include the needs for survival, freedom, power, fun, and love and belonging. Onedera and Greenwalt (2007) quoted Glasser as saying, "In a variety of countries I find that the unhappiness is all the same ... all these people are unhappy because they are trying to change the behavior of other people" (p. 81).

Some argue the needs identified in reality therapy are culturally bound, especially freedom and power. Others note some groups have limited, if any, choices due to oppression and mistreatment. Reality therapists have made a significant effort to modify choice theory to several cultures and to study the impact of those approaches (Fall et al., 2010). For example, Kim (2008) studied the use of a reality therapy group counseling program to reduce Internet addiction levels of Korean university students. Jusoh and Ahmad (2009) considered the applicability of reality therapy with Islamic, Asian, and Australian clients and suggested the approach was adaptable to many backgrounds. Tanrikulu (2011) explained reality therapy by matching the concepts to Turkish proverbs.

Wubbolding and Brickell (2000) point out that reality therapy has been well received in Asia, the Middle East, Puerto Rica, and South Africa. Reality therapy is currently taught and successfully practiced in a diversity of countries, including Canada, Korea, Japan, China, India, Singapore, United Kingdom, Norway, Israel, Ireland, Egypt, Germany, France, Slovenia, Croatia, Italy, Columbia, Kuwait, South Africa, and Russia, and in a diversity of cultures in the United States (Wubbolding et al., 2004).

EVALUATION OF REALITY THERAPY

Building trusting relationships with others is the focus of reality therapy and the goal of making better choices. Any attention to the past becomes how it affects the future. The focus remains on what the client is choosing to do now. Practitioners of choice theory reality therapy do not deny their clients have real pain, but very little time is allowed for clients to complain about their symptoms. Counselors teach clients that the only people they can control are themselves. Glasser (2004, 2005) believes that it is no kindness to treat unhappy people as helpless, hopeless, or inadequate, no matter what has happened to them. Glasser sees kindness as having faith that people can handle the truth and to do so will be to their benefit. True compassion in his opinion is helping people help themselves.

Reality therapy and the disregard for diagnosis do not bode well for insurance reimbursement of this approach. Additionally little research has been conducted on the use of reality therapy with people who have specified mental disorders, although more is coming to light. Wubbolding (2000) talked about using reality therapy successfully with people who are incarcerated, who abuse substances, who are depressing, and who are experiencing violence. Bhargava (2013) outlined a case using reality therapy with a depressed deaf adult.

Seligman and Reichenberg (2014) suggest that reality therapy is best for people who have mild to moderate mental disorders and that severe disorders such as bipolar and psychotic problems may require medication and other treatment approaches. Yet Ellsworth (2007) used reality therapy in his work with children who had been sexually abused, focusing on their strengths, humor, and creativity to help them make decisions about choosing healthy positive decisions about healing.

Kim and Hwang (2001) identified long-term positive effects on middle school students' sense of internal control in a follow-up of their research. Her research supported the effectiveness of eight sessions of group counseling in reality therapy. Loyd (2005) concluded that exposure to reality therapy principles changed high school students' perceptions of their needs satisfaction. He discussed expanding his protocol in order to impact schools, teachers, and administrators.

SUMMARY

Perhaps the best validation of choice theory reality therapy is Glasser's success at the Ventura School for Girls. Before his tenure, the school's recidivism rate approached 90 percent; in a relatively short time, this rate fell to 20 percent. What was the secret of changing the orientation of these young women into success identities? Glasser gave them the experience of personal responsibility and success by assigning them tasks they could handle and by making each girl responsible for her own behavior. He discarded punishment in favor of logical consequences, gave generous amounts of praise, and showed sincere interest in each girl's welfare. Glasser's approach at the Ventura School included individual and group counseling conducted within the reality therapy model and framework presented in this chapter. Regardless of one's theoretical outlook, it would be difficult to argue with Glasser's formula for success.

Reality therapy is an optimistic and encouraging approach to counseling. Reality therapy is present-oriented, straightforward, and easy to understand, but difficult and demanding to implement. The key is helping people accept responsibility for what they are doing now, and many people have spent their lifetimes not taking responsibility (fulfilling their own needs in ways that respect other people's rights). A pessimistic counselor cannot be a successful reality therapist. Reality therapists lead people through a change process that facilitates their becoming aware of their needs and determining ways to improve their lives. Considerable effort, persistence, and optimism are required from both the client and the counselor to make the reality therapy process work. The definition of behavior should expand to include feelings and thoughts, as well as what we actually do. The focus remains on what the person can change about these three behavior components. Basically, according to Glasser (2005), the purpose of counseling is not to talk about the problem, but to straighten out one's life and one's day by focusing on meeting the five basic needs in healthy ways.

People use the most effective ways they know at the time to meet their needs of survival, love and belonging, fun, freedom, and power. Counseling involves looking at current behavior and determining whether it is meeting needs. If not, an alternative is planned. The change process involves a counselor building a relationship with the client based on empathy, respect, present focus, and honesty. Successful clients adopt new, more effective ways to form relationships and to meet their needs.

Glasser outlined our preferred eight steps for counselors using reality therapy, which include: (1) building rapport, (2) asking "What are you doing?" (3) collaborating with the client in evaluating their behavior, (4) helping people make a plan to do better, (5) helping them commit to the plan, (6) accepting no excuses, (7) not interfering with reasonable consequences, and (8) not giving up!

INTRODUCTION TO REALITY THERAPY

To gain a more in-depth understanding of the concepts in this chapter, visit www .cengage.com/counseling/henderson to view a short clip of an actual therapist–client session demonstrating reality therapy.

WEB SITES FOR REALITY THERAPY

Internet addresses frequently change. To find the sites listed here, visit www.cengage .com/counseling/henderson for an updated list of Internet addresses and direct links to relevant sites.

The William Glasser Institute

Reality Therapy, UK

Center for Reality Therapy

International Journal of Reality Therapy

REFERENCES

Berges, M. (1976). A realistic approach. In A. Bassin, T. E. Bratter, & R. L. Rachin (Eds.), *The reality therapy reader: A survey of the work of William Glasser*. New York: Harper & Row.

Bhargava, R. (2013). The use of reality therapy with a depressed deaf adult. *Clinical Case Studies, 12*(5), 388–396. doi: 10.1177/1534650113496869

Burns, M. K., Vance, D., Szadokierski, I., & Stockwell, C. (2006). Student needs survey: A psychometrically sound measure of the five basic needs. *International Journal of Reality Therapy, 25,* 4–8.

Deming, W. E. (1966). *Some theory of sampling*. New York: Dover.

Donato, T. (2004). Maintenance for the CT/RT student in the classroom. *International Journal of Reality Therapy, 24,* 38–42.

Ellsworth, R. (2007). *Choosing to heal: Using reality therapy in treatment with sexually abused children*. New York: Routledge.

Fall, K. A., Holden, J. M., & Marquis, A. (2010). *Theoretical models of counseling and psychotherapy* (2nd ed.). New York: Brunner-Routledge.

Fox, L., & Delgado, E. (2008). Mission accomplished: Choice theory. *International Journal of Reality Therapy, 27,* 50–51.

Fuller, G. B. (2007). Reality therapy approaches. In H. T. Prout & D. T. Brown (Eds.), *Counseling and psychotherapy with children and adolescents: Theory and practice for school and clinical settings* (pp. 332–387). Hoboken, NJ: Wiley.

Glasser, W. (1961). *Mental health or mental illness?* New York: Harper & Row.

Glasser, W. (1964). Reality therapy: A realistic approach to the young offender. *Crime and Delinquency, 10,* 135–144.

Glasser, W. (1965). *Reality therapy*. New York: Harper & Row.

Glasser, W. (1969). *Schools without failure*. New York: Harper & Row.

Glasser, W. (1972). *The identity society*. New York: Harper & Row.

Glasser, W. (1976). *Positive addiction*. New York: Harper & Row.

Glasser, W. (1981). *Stations of the mind*. New York: Harper & Row.

Glasser, W. (1984). *Control theory*. New York: Harper & Row.

Glasser, W. (1986). *Control theory in the classroom*. New York: Harper & Row.

Glasser, W. (1990). *The quality school: Managing students without coercion*. New York: Harper & Row.

Glasser, W. (1992). Reality therapy. *New York State Journal for Counseling and Development, 7,* 5–13.

Glasser, W. (1993). *The quality school teacher*. New York: HarperCollins.

Glasser, W. (1995). *Staying together*. New York: HarperCollins.

Glasser, W. (1998). *Choice theory: A new psychology of personal freedom*. New York: HarperCollins.

Glasser, W. (2000a). *Every student can succeed*. Chatsworth, CA: Author.

Glasser, W. (2000b). *Getting together and staying together*. New York: HarperCollins.

Glasser, W. (2000c). *Reality therapy in action*. New York: HarperCollins.

Glasser, W. (2002). *Unhappy teenagers: A way for parents and teachers to reach them*. New York: HarperCollins.

Glasser, W. (2004). *Warning: Psychiatry can be dangerous to your health*. New York: HarperCollins.

Glasser, W. (2005). *Treating mental health as a public health problem: A new leadership role for the helping professions*. Chatsworth, CA: William Glasser.

Glasser, W. (2011). Reality therapy and choice theory. In H. G. Rosenthal (Ed.), *Favorite counseling and therapy techniques* (2nd ed., pp. 137–144). New York: Routledge.

Glasser, W., & Wubbolding, R. (1995). Reality therapy. In R. Corsini & D. Wedding (Eds.), *Current psychotherapies* (5th ed., pp. 293–321). Itasca, IL: Peacock.

Hakak, N. (2013). Effectiveness of group reality therapy in increasing the Students' happiness. *Life Science Journal-Acta Zhengzhou University Overseas Edition, 10*(1), 577–580.

Jusoh, A. J., & Ahmad, R. (2009). The practice of Reality Therapy from the Islamic perspective in Malaysia and variety of customs in Asia. *International Journal of Reality Therapy, 28*, 3–8.

Kim, J. (2008). The effect of a R/T group counseling program on the Internet addiction level and self-esteem of Internet addiction university students. *International Journal of Reality Therapy, 27*, 4–12.

Kim, R. I., & Hwang, M. (2001). The effects of internal control and achievement motivation in group counseling based on reality therapy. *International Journal of Reality Therapy, 20*, 12–15.

Kohlberg, L. (1981). *The philosophy of moral development: Moral stages and the idea of justice*. New York: Harper & Row.

Loyd, B. D. (2005). The effects of reality therapy/choice theory principles on high school students' perception of needs satisfaction and behavioral change. *International Journal of Reality Therapy, 25*, 5–9.

Murdock, N. L. (2013). *Theories of counseling and psychotherapy: A case approach* (3rd ed.). Upper Saddle River, NJ: Merrill.

Onedera, J. D., & Greenwalt, B. (2007). Choice theory: An interview with Dr. William Glasser. *The Family Journal, 15*, 79–86.

Piaget, J. (1973). *The moral judgment of children*. New York: Free Press.

Powers, W. (1973). *Behavior: The control of perception*. New York: Aldine Press.

Seligman, L., & Reichenberg, L. W. (2014). *Theories of counseling and psychotherapy: Systems, strategies, and skills* (4th ed.). Upper Saddle River, NJ: Merrill.

Tanrikulu, T. (2011). Reality therapy in Turkish proverbs. *Milli Folklor, 12*(90), 86–92.

Wubbolding, R. (1991). *Understanding reality therapy*. New York: Harper Collins.

Wubbolding, R. (2000). *Reality therapy for the 21st century*. Philadelphia, PA: Brunner-Routledge.

Wubbolding, R. E. (2007). Reality therapy theory. In D. Capuzzi & D. Gross (Eds.). *Counseling and psychotherapy: Theories and interventions* (4th ed., pp. 289–312). Upper Saddle River, NJ: Pearson.

Wubbolding, R. (2011a). *Reality therapy*. Washington, DC: American Psychological Association.

Wubbolding, R. (2011b). Reality therapy theory. In D. Capuzzi & D. R. Gross (Eds.), *Counseling and psychotherapy: Theories and interventions* (4th ed., pp. 263–285). Upper Saddle River, NJ: Pearson.

Wubbolding, R., & Brickell, J. (2000). Misconceptions about reality therapy. *International Journal of Reality Therapy, 19*, 64–65.

Wubbolding, R., & Brickell, J. (2007). Frequently asked questions and brief answers: Part I. *International Journal of Reality Therapy, 27*, 29–30.

Wubbolding, R., & Brickell, J. (2008). Frequently asked questions and not so brief answers: Part II. *International Journal of Reality Therapy, 28*, 46–49.

Wubbolding, R., Brickell, J., Imhof, L., Kim, R., Lojk, L., & Al-Rashidi, B. (2004). Reality theory: A global perspective. *International Journal for the Advancement of Counseling, 26*, 219–228.

Yarbrough, J., & Thompson, C. (2002). Using single-participant research to assess counseling approaches on children's off-task behavior. *Professional School Counseling, 5*, 308–314.

CHAPTER 10

Brief Counseling

If you want truly to understand something, try to change it.
—KURT LEWIN

Believing that someone must understand the root of a concern, many theorists of counseling highlight the causes of a person's distress rather than the solution to the worry. That cause-and-effect relationship, however, has not been supported by research that generally suggests the complexities of humans cannot be diluted to that simple formula. Indeed many people resolve their own problems never considering the causes. Solution-focused brief therapy turns the counseling process from talking about problems to focusing on solutions in the present that will support a person's healthier and happier goals in the future. Solution-focused counseling has been evolving since the beginning of the 20th century and is gaining prominence in the 21st century. This chapter reviews the approach to counseling that focuses on solutions and progress. After reading this chapter, you should be able to:

- Outline the development of solution-focused counseling
- Explain the theory of solution-focused counseling, including its core concepts
- Discuss the counseling relationship and goals in solution-focused counseling
- Describe assessment, process, and techniques in solution-focused counseling
- Demonstrate some therapeutic techniques
- Clarify the effectiveness of solution-focused counseling

BACKGROUND

Beginnings of brief therapy can be traced to the Mental Research Institute in Palo Alto, California, where Milton Erickson worked. Seligman and Reichenberg (2014) noted the writings and contributions of Richard Fisch, John Weakland,

Paul Watzlawick, and Gregory Bateson reflected their belief that treatment should focus on direct observation, *what* is going on, *how* people continue to function, and *how* behavior could change.

In the early 1980s, the husband and wife team Steve de Shazer and Insoo Kim Berg with a group at the Brief Family Therapy Center in Milwaukee, Wisconsin, originated solution focused therapy (de Shazer, 1985, 1988, 1994; de Shazer & Dolan, 2007; de Shazer et al., 1986). Based on the communication/systems theory as well as on the work of Milton Erickson (1954; Haley, 1973), solution-focused brief counseling incorporated Erickson's use of language, metaphor, and hypnosis (Murdock, 2013). Erickson discussed the importance of clients being open to change and possibilities. He accepted the worldview and life patterns of the client. His treatment involved leading clients into trancelike conditions to evoke the client's strengths and apply them to the current problem (Stalker, Levene, & Coady, 1999). De Shazer also thought that clients would benefit more if practitioners used what the clients presented and focused on the present behavior (Seligman & Reichenberg, 2014)

Assuming people maintain their realities through social interactions, counselors carefully design therapy sessions concentrating on solutions rather than problems (Berg, 1994, 2005; Berg & de Shazer, 1993; Miller, Hubble, & Duncan, 1996). De Shazer, Berg, and the others who worked with them developed a decision tree to guide their work with clients. They often began treatment by asking clients to observe what was happening in their lives that they wanted to continue (Seligman & Reichenberg, 2014). That question allows counseling sessions to start by focusing on things that have gone right in the client's life rather than what has gone wrong, exceptions to the problem. If clients failed to complete the task, treatment became more indirect with the use of metaphors or paradoxical interventions. Counselors recognize and tap client resources toward solutions and focus on any movement toward solutions (Fall, Holden, & Marquis, 2010). Progress in counseling is measured by the results achieved instead of by the number of sessions.

Solution-focused practitioners believe that even when people are not doing well, pieces of solutions are happening (Lipchik, 2002). These counselors assume they should begin by finding out what the client is doing that works. Those effective things the client is doing become the building blocks of therapy. Solution-focused counseling is founded on the idea that talking about positive parts of the client's life builds self-worth, creates optimism, and begins a change process that starts with existing strengths and resources.

Solution-oriented therapy, developed by O'Hanlon and others, is based on the same premise but is more flexible about the time spent talking about problems. As with solution-focused brief counseling, in solution-oriented therapy most of the time is spent on solution talk. The solution-oriented counselor also believes that hearing about the client's distress should be included in therapy, so the discussions about the client's challenges may take longer than in de Shazer's approach. Empathic listening about the problem is encouraged before moving to the solution-seeking part of therapy. Bill O'Hanlon's Web site, www.billohanlon.com, contains information about what he now explains as *possibility therapy*.

Other names for brief approaches to counseling include *problem-focused therapy*, *solution-focused therapy*, or *brief therapy*. Each of those ways of counseling has particular strategies and theorists. The common characteristics have coalesced into solution-focused brief counseling, our topic for this chapter.

The Nature of People

Counselors practicing solution-focused brief counseling believe that people who are feeling bad will continue to feel bad if they do not make positive behavioral changes in their lives. Merely discussing "why" people feel as they do will not help, neither will focusing on such unobservable elements as feelings, thoughts, and motivations. The key to feeling better is to focus on "what" people are doing that seems to be helpful and to set goals with plans on how to accomplish these goals. Solution-focused brief counselors believe that their clients will do better with a present and future orientation. In fact, solution-focused brief counseling may be the only counseling theory in which a future orientation takes precedence over a present orientation. The philosophy appears to be that clients can become mired in their past unresolved conflicts and failures and blocked when focusing on present problems rather than on future solutions. Clients may also be stuck in doing more of the same by continuing to try to solve their problems with the same failed strategies, the recipe for more failure.

Solution-focused brief counselors view their clients or customers as being free to make choices and not be victimized by their heredity or environment. These counselors hold a positive view of people that rivals that held by followers of Rogers's theories. People are seen as being basically good, with the power to overcome evil and to make good behavioral choices. Solution-focused brief counselors believe that people are also basically rational, having the capacity to solve their own problems, or complaints, and overcome the irrational influences in their culture. These counselors use the language of *customer* and *complaint* to emphasize the belief of the client knowing where to go and the motivation to do so. The counselor is *hired* to help construct the solutions.

The faith solution-focused brief practitioners have in their clients' ability to work through their own problems is highlighted in the words of the old song "AC-Cent-Tchu-Ate the Positive," which proceeds with "Accentuate the positive, eliminate the negative, and say no to Mr. In-Between." In other words, people do better when they concentrate on their successes rather than on their failures. Positive and helpful changes are more likely to grow from exploring strengths rather than weaknesses or deficits. Counselors do not attribute difficulties to reinforcements, irrational beliefs, unconscious conflicts, or any other reason. The problems are the reality of the person, and counselors accept that and go from there. In addition, change is considered easy and constant rather than difficult and rare as some other theories propose. O'Hanlon and Weiner-Davis (2003) include that and other differences in traditional and brief therapy in their description of the myths of therapy.

Solution-focused brief counselors cater to whatever common sense is found in their clients' thinking. For example, the test of any good idea is whether it will work for the client. Many (Berg & Miller, 1992; de Shazer, 1986; Legum, 2005; Lipchik, 2002; Sklare, 2005; Walter & Peller, 1992) emphasize the appeal to their clients' common sense in the following pragmatic points stated in colloquial, perhaps overused, everyday language:

1. "If it works, don't fix it. Do more of it."
2. "If it works a little, build on it, and try to do more of the part that is working."
3. "If it is broken, do something different to fix it. Experiment and imagine miracles."

In other words, once you know what works and what does not work, do more of what works and stop doing what does not work.

In summary, solution-focused practitioners base their work on the following assumptions (O'Hanlon & Weiner-Davis, 2003):

1. People are viewed as basically good, capable of rational thought, able to implement positive change, and free to make choices. However, without direction from the counselor, people appear by nature to want to focus on the negative aspects of their lives.
2. Clients have the resources and strengths to solve their problems. The counselor's work is to highlight those abilities in order to identify and encourage change.
3. Change is constant. A small change is all that is needed.
4. Generally it is unnecessary to have specifics, causes, or functions of the problem in order to resolve it.
5. Once the counseling focus has shifted from the negative to the positive, people will recognize what is going well in their lives. No problem occurs all of the time.
6. People have the capacity to act on common sense if given the opportunity to identify problem-solving strategies. Clients define the goal.
7. People respond better to counseling when they make positive changes in their behavior as opposed to working on the cognitive and affective components of their situation. For children who may have difficulty in handling some of the abstract thinking involved in cognitive and affective counseling, the behavior change focus is most useful.
8. People will respond better to a present and future counseling orientation than they will to a past orientation focused on reasons they have a problem they cannot solve.

Theory of Counseling

Solution-focused practitioners might well adopt the 4-H club motto: "Make the best better." The method is based on the theory that people will respond better to building up the positive aspects of their lives. Every problem is viewed as having identifiable exceptions that can be transformed into solutions. For example, a child who is having trouble making friends in her classroom might be asked to look at those times when she was able to initiate some contact. She may say, "Well, one day Jane Ann asked me to eat lunch with her, and that made me feel good." The counselor would build on that by asking how that happened and how she could make it happen more often. The search is for clients' competencies.

Solution-focused counselors believe that people's problems result from behavior based on their view of the world. People continue these actions because they are convinced there is only one right thing to do. Counselors use the clients' ideas of having their lives free of symptoms to suggest changes. That suggestion of a new possibility or frame of reference may be enough to bring about new action. This counseling theory assumes that small solutions can lead to big changes (Seligman & Reichenberg, 2014). Small behavior changes build momentum in a person's life, much like the momentum defined in Newton's laws of motion. A body at rest tends to remain at rest, and a body in motion tends to remain in motion. Many clients come for counseling because they are bodies at rest. Small behavioral changes are used to get them moving. For example, John might be asked to complete a small portion of his math assignment rather than the entire assignment based on the idea that a little positive movement will allow him to notice and build more successes, thus gaining momentum.

In addition, solution-focused counseling methods are helpful to counselors wanting to capitalize on changes in relationships. Small shifts in role by one person in a relationship will likely lead to a role shift by others in that relationship. For example, Mary notices that when she says something nice to her brother, he is more likely to be nice to her. George may notice that his parents are more cooperative with him when he does his homework and chores without being nagged.

Solution-focused counselors believe the times when the problem is absent provide clues to solutions to the troubling situation. Finding those exceptions and combining the ingredients that created the exception will lead to more change. These "skeleton keys" that are not necessary related to the problem may help clients convert many problems into solutions (Seligman & Reichenberg, 2014).

Relationship

Counselors in solution-focused brief therapy work within a collaborative model of interaction believing that their relationship with the client is a critical element in every session. These counselors do not consider themselves experts rather they believe they cannot know more about a client's life than the client knows. De Jong and Berg (2013) advised counselors to build skills for "not knowing" what puts the clients in the position of knowing about their lives. Those skills are listening, echoing key words, asking questions, getting details, being silent, summarizing, and noticing hints of possibilities. Solution-focused counselors are active and work to create an environment that invites change.

Their primary goal is to create conversations that motivate and mobilize (Shapiro, Friedberg, & Bardenstein, 2006). These counselors do not teach, interpret, train, or give directions (Bertolino & O'Hanlon, 2001) but focus relentlessly on solutions. They establish an environment of conversation in which strengths and ideas receive attention. Solution-focused practitioners use active listening, empathy, questions, explanation, reassurance, and suggestions (Seligman & Reichenberg, 2014).

Gunn, Haley, and Lyness (2007) explained that counselors have three foci in solution-focused work. They need to acknowledge and validate their clients' experiences. Counselors need to guide clients as they change their behavior or their perceptions. Finally, they need to build on their clients' existing strengths, resources, and successes.

Saleebey (2012) reviewed writing about the strengths perspective and identified the following as critical understandings about it:

- Life contains struggles, but all people have strengths that they can use to improve their lives. Counselors should respect the strengths and the directions clients choose.
- Motivation increases when counselors consistently emphasize strengths.

- Discovering strengths takes a cooperative exploration between clients and counselors. Helpers do not decide by themselves what clients need to improve in their lives.
- Counselors who focus on strengths are less likely to judge or blame people for their problems. Instead, they can discover how the clients have managed to survive.
- All environments, no matter how distressing, have some resources.

Solution-focused counselors assume people have the capacity to change but have lost confidence. Counselors spend little time trying to determine why people have not been able to solve their problems but presume that people are doing the best they can. The substance of counseling is to increase hope and optimism by building the anticipation of change, no matter how small. Counselors look for the patterns of success in the lives of their "customers." After listening for the subtle hints about success and then expanding talk about those areas, counselors ask for more and more information about these exceptions to the problem. They ask about time, place, other people, and any other factor that could be associated with success (Shapiro et al., 2006).

Solution-focused brief counselors believe change is inevitable and constant. They help people navigate a problem (O'Hanlon & Weiner-Davis, 2003) rather than continually talking about past disappointments. Difficulties are seen as a function of unsuccessful relations with others or mistakes in everyday situations. People may fail to take action, take action when none is needed, or act in the wrong way. Solution-focused counselors assume that if actions and interactions change, complaints will lessen (Seligman & Reichenberg, 2014). Additionally, solution-focused counselors believe that the right kind of talk can begin a movement toward attending to possibilities and positive direction (Shapiro et al., 2006).

De Jong and Berg (2013) offered solution-focused brief counselors tips for working with clients. Those ideas included being respectful and curious about the client's perception of life. Counselors hold clients accountable for their ideas. De Jong and Berg remind counselors to pay attention to how the client got to counseling. Finally these authors tell counselors to listen to and build on what the client wants.

Solution-focused counselors are active, gently guiding clients to strengths and solutions. Clients determine the goals they want but the practitioners are experts on the process and structure of therapy. Clients are experts on themselves and build a solution with the help of the expert clinician (Prochaska & Norcross, 2014). De Shazer (1988) writes that solution-focused counseling is special kind of intimacy and harmony as the clinician's helps the person expand options for solutions.

Goals

Solution-focused brief counseling is based on the theory that goals need to be stated in positive and observable terms to be effective. Goals are what the client wants and the counselor works to help develop specific, attainable, and concrete goals. People do better in attaining goals that are quantifiable and specific. For example, a more specific goal than "to study harder" would be "read the entire chapter that is assigned." Behavioral counselors and reality therapists would concur that clients respond better to accomplishments they can observe and record.

De Jong and Berg (2013) discussed the characteristics of well-formed goals in solution-focused brief counseling. First, the goals must be important to the client, what they want to happen. Saleebey (2012) explained that when counselors work to understand what people want for their lives, clients feel respected, are more motivated, and feel better about themselves. De Jong and Berg continue by stating that goals should be stated in interactional terms. This can be accomplished by asking the client what other people will notice as different when the problem is solved. Goals should include situational features to make them seem more possible. Clients will make choices to narrow down what they want to be different in a certain place and time.

The goals of solution-focused practitioners include the following:

- Change the *doing* of the problem situation
- Change the *viewing* of the problem situation
- Elicit *resources*, *strengths*, and *solutions* to use

(O'Hanlon & Weiner-Davis, 2003, p. 126)

Counseling Method

ASSESSMENT   Solution-focused brief counselors consider diagnosis irrelevant (Shapiro et al., 2006). O'Hanlon and Beadle (1997, p. 56) say that counselors focus discussions on "the human world of actions and changes and choices" instead of syndromes and disorders. The most basic solution-oriented question according to Shapiro et al. (2006) is "When do things go better than usual?" (p. 142).

PROCESS   De Shazer (1985) outlined seven stages for solution-focused brief counseling, which follow:

1. *Finding a solvable complaint.* The first step leads to developing goals and interventions that promote change. People's problems are considered normal and changeable. Counselors and clients work to find images of the complaint that are within the client's control. Counselors ask questions that relay optimism and encouragement. Difficulties are viewed as normal parts of life and changeable. Berg and Miller (1992) suggested scaling questions to establish where the client is beginning and to check possibilities and progress. O'Hanlon and Weiner-Davis (2003) suggest counselors ask clients to put problems and hopes into video talk, as though someone else were watching a videotape of the troubling experiences. Those authors explain that video talk allows a clearer picture of the problem and of the desired solutions.
2. *Determining goals.* Counselors work with clients to identify goals that are specific, observable, measurable, and concrete. Three common forms for goals are (1) to change the doing of the problem situation, (2) to change the viewing of the problem situation or frame of reference, and (3) to access resources, solutions, and strengths (O'Hanlon & Weiner-Davis, 2003). Questions such as "What will be the first sign of change?" and "How will you know when counseling has been helpful to you?" elicit discussion of positive change and what a solution might be. Counselors may use this miracle question (de Shazer, 1991,

p. 113) "Suppose that one night there is a miracle and while you were sleeping the problem that brought you to therapy is solved. How would you know? What would be different?" The question stimulates problem solving, hope, and a discussion of making the miracle a reality. Murdock (2103) explains that delivery of the question should be slow and soft. Berg and Miller (1992) suggest counselors may substitute other images such as a magic pill, divine intervention, a silver bullet, or a magic wand, depending on the client's belief system. Solution-focused counselors accept and use whatever clients present as the result of the miracle question.

3. *Planning an intervention.* Counselors make use of their understanding of clients and treatment strategies to encourage change. Helpful questions are "What changes have already happened?" "What worked in the past when you faced a similar situation?" and "How did you make that happen?"

4. *Drafting strategic tasks.* The tasks are written so clients can understand and agree to them. The tasks are chosen to build cooperation and success. De Shazer (1988) talked about three types of tasks that link to motivation:

   a. *Visitors or window shoppers* have not presented clear problems or expectations of change. In this case, counselors only give compliments.

   b. *Complainants* have concerns and expect change but think others should be doing the work. Counselors should suggest observations so that people become more aware of themselves and their situations. A homework assignment for this type client would be to find things that are happening in the person's life to do more often, thus eliciting more self-awareness.

   c. *Customers* are ready to take action to find solutions to their concerns.

5. *Focusing on positive new behaviors and changes.* As clients return and report on their task, counselors focus on change, progress, and possibilities. The problem is viewed as external to the client and may be referred to as "it" or "that." Questions that help at this stage of treatment are "How did you make that happen?" and "Who noticed the changes?" Counselors highlight strength and competence; they are cheerleaders for the client.

6. *Maintaining.* The focus in this stage is on consolidating gains. Counselors give clients adjustment time to promote further success. Counselors also help clients stay hopeful if change happens slower than they would like.

7. *Ending.* When the goals are accomplished, clients often initiate the ending of the relationship. Clients may return for future concerns. Clients have improved by developing confidence, being heard and praised, and finding strengths and resources.

The emphasis in solution-focused brief counseling is on creating concrete word pictures to describe the problem and the problem setting. Clients are asked to describe exactly what happens, who is there, and what is said and done. Bruce (1995) has detailed four useful intervention tasks:

1. "Do something different" for the client who tends to repeat the same ineffective reaction in problem situations.

2. "Pay attention to what you do when you overcome the urge to ..." for the client who has trouble controlling impulsive behaviors.

3. "Tell me about a time when you had a good day at school" for clients who have taken on the victim mentality of believing that nothing good ever happens to them.

4. "Observe and take notes" for clients who have trouble avoiding problem situations and interactions. The observations help the client identify the good and bad things that happen in the problem setting; however, the most beneficial outcome is the client's role shift from someone who interacts to someone who observes. A role shift by one person in a group leads to role shifts by the other interacting members.

ORIENTATION STATEMENT   Solution-focused brief counseling generally requires more structuring than most methods because it differs radically in counselor activity and the number of sessions required. Although it is of prime importance to clarify any counseling process to new clients and to children, it is mandatory as a first step in solution-focused counseling. The focus and goal-setting strategies begin to take shape with the counselor's orientation statement about how the process works. For example, a counselor's opening statement might be:

> Our purpose in talking together will be to help you find out what you need to do to solve a problem. We will look at some things you do well and see if we can use them to figure out what you want to do and what steps you should take next. I will be asking you several questions. Some of these questions will be hard to answer. I will be writing things down about what we are talking about. After we finish our talk, I will leave for a few minutes and write you a message from the notes I have been taking. I will make a copy for you and keep a copy for me. Does all of this sound okay with you?

STATEMENT OF THE PROBLEM   As is true with any other approach to counseling, we recommend that counselors use active listening from person-centered counseling before embarking on the preferred counseling interventions. Active listening helps the counselor and client know each other well enough to be working on the correct problem; therefore, we suggest that counselors remain in the active listening mode until clients agree that their counselors understand four important things about their situation:

1. The problem
2. The feelings associated with the problem
3. The intensity of those feelings on a 0 to 10 scale (10 is best [high] and 0 is worst [low])
4. The client's expectations of what he or she would like to happen in counseling and the goals the client would like to accomplish

Regarding the third point, rating intensity of feelings on a ten-point scale, this activity can result in a goal statement. When the client says, "I am about a six on a ten-point scale in feeling good," the counselor can focus the interview on those good things the client is doing and the things that are happening in the client's life that make the client's rating as high as a 6. Then, the interview can be directed toward discovering how the client can make more of these good things happen.

Children may need visual presentations of such a rating scale. Five smiley faces ranging from a very happy smile to a deeply frowning, unhappy face help younger children identify how good or bad they are feeling. Some counselors use a "feel-o-meter" constructed like a regular outdoor thermometer and let the child color in how high the mercury level has risen on the feelings scale. Smiling and frowning faces also can be used on the feel-o-meter to depict how the child is feeling. Computer-generated sliding scales may also be used to illustrate the degree of distress or success children report.

The same rating scale can be used throughout the solution-oriented process for setting goals and measuring the child's progress. Note that many children set behavioral goals to jump all the way from a low rating of a 3 to a high rating of 10 in just a day or two. Counselors will do well to focus on helping children move from a 3 to a 4 on goals (what the child will actually be doing at level 4) to ensure early success with the solution-oriented process. Gains of 10 percent are good when they are defined in observable, positive behavioral changes.

Setting Counseling Goals

The heart of many counseling methods is to set good or productive goals, and that is essential in solution-focused counseling. Good goals have some of the following common properties:

1. Goals owned or set by the client work best because clients are more likely to achieve the goals for which they hold ownership.
2. If clients need assistance in goal setting—and they probably will with solution-oriented brief counseling—be sure that the goals are cocreated and are not the counselor's goals.
3. Behaviorally oriented goals that are observable help clients. Goals work best when they are positive, concrete, attainable, and reduced to small steps.
4. Goals should be stated in terms of what behavior will occur, how often it will occur, and under what conditions it will occur. Action, such as doing something, rather than inaction, such as not doing something, is preferred. For example, running around the block would be preferable to not watching television.

For example, Frank's goal is to earn an A grade in English. To earn an A, Frank has agreed to request that his seat be moved to the front row, attend class every day, complete each day's homework assignment, and answer at least one question per day during class discussion.

The Skeleton Key Question/Statement for Goal Setting

De Shazer (1985) and Berg and Shilts (2005) recommend beginning goal setting by asking clients to think about the good things rather than the bad things that have been happening in their lives; for example, "I would like to have you think about your life recently and the things that have happened to you that you would like to have happen more often in the future," or "Please think about what you would like to get done in counseling and how you will know if counseling is helping." The client's thoughts on either of these statements will help the counselor determine what the client's goals might be. Berg and Shilts use what they call the "woww" approach, which is *working on what works*.

WORKING WITH UNPRODUCTIVE CLIENT GOALS   Unproductive goals will scuttle the solution-oriented brief counseling approach before it leaves the harbor. The three most common unproductive client goals are negative goals, harmful goals, and "Beats me, I don't know" goals. Sklare (2005) has done an excellent job in describing how each of these three types of unproductive goals can be reframed into productive, positive goals.

Negative Goals   Negative goals are stated as "Thou shalt not ..." goals—that is, goals to "stop doing things" and goals to get others to stop doing things; for example, "I would like to stop getting so many detentions." All of the preceding goals need to be reframed to describe what it is the client *will be doing* rather than *not doing*; for example, "I need to raise my hand in class to get permission to speak and that will lower the number of detentions I have been getting." The refocused goal can be derived from the things the client can do; for example, "If you stop doing all those things you said caused you to fail English, what will you be doing instead?" Nature abhors a vacuum, and something is sure to rush in and fill the void in a person's life when an activity is stopped. Therefore, clients should be asked how they plan to fill the free time they will have when they stop doing an unproductive behavior such as arguing excessively with their parents.

Harmful Goals   Harmful goals are those goals that, when achieved, will bring either harm to the client or to others. More often than not, these goals also will lead to violations of the law or school rules such as selling drugs or engaging in other criminal acts. The counselor can approach harmful goal statements by exploring with clients how achieving such goals would get the clients what they want. For example:

COUNSELOR: So, dropping out of school and selling drugs to make a living is what you really want. How will this help you?

CLIENT: Well, I hate school because I don't do the work and I get Fs.

COUNSELOR: So you are saying if you did the work, you would get better grades and then you might like school a little better?

CLIENT: Maybe.

COUNSELOR: Maybe a goal for you would be to find out how you could do the work and do better on your grades just to see what would happen.

I Don't Know Goals   "I don't know goals" are most likely ploys by the client to engage the counselor in some type of resistance activity. The client usually has been sent for counseling by parents, teachers, or judges and is determined to resist any effort by the counselor to help in any way. As noted previously, to overcome a child's resistance, the counselor can begin with the following dialogue:

COUNSELOR: What would have to happen to get your parents off your back and say you don't need counseling?

CLIENT: They want me to try harder at school.

COUNSELOR: What would I be seeing you do at school that would let your parents know that you were trying harder?

By following this script, the counselor becomes an ally who is working on the same team with the client to figure out how to help her or him avoid the need for counseling.

Legum (2005), in working with involuntary clients, recommends finding out whose idea it was to come for counseling and ask if it is what the client wants. If not, ask what the client might like to have happen in counseling and explain how counseling could help with the presenting problem.

Techniques

Counselors who use solution-focused brief therapy choose interventions from behavioral and cognitive treatments. Some of the strategies specific to solution-focused brief therapy are scaling, identifying exceptions, solution talk, and the miracle question.

Scaling involves asking the client to rate something on a scale of 1 to 10. DeJong and Berg (2013) described one way to use scaling with children. The counselor makes two slash marks on opposite ends of the paper, then says something like this: "So this mark here we'll call 1 and that stands for when things are awful with your teacher, and this other mark is 10 and stands for when things are absolutely, exactly right. What number are you at today?" The visual helps the child connect the scale to the situation under discussion.

Identifying exceptions to the problem allows people to search for times when their problems were absent or less bad than they are currently. Those exceptions become sources of information when making plans for change. Some questions that might help uncover exceptions are "When the problem is not present, how are things different?" and "How did you handle this before?" and "What would you need to have that happen again?"

Solution talk is another technique used in this type of counseling. Words are chosen to convey hope and optimism, a sense of control, and openness to possibilities. Seligman and Reichenberg (2014) summarized the following tools to create solution talk.

- Ask open questions
- Use language that assumes problems are temporary and positive change will happen such as "When the problem is gone, what will you be doing?"
- Talk about the problem as something external
- Normalize the problem with phrases such as "risky behavior" or other less emotional terms
- Focus on coping behaviors
- Notice and reinforce strengths
- Create hypothetical solutions such as "If you weren't feeling scared, what would you be feeling and doing instead?"
- Concentrate on behaviors rather than thoughts and emotions
- Use these words frequently: *change, different, possibility, what,* and *how*
- Use *and* to indicate that what seems contradictory outcomes can exist together

- Offer different perspectives
- Match the clients' vocabulary or style

Using the Miracle Question to Formulate Goals

As noted earlier, the miracle question, developed by de Shazer (1991) in his frustration with some clients' inability to form good behavioral goals, is used to help clients visualize and hypothesize what their problems would be like if suddenly they were solved. For example, the counselor could say, "If you opened your woke up one morning and this problem was gone, what would be different?"

Children may respond better to the question stated in magic terms (Sklare, 2005); for example, "If I were to wave a magic wand or rub a magic lamp and wish all your problems away, what would we see you doing if we could video you for a day?" Older children, teenagers, and adults might respond better with a visualization about what their life would look like 6 months or a year from now if the problem brought to counseling was solved; for example, "If the problem you brought to counseling was solved in the next 6 months, how would you know things were okay, and what would you be doing differently?" Again, active listening is a good way to help clients put their hypotheses about their problem-free futures in good behavioral goal language. This is where the future orientation parts of solution-oriented brief counseling stand out. The counselor's job is to keep the focus on what the client *will* be doing when the problem is solved.

Frequently, clients still use ineffective goal statements and generalizations in stating their hypotheses about their problem-free futures, such as "Well, I would feel good, I would be happy, or my parents would be nicer to me." When this happens, the counselor tries to identify the client's specific behavior: A potential question would be "When you are feeling this good feeling, what are you doing that will let you know that you are feeling good, or that you are happy?" and "What are you doing that would cause your parents to be nicer to you?" Again, visualization of the "new" behavior in the client's future, problem-free environment can be assisted with the video recording metaphor of what the video would show the client doing and by asking what others would see him or her doing. Others who would be observing the client could be the counselor, family members, classmates, teachers, and friends. For example, you could ask, "What would your friends see you doing differently, and what would they say?"

Sklare (2005) points out that clients often respond to the miracle question with improbable (if not impossible) miracles and "I want others to be different" miracles. For the former, the counselor's job is to reframe the improbable answer into what might be probable. For example, in the case of a divorce, the child may say:

CLIENT: I want my Mom and Dad to get married again.

COUNSELOR: How would that help you?

CLIENT: I would feel like I was part of a real family.

COUNSELOR: So, feeling a part of your family would be a goal for you.

CLIENT: Yes, because now it doesn't seem like I am.

COUNSELOR: What would you be doing to let you know that you were a part of your family?

CLIENT: I would like to be doing things that would help Mom and Dad out, like I did before they got divorced.

COUNSELOR: So, finding out how you could help both your Mom and Dad could be another goal for you.

For the latter "I want others to be different" goal, the counselor would continue to keep the focus on what the client will be doing to cause others to behave differently. For example:

CLIENT: I would like other kids in my class to be friends with me.

COUNSELOR: Well, if that miracle occurred, what would we see on a video of what was going on in your classroom?

CLIENT: Other kids would choose me to work with them on our projects.

COUNSELOR: So, if the other kids were choosing you for a work partner, what would you start doing differently?

CLIENT: I guess I would be nice about sharing my things with them. I have really awesome markers, but I don't want them messed up. Maybe if I let my friends use them, they would let me be on the team.

COUNSELOR: That sounds like a good goal for you to have. What else would you be doing?

CLIENT: I would be working hard to do my share of the work.

COUNSELOR: That sounds like a better goal, because you would know right away if you did at least your share of the work.

Case Study

Identification of the Problem

George is an 8-year-old boy in the second grade at Mountain Springs School. His parents brought him to counseling because they who were concerned because of his anxiety about going to school.

Individual and Background Information

Academic George's school records indicated a pattern of low achievement beginning midway through the first grade, when he began to fall behind the others in reading and mathematics concepts. Testing by the school psychologist did not reveal any learning disabilities, and his verbal and performance IQ was calculated to be within the 100 to 110 range. The school psychologist concluded that George's poor academic progress was more of a case of not wanting to do the school work rather than not being able to do it.

Family George is the middle child between an older sister, age 10, and a younger brother, age 5. His parents said that George's older sister had always made top grades, and that his younger brother enjoyed going to kindergarten.

Social George's first-grade teacher had reported that he had some difficulty in making friends with other children. He seemed to gravitate toward two boys who were causing most of the classroom discipline problems, and George frequently had to be corrected because of his own misbehavior, as well as his misbehavior with the other two boys. The pattern has continued in the second grade.

Counseling Method

The counselor used solution-focused brief counseling to help George identify some specific behavioral goals for himself. After identification of the goals, the counselor had periodic follow-up sessions with him to coordinate his progress with the school counselor, who was working with George's teachers in reinforcing progress on his goals. Behavioral contingency contracts and reality therapy used by the school counselor had not been successful with George.

Transcript

After about 5 minutes of getting to know each other and giving the structuring speech about what the solution-oriented counselor does, the counselor begins:

COUNSELOR: Well, George, do you know why your parents wanted you to see me?

GEORGE: I don't know.

COUNSELOR: That is one of the hard questions I told you I would be asking. So, I would like to have you pretend for a moment that you do know why your parents brought you here.

GEORGE: Well, it's probably about school, isn't it?

COUNSELOR: That was a good guess. What do you think they want to have happen to you in school?

GEORGE: Probably make better grades on my schoolwork.

COUNSELOR: George, I have something like a rule here that goes from a low of zero to a high of five. The zero would be for very low grades, like all Fs, and the five would be for very high grades, like all As. Which number on my thermometer is most like your grades?

GEORGE: I think I am about a two, because my grades are Cs and Ds.

COUNSELOR: I wonder how good your grades will have to be to get your parents to stop bringing you here for counseling.

GEORGE: Bs and Cs might make Mom and Dad happier with me, and that would be about a three on your scale.

COUNSELOR: So raising your grade one level would be a good goal for you. I would like to do another "let's pretend" with you. Suppose I had a magic lamp like in the genie story, and I could rub it and make a wish and a miracle happened. Imagine that your parents said, "George, your grades are good enough, and you don't have to go back to see the counselor." What would you be doing in your classroom the next day?

GEORGE: I would be really happy, and so would my teacher and Mom and Dad.

COUNSELOR: If I could videotape you in your classroom, what would I see you doing that would let me know you were happy about your grades?

GEORGE: I wouldn't be getting into trouble.

COUNSELOR: That's right, George, but what would you be doing instead?

GEORGE: I would be doing my schoolwork at my desk and raising my hand before talking in class.

COUNSELOR:	These things sound like two good goals for you to work on this week. What else would you be doing that we could see on a videotape?
GEORGE:	I would be finishing nearly all of my work at school so I wouldn't have to bring it home.
COUNSELOR:	These goals are getting better all the time. Do you think this would be a good goal that you could do?
GEORGE:	Yes, I could if I could sit away from some guys who always get me into trouble.
COUNSELOR:	So changing your seat might be another goal for you. Where do you see yourself sitting?
GEORGE:	I think I would do better in the front row.
COUNSELOR:	What else would we see you doing?
GEORGE:	Making mostly B grades and no more than two C grades.
COUNSELOR:	What would that videotape show you doing to make mostly B grades and just two Cs?
GEORGE:	Well, like I said, I would be getting nearly all my work done at school, and I would be working away from the troublemakers.
COUNSELOR:	Okay, George, it looks like you have two good goals to work on this week. Would it be okay if I talked to the school counselor about getting your seat moved so that you can get your work done at school, or do you want to talk this over with your teacher?
GEORGE:	I'll ask my teacher.
COUNSELOR:	What if she asks you why you want to move?
GEORGE:	I'll tell her that it will help me get my work done.
COUNSELOR:	Well, George, I have asked you about all the questions I have for you, and you have given me some really smart answers. I am wondering if you have any questions for me. [Pause] If not, I have one last question: What other things do I need to know that might help you reach your goals? [Pause] If there isn't anything else, we need to look at what might happen to stop you from meeting your goals. [Pause] If there is nothing you can think of, I need to leave you for a few moments to think about my notes and all the answers you gave me and to write you a message that you can take with you. You can play with any of the toys in the room and read any of the magazines while I am gone for a few minutes.

While they write these messages, some counselors prefer to remain in the room with younger children. Sklare (2005) recommends that messages should contain at least three compliments, with each compliment bridged to a task that will indicate that the child has met his or her goal. In George's case, the counselor would refer to the notes taken during the session.

George's Goals

1. Raise his grades to all Bs and Cs.
2. Improve his classroom behavior by moving away from two boys and by raising his hand.
3. Do well enough in school to get out of having to go to counseling.

Miracle

- I would be completing most of my homework at school and finishing the rest of my assignments at home.
- My grades would be all Bs and Cs.

- My classroom behavior would be good.
- My parents would be happy with my school behavior and grades, and I would not have to have more counseling.

First Sign(s) the Miracle Had Happened

- I would be doing my work in a front row seat away from the guys who got in trouble with me.
- I would be completing all of my school assignments, and my teacher would notice that I am doing better.
- I would be raising my hand for permission to speak in class, and that would make my teacher happy.

Instances or Exceptions When the Miracle Has Happened a Little Bit

- When I ignore the two boys who try to get me to break the rules.
- When I do my assignments during work periods.

Scaling

- Currently at a 2 because grades are all Cs and Ds.
- To get to a 3 on a 5-point scale, all grades have to be a C or better.
- To get a 5, grades will have to be at least half Bs and half As.
- Classroom behavior is at a 2 because George had to go to three time-outs for disrupting class last week. To get to a 4, he would have to be sent to no more than one time-out each week.

The counselor's written message to George was as follows:

[Compliment] I think you were really smart in coming up with some good ways to let your parents know that you won't need to come in here for more counseling. You figured out a good way to stay out of trouble and an even better way to raise your grades. Getting your seat moved to the front row, doing most of your homework assignments at school, turning in all of your assignments, and raising your hand to get permission to speak are four excellent ideas that should help you meet all your goals. [Bridges] Because of your promise to do your four ideas at school, [Task] you thought that you could begin by asking the teacher if she would move your seat to the front and tell her why you want to do this. Then I would suggest that you start doing the three other ideas and move up to a 3 on your 5-point scale for grades and a 4 for classroom behavior.

George may have trouble reading the message, so the language may need to be simplified for him to understand the compliments and how those are bridged to the tasks he needs to do. Sklare (2005) recommends having children draw pictures of their miracles, showing what will be happening when the miracle occurs. Discussion of the events depicted in these miracle drawings provides an excellent review of the session and leads into the counselor's message. For children who are not able to read the counselor's message, it might also be a good idea to draw a picture of their messages showing the complimented behaviors and the tasks to be done. Pictures help children visualize outcome goals being met and, hence, contribute to the child's ability to meet these goals.

Techniques in Solution-Focused Brief Counseling

Practitioners of solution-focused counseling have several interventions that are designed to be adaptable to many complaints. In fact, the prudent approach to using these techniques would be to select from the menu those interventions you think will take your clients where they want to go. Our purpose here is to present a menu of those interventions discussed by several key authors on the subject, including Berg and Shilts (2005), Daughhtree and Grant (2002), Legum (2005), Lutz (2013), Murphy and Duncan (2010), Selekman (2002), and Sklare (2005). All have contributed steps and questions typically used in conducting interviews with solution-oriented counseling.

Orientation to the Solution-focused Brief Counseling Process

Counselors should prepare the child client for the process of solution-focused brief counseling by explaining part of their time together will be asking some hard questions. Counselors should let the child know notes will be taken as memory aids and that the child's answers will help in many ways, especially with a summary note to the child at the end of the talk.

Setting Goals for Counseling

Opening questions could be either, "What is your goal in coming in for counseling?" or "What would you like to have happen from our counseling?" These keep the focus on goals and positive information, rather than on problems and negative aspects of the problem.

O'Hanlon and Wiener-Davis (2003) recommend beginning each counseling session by asking, "What happened in the past week that you would like to continue to see happen?" This question focuses on and amplifies the positive actions toward change that the client has accomplished.

Compliments

These phrases are not used as positive reinforcement because they are not contingent on anything. Compliments are used to help people feel better about themselves and hope for change (Shapiro et al., 2006).

Active Listening

As with all approaches to counseling, practitioners use active listening to help clients.

1. Clarify: (a) "What my goal is and what I will be doing when my goal is reached," (b) "My feelings about my situation," and (c) "How strongly I feel about my situation."
2. Scaling: For example, "On a ten-point scale where ten is very good and zero is very bad, where are you on the scale of zero to ten?" If clients indicate they are a 4, ask what is happening that keeps their bad feelings from being a 0. Focus on how they can make more of these good things happen.

Formulate First-Session Task

Counselors may use a traditional homework assignment at the end of the first session by asking clients to observe between now and the next session what happens in (relationships, school, and play) that they want to continue to happen. This homework focuses attention on the positives and on what they want (de Shazer, 1985).

Working with Negative Goals

Negative goals are an absence of something, as in:

CLIENT:	I don't want to …
COUNSELOR:	So, what would you be doing instead? Or
CLIENT:	I want others to stop …
COUNSELOR:	What difference would this make? [Or] How will that help you? [Or] What will you do if they don't change?

Working with Positive Goals

Positive goals are the presence of something, as in:

CLIENT:	I would like to make better grades.
COUNSELOR:	What would you be doing that would show you have gotten what you want?

Coping Question

With this technique, counselors ask clients how they have managed to cope so far. The idea is that even with the problem, the client is still carrying out life and has not been totally defeated. Therefore, some kind of coping is happening. For example, a response to "I'm miserable. I'll never be able to forget how bad he hurt me. I just want to sit and cry," might be, "How are you managing to not be crying right now?" When framed carefully, the distress can be seen as motivation to change (Shapiro et al., 2006).

The Miracle Question

Clinicians can use some of the previous variations of the miracle question or the following series of questions for getting more details. "If we videotaped you after the miracle happened, what would we see you doing? Who would notice? What would they see? How would they respond? How would you respond? What would be different after this miracle?" Counselors will want to repeat this last question three or four times to get more indicators of what the counseling goals should be for the client. The counseling agenda can be set from the answers about the miracle question.

Relationship Questions

1. "What will your [parents, brother or sister, teacher, friend] say that will be different after the miracle?"
   a. "How will they act when they see you are different after the miracle?"
   b. "When they act differently toward you, what will you do differently in response to them?"

Exceptions to the Problem Situation

1. Ask about some instances when some of the miracle has already happened a little bit.
2. Encourage and reinforce these exceptions to the problem situation.
3. Use the EARS approach—which stands for Elicit, Amplify, Reinforce, and Start again—when exceptions to the problem, other positive thoughts, and positive behaviors are mentioned. Elicit—ask for positive change; Amplify—ask for details about positive change; Reinforce—make sure the client notices and values positive change; Start again—go back to the beginning and focus on client-generated change (DeJong & Berg, 2013).

Positive Blame

Counselors can use humor and positive blame when exceptions to the problem situation are identified. For example, say, "How in the world did you make that happen?"

Changing the Doing

With a vision of the solution, counseling turns to designing steps toward the goal (Lipchick, 2002). The steps include action-oriented assignments that work from the exceptions to the problem. Shapiro et al. (2006) outline a three-step process for bridging the client's competencies and the new challenge:

1. Identify an activity in which the client is successful. (You say you take good care of your dog.)
2. Give abstract definitions of the abilities involved in that success. (That takes dedication, compassion, and patience.)
3. Talk about the concrete ways those abilities would take in the problem area. (How could you use that sticking to it with your school work?)

Practitioners can help clients see approximations of change by using scaling and ten percent improvements. To anticipate barriers, clinicians can help clients identify the minefield that might impede change. Finally counselors are careful about closing the sessions and increase the continuity of treatment by writing notes about client goals.

Scaling Progress toward Goal

1. "On a scale of 0 to 10, where 0 is the worst that things could be and 10 is the day after the miracle, where are you right now?"
2. Again, if the client says 4, ask what is going on that keeps it from being a 0.
3. Focus on talking about how to make more of these good things happen.
4. Again, reinforce any indicators that the client is already doing some helpful things that can be increased.

Ten Percent Improvements

1. Ask clients what they need to do to go up one step, or 10 percent, on the scale. Modify the question for young children who may not understand the concept of percentages.
2. Develop a plan for making the 10 percent improvement in specific terms such as one assignment on two different days.

Flagging the Minefield

1. Ask clients what things might prevent them from moving up 10 percent on the scale or what might sabotage their plan.
2. Ask your clients what they could do to prevent their plan from being sabotaged.

Closing the Session

1. Ask clients to draw a picture of what will be happening after the miracle occurs (visualization).
2. Ask clients if they have any questions or if there is anything else you (the counselor) should know.
3. Sessions may end with a summary statement by the counselor in which positive exceptions to the problem are highlighted and experiments or observations to be completed before the next session are repeated (Shapiro et al., 2006).

Writing the Note

Write the client a message with at least three compliments and a bridging statement from each compliment to one of the tasks the client needs to accomplish to raise the scale score 10 percent, or one level from a 4 to a 5. The counselor has the option of drawing a picture of what the client will be doing the day after the miracle occurs.

Most solution-oriented counseling sessions will not require all of the steps mentioned in this chapter. In fact, Daughhtree and Grant (2002) use only five questions or steps in their practice of solution-oriented counseling.

1. Ask clients, "How do you experience the problem?"
2. Ask clients, "When do (or did) you not experience the problem? What were you doing then?"
3. Have clients rate their current progress on solving the problem on the 0 to 10 scale.
4. Ask the miracle question.
5. Set goals based on increasing what works for the client.

Other solution-focused brief counseling statements that assist clients in moving away from the problem impasse toward solutions.

1. *Normalizing statements.* These statements let clients know they are not alone in experiencing their problem; for example, "No wonder you are feeling ..." Although this statement appears to be in conflict with our philosophy of not using "level one, discount of feelings" statements in person-centered counseling, it does have the possibility of offering clients the hope that others have worked their way out of similar difficulties and that they are not "crazy" for experiencing the feelings they are having.
2. *Restructuring statements.* These statements are used to rephrase the impasse as directions for the future; for example, "You have reached a decision point in your life."

3. *Affirmation statements.* These statements reinforce the positive steps the client has already taken and attributes the client can marshal to achieve personal goals.
4. *Bridging statements.* These statements connect client attributes with the next steps in achieving goals.
5. *Between-session homework statements.* These statements of what the client will be doing serve to connect the sessions and remind students of when times are better. Homework will also move clients toward their goals (O'Hanlon & Weiner-Davis, 2003).

De Jong and Berg (2013) outlined modifications to solution seeking with children. They reminded counselors to prepare a child-friendly place with age-appropriate materials and toys. Counselors should build alliances with adults to help the child. These authors state that children's problems are resolved either when the behavior no longer happens or when the adult decides the action is no longer a problem. That shift in adult thinking may create more positive interactions between the adult and the child. Counselors need to get the child's perception of the difficulty, something the child may be able to draw rather than express verbally. Children's strengths include their creativity and vivid imaginations. With children and adolescents counselors should use many relationship questions and avoid "why" questions. A helpful response to the familiar "I don't know" phrase teenagers use would be "Suppose you did know, what would you (or your best friend) say?" De Jong and Berg remind counselors to assume children are competent and that hints of exceptions will be within the conversations.

SOLUTION-FOCUSED PLAY THERAPY

Nims (2011) outlines the juxtaposition of language and play therapy with solution-focused play therapy. He notes the process of goal setting, the miracle question, exceptions to the problem, scaling, and the solution message as mirroring the treatment process of solution-focused counseling with the use of play media to lead children through those steps. Selekman (2005) also explains the modified model of solution-focused work with play and art therapy.

Griffith (2007) explained the characteristics of solution-oriented counseling and play therapy that can be used in schools. The approach is pragmatic and focused on the child's strengths rather than weaknesses. Discussions are about what the child presents and about what has changed since the last meeting. The counselor questions the child about what the child sees as a solution—what it would look like, how people will know something has changed, and what will be different when the change happens.

Griffith (2007) cautioned that sometimes children understand more than they can share verbally and other times they seem to understand only to please. Counselors are patient, listen carefully, and use tracking, reflection, and encouragement. The child tells his or her story through play and the counselor learns the child's perspective and sees the situation through the child's eyes. Puppets play out problems or solutions, and other play materials can aid the child in searching for alternative actions. Griffith suggested that helping children rehearse solutions in play helps them practice what they can handle and what is a good fit for them. She reminded counselors not to give the child the solution but allow the child to discover it in order to build competencies. Techniques used in solution-oriented play therapy are scaling questions, externalizing, playing detective, trying magic tricks, experimenting, and reporting changes. Griffith's case study provides a valuable study of how this therapy builds on the child's resources, language, exceptions, and images.

Nims (2007) gave another description of solution-focused brief therapy. He used expressive play therapy techniques of art, sand tray, and puppets to help children set goals, visualize how things could be different if the goal was achieved, describe exceptions, and write the solution message. Nims includes credits, bridge, and a solution task in the solution message. Credits are affirmations of the child and the child's efforts. The bridge is the connection between the credits and the task. The task is what the child has agreed to try before the next session. Taylor (2009) and Sweeney (2011) expanded the use of the sand tray with the solution-focused brief therapy process and provided specific procedures for practitioners.

DIVERSITY APPLICATIONS OF SOLUTION-FOCUSED BRIEF COUNSELING

De Jong and Berg (2013) related that many things in solution-focused brief therapy have multicultural relevance. They suggested the flexibility and emphasis on health, resources, strengths, dignity, collaboration, empowerment, and self-determination are appropriate with diverse people. Additionally, respecting each person's view of the world, recognizing the importance of people's connections to each other, and the brief, nonintrusive approach make solution-focused brief therapy appropriate to a range of people. De Jong and Berg provided outcome data for clients that had been seen in the Brief Family Therapy Center, which supported their reasoning of effectiveness and satisfaction of solution-focused brief therapy.

Solution-focused counseling has been employed with Muslim American clients (Chaudhry & Li, 2011), African American and Mexican American clients (Corcoran, 2000), those with religious/spiritual concerns (Guterman & Leite, 2006), and clients with Asian origins (Lee & Mjelde-Mossey, 2004) as well as elder people in Mexico (Seidel & Hedley, 2008).

Brief counseling enjoys wide appeal among cultures and clients who emphasize individual responsibility over the family and the community. Sue and Sue (2013) point out that in Western cultures when one does something wrong, the most common reaction is guilt, yet in non-Western cultures, the emotion most often expressed is shame. Sue and Sue hold that guilt focuses on the individual, whereas shame appears to focus on the group, as in "I did something wrong and let down my family." Although brief counseling does take an individual approach, considerable attention is given to how the client's family, friends, and colleagues will be reacting when the problem's solution is achieved. In fact, brief counseling is being used to counsel families.

EVALUATION OF SOLUTION-FOCUSED BRIEF THERAPY

Three meta-analyses of solution-focused counseling have been completed. Kim (2008) conducted a meta-analysis to evaluate the effectiveness of solution-focused brief therapy and found small, but positive, treatment effects on behavior and relationship problems like depression and anxiety. In a study of solution-focused therapy in schools, the results were mixed (Kim & Franklin, 2009) as were those in the other meta-analysis (Corcoran & Pillai, 2009).

George, Iveson, and Ratner (2006) summarized outcome data from 44 studies on solution-focused brief therapy and concluded the results were impressive and justified claims of effectiveness and brevity of the approach. Franklin and Streeter (2006) concur.

More specific studies have positive outcomes. Perkins (2006) studied the effectiveness of one solution-focused session with children and adolescents at a mental health clinic. Parent and clinician measures indicated significant improvement in mental health problems with only one session. Smock and colleagues (2008) assigned clients to substance abuse treatment solution-focused groups or psych educational groups. After six treatment sessions, those in the solution-focused group had fewer symptoms and less distress than the other groups.

Myrick (2003) and Lines (2011) stress the importance of accountability in the school counseling program. Documentation of the counselor's success can provide support for the program and meet the compliance requirements of local, state, and federal laws. Brief counseling is particularly strong in setting specific goals and documenting progress in meeting these goals.

Other researchers have documented success with solution-focused brief therapy in schools. Corcoran and Stephenson (2000) found solution-focused brief therapy led to improvement with children who had behavior problems. Littrell (2002), using three variations of brief counseling ranging from problem-focused to solution-focused methods, reports all three to be effective in single-session counseling with high school students. Newsome (2004, 2005) who worked with a group of African American young people improved their grade point average during the treatment. Vallaire-Thomas, Hicks, and Growe (2011) outline a longitudinal study in which solution-focused brief counseling combines with positive behavioral support in schools to address student behavior problems. Finally Franklin, Moore, and Hopson (2008) studied the effectiveness of five to seven sessions of solution-focused brief therapy with 67 children who had classroom behavior problems. Students in the experimental group improved their behavior based on teacher's reports.

Brief counseling methods infused into the other approaches presented in this book can provide counselors with the tools they need to be successful in helping their clients meet their goals in the least number of sessions. Cepeda and Davenport (2006) provided just such an integration of person-centered therapy and solution-focused brief therapy.

Researchers and practitioners of solution-focused counseling also want their colleagues to succeed and have compiled valuable resources. Some of these are the informative review of solution-focused brief therapy by Franklin, Trepper, Gingerich, and McCullum (2012) and Milner and Bateman's (2011) explanations of working with children to overcome barriers with a solution-focused approach.

Additionally Hanton (2011) provides a useful overview of the skills needed to practice solution-focused brief counseling. Finally the research committee of the solution-focused brief therapy association has designed a treatment manual for working with individuals (Trepper et al., 2010).

SUMMARY

Solution-focused brief counseling has been effective with a range of problems. Solution-focused brief therapy is an optimistic, encouraging approach to change that offers people new ways of thinking about their concerns. Building on strengths, competencies, and resources, clients face their immediate problems by making small changes that lead to solutions. This approach favors a collaborative relationship in which the counselor uses language and techniques to focus on exceptions to a problem. Client and counselor create specific, meaningful goals that lead to success.

The brief counseling approaches appear to be deceptively easy to master; however, this is not the case. As is true with any other approach to counseling, therapists and counselors of all orientations need to study and practice brief counseling under expert supervisors if they are to do it well and not harm their clients.

INTRODUCTION TO BRIEF COUNSELING VIDEO

 To gain a more in-depth understanding of the concepts in this chapter, visit www .cengage.com/counseling/henderson to view a short clip of an actual therapist–client session demonstrating brief counseling.

WEB SITES FOR BRIEF COUNSELING

Internet addresses frequently change. To find the sites listed here, visit www.cengage .com/counseling/henderson for an updated list of Internet addresses and direct links to relevant sites.

Solution-Focused Brief Therapy Association

The Brief Family Therapy Center (BFTC)

Brief Therapy

REFERENCES

Berg, I. K. (1994). *Family-based services: A solution-focused approach*. New York: Norton.

Berg, I. K. (2005). The state of miracles in relationship. *Journal of Family Psychotherapy, 16*, 51–56.

Berg, I. K., & de Shazer, S. (1993). Making numbers talk: Language in therapy. In S. Friedman (Ed.), *The new language of change: Constructive collaboration in psychotherapy* (pp. 5–24). New York: Guilford Press.

Berg, I., & Miller, S. (1992). *Working with the problem drinker*. New York: Norton.

Berg, I., & Shilts, L. (2005). Keeping solutions inside the classroom. *ASCA School Counselor*, 42(6), 30–35.

Bertolino, B., & O'Hanlon, B. (2001). *Collaborative, competency based counseling and therapy*. Boston, MA: Allen and Bacon.

Bruce, M. (1995). Brief counseling: An effective model for change. *The School Counselor*, 42, 353–364.

Cepeda, L. M., & Davenport, D. S. (2006). Person-centered therapy and solution-focused brief therapy: An integration of present and future awareness. *Psychotherapy: Theory, Research, Practice, Training*, 43, 1–12.

Chaudhry, S., & Li, C. (2011). Is solution-focused brief therapy culturally appropriate for Muslim American counselees? *Journal of Contemporary Psychotherapy*, 41, 109–113.

Corcoran, J., & Pillai, V. (2009). A review of the research on solution-focused therapy. *British Journal of Social Work*, 39(2), 234–242. doi:10.1093/bjsw/bcm098

Corcoran, J., & Stephenson, M. (2000). The effectiveness of solution-focused therapy with child behavior problems: A preliminary report. *Families in Society*, 81, 468–474.

Daughhtree, C., & Grant, D. (2002). Stress management. *ASCA School Counselor*, 39, 17–19.

DeJong, P., & Berg, I. K. (2013). *Interviewing for solutions* (4th ed.). Pacific Grove, CA: Brooks/Cole.

de Shazer, S. (1985). *Keys to solutions in brief therapy*. New York: Norton.

de Shazer, S. (1986). Minimal elegance. *Family Therapy Networker*, 59, 57–60.

de Shazer, S. (1988). *Clues! Investigating solutions in brief therapy*. New York: Norton.

de Shazer, S. (1991). *Putting difference to work*. New York: Norton.

de Shazer, S. (1994). *Words were originally magic*. New York: Norton.

de Shazer, S., Berg, I. K., Lipchik, E., Nunnaly, E., Molnar, A., Gingerich, W., & Weiner-Davis, M. (1986). Brief therapy: Focused solution development. *Family Process*, 25, 207–221.

de Shazer, S., & Dolan, Y. (2007). *More than miracles: The state of the art of solution focused therapy*. New York: Haworth Press.

Erickson, M. H. (1954). Special techniques of brief hypnotherapy. *Journal of Clinical and Experimental Hypnosis*, 2, 109–129.

Fall, K. A., Holden, J. M., & Marquis, A. (2010). *Theoretical models of counseling and psychotherapy* (2nd ed.). New York: Routledge.

Franklin, C., Moore, K., & Hopson, L. (2008). Effectiveness of solution-focused brief therapy in a school setting. *Children & Schools*, 30(1), 15–26.

Franklin, C., & Streeter, C. L. (2006). Solution-focused accountability schools for the twenty-first century: A training manual for Gonzalo Garza Independence High School.

Franklin, C. G., Trepper, T., Gingerich, W., & McCullum. E. (2012). *Solution-Focused Brief Therapy: A Handbook of Evidence Based Practice*. New York: Oxford University Press.

Griffith, S. G. (2007). School-based play therapy and solution-oriented brief counseling for children in crisis: Case of Melinda, age 6. In N. B. Webb (Ed.), *Play therapy with children in crisis: Individual, group, and family treatment* (3rd ed, pp. 322–342). New York: Guilford.

Gunn, W. B., Jr., Haley, J., & Lyness, A. M. P. (2007). Systemic approaches: Family therapy. In H. T. Prout & D. T. Brown (Eds.), *Counseling and psychotherapy with children and adolescents: Theory and practice for school and clinical settings* (4th ed., pp. 388–418). Hoboken, NJ: Wiley.

Guterman, J. T., & Leite, N. (2006). Solution-focused counseling for clients with religious and spiritual concerns. *Counseling and Values*, 51, 39–52.

Haley, J. (1973). *Uncommon therapy: The psychiatric techniques of Milton H. Erickson, M.D.* New York: Norton.

Hanton, P., & Ebooks Corporation. (2011). *Skills in solution focused brief: Counselling & psychotherapy*. Thousand Oaks, CA: Sage.

Kim, J. S. (2008). Examining the effectiveness of solution-focused brief therapy: A meta-analysis. *Research on Social Work Practice, 18*(2), 107–116. doi:10.1177/1049731507307807

Kim, J., & Franklin, C. (2009). Solution-focused brief therapy in schools: A review of the outcome literature. *Children and Youth Services Review, 31*, 464–470.

Lee, M. Y., & Mjelde-Mossey, L. (2004). Cultural dissonance among generations: A solution-focused approach with East Asian elders and their families. *Journal of Marital and Family Therapy, 30*(4), 497–513. doi:10.1111/j.1752-0606.2004.tb01258.x

Legum, H. (2005). Finding solutions. *School Counselor, 42*(5), 33–37.

Lines, D. (2011). *Brief counseling in schools* (3rd ed.). London: Sage Publications.

Lipchik, E. (2002). *Beyond technique in solution-focused therapy*. New York: Guilford.

Littrell, J. (2002). Single-session brief counseling in a high school. *Journal of Counseling & Development, 73*, 451–459.

Lutz, A. B. (2013). *Learning solution-focused therapy: An illustrated guide*. Arlington, VA: American Psychiatric Publishing.

Miller, S. D., Hubble, M. A., & Duncan, B. L. (1996). *Handbook of solution-focused brief therapy*. San Francisco, CA: Jossey-Bass.

Milner, J., & Bateman, J. (2011). *Working with children and teenagers using solution focused approaches: Enabling children to overcome challenges and achieve their potential*. London; Philadelphia: Jessica Kingsley Publishers.

Murdock, N. L. (2013). *Theories of counseling and psychotherapy: A case approach*. Upper Saddle River, NJ: Pearson.

Murphy, J., & Duncan, B. (2010). *Brief interventions for school problems* (2nd ed.) New York: Guilford.

Myrick, R. (2003). Accountability: Counselors count. *Professional School Counseling, 6*, 174–179.

Newsome, W. S. (2004). Solution-focused brief therapy group work with at-risk junior high school students: Enhancing the bottom line. *Research on Social Work Practice, 14*, 336–343.

Newsome, W. S. (2005). The impact of solution-focused brief therapy with at-risk junior high school students. *Children & Schools, 27*, 83–90.

Nims, D. R. (2007). Integrating play therapy techniques into solution-focused brief therapy. *International Journal of Play Therapy, 16*, 54–68.

Nims, D. (2011). Solution-focused play therapy: Helping children and families find solutions. In C. E. Schaefer & Ebooks Corporation, *Foundations of play therapy* (pp. 297–309). Hoboken, NJ: Wiley.

O'Hanlon, W. H., & Beadle, S. (1997). *A guide to possibility land: Fifty-one methods for doing brief, respectful therapy*. New York: Norton.

O'Hanlon, W. H., & Weiner-Davis, M. (2003). *In search of solutions: A new direction in psychotherapy* (Rev. Ed). New York: Norton.

Perkins, R. (2006). The effectiveness of one session of therapy using a single-session therapy approach for children and adolescents with mental health problems. *Psychology and Psychotherapy: Theory, Research and Practice, 79*, 215–227.

Prochaska, J. O., & Norcross, J. C. (2014). *Systems of psychotherapy: A transtheoretical analysis* (8th ed.). Pacific Grove, CA: Cengage.

Saleebey, D. (Ed.). (2012). *The strengths perspective in social work practice* (6th ed.). Boston: Allyn & Bacon.

Seidel, A., & Hedley, D. (2008). The use of solution-focused brief therapy with older adults in Mexico: A preliminary study. *The American Journal of Family Therapy, 36*(3), 242–252.

Selekman, M. (2002). *Solution-focused therapy with children: Harnessing family strengths for systematic change*. New York: Guilford.

Selekman, M. D. (2005). *Children in therapy: Using the family as resource*. New York: Norton.

Seligman, L., & Reichenberg, L. W. (2014). *Theories of counseling and psychotherapy: Systems, strategies, and skills* (4th ed.). Upper Saddle River, NJ: Merrill.

Shapiro, J. P., Friedberg, R. D., & Bardenstein, K. K. (2006). *Child and adolescent therapy: Science and art*. Hoboken, NJ: Wiley.

Sklare, G. (2005). *Brief counseling that works: A solution-focused approach for school counselors and administrators* (2nd ed.). Thousand Oaks, CA: Corwin.

Smock, S. A., Trepper, T. S., Wetchler, J. L., McCollum, E. E., Ray, R., & Pierce, K. (2008). Solution-focused group therapy for level 1 substance abusers. *Journal of Marital and Family Therapy, 34*(1), 107–120. doi:10.1111/j.1752-0606.2008.00056.x

Stalker, C. A., Levene, J. E., & Coady, N. F. (1999). Solution-focused brief therapy—one model fits all? *Families in Society: The Journal of Contemporary Human Services, 80*, 468–489.

Sue, D., & Sue, D. (2013). *Counseling the culturally diverse: Theory and practice* (6th ed.). Hoboken, NJ: Wiley.

Sweeney, D. (2011). Integration of sand tray therapy and solution-focused therapy techniques for treating noncompliant youth. In A. A. Drewes, S. Bratton, C. E. Schaefer, & Ebooks Corporation (Eds.), *Integrative play therapy*. Hoboken, NJ: John Wiley & Sons, Inc.

Taylor, E. R. (2009). Sand tray and solution-focused therapy. *International Journal of Play Therapy, 18*, 56–68.

Trepper, T. S., McCollum, E. E., DeJong, P., Korman, H., Gingerich, W., & Franklin, C. (2010). *Solution focused therapy treatment manual for working with individuals*. Retrieved from http://www.solutionfocused.net/treatmentmanual.html

Vallaire-Thomas, L., Hicks, J., & Growe, R. (2011). Solution-focused brief therapy: An interventional approach to improving negative student behaviors. *Journal of Instructional Psychology, 38*(4), 224.

Walter, J., & Peller, J. (1992). *Becoming solution-focused in brief therapy*. New York: Brunner/Mazel.

CHAPTER 11

Individual Psychology

One of the most beautiful gifts in the world is the gift of encouragement. When someone encourages you, that person helps you over a threshold you might otherwise never have crossed on your own.

—JOHN O'DONOHUE

If Freud had done nothing more than stimulate thinking and reactions in other theorists, he would have made a significant contribution to counseling and psychotherapy. Like many others, Adler reacted to Freud's ideas by developing a new theory that emphasized the social nature of human beings and rejecting the emphasis on sexuality he felt Freud supported. Adler proposed a philosophical approach that focused on responsibility, creativity, purposeful behavior, and social connections. He called his work "individual" psychology to refer to understanding a person in totality—a unity of thinking, feeling, and acting, in every expression of self. Adler talks about striving for perfection as an innate, primary motivator of life. For Adler, each person creates a life path and has the capacity to triumph over struggles and make a meaningful contribution to society. After reading this chapter, you should be able to:

▶ Outline the development of individual psychology and the impact of Alfred Adler
▶ Explain the theory of individual psychology including its core concepts
▶ Discuss the counseling relationship and goals in Adlerian counseling
▶ Describe assessment, process, and techniques in individual assessment
▶ Demonstrate some therapeutic techniques of individual psychology
▶ Clarify the effectiveness of Adlerian counseling
▶ Discuss Adlerian play therapy

ALFRED ADLER
(1870–1937)

Alfred Adler, the founder of individual psychology, was born in Vienna. His mother coddled him until the birth of another child, which led to his subsequent interest in birth order. As a result of his suffering from rickets, pneumonia, poor eyesight, and several accidents, Adler had frequent contact with doctors, which influenced him to study medicine.

Adler received his medical degree from the University of Vienna in 1895. He worked as an eye specialist, a general physician, and a neurologist. In addition to medicine, Adler was also knowledgeable in psychology, philosophy, the Bible, and Shakespeare. Two years after his graduation, Adler married Raisa Timofeyeuna Epstein, an intellectual and a friend of Freud's who had moved from Russia to study at the University of Vienna (Alexander, Eisenstein, & Grotjahn, 1966).

In the fall of 1902, Adler accepted an invitation to join Sigmund Freud's discussion group, which was to become the first psychoanalytic society. Adler was not a proponent of Freud's psychosexual theory, and Adler's writings about "feelings of inferiority" in 1910 and 1911 initiated a disagreement with Freud. In 1910, in an attempt to reconcile the gap between himself and the Adlerians, Freud named Adler president of the Viennese Analytic Society and coeditor of a journal that Freud published. Nevertheless, Adler continued to disagree with Freud's psychosexual theory. Adler was the first psychoanalyst to emphasize human nature as being fundamentally social. On Freud's demand that his entire staff accept his theory without any conditions, Adler resigned, together with seven others, and founded the Society for Free Psychoanalytic Research. In 1912, Adler changed the name to the Society for Individual Psychology.

Adler served for two years as a military doctor in World War I and later was appointed to head a large hospital for the wounded and those suffering from shell shock. In 1926, Adler accepted a visiting professorship at Columbia University in New York; and in 1935, he moved his family to the United States. His children, one son and one daughter, became psychiatrists and worked within the principles of individual psychology. In 1937, while giving a series of lectures in Scotland, Adler suddenly collapsed on the street and died of heart failure.

Seligman and Reichenberg (2014) explained that Adler's professional development had four distinct parts. The first came after his graduation from medical school during which he determined his interests centered on the mind rather than the body. The second phase came when he joined Freud and was able to promote the idea of healthy emotional development. The third occurred after he became disillusioned with Freud's ideas and advanced his own ideas of understanding and helping individuals. The final stage occurred after he served in World War I as a psychiatrist where he was convinced people's drive toward social interest outweighed other motivations.

Adler's achievements included founding *Zeitschrift für Individualpsychologie* (1912), introducing the term *inferiority feelings*, and developing a flexible, supportive psychotherapy to direct those emotionally disabled by inferiority feelings toward maturity, common sense, and social usefulness. Individual psychology originated from the German word *Individualpsychologie*, meaning "psychology of the whole that cannot be divided." Basically, it is a psychology that is concerned both with individuals as they are in themselves and in their relationships with others.

In 1919, Adler originated the network of child-guidance clinics called *Erziehungsberatungsstellen*, which means literally "places to come for questions about education," or parent-education centers. Their staffs included physicians, psychologists, and social workers. His idea of group discussions with families caused many people to believe Adler was 50 years ahead of his time. The current emphasis on group counseling, parent education, and full-service schools supports this claim.

Adler favored efforts directed toward prevention of mental illness through parent-education programs. He recognized the difficulty of undoing in adulthood the wrongs done to individuals in their childhood.

Rudolf Dreikurs contributed perhaps the most helpful adaptations and development to Adler's work. A leading proponent of individual psychology until his death in 1972, Dreikurs was a pioneer in music therapy and group psychotherapy, which he introduced into private psychiatric practice in 1929. His most significant contribution to counseling children was his ability to translate theory into practice. Dreikurs developed many of Adler's complex ideas into a relatively simple applied method for understanding and working with the behavior of children in both family and school settings.

THE NATURE OF PEOPLE

According to Adler, people are responsible, creative, connected, social beings who behave with purpose toward a goal. While Freud attempted to interpret all behaviors and problems as extensions of sex, pleasure, and the death instinct, Adler believed that all people develop some sense of inferiority because they are born completely helpless and remain that way for a rather long childhood. Such feelings of inferiority may be exaggerated by body or organ defects (real or imaginary); by having older and more powerful siblings; or by parental neglect, rejection, or pampering. One way to cope with feelings of inferiority is compensation or gaining power to handle the sense of weakness. The effects of organ inferiority are reduced through development of skills, behaviors, traits, and strengths that replace or compensate for these thoughts of weakness and powerlessness. This innate drive Adler called *striving for superiority*, the core personality motivation that lasts throughout life (Prouchaska & Norcross, 2014).

According to Adler, being superior means being more that we currently are—not necessarily becoming socially distinctive or dominate or a leader. Rather striving for superiority refers to trying to build a more perfect and complete life (Prouchaska & Norcross, 2014). Mosak and Maniacci (2011) explain that as children grow, they develop conclusions about how to strive for superiority based on their subjective experiences. Each child considers members of his family and makes decisions about how to fit in, how to earn love, and what the rules about relationships are. From those observations, the child forms conclusions which, by around the age of 6, have developed into a lifestyle and specific goals of living (Kottman, 2009). Maniacci, Sackett-Maniacci, and Mosak (2014) explain lifestyle as a person's "use of personality, traits, temperament, and psychological and biological process in order to find a place in the social matrix of life" (p. 66).

The child behaves as though the convictions that make up his or her lifestyle are true. Each person forms decisions based on this private logic that others may not comprehend. If the child cannot find a way to belong in a positive way, she or he will find a way to belong in a negative way, therefore developing either a constructive or destructive lifestyle (Kottman, 2010). Maniacci et al. (2014) explain that private logic may contain mistaken beliefs about how to gain superiority that are accepted *as if* the beliefs are true. Private logic includes lifestyle goals, hidden reasons, and immediate goals. Children build this cognitive map or lifestyle to help them cope with the world. The lifestyle incorporates dreams, goals, and conditions that the individual needs to be secure. Four groups of lifestyle convictions are those about who I am (self-concept), what I should be (self-ideal), picture of the world (about other people and what the world demands), and personal right–wrong code (ethical convictions). Discrepancies between any of these convictions lead to inferiority feelings.

Adler viewed human behavior as falling on a continuum between his concepts of masculinity, representing strength and power, and femininity, symbolizing weakness and inferiority. What he called *masculine protest*—a striving for power—was common to both sexes, particularly women. Adler replaced Freud's concept of sexual pleasure as the prime motivator of behavior with the search for power.

According to Adler, personality development progresses along a road paved with evidence of either personal superiority or inferiority. As infants—small, helpless, inexperienced—we are especially subject to others' whims and vulnerable to feelings of inferiority. As we grow older, both family and society emphasize the advantages of size, beauty, and strength. Therefore, our wishes and dreams for superiority, our attempts to achieve it and the social realities that make us feel inferior are in continual conflict. This striving for power (masculine protest) occupies a place in his theory similar to that of the Oedipus situation in Freudian theory. A person develops into a normal, neurotic, or psychotic adult as the result of this struggle between the masculine protest and social reality. For Adlerians, our most fundamental motivation is to gain a sense of superiority, competence, belonging, and significance (Fall, Holden, & Marquis, 2010).

The second innate motivation that Adler proposed was *social interest,* the desire to contribute to others and to society, trying to gain superiority in ways that positively contribute to others. Adler theorized that everyone is born with the potential to develop social interest but that desire must be cultivated by parents, siblings, and others. Actions related to social interest are sharing, helping, participating, compromising, and cooperating (Fall et al., 2010).

Freud believed that love and work were the two important indexes of mental health in that a person's mental health depends on how well these two areas are progressing. In a similar vein, Adler believed that problems brought to therapy reside in the areas of career (occupation), love relationships (intimacy), and friendships.

The following points summarize the Adlerian view on the nature of people:

- Beginning in childhood, people develop feelings of inferiority stemming from being totally dependent on their parents. Life becomes a process of believing in ways to become less inferior and more independent. People behave in ways to give themselves feelings of perfection or superiority.
- The future determines the present as people behave in ways to become the fictionalized ideal person they have established as a goal in their future. All parts of the person are directed toward achieving the goal of becoming the ideal self: cognitive, affective, behavioral, conscious, and unconscious. Psychological goals are often unknown and have to be identified and explained to clients by their counselors as they examine the purposes of their clients' behaviors.
- Individual perceptions of events and relationships are governed by one's own unique view of the world and its people. Understanding one's relationship to others is a first step to understanding oneself.
- People need to be educated to value and exhibit social interest. Children and adults make contributions to social interest when they make their neighborhood (and world) a better place to live.
- Unsolved problems of an individual may become problems for society if they are not treated before they become too difficult to solve.

Kelly and Lee (2007) explained six primary propositions of individual psychology according to Adler. The first involves the basic motivational force as striving from a feeling of inferiority to one of significance, completion, and perfection. Another principle is that human behavior is goal directed. Viewing personality as a unified, holistic, and self-consistent pattern is another belief in individual psychology. Behavior happens in a social context so actions have social meaning in a social system that judges behavior. Finally, Adlerians propose that the actions of human beings are understood by universal principles.

CORE CONCEPTS

Health

Adler considered social interest the barometer of healthy functioning. He explained that the healthy person courageously faces the tasks of life with strategies that consider not only self-interest but also the welfare of others. One does not achieve health but continues to strive for it (Fall et al., 2010).

In the Adlerian view, the ideal or well-adjusted child exhibits the following qualities:

1. Respect for the rights of others
2. Tolerance for others
3. Interest in others
4. Cooperation with others
5. Encouragement of others
6. Courteous to others
7. Strong, positive self-concept
8. Feeling of belonging
9. Socially acceptable goals
10. Exertion of genuine effort
11. Willingness to share with others
12. Concern with how much "we" can get rather than how much "I" can get

The Need for Success

Adler was struck by the importance of the hunger for success in human life—that is, the ways people seek power and prestige and strive for goals associated with social approval. He was concerned with the problems of competition, blocked ambition, feelings of resentment and hostility, and impulses to struggle and resist or to surrender and give in. Adler shifted his clinical attention from a primary focus on clients' psychosexual history to an examination of their success/failure pattern, or style of life. Adler's term *style of life* emphasizes the direction in which the individual is moving. Style-of-life analysis involves an assessment of children and adolescents for their habitual responses to frustration, to assumption of responsibility, and to situations that require exercising initiative.

Goals of Behavior

Adler's individual psychology emphasizes the nature of human strivings as having purpose. All behavior, including emotions, is goal directed (Carlson & Glasser, 2004). According to Adlerian theory, the issue is not the cause of the behavior but determining what children want to accomplish, either in the real world or in their own minds. Behaviors do not continue over time unless they "work" for children. By looking at the consequences of children's behaviors, adults can determine their goals. Adler's conception was that people are guided by a striving for ideal masculinity. Adler described what Horney (1950) termed the *neurotic search for glory*: Neurotics are characterized by an unrealistic goal of masculinity and mastery that they strive to overcome or attain. Adler also anticipated later psychoanalytic groupings in his emphasis on the social and constitutional determinants of one's style of life. To Adler, the term *individual psychology* emphasized the unity of personality as opposed to Freud's emphasis on instincts common to all people. An individual builds a style of life from interactions between heredity and environment; these lifestyle building blocks fit a person into life as that person perceives it.

Lifestyle

Adler believed that a person's behavior must be studied from a holistic viewpoint. Usually by around 6 years, children have drawn general conclusions about life and the "best" way to meet the problems life offers. They base these conclusions on their biased perceptions of the events and interactions that go on around them and form the basis for their lifestyle. The style of life, unique for each individual, is the pattern of behavior that will predominate throughout that person's life. Only rarely does a person's lifestyle change without outside intervention. Understanding their lifestyle—that is, the basic beliefs they developed at an early age to help organize, understand, predict, and control their world—is important for adults, but children who have not reached the formal stage of cognitive development have trouble understanding their lifestyles. Therefore, in working with children, Adlerians focus on the immediate behavioral goals rather than on long-term goals. Socratic questioning methods help children learn their current lifestyle and goals through self-discovery.

Adlerians think that style of life can be structured around themes or personality priorities that are pleasing, superior, comfortable, and control of self or others (Fall et al., 2010). The following sections contain more information about those themes. The assumptions of a person's lifestyle include private rules of interaction that connect a person's actions, or the personality priorities. Everyone has a number-one priority and has access to the other priorities they use to work for the number-one priority. When someone is stressed, the number-one priority is the most obvious. Finally, no priority is better than any other one; all have advantages and disadvantages (Fall et al., 2010).

Maniacci et al. (2014) discuss lifestyle as a client's self-concept, self-ideal, worldview, and ethical convictions. They provide this shorthand example of these connections:

I am small and weak (self-concept).

I should be big and strong (self-ideal).

The world is a tough place where only real mean survive (worldview).

It is better to be the top dog than to be eaten by the other dogs (ethical convictions) (pp. 67–68).

Stiles and Wilborn (1992) developed a lifestyle instrument for children. That assessment describes those who responsibly cope with and solve problems and those who engage in social interest activities that help others. Based on Adler's four lifestyle types, the scale reflected six lifestyle themes: *pleasing, rebelling, getting, controlling, being inadequate, and being socially useful.* They found that boys (ages 8 to 11) scored higher than girls of the same age on rebelling; girls scored higher on pleasing.

Social Interest

Gemeinschaftsgefuhl, Adler's term for social connectedness, has been translated as social interest but Ansbacher (1992) said that community connectedness is a better translation. Social interest is a feeling for and cooperation with people—that is, a sense of belonging and participating with others for the common good. Ansbacher (1992) and Mosak (1991) talked about social interest as a cluster of feelings, thoughts, and actions. Feelings connected to social interest include optimism, faith in others, and courage to be imperfect. Thoughts attached to social interest include these beliefs: (1) assuming personal goals do not have to interfere with social welfare, and (2) others deserve to be treated as I would like to be. Community connectedness is the sense of participating in a larger community in productive ways. Watts (2007) suggested using both terms to capture Adler's meaning. He explained that *social interest* is the behavioral aspects of the concept because it relates to ways the individual handles the life tasks of love, friendship, and work in the social context. Social interest is the more concrete, workable term, whereas *community feeling* deals with the spiritual, universal order of a person's life and the emotional, motivational aspects of *gemeinschaftsgefuhl.*

Everyone has a need to belong to a group. Although social interest is inborn, it does not appear spontaneously, but rather must be encouraged and trained, beginning with the relationship between the newborn infant and his or her mother. Children who feel they are part of a group do useful things that contribute to the well-being of that group; those who feel left out—and therefore inferior—do useless things to prove their own worth by gaining attention. From this concept comes the idea that misbehaving children are discouraged children—that is, children who think that they can be known only in useless ways. Children behave within the social context. Accordingly, their behavior cannot be studied in isolation. The study of human interaction is basic to individual psychology.

Many of life's problems center on conflicts with others. Solutions for these problems involve cooperating with people in the interest of making society a better place to live. A strong point in Adler's theory is his understanding of the implications of the social structure of life. Because every individual depends on other people for birth and growth; for food, shelter, and protection; and for love and companionship, a great web of interdependence exists among people. Thus, the individual, Adler pointed out, owes a constant debt to society. Each person is responsible to the group, and those who do not learn to cooperate are destroyed. Adler thought social interest was exhibited through such qualities as friendliness, cooperation, and empathy. He believed that a person cannot violate the love and logic that bind people together without dire consequences for the health of one's personality. Pronounced egocentricity (the opposite of social interest) leads to neurosis, and the individual becomes healthy again only when this egocentricity is renounced in favor of a greater interest in the well-being of the total group. Critics of Adlerian theory who hold a less positive view of human nature point out that people know they should cooperate but ordinarily do not do so until forced.

ENVIRONMENTAL FACTORS

Three environmental factors affect the development of a child's personality: family constellation, family atmosphere, and relationships. Through the family atmosphere, children learn about values and customs and try to fit themselves into the standards their parents set. Family atmosphere refers to the tone of the family and includes the qualities of mood, order, and relationships. Mood is the emotional style such as where families fit on the ranges between sad–happy, cold–warm, tense–relaxed, or pessimistic–optimistic. Order means the stability and structure of the relationships and the activity patterns of the family that can range from predictable to unpredictable, rigid to flexible, arbitrary to rational, and confusing to clear. Relationships refer to the patterns of interactions between members of the family that may extend from dominant to submissive, superior to inferior, distant to close, or accepting to rejecting (Kelly & Lee, 2007).

The Family Constellation

Children also learn about relationships by watching how their family members interact and about sex roles by seeing the patterns adopted by their parents. The family constellation is important in that children formulate personalities based on how they interpret their positions in the family relative to other siblings. The firstborn child dethroned by a new baby tries very hard to maintain the position of supremacy and seeks recognition by whatever means possible. The second child feels inadequate because someone is always ahead and seeks a place by becoming what the older child is not; this second child may feel squeezed out by a third child and adopt the position that life is unfair. The youngest child may take advantage of being the youngest and become outstanding in some respect, good or bad, even by becoming openly rebellious or helpless. Kottman (2010) describes these child dynamics as "boxes" or categories in which the child places self—examples are the smart child, the lazy child, the good child, the bad child, the sick child, and so on.

Although certain characteristics are associated with each child's *birth order* (one of the Adlerian birth positions: first, second, middle, youngest, and only), there are many exceptions; thus, not all firstborns are alike. Maniacci et al. (2014) discuss the study of birth order and ordinal position having limited value because of the confounding variables of family size and number of children; for example, the second-born child is the youngest in a two-child family and the middle child in a three-child family. Those authors note that parents profoundly affect these birth-order priorities and that sibling relationships are crucial, even if those connections do not fit into these traditional birth-order roles.

Mosak and Maniacci (2011) more fully explain that Adlerians view family constellation in terms of psychological birth-order position, a person's perception about birth position. Adlerians do not assume a one-to-one relationship between family position and traits. They recognize that whatever relationship exists must be understood in terms of the family climate and total family context. Yet Adlerians do accept that in an effort to find their special place in the family, children tend to select different roles, behaviors, and interests. In general, some stereotypical behaviors based on birth order have been cataloged by Adlerians over the past century.

ONLY CHILDREN   Only children are little people in a world of big people. The only child enjoys some intellectual advantages by not having to share his or her mother and father with any siblings. Only children may feel very competent and not be compelled to compete with other children. This advantage may help them form responsible and helpful life patterns (Fall et al., 2010). They may mature early. They may also experience difficulties outside the home when peers and teachers do not pamper them, and only children may be skillful in getting along with adults, but not in making friends with their peers. They may feel threatened that their significance is less with other children around. They may withdraw as a result. Generally, they enjoy being the center of attention and they may combine the achievement push of older children with the creativity of later-born (Seligman & Reichenberg, 2014). Observing how they gain the approval and attention to maintain their center-stage position can help a counselor understand these children. Have they developed skills? Do they elicit sympathy by being helpless? Or, do they act shy?

FIRSTBORN CHILDREN   Often considered the special child by the family, especially if a male child, firstborns enjoy their number-one ranking but often fear dethronement by the birth of a second child. Firstborns work hard at pleasing their parents. They are likely to be conforming achievers, defenders of the faith, introverted, and well behaved. Twenty-three of the first twenty-five astronauts were firstborn men. The National Aeronautics and Space Administration (NASA) was interested in recruiting high-achieving followers for the space program; it had no need for "creative astronauts" who might decide to take the scenic route home. Firstborns often find themselves functioning as substitute parents in larger families. Dependable, well-organized, and responsible, the oldest child may be fairly traditional (Seligman & Reichenberg, 2014). Fall et al. (2010) stated that when the second child comes, the secure oldest may try even harder to be the best, the star, the responsible, achievement-oriented exemplar, and the person in charge of the family ideals. The less secure child may become hostile or take on infantile behaviors. Dealing well with the birth of the next child will help firstborns be more affiliative and confident (Seligman & Reichenberg).

SECOND-BORN CHILDREN   Second-born children may be those extroverted, creative, free-thinking spirits that NASA was trying to avoid. More often than not, second-born children look at what is left over in the way of roles and behavior patterns that the firstborn child has shunned; picking another role is easier than competing with an older sibling who has a head start. Second-born children may get lower grades in school, even if they are brighter than their older sibling. Parents are often easier on second-born children and show less concern with rules. In fact, second-born children may be the family rebels—with or without a cause! In any case, a second-born is usually the opposite of the first child. Second-born children are easily discouraged by trying to compete with successful, older, and bigger firstborns. The more successful firstborns are, the more likely second-born children are to feel unsure of themselves and their abilities. They may even feel squeezed out, neglected, unloved, and abused when the third child arrives. The pressure to catch up and compete may lead second-born children to succeed in more creative and less conventional areas and to emphasize social over academic success. They tend to be caring, friendly, and expressive (Seligman & Reichenberg, 2014).

MIDDLE CHILDREN   Some of the idiosyncrasies common to the middle-child position may affect second-born children. Middle children are surrounded by competitors for their parents' attention. They have the pace-setting standard-bearers in front and the pursuers in the rear. Middle children often label themselves as squeezed children. They may search for a way to be special. However, many younger children increase their skills in academic, athletic, and other pursuits through competition with older siblings. With positive parents who encourage and value their individual strengths, these children become well-adjusted, friendly, creative, and ambitious (Seligman & Reichenberg, 2014).

YOUNGEST CHILDREN   Often referred to as Prince or Princess Charming, the youngest child could find a permanent lifestyle of being the baby in the family and being pampered by all. Youngest children often get a lot of service from all the other family members, and they may feel they should always be cosseted. They may become dependent or spoiled and lag in development. Youngest children readily develop real feelings of inferiority because they are smaller, less able to take care of themselves, and often not taken seriously. The really successful charmers may learn ways to manipulate the entire family. They decide either to challenge their elder siblings or to evade any direct struggles for superiority. Then again, the path is marked and the trail is broken for the youngest child. Family guidelines are clear, and the youngest children always retain their position. Perhaps the downside is the child's perception that a lot of catching up is necessary to ever find a place in the family. Nonetheless, these late born children often become adventurous, easygoing, empathic, social, and innovative, pursuing interests different from their siblings (Seligman & Reichenberg, 2014)

"Belonging," in Adlerian thought, means finding one's place in the family (Fall et al., 2010). With a 5-year difference between two children in a family, the situation changes and the next-born child often assumes the characteristics of a firstborn; apparently, the gap removes the competitive barriers found between children who are closer in age.

Large families appear to offer some advantages in child rearing by making it tough for parents to over-parent each child. Children in large families frequently learn how to solve their own problems, take care of themselves, and handle their own conflicts because their parents cannot give personal service and attention to each and every problem. Large families are probably good training grounds for learning how to be independent.

The following factors influence the perceptions children have of their particular roles in their family:

1. The parents may have a favorite child.
2. The family may move.
3. Parents become more experienced and easygoing as they grow older.
4. Some homes are single-parent homes.
5. The children may have a stepparent living in the home.
6. The family climate changes with each addition to the family.
7. Chronic illnesses or handicaps may be a problem in the family.
8. A grandparent may live in the home.
9. Some families are blended families.

In summary, too much emphasis on birth-order and ordinal position works in opposition to the Adlerian principle of free choice. People with the same birth order may share some commonalities, but they are not predestined to have the identical life scripts. Predicting a child's temperament or lifestyle or anything else based on anything other than the child's words and behaviors weakens the bond and understanding counselors need to work effectively with children. The key question for counselors is not birth order, but rather how each child finds his or her place in the family.

The Family Atmosphere and Relationships

Adlerians stress the importance of the family atmosphere in the development of the child. Whereas the family constellation is a description of how family members interact, the family atmosphere is the style of coping with life that the family has modeled for the child. It is the emotional tone that families demonstrate. The following 12 family atmosphere profiles are indications of how a negative family atmosphere can adversely affect children:

1. *Authoritarian.* The authoritarian home requires unquestioned obedience from the children. Children have little or no voice in family decisions. Although these children are often well behaved and mannerly, they also tend to be more anxious and outer directed. The child who once was shy may turn into a rebel with a cause in later life.
2. *Suppressive.* In tune with the authoritarian home is the suppressive family atmosphere, in which children are not permitted to express their thoughts and feelings. Expression of opinion is limited to what the parents want to hear. Frequently, children from such a family cannot express their ideas or feelings when they are allowed to in situations outside the home such as counseling. This type of family atmosphere does not encourage close relationships or independence.
3. *Rejecting.* Children feel unloved and unaccepted in this family atmosphere. some parents do not know how to show love and frequently cannot separate the deed from the doer. Children and parents need to know and understand that

love can be unconditional and not tied to unacceptable behavior; for example, "I love you, but I am still angered by your irresponsibility." A child can easily become extremely discouraged in the rejecting family.

4. *Disparaging.* A child criticized by everyone else in the family often turns out to be the "bad egg" everyone predicted. Too much criticism generally leads to cynicism and inability to form good interpersonal relationships.

5. *High standards.* Children living in the high-standards atmosphere may think such things as "I am not loved unless I make all As." Fear of failure leads to the considerable distress perfectionist people experience. The tension and stress these children have often prevent them from performing as well as they are able.

6. *Inharmonious.* In homes with considerable quarreling and fighting, children learn the importance of trying to control other people and keeping others from controlling them. Power becomes a prime goal for these children. Discipline may be inconsistent or harsh in these homes, depending on the mood of the parents.

7. *Inconsistent.* Inconsistent methods of discipline and home routines are often sources of confusion and disharmony in the home. Lack of self-control, low motivation, self-centeredness, instability, and poor interpersonal relationships are often attributed to inconsistency in parenting practices.

8. *Materialistic.* In the materialistic type of home, children learn that feelings of self-worth depend on possessions and on comparisons with what peers own. Interpersonal relationships take a backseat to accumulating wealth.

9. *Overprotective.* Overprotective homes often prevent children from growing up because parents do too much for them. They protect the children from the consequences of their behavior and, in doing so, deny the reality of the situation. This parental overindulgence leads to a child who feels helpless and dependent. Dependent children fall into the class of outer-directed people who rely on others for approval.

10. *Pitying.* Like overprotectiveness, pitying also prevents children from developing and using the resources they have for solving their problems. Such may be especially the case with handicapped children, who may be encouraged to feel sorry for themselves and to expect favors from others to make up for their misfortunes.

11. *Hopeless.* Discouraged and "unsuccessful" parents often pass on these attitudes to their children, who make hopelessness a part of their lifestyle. A pessimistic home atmosphere may be due to economic factors, especially if the breadwinners lack financial resources.

12. *Martyr.* People experiencing low self-esteem, hopelessness, and discouragement may have another pessimistic viewpoint, martyrdom. Once again, children may learn that life is unfair and that people should treat them better; martyrdom is a breeding ground for dependency.

Families may exhibit more than one set of these characteristics over time and across different situations. Children will assume the primary atmosphere based on what they consider happens more often or what makes the most impact on them or what they can best predict. Their behavior then is most influenced by their perception of family atmosphere. Unpredictable family atmosphere in childhood may produce adults who are anxious, believing that is the way to prepare for the future (Maniacci et al., 2014).

THEORY OF COUNSELING

Adler (1938, 1964) held that four ties create reality and meaning in people's lives:

1. People are on earth to ensure the continuance of the human species.
2. Our survival depends on our need to cooperate with our fellow human beings.
3. Human beings have a masculine and a feminine side of their personalities.
4. Human problems can be grouped into three categories: relationships, work life, and love life.

Likewise, all people have the life tasks of occupation, society, and love. Occupation involves ways people use their abilities to contribute to society. Children's occupation task occurs first in play and then in school. The task of society incorporates the quality of connections to others. This task is extremely important to children and adolescents who strive for friendships and connections. The task of love means the ability to establish and maintain satisfying intimate relationships such as a child with parents or with a love partner.

As noted earlier, the psychologically healthy person has developed a social interest and commits to the tasks of life. That person has confidence and optimism, a sense of belonging and contributing, and the courage to be imperfect (Maniacci et al., 2014).

Adler viewed the counselor's job as helping the child substitute realistic goals for unrealistic life goals as well as instilling social interest and concern for others. To be healthy, children need to recognize and develop a sense of meaning in giving to others, to work through feelings of inferiority with courage, and to believe they belong. Parents are instrumental in creating an environment that allows children to develop those goals in order to become healthy adults.

Maladjustment, to Adlerians, does not mean someone is mentally ill but rather the person is discouraged. Those troubled humans have not found useful ways of belonging and being significant. They cannot cope with feelings of inferiority or other problems they encounter in life (Oberst & Stewart, 2003). They are people who see themselves as inadequate and may create symptoms to escape the tasks of life or accomplish superiority at the expense of others. Kelly and Lee (2007) discussed three factors as the root of discouragement: (1) being overambitious, (2) lacking courage, and (3) having a pessimistic attitude. Typical challenges for children and adolescents who are discouraged revolved around inferiority feelings in school, friends, and/or family.

Basic inferiority, to Adler, characterizes every person at birth and to different degrees across life during which people try different strategies to compensate for that state. Inferiority feelings refer to self-evaluation, every person's emotions about being inferior. Inferiority complex means the ways a person acts due to the belief one is inferior (Fall et al., 2010).

Children try to protect themselves by what Adler (1983) called "self-guarding devices," which Clark (1999; Clark & Butler, 2012) outlined in four patterns: distancing, hesitating, detouring, and narrowing the path. *Distancing* refers to withdrawing from threats or challenge by doubts, indecision, and isolation. People who use the safeguard of *hesitating* confront the task of life but then explain why they cannot accomplish it. *Detouring* people protect themselves from failure by focusing on something else in order to avoid failure. Finally, in the *narrowed path* form of safeguard, a person accepts only tasks that are easy to accomplish so that they avoid failure but they also underachieve. The self-guarding devices allow people to remain in their discouraged and inferior state. The inferiority complex includes symptoms such as self-guarding devices used to evade the tasks of life and responsibility for meeting them.

Relationship

For Adlerians, counselors represent health. They are genuine, fallible, laugh at themselves, and care about others—they are models of social interest (Seligman & Reichenberg, 2014). The relationship between counselor and client is cooperative, a connection that allows the client to be open and active in challenging assumptions. The counseling relationship is in fact a training ground for the client to enhance social interest (Fall et al., 2010). The counselor emphasizes the importance of the client's involvement in the therapeutic relationship by setting goals, discussing concerns, and following through on plans.

The effective Adlerian clinician educates, collaborates, and encourages. Counselors educate about social interest and the purpose of behavior. Counselors collaborate rather than taking total control or assuming responsibility for change. The practitioner encourages the person to face the tasks of life with courage and a sense of social interest. The counselor models that healthy interest in others (Fall et al., 2010). Adler (1983) admonished counselors to see things from the client's perspective, understand the purpose of the client's behavior, and shed light on the client's style of life. With those steps in mind, Adler said counselors would never forget what to do next. Components of effective Adlerian counseling include being interested in the client's world, understanding motives, and pointing out patterns while encouraging the client.

Mosak and Maniacci (2011) considered three factors necessary for effective counseling. First, the person coming to counseling must have faith in the counselor. Practitioners may boost faith by explaining the process of counseling; being wise, strong, and assured; and listening without criticizing. Hope is another necessary component. Since Adlerians believe that people who hurt are discouraged, a critical part of counseling is encouragement. Counselors talk about their faith in the person and avoid being judgmental or overly demanding. Counseling is a "we" experience in which people do not feel alone but do feel secure in the counselor's strength and competency. The third component is love, the client knowing that the counselor cares. Mosak and Maniacci reminded counselors that the counseling relationship may be the client's first experience with a healthy interpersonal connection, a place to learn that good and bad relationships are products of people's efforts.

The establishment of the counselor–client relationship is the key step in the counseling process. The counselor's job is to re-educate children who have developed mistaken ideas about some concepts of their lives. The counseling relationship assumes that the counselor and child are equal partners in the process, and that the child is a responsible person who can learn better ways to meet personal needs. The positive view of human nature is indicated through the counselor's faith, hope, and caring attitude toward the child.

Counselors approach children understanding that no matter what children are doing, they are probably doing the best they can at the moment. Counselors may help relieve some anxiety and conflict by helping children interpret what is happening and giving the problem, child, or action a "handle." Counselors can change negative situations to positive ones by telling fables where appropriate; for example, "The Miller and the Donkey" helps children understand they can never please everyone, even by absurdly attempting the impossible like trying to carry the donkey. "The Frogs in the Milk" tells about two frogs who jumped into a barrel of milk and simply paddled until they made butter; then they were then able to jump out easily.

Goals

Mosak (1995) and Mosak and Maniacci (2011) identify six common factors as the goals of Adlerian counseling:

- Promoting social interest
- Decreasing feelings of inferiority, overcoming discouragement, and recognizing resources
- Changing lifestyle perceptions and goals
- Altering faulty motivation
- Teaching the person to realize the equality among humans and acceptance of self and others
- Encouraging the person to become a contributing person in the world community

The counselor helps the client discover the basic mistakes of private logic on which lifestyle is built. The client can then change the beliefs and bring those beliefs more in line with social interest (Fall et al., 2010).

Children may be in counseling because life is not working for them. Adlerians understand that as being discouraged, not belonging and operating from an unhealthy style of life. Children need to feel good about finding a place in life and about their progress in overcoming the unpleasant sense of inferiority associated with the dependence, smallness, and vulnerability introduced in early childhood.

Adler recognized two fundamental styles of life: through strength and power or through weakness. A person usually tries power first; if power is blocked, a person chooses another road to the goal. The second road is paved with gentleness and bids for sympathy. If both roads fail, secondary feelings of inferiority arise. These secondary inferiority feelings, which Adler considered more serious than the primary, universal inferiority feelings, are ego problems, which can be the most burning problems of all. The focus of counseling, therefore, is harnessing this drive to compensate for weakness so that positive, constructive behavior results. Freud held that the backbone of civilization was sublimation. Adler thought that talent and capabilities arise from the stimulus of inadequacy. Adlerians believe that people are pulled by their goals and priorities. Knowledge of these goals is a major key to understanding behavior for Adlerian counselors. Four personality priorities relate to the need to belong and counselors may recognize these by their own reactions to children who exhibit these ways of gaining significance:

1. *To please others:* The main objective of pleasing others is to avoid rejection. Although other people may find a "me last" person quite easy to accept, the price for this behavior may be the rejection the person is trying to avoid. The "me last" position may also limit a person's growth and opportunities for learning, personal development, and general success in life. The pleasing attitude is supported by the faulty belief that "My meaningfulness and survival depend on whether I am loved by all," or that "Life is good when my approval rating is high and bad when it is not." When working with someone who uses this method of belonging, counselors may be pleased as the client's desire to be unselfish has been accomplished.

2. *To be superior:* The main objective of trying to be superior is to avoid meaninglessness. The price for superiority may be an overloaded lifestyle. Children may become overly responsible and perfectionistic, with all the resulting worry and anxiety when things are not perfect. People holding superiority as their number-one priority attempt to avoid insignificance by influencing others through high achievement, leadership, and martyrdom. The superiority priority is supported by the faulty belief that "I am meaningful and therefore can survive only if I am better, wiser, or know more than others." With these clients, counselors may feel inadequate or inferior.

3. *To control:* The main objective of trying to control oneself, others, and the environment is to avoid unexpected humiliation. Controlling others tends to make them feel challenged, with the resulting price of increased social distance. Too much self-control results in an extremely structured life with little spontaneity. Control people are best described as uptight, and their faulty belief is that "I am meaningful and therefore can survive only if I can control my life and the events and people who are part of my life." Counselors may react to these who want to be in charge by feeling challenged, as though they were in a struggle.

4. *To be comfortable:* Avoidance of stress and pressure is the main objective of those holding comfort as their number-one priority. At their extreme, comfort seekers specialize in unfinished business and unresolved problems and conflicts. They adopt a reactive rather than proactive stance toward life. Delayed gratification is not one of their strengths; they often give way to the self-indulgent attitude of "I want what I want now." The comfort-seeking priority is supported by the faulty beliefs that "I am meaningful and therefore can survive only if I am left alone, unpressured, and free to move" and "Life is bad when I am uncomfortable." Counselors may feel irritated or impatient with these clients who want no one to "rock the boat" (Fall et al., 2010; Brown, 1976; Seligman & Reichenberg, 2014).

Each priority has a price. As is done in the practice of reality therapy, the counselor can confront children and adults with a cost analysis of their chosen priorities.

Because people are often reluctant to give up their number-one priority, counseling may focus on cost reduction by exploring how clients can manage their priorities in more cost-efficient ways. As is done in the practice of cognitive therapy, the counselor can ask clients to modify their faulty beliefs that meaningfulness and survival rest solely on the total and constant fulfillment of their number-one priority.

Goals of Misbehavior

As children grow and interact with their environment, they gradually develop methods for achieving their basic goal: belonging. Several factors, including the child's place in the family, the quality of the parents' interaction with the child, and the child's creative reaction to the family atmosphere, are critical in the development of coherent patterns of behaviors and attitudes.

Dreikurs and Soltz (1991) make an especially insightful and useful analysis of the immediate goals by which children attempt to achieve their basic goal of belonging. Children with no pattern of misbehavior have an immediate goal of cooperation and constructive collaboration. They find their places and feel good about themselves through constructive cooperation. They generally approach life with the goal of collaborating, and their usual behavior is socially and personally effective. Dinkmeyer, Mckay, and Dinkmeyer (2007) list four goals of positive behavior that mirror the above. The first goal is of attention, involvement, and contribution. The second is of autonomy and self-responsibility. The third goal of positive behavior is of justice and fairness, a child who is cooperative and responds to cruelty with kindness. The final goal of positive behavior is avoiding conflict and accepting the opinions of others.

By contrast, discouraged children with a pattern of misbehavior are usually pursuing one of four mistaken goals: attention, power, revenge, and inadequacy (or withdrawal). Understanding the goal for which a misbehaving child is striving helps put the behavior in perspective and provides a basis for corrective action. A helpful clue to the goal of the misbehavior is the reaction of the adult. For example, four children may be tapping a pencil on the desk, the teacher may be annoyed with one, ready to argue with another, hurt by the other, and ready to give up on another—those reactions signal different mistaken goals of behavior which are outlined below.

ATTENTION   All children seek attention, especially those of preschool age. However, excessive attention-getting behavior should diminish in the primary school years before it becomes a problem to teachers, parents, and peers. The child's goal is to keep an adult busy, and the adult's natural reaction is to feel annoyed and provide the service and attention the child seeks. Attention-getting behavior appears in four forms:

1. *Active constructive.* This child may be the model child, but with the goal to elevate self, not to cooperate. This is the successful student whose industrious and reliable performance is for attention only.
2. *Passive constructive.* This charming child is not as vigorous as the active-constructive child about getting attention. This child is a conscientious performer and a prime candidate for teacher's pet.

3. *Active destructive.* This nuisance child is the prime candidate for the child most likely to ruin a teacher's day—the class clown, show-off, and mischief maker.
4. *Passive destructive.* This lazy child gets a teacher's attention through demands for service and help. This child often lacks the ability and motivation to complete work.

POWER   Some children have an exaggerated need to exercise power and superiority. They take every situation, debate, or issue as a personal challenge from which they must emerge the winner; otherwise, these children think they have failed. The child's goal is to be the boss. A teacher's or parent's reaction ranges from anger to feeling threatened or defeated. The child acts in a stubborn, argumentative way and may even throw tantrums; this child leads the league in disobedience. The power struggle takes two forms:

1. *Active destructive.* This child is the rebel who has the potential of leading a group rebellion.
2. *Passive destructive.* This child is stubborn and forgetful and also could be the lazy one in the group.

REVENGE   Some children feel hurt and mistreated by life. Their goal is to get even by hurting others. They may achieve social recognition for their aggressiveness, although they usually make themselves unpopular with most other children. The child's goal, then, is to even the score, and the adult's reaction is usually to feel hurt. Revenge has two forms:

1. *Active destructive.* This child is violent and resorts to stealing, vandalism, and physical abuse to extract revenge. This child is a candidate to become a gang leader.
2. *Passive destructive.* This child is violent, but in a passive way, that is, quiet, sullen, or defiant. Both revenge types believe their only hope for alleviating hurt feelings lies in getting even.

INADEQUACY OR WITHDRAWAL   Many children often feel inferior and think they are incapable of handling life's problems. Their deficiencies may be real or imagined. By giving up, they hope to hide their inferiority and to prevent others from making demands on them. The child's goal is to be left alone, and the adult's reaction is helplessness and giving up. Inadequacy has only one form: passive destructive. These children usually are described as hopeless. They often put on an act of being stupid just to discourage the teacher from asking them to do work. They may have an unwritten contract with their teachers that says, in effect, "I'll leave you alone if you leave me alone."

Manly (1986) has adapted the four-goal questions into an informal inventory for use with students who have been referred to her for behavior or attitude problems. Manly tells her students that the goals inventory will help her know them better and know what they think. The goals inventory may be taken as a pencil-and-paper checklist or as an interview between counselor and client. Students are asked to indicate which of the following sentences are true for them:

ATTENTION

_____ I want people to notice me.

_____ I want people to do more for me.

_____ I want to be special.

_____ I want some attention.

POWER

_____ I want to be in charge.

_____ I want people to do what I want to do.

_____ I want people to stop telling me what to do.

_____ I want power.

REVENGE

_____ I think I have been treated unfairly.

_____ I want to get even.

_____ I want people to see what it is like to feel hurt.

_____ I want people to feel sorry for what they have done.

DISPLAY OF INADEQUACY

_____ I want people to stop asking me to do things.

_____ I want people to feel sorry for me.

_____ I want to be left alone. I can't do it anyway.

_____ I know I'll mess up, so there's no point in trying.

The questions may be intermixed or administered in these groupings. The four-goal labels are not included on the inventory.

As mentioned earlier, the four mistaken goals of misbehavior are pursued by students who are having difficulty finding their place in their peer group by exhibiting appropriate behaviors. All four goals are referred to as mistaken goals because they are based on faulty logic by students who resort to them to get what they want, whether it is attention, power, revenge, or avoidance of failure (withdrawal and giving up). Most misbehavior by children will be directed toward one or more of the four goals. However, adolescents begin to develop their capacity to incorporate more examples of faulty logic into their belief systems. Hence, each new faulty belief can result in a new goal of misbehavior. For example, the irrational idea "I must be perfect" could lead a student to engage in several types of perfectionistic behavior that make life miserable for the student. Most irrational messages produce failure because they lead to unattainable goals. Therefore, when counseling adolescent students, it is important to help them examine the faulty logic behind their behavior, as well as the goal of the misbehavior. Changing some language may help; for example, the word *must* to *it would be nice if* appears to help adolescents put irrational messages in a better perspective. For example, "It would be nice if I were perfect, but since I'm human and humans make mistakes, it is okay to make mistakes, and I'm okay when I do."

COUNSELING METHOD

Adler based the counseling methods he pioneered on his experience and philosophy about the nature of people. Later Adlerians, including Rudolf Dreikurs, Heinz Ansbacher, Harold Mosak, and Don Dinkmeyer, have used and modified many of Adler's original ideas.

Adlerian counseling makes no distinction between conscious and unconscious material. The counselor uses dreams, for example, to discover the lifestyle of adult clients—that is, the type of defense used to seek superiority. Many counselors use questions similar to adult lifestyle interviews with children as a means of assessing how well things are going for the child. Next, the counselor proceeds to examine the client's academic, extracurricular, and social adjustments to see how the client has maintained or achieved superiority in each of these major areas of life and to examine the inferiority feelings that may plague the client. As stated previously, the primary goal of Adlerian counseling is to point out to the client the overcompensation and defensive patterns the client is using to solve problems and to find more successful ways of solving problems related to school, play, and other social concerns.

Assessment

As noted earlier, Adlerians are emphatically holistic. The unity of the person takes priority over any part, process, or function. Lifestyle refers to the unity of the child, the person's concrete involvement with the world (DeRobertis, 2011). Dinkmeyer, Pew, and Dinkmeyer, Jr. (1979) refer to *teleoanalytic holistic theory,* which regards any troubled or troublesome behavior as a reflection of one indivisible, unified, whole organism moving toward self-created goals. Adlerian counselors support this idea of unity in people, specifically in their thinking, feeling, and behavior—in fact, in every expression of their personality (Ansbacher & Ansbacher, 1956).

Mosak and Maniacci (2011) explain a two-part investigation of the client. First, the counselor wants to understand the person's lifestyle, and next, how the lifestyle impacts current life tasks. The analysis begins when the client enters the room, stands, and chooses a seat, words, and content. Counselors understand various communications as interpersonal scripts.

Adlerians believe that children are the artists of their own personalities and are constantly moving purposefully toward self-consistent goals. An information-gathering interview based on questions used in the adult lifestyle analysis helps to reveal the pictures children have painted of their lives and their current personality development. The information interview consists of present and past (early) recollections of the children themselves and their families, how they fit into the family constellation, and how they perceive siblings and parents in relation to themselves. Eckstein and Kern (2002) provided an invaluable guide to using these assessments. Questions often used include those in the following structured, interview guide:

Information Interview Guide

a. What type of concern or problem would you like to discuss, and how did this problem develop?

b. On a five-point scale (1 or 2 = great; 3 or 4 = medium; 5 = poor), how are things going for you?

In school? _____

With your friends? _____

With your hobbies? _____

With your parents? _____

With your brothers and sisters? _____

With your fun times? _____

c. Can you tell me about your mother and father? (Separate the answers for mother and father or for any other parental figures living at home with the child.)

What do they do?

What do they want you to do?

How do you get along with them?

How are you like your parents?

How are you different from your parents?

d. What things in your family would you like to be better?

e. Can you tell me about your brothers and sisters? (Make a list of children in the family, from eldest to youngest, with their ages.) Of all your brothers and sisters, who is:

Most like you? How?

Most different from you? How?

f. What kind of child are you?

g. What kind of child did you used to be?

h. What scares you most?

i. What used to scare you most?

j. Have any of your brothers or sisters been sick or hurt?

k. What do each of the children in your family do best?

Who is the smartest?

Best athlete?

Mother's favorite?

Father's favorite?

Hardest worker?

Best behaved?

Funniest?

Most spoiled?

Best in mathematics?

Best in spelling?

Best in penmanship?

Most stubborn?

Best looking?

Friendliest?

Strongest?

Healthiest?

Best musician?

Best with tools?

The counselor uses these and other questions initially to explore the pictures children have painted of their lives. The information helps in assessing how children are developing their lifestyles. The interview also can lead older adolescents and adults to understand their lifestyles.

Process

Fall et al. (2010) outlined four phases of the Adlerian counseling process. Counselors develop the relationship, investigate and understand the style of life, help clients gain insight, and finally collaborate with the client to revise lifestyle. The first phase, fostering a cooperative relationship, provides the foundation for change. The second phase includes understanding the style of life and ways that style impacts life tasks. Counselors consider the way the client is interacting, the manner of explaining the problem, who is blamed, and other information to assess lifestyle. Insight and reorientation are the phases that involve change and redirection. Terner and Pew (1978) provide more specifics on examining the client's personality structure (the lifestyle) in the following steps. They (Fall et al., 2010; Terner & Pew, 1978) further explained the counseling process:

> *Phase I:* Relationship and Understanding: The first phase includes an examination of the formative years of the person in his or her family constellation. For younger children, this phase is an ongoing or current event; it is an early recollection (ER) of an older adolescent or an adult.

> *Phase II:* Assessment: The second phase focuses on collecting ERs from the client's past, which are detailed in the next section. The counselor may also ask about dreams, which Adler considered problem-solving activities. The dream is an extension of the patterns of the person's life and a rehearsal of possible future actions (Mosak & Maniacci, 2011).

> *Phase III:* Insight: The objective of the third phase is to illustrate for clients what they are doing in their lives and the principles under which they are operating. Clients are confronted with the goals they are attempting to reach. This phase of insight focuses on the underlying purpose of behavior. The counselor may provide tentative hypotheses about the style of life and private logic. Those guesses by the counselor may begin with "Could it be …?" or "Is it possible …?" or "I'm wondering if this fits…." (Fall et al., 2010, p. 124). The goal for this

phase is to see the basic mistakes and develop insight by looking at the thoughts, feelings, and behaviors in the maladaptive patterns.

Phase IV: Reorientation: The fourth phase is reorientation toward living through an encouragement process designed to build clients' self-confidence. The counselor assesses strengths within clients in lieu of the problems that need to be solved and attends to how clients make themselves sick and what they need to recover. The counselor identifies discouragement—that is, the loss of self-confidence—as the root of all deficiencies. Clients now translate their growing insight into action. Counselors challenge clients to act as if they were different and to challenge their old beliefs and patterns. Adlerians believe that through this process, clients learn they have choices and control over themselves.

TECHNIQUES

Early Recollections

Adler believed accidental memories do not exist but that recollections about the past are summaries of a person's current philosophy (Fall et al., 2010). Adlerians believe memories are chosen because they reinforce the way we see ourselves, others, and the world. Counselors use early recollections (ER) to understand the child's earliest impressions of life and how the child felt about them. They ask children to remember as far back as they can, particularly recollections of specific incidents, with as many details as possible, including the child's reaction at the time. "If we took a snapshot when that happened, what would we see? How did you feel?" Three to six of those ERs help to show a pattern in the lifestyle. These recollections tend to reflect a prototype that is apparent in the lifestyle analysis. Kopp and Eckstein (2004) provide two structured protocols for using early recollections as metaphors to help clients' gain insight. Disque and Bitter (2004) also offer ways to use early recollections as do Mosak and Di Pietro (2006).

Although the occurrences children relate may not be factually accurate, they are true insofar as they reflect the children's memories and feelings. The memories shed light on the child's style of life and basic mistakes. The counselor then has a clearer idea of the child's basic view of life and how some attitudes may have mistakenly formed. Kelly and Lee (2007) and Clark (2013) suggest looking for these hints in early recollections: whether the child is active or passive, observer or participant, giving or taking, approaching or withdrawing, alone or with others. Examples of themes that may appear in these recollections and the child's accompanying mistaken beliefs include the following:

1. *Early dangers*. Be aware of the many hostile aspects of life.
2. *Happy times with adults around*. Life is great as long as many people praise and serve me.
3. *Misdeeds recalled*. Be careful that they do not happen again.
4. *Pleasure versus pain*. The easy way is best.
5. *Cheerful versus depressed*. It does not pay to be happy.

6. *Pampered versus mistreated.* I need someone to take care of me.
7. *Secure versus jeopardized.* People cannot be trusted.
8. *Reward versus punishment.* Life is good only when I get my way.
9. *Benevolent versus hostile.* Doing the right thing does not pay.
10. *Obedient versus defiant.* Stay out of trouble.
11. *Participant versus observer.* When in doubt, do something; or when in doubt, do nothing.
12. *Praise versus blame.* It is never my fault.
13. *Confident versus inferior.* I will never be good at anything.
14. *We versus I.* I should be able to do it by myself.
15. *Active versus passive.* It is always better to wait and see.
16. *Success versus failure.* Nothing ever works out well for me and never will.

Myer and James (1991) present useful guidelines on ERs as an assessment technique to discern children's behavior patterns. A nonverbal child can produce ERs as drawings and in other types of play media. Counselors can make ERs a memory game or a "make up a story about when you were small" game. Modeling what the child is to do may be helpful. At least three ERs are needed to find a child's pattern of behaviors. The process should not be rushed. The counselor's job is to help the child teach the counselor about his or her situation by summarizing content and feelings. Open-ended statements are good if the counselor is not leading the child into one of the counselor's own ERs. Myer and James recommend paying attention to context (e.g., a child alone may indicate isolation), content (e.g., recurring topics such as food, water, animals, and wearing boots have special significance for the child), people (e.g., family members left in and out of the story), movement (e.g., passivity and compliance may indicate discouragement), and feelings (e.g., hot and cold feeling words tell much about the child's outlook on life). The counselor must be careful to avoid overinterpreting or underinterpreting ERs in planning interventions for children.

With the story of a person's life from the lifestyle assessment and early recollections, the counselor may begin to hear the basic mistakes in the client's life. Mosak and Maniacci (2011) classified those in the following categories:

Overgeneralizations. "No one loves me." "I never do anything right."

False or impossible goals of security. "I have to be perfect to be loved."

Misperceptions of life and its demands. "School is impossible."

Minimization or denial of one's worth. "I'm dumb."

Faulty values. "Do whatever it takes to succeed."

Stages for Children's Insight

Actual changes in children's perspectives occur in stages. First, children are limited to afterthoughts of insight: They can clearly see what they are doing to cause mistaken ideas or unhappiness to persist, but only after they have actually misbehaved. In the second stage, children become able to catch themselves in the act of misbehaving. Added awareness enables them to sensitize themselves to inappropriate behavior. In the next stage, children have developed a heightened sense of awareness that enables them to anticipate the situation and plan a more appropriate behavior or response. These three stages match the preconventional, conventional, and post-conventional stages in Piaget's theory of moral development. Stage 3 may not occur until about age 11, if it occurs at all. De Robertis (2011) has detailed those stages within an Adlerian framework of a child's goal-setting process.

Interventions for the Four Goals of Misbehavior

The four goals of misbehavior are intended to help parents, teachers, and counselors understand a child's misconduct. Adults learn that how they feel about what the child is doing most clearly explains the child's mistaken goal (Dreikurs & Soltz, 1991). The earlier descriptions included details about the goal of getting attention, gaining power, exacting revenge, or assuming inadequacy. Analysis and description of the four mistaken goals, the ways of identifying them, and the methods of correction have resulted in an impressive array of guidance and counseling approaches to help discouraged children and their discouraged families. The steps outlined for determining a child's mistaken goals—learning the adult's corrective response to mis-behavior and the child's reaction to the correction—are both penetrating and simple. The counselor who understands the child's goal can, through counseling the child and parents, help the child develop a constructive goal and appropriate behavior.

In describing and analyzing specific immediate goals, Dreikurs and his col-leagues (Dreikurs & Grey, 1993; Dreikurs & Soltz, 1991) focus primarily on pre-adolescents. Dreikurs and his coauthors note that, in early childhood, the children's status depends on the impression they make on adults. Later, they may develop dif-ferent goals to gain social significance in their peer group and, later still, in adult society. These original goals can still be observed in people of every age. However, they are not all-inclusive; teenagers and adults have additional goals of misbehavior based on irrational self-messages (see Chapter 8). Dreikurs reminds us that people often can achieve status and prestige more easily through useless and destructive means than through accomplishment.

Dreikurs advocates modifying the motivation rather than the behavior itself. When the motivation changes, more constructive behavior follows automatically.

The "four-goal technique" requires the following steps:

- Observe the child's behavior in detail.
- Be psychologically sensitive to one's own reaction.
- Confront the child with the goal of the behavior.
- Note the recognition reflex.
- Apply appropriate corrective procedures.

Remember that misbehaving children are discouraged children trying to find their place; they are acting on the faulty logic that their misbehavior will give them the social acceptance that they desire. The first goal, attention getting, is a manifestation of minor discouragement; the fourth goal, display of inadequacy, is a manifestation of deep discouragement. Sometimes a child switches from one kind of misbehavior to another, which is often a signal that the discouragement is growing worse.

To identify a young child's goals, the counselor's own immediate response to the child's behavior is most helpful; it is in line with their expectations. The following four examples of behaviors show how the adult may feel, what the child may be thinking, what alternate behaviors exist, and what questions may come to mind about the child's behavior.

ATTENTION

You are annoyed; you begin coaxing, reminding.

Charlie thinks he belongs only when he is noticed, or life is only good when he is the center of attention.

You can (1) attend to the child when he is behaving appropriately or (2) ignore misbehavior (scolding reinforces attention-getting behavior).

You can ask: *Could it be that you want me to notice you and the only way you know how to do this is to interrupt me without permission?*

POWER

You are angry, provoked, and threatened.

Linda thinks she belongs only when she is in control or the boss, or life is good only when she gets her own way.

You can withdraw or "take your sail out of her wind" by leaving the room.

You can ask: (1) *Could it be that you want to be the boss?* (2) *Could it be that you want me to do what you want and the way you do this is to break our rules?*

REVENGE

You are deeply hurt and want to get even.

Sally thinks her only hope is to get even, or the best way to handle hurt feelings is to hurt somebody back.

You can (1) use group and individual encouragement and (2) try to convince her that she is liked by building a positive relationship with her.

You can ask: *Could it be that you want to hurt me because you have been hurt, and the only way to handle hurt feelings is to hurt back?*

INADEQUACY

You are feeling helpless, hopeless, and do not know what to do.

Tom thinks he is unable to do anything and that he belongs only when people expect nothing of him, or life is only good when adults do not require him to do difficult work.

You can show genuine faith in the child and use encouragement to help Tom begin having success in class every day.

You can ask: *Could it be that you don't feel very smart and don't want people to know, and the way to hide this is to never do any work at all?*

SEQUENCE OF THE "COULD IT BE …?" QUESTIONS A counseling interview that uses the four "Could it be?" questions might go as follows:

COUNSELOR: Alice, do you know what you were trying to get when you threw down your book (the misbehavior)?

ALICE: No. [This may be an honest response.]

COUNSELOR: Would you like to work with me so that we can find out? I have some ideas that might help us explain what you are trying to get when you threw the book on the floor. Will you help me figure this out?

ALICE: Okay.

COUNSELOR: [using one question at a time, in a nonjudgmental, unemotional tone of voice]:

- Could it be that you want Mr. Marmar to notice you more and give you some special attention?
- Could it be that you would like to be boss and have things your own way in Mr. Marmar's class?
- Could it be that you have been hurt and you want to get even by hurting Mr. Marmar and others in the class?
- Could it be that you want Mr. Marmar to leave you alone and to stop asking you all those hard questions in math?

The counselor always asks all four of these questions sequentially, regardless of the child's answers or reflexes, because the child may be operating on more than one goal at a time. The counselor observes the body language and listens carefully for the response to catch the "recognition reflex." An accurate disclosure of the child's present intentions produces a recognition reflex such as a "guilty" facial expression, which is a reliable indication of his or her goal, even though the child may say nothing or even "no." Sometimes the confrontation itself helps the child change. Another indication of the child's goal is the child's response to correction. Children who are seeking attention and get it from the teacher stop the misbehavior temporarily and then repeat it or do something similar. Children who seek power refuse to stop the disturbance or even increase it. Those who seek revenge respond to the teacher's efforts to get them to stop by switching to some more violent action. Instead of cooperating, a child acting out the fourth goal remains entirely passive and inactive.

Once the counselor suspects the goal of the child's misbehavior, confronting the child is most important. The purpose of this confrontation is to disclose and confirm the mistaken goal of the child. The emphasis is on "for what purpose," not "why."

The next step after identifying the goal of misbehavior is to choose and use appropriate corrective procedures, which may range from encouragement to logical consequences.

ENCOURAGEMENT Mosak and Maniacci (2011) have written that Adler and his followers considered encouragement a crucial aspect of living, as well as a crucial part of the counseling process. Encouragement is the key to developing positive expectations in the people we counsel, which help clients engage in wider varieties of adaptive behaviors with less stress and discomfort. Conversely, according to Mosak and Maniacci, maladaptive, pathological behavior is viewed as a reflection of discouragement, which leads to a lack of confidence. Lacking confidence, clients are likely to cling to their old, unhelpful attitudes and behaviors that give them a false sense of security but get them into trouble. Encouragement becomes an important key in breaking the vicious cycle of discouragement, which causes the client to cling to unhelpful attitudes and behaviors that, in turn, perpetuate more discouragement and a repetition of maladaptive behaviors.

Dreikurs and Soltz (1991) have written that encouragement implies faith in and respect for children as they are. One should not discourage children by having extremely high standards and ambitions for them. Children misbehave only when they believe they cannot succeed by other means. In fact, one evaluation of counseling is how far the child has moved from feeling discouraged toward feeling encouraged. Children need encouragement as plants need water and sunshine. Judgments or praise indicate to children that the next product or action may be inadequate; for example, telling children they can be better implies they are not good enough as they are.

Problems with these ideas on encouragement arise when parents ask how they are supposed *not* to expect children performing below their ability levels to do better. The answer seems to be in loving children unconditionally despite their behavior and performance. However, one does not have to love or pretend to love the child's misbehavior.

Carmichael (2006) and Seligman and Reichenberg (2014) provided some tips on ways to provide encouragement. The adult can express unconditional acceptance by talking about the value of the child without expressing a need to change. People can show faith in the child's abilities by noting the child's efforts, accomplishments, and progress rather than a product. For instance, a child who shows her dad a homework paper could be told "you did every problem on this sheet." Adults should focus on the young person's strengths and emphasize the work and the joy of the task as a mother responding to a child's efforts to fold clothes with "you really enjoy matching your socks." The encourager can focus on the positive parts of the child's contributions and ignore the negative aspects with a statement like "every game you own is on the shelf" even though clothes still litter the floor. Focusing on what is being learned rather than what has been missed is encouraging. Adults can show support for the child and model fallibility, helping the child learn from mistakes and not be devastated by them.

Encouragement is advocated in place of praise and reinforcement, but bribery is strongly discouraged. Adlerians see praise as a message that tells children that, under conditions determined by the adult, they are all right. Praise focuses on the product. Encouragement, however, accepts children as they are; it focuses on the process. Encouragement may occur *before* the child completes a task or even starts it. For example:

- "I can tell you are trying your best."
- "That's a rough one, but I think you have what it takes to work it out."
- "I know you can do it; let me help you get started."

PRAISE   Praise focuses on outcomes, uses superlatives, and is conditional (Milliren, Evans, & Newbauer, 2007). Praise (reinforcement) occurs *after* the child performs a behavior or completes a task. For example:

1. "You certainly did a good job."
2. "That was great work you did in math."
3. "I like the way you handled that."
4. "You played a good game."

DISCOURAGEMENT   Milliren et al. (2007) talked about five ways to discourage. Those are setting high or unrealistic expectations, focusing on mistakes, making comparisons, providing pessimistic interpretations, and dominating. Discouragement may come before, after, or during behavior and may sound like praise but includes a judgment that could be heard by the child as "You are not good enough" such as:

"You left out the second problem. I hope you do better on the next test."

"I see you made a good grade on your reading, but how about math?"

"Let me do that for you."

"I don't want to hear that excuse again."

BRIBERY   Bribery often occurs *during* the child's misbehavior. For example:

"If you quiet down, I'll give you a candy bar."

"I'll buy you a surprise if you stop fighting."

"If you stop bothering me, you won't have to help with the dishes."

Adlerian counselors believe that extrinsic reward and illogical punishment have detrimental effects on the development of the child. Only in an autocratic society are these reward-and-punishment systems an effective and necessary means of obtaining conformity; they presuppose a certain person is endowed with superior authority and has the right to dictate. Children may see rewards as one of their rights and soon demand a reward for everything they do if they are conditioned under this type of system. Adlerians agree with Kohn (2005), who admonishes parents to move beyond rewards and punishment, an extrinsic reward system that robs the child or adult of the intrinsic reward of simply engaging in an activity for its own enjoyment. Children rewarded for practicing the piano will begin to view playing the piano as work that nobody would do without pay. Children may interpret punishment as their right to punish others. In fact, children often are hurt more by their retaliation than by the punishment. They are experts in knowing how to hurt their parents, whether by getting into trouble or by earning low grades. Therefore, Adlerians reject reward-and-punishment methods in favor of encouragement, intrinsic reinforcement, and logical consequences.

Natural and Logical Consequences

Natural and logical consequences allow children to experience the actual consequences of their behavior focusing on the Adlerian belief that people are responsible and capable of leading full, happy lives. Consequences allow the child to understand an inner message that is more likely to be remembered than punishment, which can harm the relationship with a child.

NATURAL CONSEQUENCES   Natural consequences are a direct result of a child's behavior. Careless children who touch the hot stove get burned and become more careful of stoves in the future. Natural consequences of irresponsible behavior are unfavorable outcomes that occur naturally without any prearranged plan or program. For example, if Sue leaves her baseball glove outside and it is ruined in a rainstorm, she has experienced a natural consequence. Natural consequences to irresponsible behavior happen on their own, or naturally, without being planned and administered by others.

LOGICAL CONSEQUENCES   Logical consequences, those resulting from an intervention by another person (Sweeney, 2009), teach the social rules of life (Mosak & Maniacci, 2011). Those consequences are established through rules and family policy and are fair, direct, consistent, and logical results of a child's behavior. For example, if Frank comes home late for dinner, his family has assumed that he would have been home on time to eat or he would have called. Therefore, they removed his plate from the table. He is allowed to fix any food he can as long as he cleans up after himself. Another example of a logical consequence is, if John interferes with someone else's right to learn in school, he is moved to a place where he cannot continue to do so (some form of isolation). In other words, the consequence fits the misbehavior; it is a logical consequence. Punishment, as defined by Adlerians, is any illogical consequence for irresponsible behavior. For example, if Frank is late for dinner, he gets paddled and sent to bed. The punishment or consequence does not match the crime, but it teaches children that bigger people get to overpower smaller people. Children reared under a punishment-by-power system become very impressed with power and use it whenever they can to get what they want.

Both natural and logical consequences allow children to experience the results of their behavior instead of arbitrary punishment exercised through the parent's personal authority. These two techniques direct children's motivation toward proper behavior through personal experience with the social order in which they live. We are not recommending, however, that adults *not* protect children in dangerous situations; for example, teaching children about the dangers of street traffic through personal experience!

Natural and logical consequences give children the message that they are capable of making their own decisions. They have an opportunity for growth through weighing alternatives and arriving at a decision. Given overly severe limits, however, the child is deprived of making decisions that foster self-respect and responsibility. Children and adolescents need to do for themselves what they are capable of doing.

Case Study

Identification of the Problem

J.B., a 9-year-old boy in the fourth grade at Spoonbill Elementary School, was referred to our group by the teacher because of his classroom behavior. J.B. repeatedly leaves his seat and does not complete his work.

Individual and Background Information

Academic   According to J.B.'s teacher, J.B. does less than average work. Most of his grades are **U** (unsatisfactory). He does not usually complete his assignments; when he does, he hurries and commits many errors. His teacher believes that he is not working up to his potential in many areas. His test scores support the teacher's view that J.B. is an underachiever, although J.B. loves to read. His teacher reported that J.B.'s behavior sometimes annoyed her and at other times made her angry. She mentioned that she was discouraged about his schoolwork and out of ideas about what to do.

Family   J.B. is the youngest son of an older father and stepmother. The sibling closest to his age is 19. J.B. came to live with his father last year after spending time in a home for boys because of his abusive mother. Recently, his stepmother threatened to send him back to the home for boys if he did not behave in school and bring his grades up.

Social   J.B. has a friendly personality and seems to relate well with his peers.

Counseling Method

The counselor used the Adlerian counseling method to help J.B. identify the goals of his behavior and how well he was meeting his goals. They spent considerable time on helping J.B. understand what he did to get himself in trouble at school and what he could do to make his life more pleasant at school and at home. The counselor and J.B. looked at ways J.B. could meet his goals without getting into trouble.

Transcript

COUNSELOR: Well, J.B., it is good to see you again. We need to check up on how things are going with you in Ms. Johnson's room.

J.B.:   Did she tell you I have been bad?

COUNSELOR: She is concerned and doesn't know how to help about your schoolwork.

J.B.:   Sometimes it is just too hard.

COUNSELOR: So sometimes you feel discouraged too.

J.B.:   Yeah, I sure do.

COUNSELOR: It is sort of like sometimes you don't get the help you need.

J.B.:   She won't look at me when I raise my hand to get her to help.

COUNSELOR:	That must be frustrating to you. Do you know what I mean by frustrating?
J.B.:	Yeah, I get mad and go up by her desk, and she tells me to get back in my seat.
COUNSELOR:	So a lot of bad things seem to happen, one right after another one, and you just keep getting angrier.
J.B.:	That's right!
COUNSELOR:	Well, J.B., we've got some work to do. We need to figure out what you are trying to get and if you are getting what you want.
J.B.:	What do you mean?
COUNSELOR:	If we can find out what goals you are trying to reach, we will be able to figure out what you need to do to get what you want without getting into trouble.
J.B.:	I'm not trying to get anything.
COUNSELOR:	Could be; let's check it out.
J.B.:	Okay, I guess.
COUNSELOR:	J.B., could it be when you do your work poorly or don't do it at all, you want to get Ms. Johnson to leave you alone?
J.B.:	What do you mean?
COUNSELOR:	Maybe if you convince her you can't do the work, she and your parents will get off your back about making better grades.
J.B.:	Sometimes I really do try to do it all.
COUNSELOR:	So, you really haven't given up on making better grades.
J.B.:	Oh, no, I haven't.
COUNSELOR:	Well, could it be you would like to have Ms. Johnson pay more attention to you, and the way to do that is break rules about talking out of turn and leaving your seat?
J.B.:	Yeah, sometimes she really loses it and everybody laughs.
COUNSELOR:	So, you end up getting a lot of attention, some good and some bad.
J.B.:	Yeah, but it's worth it.
COUNSELOR:	You seemed pleased with having the attention and don't mind the consequences or bad stuff that happens to you.
J.B.:	Well, I do wish I could move back to my old seat. I don't like sitting right in front of the teacher's desk.
COUNSELOR:	So attention is important to you, but sitting close to the teacher is not what you want.
J.B.:	You got that right! Can you get me moved?
COUNSELOR:	You and I can work on it. We might be able to figure out how.
J.B.:	Let's go for it!
COUNSELOR:	We have to figure out how to convince Ms. Johnson that you can be trusted to follow the class rules and do your work when you are sitting away from her desk.
J.B.:	How?

COUNSELOR:	Well, J.B., you know her a whole lot better than I do. I would like to know what you think would work.
J.B.:	Maybe I can make a deal. She likes deals.
COUNSELOR:	How would that work?
J.B.:	Well, I could ask her if I stay out of trouble and turn in all of my work for a whole week, could I move to my old seat?
COUNSELOR:	I wonder what she will say about how well your work needs to be done.
J.B.:	I could tell her that I will make at least a B in everything.
COUNSELOR:	Well, I guess you could try that. Tell me again what the deal would be?
J.B.:	I would turn in all my work for a week and get a B on everything and then I could move back to my other seat.
COUNSELOR:	Tell you what. If Ms. Johnson agrees to your plan, would you come by the office each day on your way home and give me the word on how your day went?
J.B.:	Sure.
COUNSELOR:	If it doesn't work out, come back tomorrow, and we'll try to write a plan that will work.
J.B.:	See you.
COUNSELOR:	Let's shake hands on this deal. Hope it works out. See you tomorrow.

As noted in the interview transcript, the Adlerian counseling method works well in concert with many of the other counseling approaches discussed in this chapter. Encouragement, group discussions, and logical consequences often are used with shaping (positive reinforcement and extinction) and reframing to bring about positive behavioral change.

ADLERIAN PLAY THERAPY

An expert on Adlerian play therapy, Terry Kottman (2011) emphasizes that counselors who practice Individual Psychology understand that people are social beings who need to belong. She reminded counselors about factors important in personality formation. Those personality priorities are the need to belong and to move toward goals, as well as the creativity and uniqueness of each person. In addition, counselors are reminded that people have subjective experiences of life.

In Adlerian play therapy, the counselor tries to discover children's lifestyles and explore their private logic. The counselor can help children make conscious choices about what parts of their lifestyle they want to keep and what parts they would like to change. After changing perceptions about themselves, children can learn new ways of belonging and interacting.

Kottman (2010) explained that a counselor using Adlerian play therapy begins by assuming that the children who have been referred are discouraged children. Discouraged children have negative convictions about themselves and the world. Their self-defeating goals, behaviors, and attitudes reflect those negative convictions. The goal of Adlerian play therapy is the reduction of this discouragement. Therefore, the counselor chooses play techniques to provide encouragement to accomplish four outcomes—the Critical Cs. The counselor helps the child *connect* to others, believe in self as *capable* and confident, and see oneself as valuable and important or someone who *counts*. The counselor also builds the child's *courage* to explore new experiences and face challenges (Kottman, 1999). The practitioner may use music, art, sand, clay, stories, puppets, and other media in the play therapy process (Kelly & Lee, 2007).

This type of play therapy, what Kottman (2001) has dubbed "The Encouragement Zone," has four phases similar to the ones discussed earlier and each phase has goals (Kottman, Bryant, Alexander, & Kroger, 2008). The first phase involves establishing a democratic, empathic *relationship*. The counselor then explores the child's lifestyle, highlighting the child's beliefs, attitudes, goals, emotions, and motives in the second, *exploring* phase. The counselor's goal in the third phase is to help the child gain *insight* by interpreting the lifestyle, faulty convictions, and self-defeating goals and behaviors. During the final phase, *reorientation and re-education*, the counselor's objective is to help the child use the insight and convert it into action such as behavioral and attitudinal changes. Kottman (2011) cautions the play therapist to be alert to small shifts in attitude and behavior in the playroom and in other settings.

Kottman and Johnson (1993) as well as Ashby and Noble (2011) discuss strategies to be used during the four phases of Adlerian play therapy. The counselor can use several approaches when establishing a relationship with the child. The counselor may choose to track the behavior of the child by giving a running account of what is being done and said. The counselor may also restate the content and reflect feelings so that the child knows that emotions, behaviors, and attempts to communicate are important to the counselor. The counselor also encourages the child by conveying respect for the child's strengths, faith in the child's abilities, and recognition of the child's attempts and improvement. During the first phase of Adlerian play therapy, the counselor sets limits to protect the child and others, to prevent toys or other things from being damaged, and to deter destructive behavior. In the second phase, the counselor explores the lifestyle of the child, examining the goals of the child's behavior. Considerations of the family atmosphere, family constellation, and the ERs of the child also are important in this phase. Based on this information, the counselor begins to form a hypothesis about the child's beliefs and shares this understanding with the child. The third phase includes a deepening insight into the child's lifestyle. The counselor shares hypotheses and interpretations with the child and may use therapeutic metaphors. During the fourth phase, the counselor helps the child develop alternative behaviors that are practiced and encouraged. The counselor also consults with the adults in the child's life.

Meany-Walen, Bratton, and Kottman (2014) found significant positive outcomes on classroom disruptive behaviors after children participated in Adlerian play therapy. The emphasis on belonging and social interest creates a springboard for using Adlerian interventions in the school with children who have attention-deficit/hyperactivity disorder (ADHD). Portrie-Bethke, Hill, and Bethke (2009) integrated adventure-based counseling with Adlerian play therapy to work with children who have ADHD. Kottman (2011) suggests that Adlerian play therapy seems particularly effective for children with problem behaviors, difficulty with peers and difficult life situations such as divorce or death, as well as children with power and control issues, who have had traumatic experiences, with poor self-concepts, with family problems, and those who have poor social skills.

ADLERIAN FAMILY COUNSELING

Adlerian methods are well suited for counseling the entire family. The goals of family counseling are for members to live in social equality and to solve problems cooperatively. The tasks of Adlerian family therapy are to demonstrate mutual respect, identify problems to be resolved, develop alternative viewpoints, and participate in decision making and reaching new agreements (Kelly & Lee, 2007). The following interview guide is suggested:

Interview the parents on the following topics (while their children are observed in a playroom situation):

Describe your children—their respective ordinal positions, schoolwork, hobbies, athletics, and so on.

How does each child find his or her place in the family?

What problems revolve around getting up? Mealtime? TV? Homework? Chores? Bedtime?

Does something in your family need to be better?

Would you like to make a change? (Before the counselor gives suggestions, it is preferable that the parents admit they are bankrupt in child-rearing ideas; that is, nothing has worked in improving the particular family concern.)

Interview the children on the following topics with the parents not present. (Use "Could it be?" questions when appropriate. Ask who is in charge of discipline.)

Do you know why you are here today?

Does anything bother you in the family that you would like to change?

How can we make things better at home?

Who is the good child?

Who is Father's favorite?

Who is Mother's favorite?

Who is best in sports?

What do each of you do best?

Which are your best school subjects?

Which are your worst school subjects?

Interview the entire family. Summarize plans for the coming week, clarifying roles, behaviors, and expectations. Recommendations for each family generally include the following:

Provide individual parent time for each child, each day.

Have one family conference per week. Use collaboration and/or compromise to reach family consensus in making decisions. *No voting.* Three-to-two votes split the family, with the losing voters dragging their heels and not being enthusiastic supporters of the issue supported by the "winning" side.

Do one family activity per week.

Each family member does chores.

Dreikurs, Dinkmeyer, and others have provided a foundation for teaching parenting skills, improving family time, and helping parents raise healthy children. Dreikurs (Dreikurs, Cassell, & Ferguson, 2004) focuses on families that communicate, demonstrate respect for each other, and encourage each other. He supports education, the use of natural and logical consequences and shared responsibilities in the family, and notes that having fun together is paramount. Dreikurs discusses a family council weekly meeting to talk about concerns or difficulties that fosters a sense of belonging, responsibility, cooperation, and participation. The Active Parenting and Systematic Training for Effective Parenting (STEP) educational programs provide parents with tools to implement these ideas (Dinkmeyer, McKay, & Dinkmeyer, 2007).

DIVERSITY APPLICATIONS OF INDIVIDUAL PSYCHOLOGY

Individual psychology by title alone would seem to suggest a focus on the individual above the family, group, or society in general. This is far from the truth, however. Social interest development and the need to feel part of a group have always been main pillars supporting the practice of individual or Adlerian psychology (Sakin-Wolf, 2003). Therefore, cultural groups favoring a family, group, and/or community emphasis in counseling will find individual psychology to be a comfortable and compatible way to examine their lives and behavioral patterns for possible change. Adlerians work from an appreciation of each person's subjective view of the world. Maniacci et al. (2014) report have done detailed lifestyle assessment over the years with many clients in China, Ghana, Israel, Ireland, Iraq, Iran, South Africa, Belize, Thailand, Vietnam, Korea, Japan, France, England, Canada, Italy, Columbia, Turkey, and Germany. Those authors explain that working with people from these diverse cultures compares to having a personal tutorial in multiculturalism provided by each individual person they met. Birth order, goals of behavior, ERs, lifestyles, and faulty reasoning problems transcend most cultures, and the client is never asked to fit a certain model described by the counselor (Carlson & Carlson, 2000; Carlson, Watts, & Maniacci, 2006).

EVALUATION OF ADLERIAN THERAPY

The challenges of connecting Adlerian therapy to the movement for evidence-based practices include the focus on the individual person and complexity of the issues. Thus a case study approach rather than a randomized controlled trial method of research is needed as is a movement from the prescriptive treatment to an acknowledgement of the symptom patterns as a focus in therapy. However, many of the ideas of this therapy have been studied. Birth order (Eckstein et al., 2010), early recollections (Mosak & Di Pietro, 2006), and lifestyle themes (Kerns, Gormley, & Curlette, 2008) have considerable support as valid constructs. Baumeister and Leary (1995) validated the "need to belong" construct so relevant in Adlerian philosophy. Similarly Brown (2007) found support for the idea that people are motivated to more from a feeling of less than (inferiority) to a feeling of more than (superiority).

In addition, Adlerian counselors have modified this approach for fewer treatment sessions. Wingett and Milliren (2004) propose a brief form of Adlerian counseling quite similar to solution-focused counseling. Clients are asked to (1) describe the problem, (2) describe a time when they encountered a similar problem, (3) identify successful components of the past problem-solving strategy, and (4) apply their previously effective methods to the current problem. Their cornerstone or "miracle" question for clients is, "What would you do if I cured you immediately?" The counseling agenda can be built from their answers to this question.

Milliren et al. (2007) talked about "thin-slicing" data to get a sense of lifestyle in brief Adlerian therapy. The questions for that briefer analysis include the following:

Finish this statement: "I am the child who always...."

Which sibling is the most different from you? How? (If an only child, ask how different from other children).

What is the most positive thing about your mother? Father? What is the most negative?

What is your most unforgettable memory?

Talk about two early memories (p. 151).

The support for the effectiveness of Adlerian counseling centers then on the evidence of some of the constructs associated with the treatment and on the modification for shorter-term counseling.

SUMMARY

Seligman and Reichenberg (2014) advise that whether or not practitioners call themselves Adlerians, almost all counseling reflects some of those concepts such as the roles of early experiences on current functioning, the need to understand people in their multiple contexts, and the view of therapy as educational and growth-promoting as well as remedial.

The term *individual psychology* suggests Adler's conviction in the value, worth, and dignity of each person. Adlerian counselors assume that each person is unique, self-consistent, responsible, and capable of choices which can be constructive or destructive. Lifestyle, the system of convictions a person holds about self, others, and the world, determines the person's behaviors and goals. People become discouraged when they have not learned to meet their life tasks. Counseling is a re-education process in which clients and counselors investigate faulty perceptions and goals. The immediate goal is to encourage the client, and the ideal goal is to develop a person's social interest.

Adlerian counselors have a 100-year history of supporting a preventive approach to treating mental health problems. Adler himself proposed to school administrators in Vienna to establish child-guidance centers (Mosak & Maniacci, 2011). He also created parent-education groups that met regularly to discuss managing family problems regarding child-rearing practices and interventions. Adler emphasized problem prevention, group counseling, and educational skill building in practices which individual psychology practitioners continue to use in their work.

Lifestyle analysis is especially effective in helping people analyze their lives in light of how well their current behaviors are helping them get what they want. The Adlerians use a cognitive approach to help their clients identify the faulty logic underlying behavioral goals that get them into trouble. Clients also receive some insight on how they got to be the way they are and what they need to do to break the cycle of their ineffective or self-defeating behavioral patterns.

INTRODUCTION TO INDIVIDUAL PSYCHOLOGY

To gain a more in-depth understanding of the concepts in this chapter, visit www .cengage.com/counseling/henderson to view a short clip of an actual therapist–client session demonstrating individual psychology.

WEB SITES FOR INDIVIDUAL PSYCHOLOGY

Internet addresses frequently change. To find the sites listed here, visit www.cengage .com/counseling/henderson for an updated list of Internet addresses and direct links to relevant sites.

Adler School of Professional Psychology, Chicago

International Association of Individual Psychology

North American Society of Adlerian Psychology

New York Institute for Adlerian Therapists

REFERENCES

Adler, A. (1983). *The practice and theory of individual psychology.* Totowa, NJ: Littlefield, Adams.

Adler, A. (1964). *Social interest: A challenge to mankind.* New York: Capricorn. (Original work published 1938).

Alexander, F., Eisenstein, S., & Grotjahn, M. (1966). *Psychoanalytic pioneers.* New York: Basic Books.

Ansbacher, H. (1992). Alfred Adler's concepts of community feeling and social interest and the relevance of community feeling for old age. *Individual Psychology: The Journal of Adlerian Theory, Research, and Practice, 48,* 402–412.

Ansbacher, H., & Ansbacher, R. (1956). *The individual psychology of Alfred Adler: A systematic presentation in selections from his writings.* New York: Basic Books.

Ashby, J. S., & Noble, C. (2011). Integrating cognitive-behavioral play therapy and Adlerian play therapy into the treatment of perfectionism. In A. A. Drewes, S. C. Bratton, & C. E. Schaefer (Eds.), *Integrative play therapy* (pp. 225–240). Hoboken, NJ: Wiley.

Baumeister, R. F., & Leary, M. R. (1995). The need to belong: Desire for interpersonal attachments as fundamental human motivation. *Psychological Bulletin, 117*, 497–529.

Brown, B. (2007). *I thought it was just me (but it isn't): Telling the truth about perfectionism, inadequacy, power.* New York: Gotham Books.

Brown, J. F. (1976). *Practical applications of the personality priorities: A guide for counselors* (2nd ed.). Clinton, MD: B & F Associates.

Carlson, M., & Carlson, J. (2000). The application of Adlerian psychotherapy with Asian American clients. *Journal of Individual Psychology, 56*, 214–225.

Carlson, J., & Glasser, W. (2004). Adler and Glasser: A demonstration and dialogue. *The Journal of Individual Psychology, 60*(3), 308–324.

Carlson, J., Watts, R., & Maniacci, M. (2006). *Adlerian therapy: Theory and practice.* Washington, DC: American Psychological Association.

Carmichael, K. D. (2006). *Play therapy: An introduction.* Upper Saddle River, NJ: Merrill.

Clark, A. J. (1999). Safeguarding tendencies: A clarifying perspective. *Journal of Individual Psychology, 36*, 53–64.

Clark, A. J. (2013). *Dawn of memories: The meaning of early recollections in life.* Lanham, MD: Rowman & Littlefield Publishers, Inc.

Clark, A. J., & Butler, C. M. (2010). Degree of activity: Relationship to early recollections and safeguarding tendencies. *Journal of Individual Psychology, 68* (2), 136–148.

De Robertis, E. M. (2011). Deriving a third force approach to child development from the works of Alfred Adler. *Journal of Humanistic Psychology, 51*(4), 492–515. doi:10.1177/0022167810386960

Dinkmeyer, D., McKay, K., & Dinkmeyer, D. (2007). *The parent's handbook: Systematic training for effective parenting.* Fredericksburg, VA: STEP Publishing.

Dinkmeyer, D., Pew, W., & Dinkmeyer, D., Jr. (1979). *Adlerian counseling and psychotherapy.* Monterey, CA: Brooks/Cole.

Disque, J. G., & Bitter, J. R. (2004). Emotion, experience, and early recollections: Exploring restorative reorientation processes in Adlerian therapy. *Journal of Individual Psychology, 60*, 115–131.

Dreikurs, R., Cassell, P., & Ferguson, E. D. (2004). *Discipline without tears* (Rev. ed.). Hoboken, NJ: Wiley.

Dreikurs, R., & Grey, L. (1993). *A new approach to discipline: Logical consequences.* New York: Plume.

Dreikurs, R., & Soltz, V. (1991). *Children: The challenge (reissue edition).* New York: Hawthorn/Dutton.

Eckstein, D., Aycock, K. J., Sperber, M. A., McDonald, J., Van Wiesner III, B., Watts, R. E., & Ginsburg, P. (2010). A review of 200 birth-order studies: Lifestyle characteristics. *Journal of Individual Psychology, 66*, 402–434.

Eckstein, D., & Kern, R. (2002). *Psychological fingerprints: Lifestyle assessments and interventions* (5th ed.). Dubuque, IA: Kendall/Hunt.

Fall, K. A., Holden, J. M., & Marquis, A. (2010). *Theoretical models of counseling and psychotherapy* (2nd ed.). New York: Brunner-Routledge.

Horney, K. (1950). *Neurosis and human growth.* New York: Norton.

Kelly, F. D., & Lee, D. (2007). Adlerian approaches to counseling with children and adolescents. In H. T. Prout & D. T. Brown (Eds.), *Counseling and psychotherapy with children and adolescents: Theory and practice for school and clinical settings* (4th ed., pp. 131–179). Hoboken, NJ: Wiley.

Kerns, R. M., Gormley, L., & Curlette, W. L. (2008). BASIS-A inventory empirical studies: Research findings from 2000 to 2006. *Journal of Individual Psychology, 64*, 208–309.

Kohn, A. (2005). *Unconditional parenting: Moving from reward and punishment to love and reason*. New York: Atria Publishing.

Kopp, R., & Eckstein, D. (2004). Using early memory metaphors and client-generated metaphors in Adlerian therapy. *Journal of Individual Psychology, 60*, 163–174.

Kottman, T. (1999). Integrating the crucial Cs into Adlerian play therapy. *Journal of Individual Psychology, 55*, 288–297.

Kottman, T. (2001). Adlerian play therapy. *International Journal of Play Therapy, 10*, 1–12.

Kottman, T. (2009). Adlerian play therapy. In K. J. O'Connor & L. D. Braverman (Eds.), *Play therapy theory and practice: Comparing theories and techniques* (2nd ed., pp. 237–282). Hoboken, NJ: Wiley.

Kottman, T. (2010). *Partners in play: An Adlerian approach to play therapy* (2nd ed.). Alexandria, VA: American Counseling Association.

Kottman, T. (2011). Adlerian play therapy. In C. E. Schaefer (Ed.) *Foundations of play therapy* (2nd ed., pp. 87–104). Hoboken, NJ: Wiley.

Kottman, T., Bryant, J., Alexander, J., & Kroger, S. (2008). Adlerian play therapy in the schools. In A. Vernon & T. Kottman (Eds.), *Counseling theory applied to school counseling*. Denver, CO: Love.

Kottman, T., & Johnson, V. (1993). Adlerian play therapy: A tool for school counselors. *Elementary School Guidance and Counseling, 28*, 42–51.

Maniacci, M. P., Sackett-Maniacci, L., & Mosak, H. H. (2014). Adlerian psychotherapy. In D. Wedding & R. J. Corsini (Eds.), *Current psychotherapies* (10th ed., pp. 55–94). Belmont, CA: Thomson.

Manly, L. (1986). Goals of misbehavior inventory. *Elementary School Guidance and Counseling, 21*, 160–161.

Meany-Walen, K. K., Bratton, S. C., & Kottman, T. (2014). Effects of Adlerian play therapy on reducing students' disruptive behaviors. *Journal of Counseling & Development, 92*(1), 47–56. doi:10.1002/j.1556-6676.2014.00129.x

Milliren, A. P., Evans, T. D., & Newbauer, J. F. (2007). Adlerian theory. In D. Capuzzi & D. R. Gross (Eds.), *Counseling and psychotherapy: Theories and interventions* (4th ed., pp. 123–163). Upper Saddle River, NJ: Pearson.

Mosak, H. H. (1991). "I don't have social interest": Social interest as a construct. *Individual Psychology, 47*, 309–320.

Mosak, H. (1995). Adlerian psychotherapy. In R. J. Corsini & D. Wedding (Eds.), *Current psychotherapies* (5th ed.). Itasca, IL: F. E. Peacock.

Mosak, H. H., & Di Pietro, R. (2006). *Early recollections: Interpretative method and application*. New York: Routledge.

Mosak, H. H., & Maniacci, M. (2011). Adlerian psychotherapy. In R. J. Corsini & D. Wedding (Eds.), *Current psychotherapies* (9th ed., pp. 67–112). Belmont, CA: Thomson.

Myer, R., & James, R. (1991). Using early recollections as an assessment technique with children. *Elementary School Guidance and Counseling, 25*, 228–232.

Oberst, Y., & Stewart, A. (2003). *Adlerian psychotherapy: An advanced approach to individual psychology*. New York: Brunner-Routledge.

Portrie-Bethke, T. L., Hill, N. R., & Bethke, J. G. (2009). Strength-based mental health counseling for children with ADHD: An integrative model of adventure-based counseling and Adlerian play therapy. *Journal of Mental Health Counseling, 31*(4), 323.

Prouchaska, J. O., & Norcross, J. C. (2014). *Systems of psychotherapy: A transtheoretical analysis* (8th ed.). Stamford, CT: Cengage Learning.

Sakin-Wolf, S. (2003). Adler: East, West, and beyond. *The Journal of Individual Psychology, 59*(1), 72–83.

Seligman, L., & Reichenberg, L. W. (2014). *Theories of counseling and psychotherapy: Systems, strategies, and skills* (4th ed.). Upper Saddle River, NJ: Pearson.

Stiles, K., & Wilborn, B. (1992). A lifestyle instrument for children. *Individual Psychology, 48,* 96–105.

Sweeney, T. (2009). *Adlerian counseling and psychotherapy.* New York: Routledge.

Terner, J., & Pew, W. (1978). *The courage to be imperfect: The life and work of Rudolf Dreikurs.* New York: Hawthorn.

Watts, R. E. (2007). Counseling conservative Christian couples: A spiritually sensitive perspective. In O. J. Morgan (Ed.), *Counseling and spirituality: Views from the profession.* Boston, MA: Houghton-Mifflin

Wingett, W., & Milliren, A. (2004). "Lost? Or Stuck?" An Adlerian technique for understanding the individual's psychological movement. *Journal of Experimental Psychology, 60*(3), 265–276.

CHAPTER 12

Rational Emotive Behavior Therapy

We do not see things as they are; we see things as we are.
—THE TALMUD

Buddha (563–483 B.C.) said, "What we think, we become." Counselors who choose the rational emotive behavioral approach agree. Cognitive counselors believe that thoughts lead to emotions and behavior. Therefore, the awareness of thoughts and the decision to change what you are thinking leads to change. Albert Ellis has outlined the process for helping people discover and modify the thoughts that impact their lives.

After reading this chapter, you should be able to:

▶ Outline the development of rational emotive behavioral counseling
▶ Explain the theory of rational emotive behavior therapy including its core concepts
▶ Discuss the counseling relationship and goals in rational emotive behavior therapy
▶ Describe assessment, process, and techniques in rational emotive behavior therapy
▶ Demonstrate some therapeutic techniques
▶ Clarify the effectiveness of rational emotive behavior therapy

ALBERT ELLIS (1913–2007) Albert Ellis (1913–2007), the father of rational emotive behavior therapy (REBT), was born in Pittsburg but moved to New York and lived there for most of his life. He described his family as a mother who was independent, a father who cared about the family but was often away, and a younger brother and sister (Bernard, 2011). Ellis (2009) said his family was "pretty crazy" and that he raised himself. During his childhood he struggled with kidney disease and noted that he would work himself into a miserable state of mind and therefore learned at a young age that what people think affects their approach to life.

He earned a degree in Business Administration from the City College of New York in 1934. During the Depression, he earned his living first by working with his brother in a business that located matching pants for still usable suit coats, and then as the personnel manager in a gift and novelty firm.

Ellis's ambition was to write, which he did in his spare time. He collected material for two books on sexual adjustment that were eventually published, *The American Sexual Tragedy* (1954) and *The Case for Sexual Liberty* (1965). His friends began to regard him as an expert on the subject and often asked his advice. He discovered he enjoyed counseling people as much as writing and decided to return to school. In 1942, Ellis entered the clinical psychology program at Teachers College at Columbia University; in 1947, he was awarded his doctorate.

Ellis's early professional work as a therapist in state institutions in New Jersey applied classical psychoanalytic methods. He became dissatisfied with analytical therapy and began to experiment with briefer types of analysis. His change in philosophy came about when he discovered that clients treated once a week or even every other week progressed as well as those he treated daily. Ellis found that a more active role, interjecting advice, and direct interpretation yielded faster results than passive psychoanalytic procedures. Thus, Ellis's theory of counseling emerged after he had received training as a traditional psychoanalytic therapist. Consequently, some of the origins of REBT can be traced to Freud and others to disillusionment with Freudian psychoanalysis.

After discovering that rationalist philosophy fits his temperament and taste, Ellis began concentrating on changing people's behavior by confronting them with their irrational beliefs and persuading them to adopt more rational ones. In 1956, he introduced rational therapy at the American Psychological Association, a form of therapy that encouraged clients to learn how to dispute and overcome their maladaptive thinking. Ellis became unhappy that some people thought that rational therapy meant disregarding emotions, so he changed the name to rational emotive therapy. He reported that the name rational emotive behavior therapy captured the "highly cognitive, very emotive, and particularly behavioral" form of counseling he had developed (Ellis, 1993). Ellis considered himself a philosophical or educational therapist and saw REBT as uniquely didactic, cognition oriented, and explicative. He believed that REBT places people at the center of the universe and gives them almost full responsibility for their fate.

More than 700 books and articles, in addition to his Albert Ellis Institute, have proceeded from Ellis's conceptualization of REBT. Writing in 1977, Ellis noted that REBT, once a limited rational-persuasive therapy, had grown into a therapy that consciously used cognitive, emotive, and behavioral techniques to help clients (Ellis, 1977). In 1957, he published his first REBT book, *How to Live with a "Neurotic"* (1957/1975), and in 1960, his first successful book, *The Art and Science of Love* (1960/1969), was published. Other books by Ellis include *Reason and Emotion in Psychotherapy* (1994); *Better, Deeper, and More Enduring Brief Therapy* (1996); *The Practice of Rational Emotive Behavior Therapy* (1996) (with W. Dryden); *Rational Emotive Behavior Therapy: A Therapist's Guide* (1998) (with C. MacLaren); *Overcoming Destructive Beliefs, Feelings, and Behaviors* (2001); and *Overcoming Resistance* (2007).

THE NATURE OF PEOPLE

Ellis based REBT on the philosophy of Epictetus (ca. A.D. 55–135): "What disturbs men's minds is not events, but their judgment of events." REBT is based on the assumption that knowledge is founded on a selective, personal interpretation of the world. How someone perceives events and people impacts the way that person thinks, feels, and acts. Generally speaking, very young children have limited emotional repertoires and tend to express emotions in a quick, unsustained manner. When children grow old enough to use language effectively, they acquire the ability to sustain their emotions and possibly keep themselves emotionally upset. That emotional disturbance is the result of the innate predisposition to irrational thought and life experiences. Rather than concentrating on past events, REBT practitioners emphasize present events and how people react to them.

According to REBT, people have an innate desire to survive, to feel pleasure, and to move toward self-actualization. Ellis identified two innate biological propensities that compound with that growth potential. One is the tendency to think and behave irrationally. He discussed self-evaluation and criticism and the inclination to accept untested assumptions about self, others, and the world as inborn capacities. Likewise, the ability to think rationally and be proactive in detecting and disputing irrational beliefs to live a more self-actualizing life is also natural. This biological capacity gives each person power and responsibility for changing. Thus irrationality and rationality exist within each person, allowing each to choose to follow a rational or an irrational life (Ellis, 2001). DiGiuseppe (2007) explained that people would be emotionally healthier if they realized that all their beliefs and thoughts could be wrong. People need to check the truth, usefulness, and logic of beliefs. Certain values promote adjustment and mental health and others do not help in developing healthy attitudes and behaviors.

Therefore, the theory of REBT stresses that, as human beings, we have options. We control our ideas, attitudes, feelings, and actions, and we arrange our lives according to our own dictates. We have little control over what happens or what actually exists, but we do have both choices and control over how we view the world and how we react to difficulties, regardless of how we have been taught to respond.

People are neither good nor bad, according to REBT theory, if they respond to others with a rational belief system. If individuals react with irrational beliefs, however, they view themselves and others as evil, awful, and horrible whenever they or others fall short of their expectations. Ellis (1987, 1997) viewed people as naturally irrational, self-defeating individuals who need to be taught to be otherwise. They think crookedly about their desires and preferences and escalate them in a self-defeating manner into musts, shoulds, oughts, and demands. In assimilating these irrational beliefs, people become emotionally disturbed and feel anger, anxiety, depression, worthlessness, self-pity, and other negative feelings that lead to destructive behavior. However, Ellis also stated that people can be "naturally" helpful and loving *as long as they do not think irrationally*. In other words, Ellis described a circular process, as depicted in Figure 12-1. Irrational thinking leads to self-hate, which leads to self-destructive behavior, and eventually to hatred of others, which, in turn, causes others to act irrationally toward the individual, thus beginning the cycle again.

In the early years of the development of civilization, our very survival undoubtedly depended on our ability to face the environment, always expecting and preparing for the worst to happen. Although it was a good way to survive, it was not a happy way to live. We may carry on this pessimistic way of life inherited from the Stone Age when we tend to "catastrophize" the events that happen to us as a defense against being unprepared or caught off guard when the next "disaster" strikes. However, Ellis believed that we do have the potential to think rationally if we can master the ABC steps of REBT.

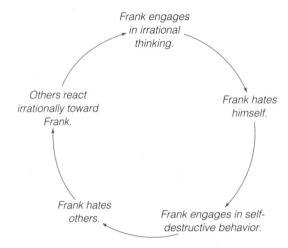

Frank engages in irrational thinking.

Others react irrationally toward Frank.

Frank hates himself.

Frank hates others.

Frank engages in self-destructive behavior.

FIGURE 12-1   THE CIRCLE OF IRRATIONAL THINKING

THEORY OF COUNSELING

Some counselors concentrate on either the developmental events in one's life or one's feelings about these events. Ellis does not believe these two methods to be totally erroneous, but he did not find either approach effective. Neither approach explained why some people are rather well adjusted (i.e., not too unhappy too much of the time, regardless of the passage of events) and others are emotionally dysfunctional much of the time with the same passage of events. REBT concentrates on people's current beliefs, attitudes, and self-statements and is based on the belief that those messages contribute to or cause as well as maintain people's emotional and behavioral disturbances. Basically REBT "holds that when a highly charged emotional consequence (C) follows a significant activating event (A), the event A may seem to, but actually does not, cause C. Instead, emotional consequences are largely created by B—the individual's belief system" (Ellis, 2008, p. 187).

Ferguson (2006) commented that appropriate emotions follow rational beliefs and inappropriate emotions come after irrational beliefs. Ellis and Ellis (2014) refer to those as "emotional upsets." Dryden (2011) named eight emotional problem—guilt, shame, jealousy, hurt, anxiety, depression, envy, and unhealthy anger. Those self-destructive emotions are enduring, immobilizing, and nonproductive; demonstrate overreactions to stimuli; and lead to negative self-image and action (Ellis, 1986). Therefore, in REBT the rational belief system is directly correlated to a person's mental health. On the other hand, appropriate emotions are transient, manageable, in proportion to the event, and create self-acceptance. The positive emotions include joy, satisfaction, peacefulness as well as appropriate annoyance, regret, and sadness.

A rational person is realistic and logical. They have flexible approaches and conclusions, make mistakes and learn from them, and base their interpretations and conclusions on reality. In difficult situations, rational people interpret the event as hurtful but not as catastrophic. Fall, Holden, and Marquis (2010) explain that after a disagreement with a friend, a rational person would achieve a rational evaluation of bad such as "I do not like fighting with my friend but our argument is not the end of the world." A rational person also has a sense of tolerance and is open to different points of view. A rational person knows that disagreements happen in most relationships and focusing only on the argument does not help. Finally, the authors suggest that a rational person accepts their imperfections and thinks along the lines of "I am a human being who makes mistakes. I may be wrong about this too." According to Ellis, the themes of a rational life are being free to define yourself, participating in life, accepting yourself, being fully present, acting and accepting certain limits in life.

According to REBT, unhealthy functioning occurs when people hold on to their disturbances. People live by their "crooked thinking" and the only remediation is to work through it to find the straight thought. The core of mental illness is in someone's beliefs. Ellis has described three areas in which people hold irrational beliefs: They must be perfect, others must be perfect, and the world must be a perfect place to live. The following examples summarize what people tell themselves when they interpret events with an irrational belief system. A more rational replacement thought follows each irrational self-message.

1. Because it would be highly preferable if I were outstandingly competent, I absolutely should and must be; it is awful when I am not, and I am therefore a worthless individual. *Alternative:* It would be nice if I were outstanding in whatever I do, but if I am not, it is okay, and I will try my best anyway.
2. Because it is highly desirable that others treat me considerately and fairly, they absolutely should and must, and they are rotten people who deserve to be utterly damned when they do not. *Alternative:* I would prefer people to treat me considerately. However, I realize they will not always, so I will not take it personally when they do not, *and* I will make it my business to be considerate.
3. Because it is preferable that I experience pleasure rather than pain, the world should absolutely arrange this outcome, and life is horrible and I can't bear it when the world doesn't. *Alternative:* I realize that in life there are both pleasurable moments and painful moments. Therefore, I will try to make the painful moments positive learning experiences so I can endure trials and even benefit from them.

Ellis and Ellis (2014) explain that human predispositions can be understood as tendencies to want, to need, and to condemn themselves, other people, and the world when they do not immediately receive what they purportedly need. This leads people to raise their goals, desires, and preferences into absolute and unrealistic *shoulds*, *oughts*, and *musts* that lead to difficulties.

Those shoulds, oughts, and musts emerge in three categories: self-, other-, and world-demandingness according to Dryden, DiGiuseppe, and Neenan (2010). Self-demandingness stands for the idea that we must always perform well and have everyone's approval; if not, we are incompetent and unworthy. The results of self-demanding are negative feelings and behaviors directed at self, such as self-hatred, anxiety, depression, procrastination, withdrawal, and obsessiveness. Other-demandingness refers to the idea that people we encounter must always be considerate and fair; if they are not, they are unworthy, bad, and deserve to be punished. The effects are anger, hurt, jealousy, vindictiveness, and violence. World-demandingness implies that our life conditions should be enjoyable, hassle-free, and safe; if not, the world is horrible and unbearable. Anger, depression, self-pity, low tolerance, withdrawal, phobias, and addictions result (Ellis, 1994). These ideas of demands, thoughts, and results are summarized in Table 12-1.

TABLE 12-1   DEMANDINGNESS

Demands	Thoughts	Results
Self-	Must perform well	Anxiety
	Must have approval of all	Depression
		Procrastination
		Withdrawal
		Self-hatred
		Obsessiveness
Other-	People must be considerate, fair	Anger
	If not, they are unworthy, bad	Hurt
		Jealousy
		Vindictiveness
		Violence
World-	Life should be enjoyable, hassle-free, safe	Anger
	If not, world is horrible and unbearable	Depression
		Self-pity
		Low tolerance
		Withdrawal
		Phobias
		Addictions

Adapted from Ellis, A. (1994). *Reason and emotion in psychotherapy* (Rev. ed.). New York: Birch Lane.

People have varying degrees of *demandingness*; nonetheless, changing from demanding to desiring is challenging no matter what degree exists. Yet people have the choice of changing and REBT shows them ways to do so.

Ellis (1998) postulated a system of inherently irrational beliefs or philosophies common to our culture that are conducive to maladjustment. When interpreting daily events with one or more irrational philosophies, the individual is likely to feel angry or hostile toward others or to internalize these feelings with resulting anxiety, guilt, or depression. In their *A Guide to Rational Living*, Ellis and Harper (1997) write that, because humans naturally and easily think crookedly, express emotions inappropriately, and behave in a self-defeating manner, it seems best to use all possible educational modes dramatically, strongly, and persistently to teach them how to do otherwise. Ellis and Harper compiled the following list of irrational beliefs that cause people trouble:

1. I must be loved or approved from all significant people.
2. I must be thoroughly competent, adequate, and achieving in all possible respects.
3. Certain people are bad, wicked, or villainous, and they should be severely blamed and punished for their sins.
4. Things are awful, terrible, and catastrophic when I am frustrated, treated unfairly, or rejected.
5. Human unhappiness is externally caused, and I have little or no ability to control or change my negative feelings.
6. If something is or may be dangerous or fearsome, I should be terribly occupied with and upset about it.
7. It is easier to avoid facing many life difficulties and self-responsibilities than to undertake more rewarding forms of self-discipline.
8. The past is all-important, and because something once strongly affected one's life, it should do so indefinitely.
9. People and things should turn out better, and I must view things as horrible and awful if I don't find good solutions to life's grim realities.
10. Maximum human happiness can be achieved by inertia and inaction or by passively and noncommittally enjoying oneself.
11. My child is delinquent (or emotionally disturbed or mentally retarded); therefore, I'm a failure as a parent.
12. My child is emotionally disturbed (or mentally retarded); therefore, he or she is severely handicapped and will never amount to anything.
13. I cannot give my children everything they want; therefore, I am inadequate.

These rigid systems of thought have patterns that lead to emotional problems. *Frustration intolerance* refers to the perceived inability to withstand the frustration of the activating event (Ferguson, 2006). One other thought pattern that creates upset is *human worth ratings*. Those beliefs evaluate self, others, or the world as not ever enough and therefore worthless. DiGiuseppe (2007) reminds us that people cannot be rated as either good or bad because it is impossible to be completely one or the other. Some other patterns of thought that lead to problems are *I-can't-stand-it* and/or *always and never thinking*. DiGiuseppe (2007) provided a table that lists referral problems of children, behavior and emotional correlates, and the irrational beliefs that accompany the problems.

In his chapter "Rational Emotive Behavior Therapy," Ellis (2008) outlines its main propositions:

1. People are born with the potential to be rational as well as irrational, self-constructive, and self-defeating.
2. People's tendency toward irrational thinking, self-damaging behaviors, wishful thinking, and intolerance is heightened by their culture and family.
3. People perceive, think, emote, and behave simultaneously.
4. REBT is cognitive, active, directive, homework-assigning, discipline-oriented, and likely to be effective.
5. REBT counselors value a warm relationship between client and counselor but do not believe the relationship is sufficient for change.
6. REBT counselors use role-playing, assertion training, desensitization, humor, operant conditioning, suggestion, support, and many other things to help clients change.

7. REBT maintains that most neurotic problems involve unrealistic, illogical, self-defeating thinking and that if those ideas are disputed, the thoughts can be minimized.

8. In REBT, clients learn how activating events (A) contribute to but do not cause emotional consequences (C) but the interpretation of the event—their unrealistic and overgeneralized beliefs (B)—are the causes of the upsets. Clients gain insights about the A-B-C pattern, about how they have made and keep themselves upset, and that only hard work and practice will correct irrational thoughts.

9. REBT represents the contents of the mind: rationality and emotions. REBT counselors try to change people's thinking and feeling to enable them to change behavior with a new rational understanding and a new set of emotions (pp. 188–190).

10. Do not blame, damn, denigrate, or condemn people for choosing irrational ideas, inappropriate feelings, or defeating behaviors.

11. Discourage absolutes, such as *must*, *should*, *always*, *never*, and *ought*, in clients' thinking. There are no absolutes (pun intended).

12. Therapists definitely do not determine whether clients' ideas or behaviors are rational or irrational.

Waters (1982) examined differences among the irrational beliefs of children, adolescents, and parents. Although she found some similarities among the three age-groups, she also found some beliefs more prevalent in one group or another.

The biggest commonality among groups is the resulting self-defeating emotions stimulated by the irrational beliefs leading to depression, anxiety, anger, and guilt.

COMMON IRRATIONAL BELIEFS OF CHILDREN

1. It is awful if others don't like me.
2. I am bad if I make a mistake.
3. Everything should go my way; I should always get what I want.
4. Things should come easily to me.
5. The world should be fair, and bad people should be punished.
6. I should not show my feelings.
7. Adults should be perfect.
8. There's only one right answer.
9. I must win; it's awful to lose.
10. I should not have to wait for anything.

COMMON IRRATIONAL BELIEFS OF ADOLESCENTS

1. It would be awful if other kids did not like me, and if I were a loser.
2. I should not make mistakes, especially social mistakes.
3. It's my parents' fault that I'm so miserable.
4. I cannot help being the way I am. I'll always have to be this way.
5. The world should be fair and just.

6. It is awful when things do not go my way.
7. It's better to avoid challenges than to risk being a failure.
8. I must conform to my peers.
9. I cannot stand being criticized.
10. Others should always be responsible.

COMMON IRRATIONAL BELIEFS OF PARENTS

1. It would be awful if my children did not like me.
2. I cannot stand it if others criticize my parenting.
3. I'm totally responsible for everything my children do, and if they behave obnoxiously, I must feel awful.
4. I must be a perfect parent and always know the right thing to do in every situation.
5. My children should always do what I want them to.
6. If my child has a problem, then I have to feel terrible too.
7. Children should not disagree with their parents.
8. My children make me angry, depressed, and anxious.
9. If my children do not turn out the way I think they should, then I am a failure.
10. Parenting should be fun all the time.

Counselors who recognize these beliefs will be well situated to help children, adolescents, and parents.

RELATIONSHIP

DiGiuseppe (2007) pointed out that many people think REBT disregards the therapeutic relationship but that is a misperception. Practitioners' unconditional acceptance demonstrates to clients that they are acceptable people even with their unfortunate traits (Ellis, 2008). Counselors also use humor and encouragement. They create a safe environment and coach clients toward new ways of thinking about themselves. They are flexible and adapt their styles to fit the client. Vernon (2011) said that with children and adolescents, the relationship between counselor and client is especially important. She directed counselors to be patient, adaptive, and less directive, and to use a wide variety of techniques.

REBT counselors direct the process of therapy. They are skilled teachers, communicators, and problem solvers. They have a sense of humor they use appropriately in counseling. They are not afraid of taking risks such as challenging their clients. REBT counselors focus on the present as they explore and question their clients' irrational thoughts. They accept themselves as flawed and work on their own irrational beliefs. Fall et al. (2010) listed these common irrational beliefs that counselors' need to change to be effective:

- I have to succeed with every client, every time.
- I must be respected and loved by every client.
- I have to be a great counselor, more competent than any other therapist.

- I am working hard so my clients must also work hard and pay absolute attention to me.
- I must be able to have a good time in session and get something for myself out of them (p. 308).

Ellis and Dryden (2007, p. 29) explain that REBT clinicians must be structured but flexible, intellectually inclined, comfortable using instruction, untroubled by fear of failure, emotionally healthy, practical and scientific, and comfortable with a variety of interventions.

Ellis quarrels with the practice followed by the majority of psychotherapy systems that appear directed toward strengthening people's self-esteem. He took issue with Rogers's practice of trying to increase clients' self-esteem by providing them with vast amounts of unconditional positive regard. Ellis points out that self-acceptance would still be conditional on the therapists' uncritical acceptance of their clients. Ellis believes that we are more than our behavior and performances, and to rate ourselves bad because we had a bad performance would lead to an unhappy life. Ellis's goal for the people of the world is what he termed *unconditional self-acceptance*—that is, we are worthwhile individuals regardless of how we did on the last test or in the last game. Unconditional self-acceptance works better when it includes what Ellis called unconditional other acceptance, or acceptance of others. Ellis's (1998, 2004) view of healthy personalities is one that accepts others *and* ourselves with our virtues and our failings, with our important accomplishments and our nonachievements, simply because we are alive and because we are human.

GOALS

The goal of REBT is to teach people to think and behave in a more personally satisfying way by making them realize they have a choice between self-defeating, negative behavior and efficient, enhancing, positive behavior. It teaches people to take responsibility for their own logical thinking and the consequences or behaviors that follow it.

Ellis (1998) hypothesizes that individuals' belief systems predicate their responses or feelings toward the same events. These individual belief systems are what people tell themselves about an event, particularly an unfortunate incident. For example, 100 people may be rejected by their true loves. One of these people may respond, "I can't go on; I've lost my purpose in life. Because I've been rejected by such a wonderful person, I must really be a worthless slob. My only solution for getting rid of the unbearable pain I feel is to kill myself." Another person may respond, "What a pain in the neck! I had dinner reservations and tickets for the show. Now I have to get another date for Saturday night. This surely sets me back. What an inconvenience!" Between these two extreme reactions are several other degrees of bad feelings growing from the various self-messages of the 100 rejected people. Such a wide variety of reactions to the same basic event suggests that one's view of the event and consequent self-message provide the key to the counseling strategy. The same process happens to children who experience bad feelings from school failure, peer conflicts, conflicts with adults, or rejection.

The main goal of REBT is to increase happiness and decrease pain. REBT has two main objectives to achieve a prevailing happier state. The first is to show the emotionally disturbed client how irrational beliefs or attitudes create dysfunctional consequences. These consequences might include anger, depression, or anxiety. The second objective is to teach clients how to dispute or crumble their irrational beliefs and replace them with rational beliefs. Once counselors lead the clients to dispute the irrational ideas, they guide them into adopting new expectations for themselves, others, and the environment. Ellis reasons that if the irrational, absolute philosophies and resultant feelings are replaced with more rational, productive thoughts, clients will no longer be trapped in a repetitious cycle of negative feelings. When children are no longer incapacitated by dysfunctional feelings, they are free to choose behaviors that eliminate the problem or at least lessen its disappointing impact.

Three insights help children improve their adjustment (Dryden et al., 2010). The first is that events do not cause disturbance but beliefs about the event do. The second insight is that people hold on to their beliefs. Finally, insight alone is not sufficient to change irrational thinking. People must make repeated efforts to challenge the beliefs, build new ones, and rehearse the rational beliefs.

COUNSELING METHOD

REBT is an active, directive therapy. Practitioners are highly involved and use their influence to help children change. The client must cooperate and interact in order to explore belief systems and learn the REBT process. Ellis and Ellis (2014) explain that a client must realize there is a problem, discover the irrational belief that underlies the problem, understand the belief is irrational, and realize the rational alternative by challenging the irrational and learning to think and do differently.

Assessment

As noted earlier, REBT is didactic, confrontational, and verbally active counseling. Initially, the counselor seeks to detect the irrational beliefs that are creating the disturbance. Seven factors help to detect irrational thinking:

1. Look for *overgeneralizations:* "I made an F on the first math test; therefore, I always will do poorly on math tests."
2. Look for *distortions:* sometimes referred to as all-or-nothing thinking or black-and-white categorizing of things as all good or all bad. "I did not make all As on my report card; therefore, I will never be a good student."
3. Look for *deletions:* the tendency to focus on negative events or disqualifying positive events. "I struck out two times and got one hit; therefore, I will probably strike out the next time I bat."
4. Look for *catastrophizing:* mistakes are exaggerated, and achievements are minimized. "I was just lucky to get that A on my last test."
5. Look for the use of absolutes such as *should, must, always, ought,* and *never:* "I should not make mistakes."

6. Look for statements *condemning* something or someone clients think they cannot stand: "He should be punished and should not be allowed to get away with that!"
7. Look for *fortune-telling* or future predictions: "I just know my friends will not have fun at my party."

Once the irrational beliefs are recognized, the counselor disputes and challenges them. Ultimately, the goal is for children and adolescents to recognize irrational beliefs, think them through, and relinquish them. As a result of this process and therapy, clients, it is hoped, reach three insights. First, the present neurotic behavior has antecedent causes. Second, original beliefs keep upsetting them because they keep repeating these beliefs. Third, they can overcome emotional disturbances by consistently observing, questioning, and challenging their own belief systems.

People hold tenaciously to their beliefs, rational or not; consequently, the counselor vigorously attacks the irrational beliefs in an attempt to show the children how illogically they think. Using the Socratic method of questioning and disputing, the counselor takes a verbally active part in the early stages of counseling by identifying and explaining the child's problem. If counselors guess correctly, which happens often, they argue with and persuade the child to give up the old irrational view and replace it with a new, rational philosophy.

Process

REBT is often referred to as the "A, B, C, D, and E" approach to counseling. A, B, and C show how problems develop; D and E are the treatment steps:

A is the activating event: "I failed my math test."

B is how you evaluate the event: (1) irrational message: "I failed the test; therefore, I'm a total failure as a person"; (2) rational message: "I failed the test. This is unpleasant and inconvenient, but that is all it is. I need to study more efficiently for the next exam."

C represents the consequences or feelings resulting from your self-message at the B stage. The irrational message (B1 stage) will cause you to feel very depressed. The rational message (B2 stage) will not make you feel great, but it will not be so overwhelming as to inhibit your performance on the next test.

D represents the disputing arguments you use to attack the irrational self-messages expressed in the B1 stage. The counselor's function is to help you question these irrational self-messages once they have been identified.

E represents the answers you have developed to the questions regarding the rationality of your B1 stage self-messages.

For example, counseling would proceed through the following steps:

A—Something unpleasant happens to you.

B—You evaluate the event as something awful, something that should not be allowed to happen.

C—You become upset and nervous.

D—You question your B self-message:

1. Is it really as awful as I believe?
2. What evidence do I have to support these beliefs?
3. Are these beliefs helping or hurting me?

E—You answer:

1. It is a disappointment.
2. It is a setback but not a disaster.
3. I can handle it.
4. I would like things to be better, but that doesn't mean I'm always supposed to get things done my way.

Bernard, Froh, DiGiuseppe, Joyce, and Dryden (2010), DiGiuseppe (2007), Vernon (2011), and Dryden and colleagues (2010) listed the steps of REBT. These authors stated that the steps can be used with any age group, but techniques may differ. They recommended that counselors follow this procedure or identifying, assessing, disputing, and modifying irrational beliefs to assure all the important parts of the counseling model are followed. Table 12-2, modified from the above works, outlines these steps in a session note format.

Counselors begin by asking the child to talk about the problem (Step 1) and then reaching agreement on the goal of the session (Step 2). DiGiuseppe (2007) alerted practitioners that conflicts may arise because clients may want to change the activating event, whereas counselors may want to focus on the consequence. Client and counselor need to reach consensus at the second step. Counselors then ask for a specific example of the problem and assess the activating event (Step 3), the consequences (Step 4), and any secondary disturbances (Step 5). At Step 6, counselors teach the client to see the connection between beliefs, feelings, and behaviors followed by an assessment of irrational beliefs (Step 7) with techniques such as offering hypotheses or inference chaining (a series of follow-up questions to what were you thinking) until the irrational belief is uncovered. When that happens, counselors would hear a "must," "awfulizing," "I can't stand it," or a global evaluation (DiGiuseppe, 2007).

The next steps include linking the irrational belief to the disturbed emotion and behaviors and connecting healthy emotions and behaviors (Step 8) and disputing the irrational belief (Step 9) by challenging its logic, its validity, or the purpose of the consequences that follow it. Vernon (2011) added that offering alternative rational ideas and direct teaching could also be parts of this step. Strategies for disputation include logical, empirical, functional disputing, or rational alternative beliefs. Counselors may use different styles in disputing: didactic, Socratic, metaphorical, or humorous (Seligman & Reichenberg, 2014). Step 10 focuses on deepening the client's conviction in the rational belief by continued disputing and by asking how the person would behave differently with the rational belief (Step 11). The client agrees to practice or rehearse new learning with REBT homework sheets that lead

TABLE 12-2   RATIONAL EMOTIVE BEHAVIORAL PROCESS NOTES

Name: _____ Date: _____

Step 1: Ask the child to talk about the problem _____

Step 2: Agree on the goal of the session _____

Step 3: Ask for a specific example of the problem _____

Step 4: Assess the activating event _____

Step 5: Assess the consequences _____

Step 6: Assess if there are any secondary disturbances _____

Step 7: Teach the client to see the connection between beliefs, feelings, and behaviors (A, B, C)

_____

Step 8: Assess the presence of irrational beliefs _____

Step 9: Connect the irrational belief to the disturbed emotions and behaviors and rational beliefs to the healthy emotions and behaviors _____

Step 10: Dispute the irrational belief _____

Step 11: Deepen the conviction in the rational belief _____

Step 12: Encourage the practice of or rehearse new learning _____

Modified from DiGiuseppe, R. (2007). Rational emotive behavioral approaches. In H. T. Prout & D. T. Brown (Eds.), *Counseling and psychotherapy with children and adolescents: Theory and practice for school and clinical settings* (4th ed., pp. 279–331). Hoboken, NJ: Wiley.

people through a disputing process or various behavioral activities. Following these steps throughout REBT sessions allows counselors to teach clients to do this for themselves.

Solutions

REBT practitioners distinguish between practical and emotional solutions (Ellis, 1994). Practical solutions focus on the child using problem solving or skill development to change the activating event. Emotional solutions center on changing the child's reaction to the event. DiGiuseppe (2007) illustrated this with the case of Serge, a child who thought his teacher disliked him. A practical solution would be to help Serge win over his teacher; an emotional solution would be to help Serge calm his anger. REBT seeks emotional solutions first so that people have a greater chance of leading happier lives by handling the hassles of life. Helping children change A is also an acceptable goal, but after the emotional solution, so that clients have lessened their disturbance before considering the practical solution.

Another consideration with solutions is the difference between elegant solutions versus inelegant solutions. REBT counselors think the best way to reach an emotional solution is to change a core irrational belief. This provides a coping strategy that people can use in similar negative activating events. REBT practitioners advise not to use interventions that attempt to change attributions or try to reframe that negative automatic thought. Those interventions may create a temporary coping mechanism but do not provide the generalizability of an elegant solution (DiGiuseppe, 2007).

Techniques

Ellis (2008) explained that REBT practitioners use cognitive, emotive, and behavior procedures to try to minimize clients' "musting," perfectionism, grandiosity, and frustration intolerance. Practitioners teach clients to recognize their *shoulds, oughts, and musts*, how to be logical, and how to accept reality. Counselors may use role-playing to demonstrate accepting new ideas, humor to reduce disturbing ideas to absurdities, and strong disputing to move people from irrational to more efficient ideas. Some of the behavioral techniques used focus on taking risks such as asking someone for a date or applying for a job.

DiGiuseppe (2007) suggested that REBT can be used with children as young as five, though techniques need to be different for children between 5 and 11 than for those who are older. DiGiuseppe and Kelter (2006) stated that children who are at Piaget's concrete operations stage and beyond can benefit from disputing. Children who have not reached that stage will have difficulty thinking about their thinking. The counselor should check to determine if the child can distinguish between thoughts and feelings (DiGiuseppe). Determining the readiness of a child to change is an early part of any type of counseling. Most children are referred to counseling. Therefore, counselors can assume they may not want to change. DiGiuseppe presented a motivational syllogism as one way to establish an alliance with an unwilling child. Counselors work through this sequence of logic to reach the goals and tasks of therapy.

1. Help the child see the present emotion is dysfunctional by using Socratic questions.
2. Identify alternative acceptable emotions for the activating event by reviewing possibilities.
3. Ask questions to help the child see it would be better to abandon the dysfunctional emotion and work toward an alternative. This step should allow the counselor and child to reach agreement on the counseling goals.
4. Begin to teach the child that beliefs influence emotions so the tasks of counseling involve the examination and alteration of thinking.

Counselors may need to explain and show how thoughts cause feelings and how irrational thoughts create disturbed emotions. Counseling includes the child identifying and labeling various thoughts and emotions as well as learning to tell those that are helpful from those that are not helpful. Counseling also incorporates disputing beliefs and replacing them with rational ones. Counselors use modeling, role-playing, and homework in therapy. With younger children, the activities and materials should be concrete. Counselors working with adolescents can focus more on insight. DiGiuseppe (2007) commented that Socratic disputing works well with adolescents and that counselors may want to ask teens to recall rational beliefs endorsed by their peers.

Counselors can dispute an irrational belief by contesting the logic, by testing the truth of it, or by calculating the impact of holding the belief. Ferguson (2006) explained more about these techniques for disputing irrational thoughts.

- Logic questions lead people to evaluate the logical consistence or clarity in their thoughts such as "Let me see. You said she doesn't love you. How does that follow from what you said?"
- Reality-testing questions ask people to gauge whether their beliefs are consistent with reality such as "What evidence do you have?" or "What would happen if …?" or "What would the scientists say?"
- Pragmatic questions aim at getting people to assess the value (pleasure or pain) of their belief system such as "How does thinking that keep you from hurting?" (pp. 345–346).

The counselor also needs to suggest an alternative rational idea and challenge it the same way.

DiGiuseppe (2007) has detailed a method for using inference chaining as a technique for helping children re-evaluate their irrational beliefs. He said that the question "What were you thinking when you got upset?" will uncover automatic thoughts rather than irrational ones. In order to determine irrational thoughts, practitioners can use inference chaining by starting with the automatic thought and following the logic by a series of follow-up questions. Children are asked to imagine or to think about what would happen next if the automatic thought (e.g., "I'm going to mess up.") were true and what it would mean to them. The counselor asks the child to imagine the chain of events that would follow the belief. The counselor continues until an irrational belief—the must, awfulizing, can't stand it, or global evaluation is uncovered. The following is modified from DiGiuseppe's example:

COUNSELOR: And what would happen if you did?

CHILD: Well, everyone would know I'm stupid.

COUNSELOR: Well, suppose that does happen. What would you be thinking then?

CHILD: I guess I would think I'm dumb.

COUNSELOR: What would it mean to you if you were not as smart as you would like to be?

CHILD: It would be awful.

DiGiuseppe also recommends deductive interpretation with children. In this method, the counselor and the child form and test hypotheses concerning the irrational belief. The hypotheses are presented as possible explanations and are revised based on the child's feedback. To do this well, counselors phrase the statement as a guess and then change their words based on the response of the child. Both inference chaining and deductive interpretation allow self-discovery by the child.

To the usual psychotherapeutic techniques of exploration, ventilation, excoriation, and interpretation, REBT therapists add techniques of confrontation, indoctrination, and re-education. Counselors are didactic in that they explain how children's beliefs (which intervene between an event and the resultant feelings), rather than events themselves, cause emotional disturbances. Because the counselor honestly believes that children and adolescents do not understand the reason for their disturbance, the counselor enlightens and teaches. Counselors frequently assign homework—reading, performing specific tasks, and taking risks—for the child as an integral part of therapy.

REBT counselors believe that the development of a person's belief system (which is defined as the meaning of facts) is analogous to the acquisition of speech. Just as children learn language by imitation and modeling, they learn a belief system. Therefore, the belief system and attitudes children acquire are largely a reflection of the significant people in their lives. Furthermore, the belief systems incorporated into children's minds determine whether they think rationally about facts. Continuing the analogy, just as one continues to build one's vocabulary and modify one's speech, one also can change or replace one's belief system. Deficient thinking results from the lack of the information-processing capacities needed to solve the problem. Distortions in thinking occur when the child has the capacity to solve the situation but thinks about the problem in an irrational way. To work successfully, the counselor must clarify whether the child needs to develop cognitive skills, correct ways of thinking, or both.

Role reversal is an effective technique with children. In this technique, the child describes the activating event and the emotional consequences. Next, the counselor explains that thoughts are upsetting the child. Then, they role-play the activating event, with the counselor playing the child. While acting out the event, the counselor demonstrates the appropriate behavior while uttering rational self-statements aloud. The roles are reversed again, with the child trying new thoughts and being rewarded, preferably with social approval, as reinforcement for rational statements and behaviors. The child may need successive approximations of the appropriate REBT behaviors reinforced before the concept is learned. Adolescents with abstract reasoning ability and an understanding of cause and effect may be more comfortable with REBT.

Rational Emotive Behavioral Education

An offspring of REBT is rational emotive behavioral education (REBE). Its objectives are to teach how feelings develop, how to discriminate between valid and invalid assumptions, and how to think rationally in "anti-awful" and "antiperfectionist" ways.

1. Students learn best through actively participating in educational experiences that involve constructive problem-solving activities.

2. Attitudes, beliefs, and emotions play a significant role in the teaching and learning process. Students can harness fact-based personal constructs and emotive motivations to shape productive directions in their lives.

3. Students who build upon realistic self-knowledge are better able to translate this knowledge into purposeful and productive activities.

4. The development of realistic self-knowledge, coupled with psychological problem-solving skills, increases the likelihood of positive school progress, career satisfaction, and a fulfilling life.

THEORETICAL FOUNDATION

REBE programs have been effective in reinforcing rational verbal expressions with disturbed children. Children become more rational not only in their verbal expressions and belief systems but also in their behaviors, a result supported in recent studies of REBE (Opre, Buzgar, & Dumulescu, 2013; Trip, McMahon, Bora, & Chipea, 2010). As well as the effectiveness of REBE with children, researchers found that teachers emotional distress was decreased after they participated in an education program built on this theory (Bora, Vernon, & Trip, 2013). Following are examples of beliefs that can be reinforced by writing statements:

I don't like school, but I can stand it.

I did something bad, but I'm not a bad person.

I don't like being called insulting names, but being insulted is not awful.

Just because someone calls you "stupid" does not mean you are.

Ellis claims that all children act neurotically simply because they are children. He states that childish behavior cannot be differentiated from neurosis until the age of 5. At this point, many children have integrated into their belief system the irrational belief that one should be thoroughly competent, adequate, and achieving in all possible respects to be considered worthwhile. Strategies for undermining this philosophy in children can be summarized as follows:

1. Teach children the joy of engaging in games that are worthwhile because they are fun. De-emphasize the importance of winning at all costs by teaching children that you do not have to win to have fun and be a worthwhile person.

2. Teach children that significant achievements rarely come easily and that nothing is wrong with working long and hard to achieve their goals.

3. Teach children that they are not bad people when they do not meet their goals. Children must like themselves during periods of failure, even when they may not be trying their best to achieve their goals. Children also need to learn the difference between wants and needs. Wanting something we cannot get is not the same as not getting what we absolutely need.

4. Teach children that, although striving for perfectionism in performance is good, perfection is not required to be a worthwhile person. Making mistakes is not only allowed but also is a good way to learn why certain things happen and how to prevent them from happening again.

5. Teach children that popularity and achievement are not necessarily related, that to be liked by all people at all times is difficult, and that being a worthwhile person does not require 100 percent popularity.
6. In summary, teach children not to take themselves and situations too seriously by turning minor setbacks into catastrophes. Balance corrective feedback with positive reinforcement in evaluating children's performances.

A manual for REBE can be found at www.**rebt**network.org/library/**Rational_ Emotive_Education**.pdf.

Case Study

Jeff is a quiet, serious, 12-year-old seventh-grade student at Smith County Middle School. He was referred to the counselor because a failing grade on a language arts test left him very upset. After the test, Jeff seemed to be firmly convinced that he would fail the class.

Individual and Background Information

Academic School records indicate that Jeff is a high achiever. He had excellent grades (B and above) in all his classes for the first two grading periods of the year. Except for an F on the last test, he has also maintained an above-average grade in language arts this grading period.

Family Jeff is the youngest of three sons. His father is retired, and his mother works as a grocery store cashier. Both of Jeff's older brothers, one a high school senior and the other a college sophomore, are excellent students. The family expects (or appears to expect) Jeff to excel also.

Social Jeff seems to get along well with his peers. He participates in group efforts and is especially good friends with one other student, John, who is also a good student with a quiet personality.

Counseling Method

The school counselor used REBT as a counseling method to help Jeff recognize and evaluate the erroneous messages he was giving himself (and which upset him) about his low grade in language arts. The counselor also taught Jeff to replace the erroneous messages with "smart" messages and to recognize "not smart" messages when he encountered them again. The basic steps the counselor used included having Jeff examine each step along the way to becoming upset and look at the real message he was telling himself at each step.

Transcript[*]

COUNSELOR: Jeff, why do you think you're going to fail language arts?

JEFF: Because I failed the last test.

---

[*] The case of Jeff was contributed by Sharon Simpson.

COUNSELOR: You mean if you fail one test, you're bound to fail the next one?

JEFF: Well, I failed that test, and I'm stupid!

COUNSELOR: What are you telling yourself about your performance on that test?

JEFF: I remember thinking it was a really bad grade—not at all the kind I was used to getting. Then I thought how terrible it would be if I failed language arts and how my mom and dad and brothers would hate me and would think I was lazy and dumb!

COUNSELOR: It would be unpleasant and inconvenient if you failed language arts, but would this make you a hateful and dumb person?

JEFF: It makes me really worried about passing the next test that's coming up.

COUNSELOR: I can understand how you would be worried about the next test, but does a bad grade make someone a bad or hated person?

JEFF: No, but it's not the kind of grade I usually get.

COUNSELOR: Okay, so a bad grade is unpleasant, and you don't like it, but it does not make you a bad person.

JEFF: My grade was an F and most of the other kids made As, so it made me look dumb.

COUNSELOR: Okay, it *was* a bad grade compared with the rest of the class, but does this mean you are the dumbest kid around?

JEFF: No, I make mostly As, a few Bs. One bad grade does not make me a dumb kid.

COUNSELOR: So, compared with your usual grade and the class's grades, this *was* a bad grade, and that is all it is, right?

JEFF: Yeah.

COUNSELOR: What else are you telling yourself about the low test grade?

JEFF: Well, like I said, I immediately thought how terrible it would be if I failed language arts, and—

COUNSELOR: Stop there for just a minute, Jeff. Suppose you did fail language arts, even with your other high grades. It would be a bad experience, but would it be the end of the world?

JEFF: No, I guess I'd have to repeat the class, that's all.

COUNSELOR: Right, it would be inconvenient and maybe embarrassing. It would not be pleasant, but you would go on living.

JEFF: Well, I guess that's right.

COUNSELOR: Are you beginning to see what you told yourself about the consequences of *one* bad grade?

JEFF: Yeah, I guess I believed that one bad grade was awful—the end of the world—and that I shouldn't even try anymore because I would fail the class anyway.

COUNSELOR: Was that the correct information to give yourself about your grade?

JEFF: No!

COUNSELOR: Okay! Let's look at the rest of the message you gave yourself after you got that bad grade. Remember what was next?

JEFF: I think I thought my family would hate me and think I was dumb and lazy because I failed that test and would probably fail language arts.

COUNSELOR: Do you think your family's love depends on your grades?

JEFF: No, Jimmy made an F on a chemistry test the first part of the school year, and nobody hated him.

COUNSELOR: What did your parents do?

JEFF: Let's see. Oh yeah, they got him a tutor—a friend of Dad's knew a student who was majoring in chemistry.

COUNSELOR: What did your brother in college do when Jimmy failed the test?

JEFF: He offered to help Jim on weekends. He's a brain—a physics major!

COUNSELOR: So when your brother failed a test, your family helped him out. They didn't say he was "dumb" or "lazy" or that they hated him for it!

JEFF: No, they didn't. And I guess they wouldn't say it to me, either; in fact, Dad and Jim ask every night if I need help with my homework. I can usually do it okay by myself.

COUNSELOR: Okay. Let's go back over some of these bad messages you've been giving yourself about your bad grade.

JEFF: I got a bad grade. I thought I would fail language arts no matter what I did. I decided my family would hate me and think I was dumb and lazy.

COUNSELOR: Do you *still* believe those "not smart" messages you told yourself about failing and the way your family would react?

JEFF: No!

COUNSELOR: Next time you mess up on something—maybe a ball game, maybe a test—what message will you give yourself?

JEFF: Well, I'm not exactly sure what I'll say, but I *won't* tell myself that it's a disaster and I'll never be able to do anything else. I'll probably say that I don't like what happened and that I'm not happy about it. That's all. Now I guess I'll go study and try to ace that next language arts test. Thanks a lot!

DIVERSITY APPLICATIONS OF REBT

REBT is especially appealing to those cultures and to those individuals in all cultures who prefer strong, directive counseling and an active counselor who favors dispensing information about the "A, B, C, D, and E" philosophy and approach to helping people think, feel, and behave better. REBT counselors are not shy in telling clients what they are doing wrong and what they need to do to correct their behavior. REBT is an education or re-education method that teaches clients what they are doing to themselves to make themselves feel bad and what to do to make themselves feel better. This therapy is especially effective with those individuals who prefer to focus on reason and thinking rather than on affect or behavior to bring about a positive change in their lives. Likewise, the approach is favored by cultures and individuals who want their counselor to be a strong and active consultant. Sue and Sue (2012) suggest this short-term, active and directive therapy matches many cultural expectations. In other words, these clients prefer reason over emotion and reason over behavior in solving their problems and resolving conflicts. In fact one of the criticisms of this theory is the focus on the intellectual aspects of life.

Vernon (2007) noted that Ellis stressed the need for counselors to be open-minded about cultures and learn as much as possible about the rules of minority culture. She said that Ellis reminded counselors to accept clients unconditionally regardless of religion, culture, or politics and that teaching clients to accept others might diminish oppression.

Ellis and Ellis (2014) identified three REBT principles applicable to diverse clients. First, clients can unconditionally accept themselves and others and can build their frustration tolerance when facing adversities. Second, if the counselor encourages clients to follow those guidelines and lead a flexible life, problems can be resolved with little intercultural or intracultural bias. Finally, Ellis emphasized that most multicultural issues contain bias and intolerance which REBT works against.

EVALUATION OF RATIONAL EMOTIVE BEHAVIOR THERAPY

Gonzalez and colleagues (2004) reviewed 30 years of published studies of REBT with children and adolescents. The conclusion of their meta-analysis of the research was that REBT produced positive and significant outcomes. REBT appeared to be equally effective with children and adolescents who came to counseling with or without identified problems and the longer the duration of counseling, the greater the impact. Esposito (2009) explains that REBT has a long history of use with counselors who find the ABCDE technique appropriate for children in disputing irrational beliefs, and Knaus (2005) discusses the Frustration Tolerance Training for Children as a method for helping children accept unpleasant feelings without magnifying them. Banks and Zionts (2009) worked with adolescents with behavior problems, and Vernon (2006a, 2006b) has written manuals for using REBT with adolescents and their parents. Stories, plays, films, and other resources have been developed to aid this process.

Silverman, McCarthy, and McGovern (1992) completed an inclusive review of published and unpublished studies of REBT with children, adolescents, and adults. They expressed positive results in therapy and concluded that no other type of treatment was significantly better. DiGiuseppe (2007) asserts that REBT studies support its efficacy in treatment of a range of problems including test anxiety, performance anxiety, stress, depression, anger, burnout, obsessive compulsive disorder, school discipline problems, and school underachievement among others. Bernard's (2006) chapter on working with underachieving students provides an excellent example of the process and effectiveness of REBT. Finally, REBT lends itself to the use of technology with mobile mind maps (Warren, 2012).

SUMMARY

Ellis (2008) explained that an elegant system of counseling would have these characteristics: "a) economy of time and effort, b) rapid symptom reduction, c) effectiveness with a large percentage of different kinds of clients, d) depth of solution of presenting problems, and e) lastingness of the therapeutic results" (p. 202). He asserted that REBT matched those criteria.

Replying to articles critical of REBT, Ellis (1998, 2003) writes that REBT remains within the field of science while resting on some evaluative assumptions. For example, the REBT concept of unconditional humanistic self-acceptance is still valid, even though it requires an operational definition. The REBT concept of self-acceptance means that a person is more than a set of behaviors; that is, people are better off negating specific behaviors without labeling their entire selves as good or bad. Albert Ellis (1993) traced the development of his REBT from 1955 to 1993, and he suggests directions where REBT may be taken in the future. He points out that, in 1955, REBT, the first of today's cognitive therapies, was highly cognitive, largely positivist, and very active directive. Its ABC theory of human disturbance held that people experience undesirable activating events (A), that they have rational and irrational beliefs (B) about these events, and that they create *appropriate* emotional and behavioral *consequences* (aC) with their *rational beliefs* (rB) or they create *inappropriate* and dysfunctional *consequences* (iC) with their *irrational beliefs* (iB). Thus, REBT is directed to the client's belief system, which is the cause of the problem, not the activating event.

In summary, Ellis's objective for all people is that they rate their performance in relation to the goals they have set. It is *healthy* to believe "It is good when I succeed and am loved" or "It is bad when I fail and am rejected." It is *unhealthy* to believe "I am good for succeeding" and "I am bad for getting rejected." Regarding unconditional positive regard, Ellis points out that REBT therapists try to give this type of acceptance to all clients, but also teach them how to give it to themselves. Ellis (2008) admonished REBT practitioners to show clients how to (a) minimize anxiety, guilt, and depression by accepting themselves; (b) ease their anger, hostility, and violence by accepting other people; and (c) decrease their frustration intolerance by accepting life even when things are difficult.

WEB SITES FOR RATIONAL EMOTIVE BEHAVIOR THERAPY

Internet addresses frequently change. To find the sites listed here, visit www.cengage.com/counseling/henderson for an updated list of Internet addresses and direct links to relevant sites.

Albert Ellis Institute

Ellis REBT

Rational Emotive Behavior Therapy Network

REFERENCES

Banks, T., & Zionts, P. (2009). REBT used with children and adolescents who have emotional and behavioral disorders in educational settings: A view of the literature. *Journal of Rational-Emotive and Cognitive-Behavior Therapy, 27,* 51–65.

Bernard, M. E. (2006). Working with the educational underachiever: A social and emotional developmental approach. In A. Ellis & M. E. Bernard (Eds.), *Rational emotive behavioral approaches to childhood disorders* (pp. 316–360). New York: Springer.

Bernard, M. E. (2011). *Rationality and the pursuit of happiness: The legacy of Albert Ellis.* New York: Wiley.

Bernard, M. E., Froh, J. J., DiGiuseppe, R., Joyce, M. R., & Dryden, W. (2010). Albert Ellis: Unsung hero of positive psychology. *The Journal of Positive Psychology, 5,* 302–310.

Bora, C., Vernon, A., & Trip, S. (2013). Effectiveness of a rational emotive behavior education program in reducing teachers' emotional distress. *Journal of Cognitive and Behavioral Psychotherapies, 13 (2A),* 585–604.

DiGiuseppe, R. (2007). Rational emotive behavioral approaches. In H. T. Prout & D. T. Brown (Eds.), *Counseling and psychotherapy with children and adolescents: Theory and practice for school and clinical settings* (4th ed., pp. 279–331). Hoboken, NJ: Wiley.

DiGiuseppe, R., & Kelter, J. (2006). Treating aggressive children: A rational emotive behavior system approach. In A. Ellis & M. E.Bernard (Eds.), *Rational emotive behavioral approaches to childhood disorders* (pp. 257–281). New York: Springer.

Dryden, W. (2011). *Dealing with emotional problems using rational emotive behavior therapy: A training handbook* (2nd ed.). New York: Routledge.

Dryden, W., DiGiuseppe, R., & Neenan, M. (2010). *A primer on rational emotive behavior therapy* (3rd ed.). Champaign, IL: Research Press.

Ellis, A. (1954). *The American sexual tragedy.* New York: Twayne.

Ellis, A. (1965). *The case for sexual liberty.* Tucson, AZ: Seymour Press.

Ellis, A. (1975). *How to live with a "neurotic"* (Rev. ed.). New York: Crown.

Ellis, A. (1977). *How to live with and without anger.* New York: Reader's Digest Press.

Ellis, A. (1969). *The art and science of love* (2nd ed.). New York: Lyle Stuart/Bantam.

Ellis, A. (1986). An emotional control card for inappropriate and appropriate emotions using rational-emotive imagery. *Journal of Counseling and Development, 65,* 205–206.

Ellis, A. (1987). The impossibility of achieving consistently good mental health. *American Psychologist, 42,* 364–375.

Ellis, A. (1993). Reflections on rational-emotive therapy. *Journal of Consulting and Clinical Psychology, 61,* 199–201.

Ellis, A. (1994). *Reason and emotion in psychotherapy* (Rev. ed.). New York: Birch Lane.

Ellis, A. (1996). *Better, deeper, and more enduring brief therapy.* New York: Brunner/Mazel.

Ellis, A. (1997). Must musterbation and demandingness lead to emotional disorders? *Psychotherapy, 34,* 95–98.

Ellis, A. (1998). *REBT diminishes much of the human ego.* New York: Institute for Rational-Emotive Therapy.

Ellis, A. (2001). *Overcoming destructive beliefs, feelings, and behaviors.* New York: Prometheus Books.

Ellis, A. (2003). Early theories and practices of rational emotive therapy and how they have been augmented and revised during the last three decades. *Journal of Rational-Emotive & Cognitive-Behavior Therapy, 21,* 219–234.

Ellis, A. (2004). Why rational emotive behavior therapy is the most comprehensive and effective form of behavior therapy. *Journal of Rational-Emotive & Cognitive-Behavior Therapy, 82,* 439–442.

Ellis, A. (2007). *Overcoming resistance; A rational emotive-behavior therapy integrative approach* (2nd ed.). New York: Springer.

Ellis, A. (2008). Rational emotive behavior therapy. In R. J. Corsini & D. Wedding (Eds.), *Current psychotherapies* (8th ed., pp. 187–221). Belmont, CA: Thomson.

Ellis, A. (2009). *All out! An autobiography.* New York: Prometheus Books.

Ellis, A., & Dryden, W. (1996). *The practice of rational emotive behavior therapy* (Rev. ed.). New York: Springer.

Ellis, A., & Dryden, W. (2007). *The practice of rational emotive behavior therapy* (2nd ed.). New York: Springer.

Ellis, A., & Ellis, D. J. (2014). Rational emotive behavior therapy. In D. Wedding & R. J. Corsini (Eds.), *Current psychotherapies* (10th ed., pp. 151–191). Belmont, CA: Thomson.

Ellis, A., & Harper, R. (1997). *A new guide to rational living.* North Hollywood, CA: Melvin Powers.

Esposito, M. A. (2009). *REBT with children and adolescents: A meta-analytic review of efficacy studies.* New York: St. John's University.

Fall, K. A., Holden, J. M., & Marquis, A. (2010). *Theoretical models of counseling and psychotherapy* (2nd ed.). New York: Brunner-Routledge.

Ferguson, K. E. (2006). Intermittent explosive disorder. In J. E. Fisher & W. T. Donohue (Eds.), *Practitioner's guide to evidenced-based psychotherapy* (pp. 335–351).New York: Springer.

Gonzalez, J., Nelson, J., Gutkin, T., Saunders, A., Galloway, A., & Shwery, C. (2004). Rational emotive therapy with children and adolescents: A meta-analysis. *Journal of Emotional and Behavioral Disorders, 12*(4), 222–235.

Knaus, W. J. (2005). Frustration tolerance training for children. In A. Ellis & M. E. Bernard (Eds.), *Rational emotive behavioral approaches to childhood disorders: Theory, practice and research* (pp. 133–155). New York: Springer.

Opre, A., Buzgar, R., & Dumulescu, D. (2013). Empirical support for self-kit: A rational emotive education program. *Journal of Cognitive and Behavioral Psychotherapies, 13 (2A),* 557–573.

Seligman, L., & Reichenberg, L. W. (2014). *Theories of counseling and psychotherapy: Systems, strategies and skills* (4th ed.). Upper Saddle River, NJ: Pearson.

Silverman, M. S., McCarthy, M., & McGovern, T. (1992). A review of outcome studies of rational emotive therapy from 1982 to 1989. *Journal of Rational-Emotive and Cognitive-Behavior Therapy, 10,* 111–175.

Sue, D. W., & Sue, D. (2012). *Counseling the culturally different* (6th ed.). Hoboken, NJ: Wiley.

Trip, S., McMahon, J., Bora, C., & Chipea, F. (2010). The efficiency of a rational emotive and behavioral education program in diminishing dysfunctional thinking, behaviors and emotions in children. *Journal of Cognitive and Behavioral Psychotherapies, 10*(2), 173–186.

Vernon, A. (2006a). *Thinking, feeling, behaving: An emotional education curriculum for adolescents: Grades 7–12.* Champaign, IL: Research Press.

Vernon, A. (2006b). *Thinking, feeling, behaving: An emotional education curriculum for adolescents: Grades 1–6.* Champaign, IL: Research Press.

Vernon, A. (2011). Rational emotive behavior therapy. In D. Capuzzi & D. R. Gross (Eds.), *Counseling and psychotherapy: Theories and interventions* (5th ed., pp. 237–262). Alexandria, VA: American Counseling Association.

Warren, J. M. (2012). Mobile mind mapping: Using mobile technology to enhance rational emotive behavior therapy. *Journal of Mental Health Counseling, 34,* 72–82.

Waters, V. (1982). Therapies for children: Rational-emotive therapy. In C. R. Reynolds & T. B. Gutkin (Eds.), *Handbook of school psychology.* New York: Wiley.

CHAPTER 13

Cognitive-Behavioral Therapy

Nothing is so terrible as activity without thought.
—JOHANN WOLFGANG VON GOETHE

Cognition comes from the Latin word that means to know. Cognition refers to the ways people use to understand their environment and themselves, such as their perceptions, sensations, learning, memory, and other psychological processes. Beck explains that if humans did not have the capacity to take in relevant information, synthesizing it, and building a plan of action based on the synthesis, they would not survive. Cognitive therapy, which is a theory, set of techniques, and system of strategies, focuses on people's thinking as the primary pathway to change. After reading this chapter, you should be able to:

▶ Outline the development of cognitive-behavioral therapy (CBT) and Aaron Beck's contributions
▶ Explain the theory of cognitive-behavioral therapy including its core concepts
▶ Discuss the counseling relationship and goals in CBT
▶ Describe assessment, process, and techniques in CBT
▶ Demonstrate some therapeutic techniques
▶ Clarify the effectiveness of CBT

AARON BECK (1921–)

Aaron T. Beck, the man who developed cognitive therapy, was the youngest of five children born to Russian Jewish immigrants. Beck was often sick during his childhood. When he broke his arm in an accident, an infection from the bone moved to his blood resulting in a traumatic surgery he barely survived. He missed so much school that he had to repeat a grade, leading to his conclusion that he was stupid. He also developed many fears as a result of his illnesses. He had a blood/injury phobia and fears of public speaking and of being suffocated. Beck used reasoning to ease his anxieties and to make a plan to catch up in school. His early experiences likely motivated his work with cognitive therapy focusing on anxiety and depression.

Beck graduated from Brown University and Yale Medical School. He studied psychiatry and was trained as a psychoanalyst. Working at the University of Pennsylvania Medical School, Beck studied psychoanalytic principles and tried to substantiate Freud's theory of depression as "anger turned on the self." Eventually his research led him to formulate cognitive therapy, the focus of his career at the University of Pennsylvania where the Beck Institute for Cognitive Therapy and Research is housed.

Beck contended that various mental disorders have particular cognitive patterns and that the most effective and lasting therapy involves intervention into those patterns. In 1976, he published his groundbreaking book *Cognitive Therapy and Emotional Disorders* and has continued scholarly contributions throughout his career.

Albert Ellis and Aaron Beck worked independently during the same time period developing their approaches to cognitive therapy. Both Ellis and Beck believed that people can adopt reason and both considered a person's underlying assumptions as the focus for interventions. Ellis confronted patients and disputed their beliefs in order to convince them that their philosophies were unrealistic. In contrast, Beck's approach is a cooperative relationship with patients to identify and solve problems, overcoming their difficulties by altering thinking, behaviors, or emotional responses (Beck & Weishaar, 2014).

THE NATURE OF PEOPLE

Beck (1996) explained that infants are born with the disposition to survive. Later in life humans develop the desire to procreate. To accomplish these primal goals of survival and reproduction as well as any other goal, people must process information. Using the innate feelings of pleasure and pain as guides throughout life, people perceive, interpret, and learn from experiences. They draw conclusions, make predictions, and generate goals (Fall, Holden, & Marquis, 2010). Cognitive therapists acknowledge that children have different temperaments that push them in diverse directions. Therefore, children and adults are more likely to perceive the same event differently. Beck and Weishaar (2014) noted that people are not passive victims of their inborn tendencies but are actively creating and moving toward goals that are vital to them.

Personality emerges from the interactions between a person's innate disposition and that person's environment. Individuals have to discern what is important, how to understand it, and then construct an appropriate response. When a person realizes a situation needs a response, a set of cognitive, emotional, physiological, motivational, and behavioral schemes go into action (Beck & Weishaar, 2014). That information processing includes the following components in cognitive theory. *Cognitive structures* of a person represent the organization of information stored in memory. Cognitive structures serve as filters, screening the ongoing experiences of life. *Cognitive content* relates to the information that is stored—the substance of cognitive structures. More about that content follows. Together cognitive structures and content comprise what is known as a *schema* which grows from the processing of life experiences. A schema acts as a person's core philosophy, influencing expectations and screening information based on that core philosophy. The schema then affects the consistency in the person's cognition, behavior, and affect (Hayden & Mash, 2014). Furthermore, those schemas exist on a continuum of adaptive to maladaptive.

Beck and Haigh (2014) explain the adaptive functioning:

> When we are adapting well to life situations, our ability to function in our various roles is not impaired by errors in thinking, emotional distress is not disproportional to our realistic problems, and our behavioral strategies facilitate rather than impede attainment of our goals. Our cognitive, affective, motivational, and behavioral systems function to meet basic needs and equip us with strategies to protect from physical or interpersonal harm. The affective system provides the emotional fabric of our lives: affection to forge and maintain relationships, pleasure to reward enhancing activities, anxiety to signal danger, sadness to underscore loss or defeat, and anger to counter offenses (p.3).

However, a biased information-processing system produces thinking errors, inaccurate meaning, content, and information. According to Beck's model, maladaptive schemas develop in childhood and may not interfere with a person's thinking until a trigger is encountered in adulthood. The risk for negatively biased schemas includes genetic influences (Gibb, Beever, & McGeary, 2013) and environmental effects that shape attention and interactions.

Beck and Weishaar (2014) describe four levels of cognition, or cognitive content, within a person that are hierarchically organized based on a person's awareness of the thoughts and the stability of the thought: automatic thoughts, intermediate beliefs, core beliefs, and schemas. Cognitive counseling usually starts with the automatic thoughts and moves to identifying, evaluating, and changing intermediate and core beliefs, then to modifying schemas.

Automatic thoughts, a person's habits of the mind that are immediate, and self-talk, a person's private everyday commentary, are one level of the cognitive model. An example from a psychologically healthy person would be something like this: "I made a goal in the soccer match. I practiced really hard and all that work paid off." Automatic thoughts connect a situation and an emotion and reflect the meaning a person gives the situation.

Intermediate beliefs reflect the absolute rules and attitudes that influence a person's automatic thoughts. For the example above, an intermediate thought might be that working hard pays dividends or a less healthy approach would be "I got lucky."

Core beliefs are the significant ideas about ourselves from which many automatic thoughts and many intermediate beliefs grow. Judith Beck (2011) explained that core beliefs are global, overly generalized, and absolute but are not necessarily true. The beliefs may have started in childhood. Core beliefs reflect a person's view of the world, people, and the future as well as the sense of self and apply those across events in a person's experiences. Core beliefs can be modified and may be healthy such as "I am capable." Many negative core beliefs are either helpless beliefs ("I am a failure"; "I am weak") or unlovable beliefs ("I am not good enough"; "People will always abandon me"). As counselors hear automatic thoughts, they can begin to discern patterns of core beliefs and build hypotheses to be shared with the client when it is appropriate. Clients learn to consider core beliefs as ideas rather than as truth and to evaluate and change those beliefs if such modification is needed.

Schemas, again, are the cognitive structures within the mind that integrate the core beliefs (Beck, 2011). They go beyond core beliefs and include emotions, thoughts, and actions. Schemas lead to expectations and can act as mental filters to perceptions of the world. Each person processes information by using survival-supporting schemas of cognitions, emotions, physiology, motivation, and behavior. Cognitive schemas are core beliefs, such as danger, violation, loss, and gain; emotional schemas are core emotions, such as anxiety, anger, joy, and sadness. Motivational schemas are the core impulses: to escape or avoid, to attack, to grieve, or to approach. Physiological schemas are the body's autonomic, motor, and sensory systems. Finally, behavioral schemas are core actions such as smiling, shaking, and crying.

Young, Klosko, and Weishaar (2006) explain those interconnected themes and schemas. The theory of modes refers to an organization of schemas that connects beliefs, memories, reflections, and self-evaluations. That network of cognitive, affective, motivational, and behavioral components are used in the pursuit of goals. Modes represent those connections across the network. These systems have overlapping components such as the cognition of danger, the emotion of fear, the motivation to escape, and the behavior of fleeing—all of these components form the anxiety mode. The thoughts with which people consider their circumstances powerfully influence their emotional-motivational-behavioral responses (Fall et al., 2010).

Friedberg and McClure (2015) provide an example. Cognitive distortions are the processes in the model. Distortions convert incoming information to keep cognitive schema intact. They use the assimilation process to maintain homeostasis. For example, Miguel's schema reflects his perception of incompetence: he believes he cannot do anything well (schema). He feels anxious (emotion). He makes the honor roll one grading period (situation) and thinks the grades do not count because his classes are too easy (automatic thought). He is discounting his achievement (cognitive distortion). The information contrary to his core belief is canceled out by the distortion process, and he cannot identify any disconfirming evidence from his environment.

Cognitive-behavioral therapists have three fundamental assumptions. One is that cognitive activity impacts behavior. The next is that cognitive activity can be monitored and changed. The third idea critical to CBT is that a desired change in behavior can be accomplished through changing cognitions (Gilman & Chard, 2007). Based on these assumptions, cognitive-behavioral counselors work to help the child become aware of their distorted thinking, identify ways the distorted thinking relates to negative feelings and behaviors, and then change their thoughts and behaviors (Gilman & Chard).

THEORY OF COUNSELING

Beck, Freeman, and Davis (2006) identify the principles of cognitive therapy. It is based on the premise that changes in thoughts will lead to changes in feeling and acting. Treatment requires a strong collaborative relationship between client and counselor. Treatment is usually short, problem-focused, and goal oriented. It is an active, structured approach to counseling that focuses on the present. Counselors carefully assess, diagnose, and plan treatment based on that information. Counselors use a range of strategies to help clients evaluate and change their cognitions, particularly Socratic questioning and inductive reasoning. The model promotes emotional health and prevents relapse by teaching clients to identify, evaluate, and modify their thoughts. Homework, follow-up, and client feedback contribute to the success of the treatment.

Beck and Weishaar (2014) explain that cognitive therapists see personality as a reflection of the person's cognitive organization and structure, which are both biologically and socially influenced. Within the constraints of each person's neuro-anatomy and biochemistry, personal learning determines how a person develops and responds. The difference between health and dysfunction is in the way new experiences are assimilated into schemas. Mental health problems are the result of cognitive biases, maladaptive thinking styles that cause misinterpretations of events, irrational beliefs, and failure to see the world or self in a realistic way (Beck, 2011). Minor cognitive biases do not impede a person's functioning and are not problems requiring interventions. However, if unrealistic thinking causes either internal pain such as depression or anxiety or problem behavior such as aggression, therapeutic intervention is needed. Beck and Haigh (2014) recognize the theory of mode as particularly relevant to psychological disorders.

Cognitive distortion incorporates a person's sense of self, environment, and future (the cognitive triad). Gilman and Chard (2007) and Young et al. (2006) explain that in psychiatric disorders, distortions are apparent in each component. The example those authors provide is that depressed individuals view themselves as lacking personal competence, see their past and current failures as evidence of that incompetence, and have little hope for a more pleasant future. Anxious individuals consider themselves unable to deal with their distress, see elements in the environment as dangerous and threatening, and look at the future with fear and apprehension. People with externalizing disorders like conduct disorders see themselves as being treated unfairly or abused in some way, think other people are interfering with their personal goals, and that any future goal will be impeded by others.

Fall et al. (2010) outline these phenomena into four major modes: anxiety mode with cognitive perception of danger; anger mode with the perception of being violated; sadness mode with a perception of loss; joy mode with perception of gain. The accompanying schemas are outlined in the following table:

MODE	Danger	**Sadness**
COGNITION: Core beliefs	**Violation**	Happiness
EMOTION:	Loss	Escape/avoid
Core emotions	Gain	Attack
MOTIVATION: Core impulses	Fear	**Grieve**
Anxiety	**Anger**	Seek/approach
Danger	Sadness	Joy
Violation	Happiness	Danger
Loss	Escape/avoid	Violation
Gain	**Attack**	Loss
Fear	Grieve	**Gain**
Anger	Seek/approach	Fear
Sadness	Sadness	Anger
Happiness	Danger	Sadness
Escape/avoid	Violation	**Happiness**
Attack	**Loss**	Escape/avoid
Grieve	Gain	Attack
Seek/approach	Fear	Grieve
Anger	Anger	**Seek/approach**

Cognitive therapists look for these patterns and connections among events, thoughts, emotions, and behavior. They attempt to identify a person's internal picture of self and situation to understand how the person's feelings and actions make sense. Psychological disorders have profiles that reflect and maintain biases in information processing. J. Beck (2011) and Beck and Weishaar (2014) offer terms for some of the cognitive distortions that are associated with distressing emotions and maladaptive behaviors:

- Catastrophizing: expecting disastrous events
  - "I'll mess up the speech and everyone will laugh at me."
- Mental filtering: seeing an entire situation based on one detail with all else ignored
  - "I got a bad grade. I'm going to fail my course."
- Blame or assigning internal responsibility entirely to external events
  - "If I had a good instructor, I'd be a great gymnast."
- All-or-nothing thinking: the person thinks in terms of two opposite categories
  - "If I don't get to be team captain, I'm a total failure."
- Discounting the positive: person says positives do not count
  - "I played a good game but that doesn't mean anything. I just got lucky."
- Overgeneralization: a sweeping negative conclusion that goes beyond facts
  - "All teachers hate me."

Counselors help clients identify and change that faulty information processing (Beck & Weishaar, 2014) by getting clients to examine thought processes and develop cognitive therapy explanations for their feelings and behaviors.

Relationship

Beck and Weishaar (2014) describe the cognitive-behavioral therapeutic relationship as collaborative, working *with,* not *on* a person. The counselor is a warm, empathic, and genuine person and appreciates the client's personal worldview. She is flexible, sensitive, and supportive. She specifies problems, focuses on important areas, and teaches cognitive techniques. Counselors ask about the thoughts, images, and beliefs that occur within clients during situations as well as the emotions and behaviors that go along with the cognitions. The counselor finds sources of distress and dysfunction and helps the child clarify goals. In cases of severe depression or anxiety, the therapist will be very directive. The practitioner serves as a guide to help the client understand how beliefs and attitudes interact with emotions and behavior. The counselor is also a catalyst promoting corrective experiences, leading to cognitive change, and building skills. Counselors explain any intervention by giving a reason for using the procedure. In CBT, the counselor asks the client for feedback about what has been helpful or not helpful, whether the client has concerns about the counselor, and whether the client has any questions. The therapist may also summarize the session or ask the client to recap their time together. Finally, counselors make frequent use of homework to allow the client opportunities to practice new skills and perspectives.

Goals

Gilman and Chard (2007) divide cognitive-behavioral therapies into three categories with goals specific to the type: coping-skills therapies, cognitive-restructuring therapies, and problem-solving therapies. Coping-skills therapies revolve around developing specific skills that help the client deal with stressful events; for example, skills like relaxation strategies or social skills like eye contact. Cognitive-restructuring therapies include modifying and replacing dysfunctional thoughts with more adaptive cognitive patterns. The assumption is that changing the thoughts will lead to positive behavior change. Problem-solving approaches combine those two components—modifying thoughts and creating strategies to promote behavioral change. CBT falls into the problem-solving category.

COUNSELING METHODS

Judith Beck (2011) outlined counselor's responsibilities in CBT:

- Base counseling on an ever-evolving understanding of the person and his or her problems in cognitive terms
- Build a strong therapeutic alliance
- Stress collaboration and active participation
- Be goal oriented and problem focused
- Begin by highlighting the present
- Teach the client to be his or her own counselor and emphasize relapse prevention
- Try to be time-limited
- Structure sessions
- Teach clients to name, evaluate, and respond to their dysfunctional thoughts and beliefs
- Use a variety of techniques to change thinking, mood, and behavior

Kalodner (2011) explained that cognitive-behavioral counselors begin by developing an understanding of the case. That case formation is a dynamic process that requires the counselor to generate and test their hypotheses. It involves five parts: problem list, diagnosis, working hypothesis, strengths and assets, and treatment plan. The **problem list** is a comprehensive inventory of the difficulties that are explained in concrete behavioral terms. Five to eight problems may be listed in a variety of areas such as psychological, interpersonal, school, and leisure. The connections between the problems may become apparent as the list is constructed. Counselors may use a structured interview along with the child's explanation of the problem to compile the problem list. The second part is **diagnosis** or the issue which predominates. The diagnosis will be linked to the treatment plan. The **working hypothesis** allows the counselor to connect the issues on the problem list. Subsections of the hypothesis are the core beliefs, precipitating or activating situations, and origins. Core beliefs are the person's negative thoughts about self, the world, others, or the future. Precipitating situations refer to the external events that caused the symptom or problem, and origins refer to history that might be related. **Strengths and assets** are the positive parts of the person's situation, what is not a problem. Things like good friends, health, a sense of humor, school success, and a strong family bond may be assets. The **treatment plan** is the product of case conceptualization. It is related to the problem list and working hypothesis. The treatment plan describes the sequence and timing of interventions. It contains the goals for counseling, the obstacles to those goals, and the strategies to be used. These elements of case conceptualization provide a recipe for putting together a plan for the counseling process, giving a guide to adapting techniques for the individual child (Friedberg & McClure, 2015).

As discussed earlier, three concepts fundamental to cognitive therapy are collaborative empiricism, Socratic dialogue, and guided discovery. **Collaborative empiricism** defines the cooperative working relationship as focused on jointly determining goals and seeking feedback. Counselor and child are co-investigators of evidence supporting or rejecting cognitions by comparing them to observations, evidence, and facts gathered from everyday life. **Socratic dialogue** is a type of questioning designed to promote new learning. Questions are used to clarify or define, to assist in identifying thoughts, to examine meanings, and to test the consequences of thoughts and actions. Counselors avoid questions for which they already have answers. Friedberg and McClure (2015) explain that Socratic method includes systematic questioning, inductive reasoning, and constructing universal definitions. The method helps counselors uncover the database for children's beliefs but must be modified based on the children's responses and level of distress. Counselors use a gentle, curious stance rather than allowing the questions to become more like an inquisition. The purpose is to encourage children to test their inferences, judgments, conclusions, and appraisals. The categories for the questions are these:

What's the evidence?

What's an alternative explanation?

What are the advantages and disadvantages?

How can I problem solve?

Decatastrophizing or reducing the perceived degree of impact to something more manageable (Beck, 2011).

The outline for Socratic dialogues includes a five-part process.

1. Counselors elicit and identify the automatic thought.
2. Next, the thought is tied to the feeling and behavior.
3. Counselors then link the thinking-feeling-behavior sequence together with an empathic response.
4. Counselors collaborate with clients on the first three steps and reach an agreement to proceed.
5. The fifth step is to test the belief.

An example based on Friedberg and McClure (2002) follows:

TRACY: I never should have tried out for cheerleading.

COUNSELOR: What goes through your mind about trying out? [Identifying automatic thought]

TRACY: I made a fool of myself.

COUNSELOR: Hmm. What makes you see yourself that way? [Continuing with automatic thought]

TRACY: Only a stupid person would fall during her flip.

COUNSELOR: So you fell and thought it was because you were a terrible cheerleader choice.

TRACY: Yes.

COUNSELOR: How does that make you feel? [Tying automatic thought to feeling]

TRACY: Sad.

COUNSELOR: Let me see if I have this right. You are sad that you fell and I guess that would mean you don't want to try any more to be a cheerleader. [Connecting thought, feeling, and behavior in an empathic way]

TRACY: That's it.

COUNSELOR: What we need to do now is figure out whether people who fall in tryouts are stupid, foolish, and terrible cheerleader choices? Would you be willing to check this out? [Collaborating with client and getting agreement to go forward]

TRACY: Do you think it would help?

COUNSELOR: Well, we can give it a try and check to see as we go along.

TRACY: Okay.

Okay.

COUNSELOR: Let's see. How sure are you that falling once means you can't be a cheerleader? [Thought testing begins and continues.]

Guided discovery occurs when the counselor coaches the child in a voyage of self-discovery in which the child does his or her own thinking and draws his or her own conclusions. Guided discovery has many ingredients that vary from child to child. Those parts may be empathy, Socratic questioning, behavioral experiments, and homework. The process is designed to cast doubt on the certainty of children's beliefs and to encourage them to discover more adaptive and functional explanations for themselves. It requires patience and artful questioning to allow clients to build new appraisals for themselves (Friedberg & McClure, 2002).

Assessment

Assessment information is gathered through many sources such as interviews, objective self-reports, objective parent and teacher checklists, observations, and test data such as cognitive functioning, academic skills, and others.

Two self-report measures useful in school settings are the *Behavior Assessment System for Children-Second Edition, Self-Report of Personality* [BASC-2] (Reynolds & Kamphaus, 2004) and the *Beck Youth Inventories of Emotional and Social Impairment* (Beck, Beck, & Jolly, 2001). The *Beck Youth Inventories-Second Edition* (Beck, Beck, Jolly, & Steer, 2005) are founded on cognitive theory and diagnostic criteria. These well-established measures have documented reliability, validity, and normative information. The questionnaires are written at the second-grade reading level and can be used with children from 7 to 14 years. The self-report inventories are screening measures for anxiety, anger, disruptive behavior, and self-concept.

Process

The cognitive counselor helps the child learn how to shift out of the dysfunctional mode into a more functional way of thinking and doing, what

Leahy (1996) calls *power of realistic thinking*. The counselor and client share responsibility for setting the agenda, describing problem situations, and providing information about distressing emotions, behaviors, and associated thoughts. Again, the goals of cognitive therapy are to correct faulty information processing and to modify assumptions that maintain dysfunctional emotions and behaviors (Beck & Weishaar, 2014). One way to introduce the cognitive model to children is to use a story about a situation in which people may be thinking differently, such as riding a roller coaster (Creed, Reisweber, & Beck, 2011). Stories, pictures, or other examples make the explanation more fun, engaging, and more connected to the child's world.

Shapiro, Friedberg, and Bardenstein (2006) suggested asking children to think and talk about problems in general terms with these basic questions:

"What goes through your mind when _____ happens?"

"What goes through your mind when you feel _____?"

Other suggested questions for understanding children's cognitions are as follows:

"What do you make of this? What does it mean about you?"

"Why do you think _____ happens? How do you explain it?"

"What are your reasons for believing this? What is the evidence for that belief? What is the evidence against that belief?"

"What is another way to look at what happened?"

"How likely is it that _____ will happen?"

"What are the advantages of looking at things this way? What are the disadvantages?"

Cognitive therapy sessions typically follow an established framework according to Judith Beck (2011) even though the content of the session will change depending on the client. For the initial session she suggests these steps:

- Build an agenda that has meaning for the client
- Ascertain and measure the intensity of the person's mood
- Identify and review presenting problems
- Ask about the client's expectation for counseling
- Teach the person about cognitive therapy and the client's role in it
- Give information about the person's difficulties and diagnosis
- Establish goals
- Recommend homework
- Summarize
- Obtain the client's feedback (Beck, 2011, p. 60).

All of the following sessions have a similar format to the one above. Each session embodies a collaborative problem-solving focus with both the counselor and client actively involved with the use of *collaborative empiricism*. In collaborative empiricism, the situation experienced by the child is tested next to the child's interpretation of self, the world, and the future. In an example of a child who has been turned away from a play group and sees herself as friendless, the counselor would help the child check her interpretation of the situation against opposing or confirming evidence such as "Was there ever a time when someone asked you to play with her?" "Have you never been a part of a play group?" The counselor asks about each element in the cognitive triad like how important the friendship is to the child's sense of self, how true are the child's ideas about being isolated, and how deep is her belief that she will never have a friend. Counselors listen for and challenge words like *always*, *never*, and *should*.

CBT may be structured through the use of a manual. Sessions start with a check-in, a brief report of the child's emotional state. Counselor and child *set the agenda* or discuss what will be covered during their time together. Next, they *review homework* and examine any obstacles that interfered with completing the assignment. *Goal setting* for the current session often follows the review and a *new skill* is taught and practiced. The skill comes from what was learned previously and is taught by didactic methods, role-playing, and other methods. The session content or therapeutic techniques fill the rest of the time. Homework assignments give children ways to find evidence, face challenges, or practice skills they have learned. Finally, the counselor asks for *feedback* about the child's reaction and concerns.

Techniques

The practice of CBT combines behavior-change methods with thought-restructuring methods to produce behavior and feeling change in clients. Cognitive therapy has specific learning experiences designed to help clients monitor their negative, automatic thoughts; recognize the connections between cognition, emotion, and behavior; examine the evidence that supports and disputes automatic thoughts; substitute more reality thinking for biased cognitions; and learn to identify and alter distorted beliefs (Beck & Weishaar, 2014).

Cognitive counselors use verbal techniques to extract automatic thoughts, analyze the logic behind the thoughts, identify the assumptions underpinning the thoughts, and examining the validity of those assumptions. Gilman and Chard (2007) reviewed some common techniques of Socratic questioning, previously described, problem-solving, cognitive restructuring, self-monitoring, modeling, and role-playing.

Socratic questioning is widely used. The counselor questions and questions and questions to get the client's complete knowledge about a topic. Incomplete or inaccurate ideas can be corrected in follow-up questions and the client can replace misinterpretations with more realistic thoughts.

Problem-solving starts when the client and counselor create a problem list that is described with concrete, clear, and goal-oriented terms. The counselor teaches problem-solving skills to children and eventually encourages them to generate their own strategies. Socratic questioning, a problem-solving worksheet, and role-playing are used to help problem-solving. The basic steps in problem solving involve first (Step 1) identifying the problem in specific, concrete terms and then (Step 2) generating solutions to the situation. This brainstorming phase helps the child produce several alternatives. Step 3 involves evaluation of the option by looking carefully at short-term and long-term consequences of each possibility. Recording those ideas on paper makes them more concrete for the child. After deliberating the options and consequences of each solution, the counselor and child develop an implementation plan for the best option. The final step is the child rewarding himself or herself for trying out the solution (Friedberg & McClure, 2002).

Cognitive-restructuring is used to reduce, modify, or replace a person's cognitive distortions. It can be done in many ways such as challenging the distortion, examining the logic, testing the truth of the thoughts, and finding alternative explanations for situations. The counselor may want to use a sheet that has two columns, one for "evidence for" and the other column for "evidence against" the thoughts. This cognitive technique helps in testing automatic thoughts by direct evidence or by logical analysis.

Self-monitoring requires the client keep a log of their thoughts, emotions, and behaviors in response to events.

Modeling and role-playing are two common techniques in many forms of counseling. In modeling, the counselor shows the child how to do something and the child imitates the behavior. This can also be used to help parents learn positive behaviors with children. In role-playing, the child and counselor enact a situation and the child practices a newly learned behavior.

Beck and Weishaar (2014) define other techniques such as de-catastrophizing, reattribution, redefining, and decentering. Behavioral techniques such as homework, hypothesis testing, exposure therapy, behavioral rehearsal and role-playing, diversion techniques, and activity scheduling are also part of cognitive counseling.

De-catastrophizing is also called the "what if" technique. Clients state their feared consequences and identify problem-solving strategies to cope with the concerns.

Reattribution tests automatic thought by considering alternative reasons for the events. Clients may see themselves as the cause of a situation, an unreasonable assumption since a single person is rarely the sole reason for something happening. Reattributions use reality testing and appropriate assigning of responsibility by examining all the factors that affect a situation.

Redefining includes making a problem more concrete, specific, and restated in terms of the client's behavior. For example, a lonely person would switch "Nobody likes me" to "I need to reach out to people" (Burns, 1985).

Decentering occurs most often with anxious clients who think they are the focus of everyone's attention. The logic is examined and behavioral experiments are designed to test the beliefs. An example Beck and Weishaar (2014) provide is of a student who was afraid to speak in class because he thought his classmates always watched him and saw his anxiety. When he focused on them, he saw students looking at the teacher, taking notes, and daydreaming. He decided they had concerns other than him.

Behavioral techniques, as described by Beck and Weishaar (2014), are used to modify automatic thoughts and maladaptive assumptions. The behavioral experiments are designed to challenge beliefs and promote learning. Behavioral techniques are also employed to expand skills with training exercises, to help clients relax with progressive relaxation, to make them more active with activity scheduling, or to prepare clients for something they fear with exposure therapy or behavioral rehearsal.

Meichenbaum (1985) developed stress-inoculation training, one of the most successful cognitive-behavioral procedures. Stress-inoculation methods combined with role-playing to provide an example of a cognitive-behavioral technique. In cases of test anxiety, the client might be asked to practice the following examples of self-talk: (1) "Tests are no fun, but all I want is to do the best I can"; (2) "Though it would be nice to make an A, it is not required for me to be a good and worthwhile person"; (3) "All I need to do is prepare for the test and do the best I am able to do. If I fail, it will be inconvenient and no fun at all, but that is all it will be. For the moment, I just will not be getting what I want." Combining the self-talk with taking practice tests and visualization practice of the steps in the client's test-taking stimulus hierarchy (systematic desensitization) represents a typical CBT treatment plan.

Other stress-inoculation techniques include relaxation training, deep-breathing exercises, and reframing exercises that help children replace their anxiety with relaxation. Such reframing exercises help children perceive anxiety-provoking situations in a less threatening light. Rather than having the child focus on school as a place of potential failure and frightening teachers, for example, the counselor teaches the child to focus on the friends and fun available at school.

Stress-inoculation training programs, such as those designed by Meichenbaum (1977, 1985), have four categories of self-talk designed to help people master difficult and highly stressful situations and events. The categories are:

1. *Preparation for a stressor*: "What is it you have to do? You can develop a plan to deal with it. Don't worry."
2. *Confrontation and management of a stressor*: "One step at a time; you can handle the situation. Relax, you are in control. Take a slow, deep breath."
3. *Coping*: "Don't try to eliminate fear totally; just keep it manageable. Keep the focus on the present; what is it you have to do?"
4. *Reinforcing self-statements*: "It worked; you did it. It wasn't as bad as you expected. It's getting better each time."

Watkins (1983) adapted Maultsby's (1976) rational self-analysis format to fit the developmental level of children (Table 13-1). In Step 1, children write down what happened ("Jimmy called me a name because he doesn't like me."). In Step 2, children are asked to write, from the vantage point of a digital camera, what they would see and hear ("Jimmy didn't like it when I didn't choose him for my team."). With the increased objectivity obtained in Step 2, children are then asked in Step 3 to write down their thoughts about what happened ("It's terrible when people talk mean to me," or "If people get angry at me, I'm a bad person."). In Step 4, children are asked to write how they felt (hurt, angry) and what they did ("I hit him."). In Step 5, children are asked to find out if they have been thinking "smart" thoughts by testing their thoughts with the five questions listed in Step 6 (e.g., "Does my thought help me stay out of trouble with others?"). The answers are tabulated in the Step 5 box. If "no" wins, the children go to Step 7 and list some of the feelings they want to feel (e.g., a child may prefer to feel sad or disappointed instead of hurt, irritated, or angry). In Step 8, children are asked to write "smarter" thoughts that would help them feel better feelings ("I don't like it when others get upset with me, but things could be worse, and I don't have to let others control how I act."). Step 9 is reserved for a plan of action children can use the next time somebody does something to make them feel bad.

TABLE 13-1 COGNITIVE SELF-ANALYSIS FOR CHILDREN

Step 1. Write down what happened.	**Step 2.** Be a video camera. If you were a video camera and recorded a videotape of what happened, what would you see and hear?	**Step 3.** Write down your thoughts about what happened. What did you think? A. B. C.

Step 4.
A. How did you feel?
B. What did you do?
	Step 5. Decide if your thoughts are "smart." To do this, look at each thought you had and ask yourself the five questions in Step 6. Answer yes or no to each question and write your answers below.
	
	   A. 1. B. 1. C. 1.
	      2. 2. 2.
	      3. 3. 3.
	      4. 4. 4.
	      5. 5. 5.
		Step 6. How do you know if you're thinking "smart" thoughts? Ask:
		1. Is my thought really real, say if I were a video camera, what would I see?
		2. Does the thought help me stay alive and in good physical shape?
		3. Does the thought help me get what I want?
		4. Does the thought help me stay out of trouble with others?
		5. Does the thought help me feel the way I want to?

Step 7. How do you want to feel?	**Step 8.** Write down thoughts you could have that would be "smarter" than those listed. A. B. C.	**Step 9.** What do you want to do?

Source: Watkins, (1983); adapted from Maultsby (1976).

Counselors may be confused about which of these strategies to use. J. Beck (2011) provides these guidelines. Before the session, cognitive practitioners need to consider the client's problem and the cognitive formulation of that problem; effective counseling practices with this concern; and an overall understanding of the client, the strength of the alliance, and the treatment stage among other things. During the session, clinicians should think about the recent, specific example of the problem empathy and on which part of the cognitive model to focus the session. Her examples of those parts are designing a solution to the problem, addressing automatic thoughts, teaching emotional regulation skills, working on behavior change, or decreasing physiological distress. She notes the decision about which technique should be collaborative using a question such as "do you think it would be more helpful if we did _____ or _____?" With that information the counselor can make an informed decision about the strategy to use in that session.

APPLICATIONS OF COGNITIVE-BEHAVIORAL THERAPY

Kendall and Hollon (1979) said many years ago and Benjamin and colleagues (2011) more recently that CBT targets multiple areas of vulnerability and uses many strategies for intervention. Some examples follow.

Middle school children who witnessed traumatic events and who had symptoms of PTSD improved with cognitive interventions (Stein et al., 2003) in a 10-session cognitive therapy group. The sessions followed this sequence:

1. Introduction, explanation of treatment, information on stress and trauma;
2. Education on responses to stress and trauma, relaxation training;
3. Introduction to cognitive therapy, connecting thoughts and feelings, measuring fear, and the ways of fighting negative thoughts;
4. Fighting negative thoughts;
5. Coping strategies, fear hierarchy;
6. Exposure to troubling memories using imagination, drawing, writing;
7. Same as 6;
8. Social problem-solving;
9. Practicing social problem-solving;
10. Relapse prevention.

In a meta-analysis of six studies of trauma-focused CBT, the researchers concluded the treatment was an effective intervention for PTSD in children who have been sexually abused (Macdonald et al., 2012). Similarly, Silverman and colleagues (2008) analyzed 21 treatment studies of cognitive therapy. They concluded that trauma-focused CBT met the criteria for a well-established treatment. They also determined that school-based group CBT met the criteria for probably efficacious approach for children exposed to traumatic events.

Anger Control

Christner, Friedberg, and Sharp (2006) explained the cognitive distortions of angry or aggressive young people: all-or-nothing thinking, mental filtering, emotional reasoning, and personal codes. All-or-nothing thinking is a distortion that allows only absolutes so that no medium area is considered—for example, people are either for or against them, love or hate them. Mental filtering refers to their focus on the negative or potentially hostile parts of the situation. They jump to conclusions without considering all factors in the situation. A too common example is a young man who gets pushed while walking in a crowded hall. He immediately thinks the push was deliberate and meant to provoke him. This example also illustrates emotional reasoning or basing actions and thoughts only on an emotional state, which causes impulsive behavior without adequate cognitive mediation. Aggressive children also have some personal codes or rules that are rigid *should* statements like "no one treats me that way." When the rules are broken, the youngsters are enraged and try to punish the person who has violated the rule.

Christner et al. (2006) and Lochman and colleagues (2012) discussed working with angry and aggressive young people in school settings. They outlined types of aggressive behavior and the need for effective interventions in the schools. Three programs grounded in cognitive-behavioral theory were shown to be effective: anger coping, social problem-solving, and parent training programs. Garland, Hawley, Brookman-Frazee, and Hurlburt (2008) also identified common elements of evidence-based treatments for children's disruptive behavior problems as problem-solving and other cognitive-behavioral interventions. Finally, Lochman, Powell, Boxmeyer, and Jimenez-Carmargo (2011) provide a comprehensive review of CBT for children and adolescents with externalizing disorder such as antisocial behaviors.

Anxiety

Kendall, Hudson, Choudhury, Webb, and Pimentel (2005) developed a program for childhood anxiety disorders, *Coping Cat*, which involves 16 sessions and includes psychoeducation, self-monitoring, relaxation, and cognitive coping skills training. *Coping Cat* has been the most widely evaluated program for a broad range of childhood anxiety and has significantly positive results (NREPP, 2014). Five principles for the child are to:

1. Learn to recognize anxious feelings and physical reaction related to anxiety
2. Identify unrealistic expectations and distorted thoughts in the anxious situations
3. Develop a plan to cope with the anxiety-producing events
4. Be gradually exposed to the anxiety-provoking situation
5. Evaluate performance with self-reinforcement strategies (Gilman & Chard, 2007)

Gosch and Flannery-Schroeder (2006) identified school-based interventions for anxiety disorders. They taught children about identifying their somatic reactions to anxiety, modifying their anxious self-talk, problem solving, and contingency management. After skills were mastered, the CBT counselors used graded exposure or gradual contact to the feared situation, object, or event so that students could practice their new coping skills. These authors also suggested training teachers and other school personnel ways to reduce children's anxiety.

Khanna and Kendall (2010) studied the efficacy of a computer-assisted cognitive-behavioral therapy for child anxiety. The finding of the program, Camp Cope-A-Lot (CCAL), supports the feasibility, acceptability, and beneficial effects of CCAL for anxious youth. Blocher, Fujikawa, Sung, Jackson, and Jones (2013) also used a manual-based, computer-assisted cognitive-behavioral therapy intervention for children with anxiety and epilepsy. They reported significant reductions in the symptoms of anxiety and depression in children.

Depression

Beck (1976) explained a cognitive triad that characterizes depression. The depressed person has a negative view of self, the world, and the future. The depressed individual considers self as inadequate, deserted, and worthless. Beck (2008) has also connected this psychological explanation of depression to its neurobiological correlates. His explanation combines the growing evidence of brain topography with the symptoms of depression and his call for further research will be answered to clarify those connections.

Depressed children and adolescents experience distortions in attributions, self-evaluation, and perceptions of past and present events. Silverman and DiGiuseppe (2001) have found a significant correlation between self-reported depression and negative automatic thoughts in a study of 126 students in grades 4 through 8. Depressed children exhibit more external locus of control (an indication that they feel less capable) and low self-esteem resulting from a perceived inability to succeed academically and socially. Effective help for depressed children included training them in self-control, self-evaluation, assertiveness, and social skills. Their social skills training included initiating and maintaining interactions and conflict resolution. The specific cognitive-behavioral techniques included relaxation, imagery, and cognitive restructuring.

As stated earlier, cognitive-behavioral treatments for depression are based on the assumption that depression is a result of faulty thoughts and maladaptive behavior. Therefore, the child's cognitions, affect, and behaviors are targeted simultaneously (Gilman & Chard, 2007). Children are taught to distinguish between thoughts and feelings by teaching, role-play, and storytelling. After children understand that difference, discussions about the situations that bring out positive and negative moods happen. The counselor helps the child see how thoughts may have influenced behaviors. At the same time, behavioral strategies such as activity planning, social problem-solving, or interaction skills may be used. The child practices cognitive restructuring both in and outside the sessions. Setting appropriate goals, identifying distorted thoughts, and learning to replace those cognitions with constructive thoughts and management skills, like relaxation, may be included.

CBT models for depression often consist of four levels of treatment: (1) behavioral procedures, such as contingent reinforcement, shaping, prompting, and modeling, to increase social interaction; (2) CBT interventions, which include pairing successful task completion with positive self-statements and reinforcement for those self-statements; (3) cognitive interventions, which are used with social-skills training, role-playing, and self-management; and (4) self-control procedures such as self-evaluation and self-reinforcement. McLaughlin and Christner (2012) outline ways to accomplish those tasks.

One intervention, the *Adolescent Coping with Depression Course* (CWD-A), includes monitoring mood, developing social skills, increasing pleasant activities, decreasing anxiety, reducing depressive cognitions, improving communication, and resolving conflicts (Lewinsohn, Clarke, Hops, & Andrews, 1990). Cuiipers, Muñoz, Clarke, and Lewinsohn (2009) reviewed studies of this treatment plan across a 30-year span, which supported the efficacy of the approach. This intervention model is recognized in the National Registry of Evidence-based Programs and Practices (NREPP), a service of the Substance Abuse and Mental Health Services Administration (SAMHSA). CBT for Adolescent Depression (Brent & Poling, 1997) also has been identified as an effective treatment program (NREPP, 2014).

Donoghue, Wheeler, Prout, Wilson, and Reinecke (2006) provided explanations and interventions for children and adolescents who are depressed. Those authors focused on activities that may be delivered in school settings such as small groups and courses. Deblinger, Mannarino, Cohen, Runyon, and Steer (2011) studied the effectiveness of trauma-focused cognitive-behavioral therapy for children with depression had found strong positive results for children and parents. Eckstein and Gaynor (2013) conducted follow-up of treatment that combined individual cognitive-behavioral therapy and parent training for childhood depression. Their results suggested that the significant decreases in depressive symptoms observed after treatment were maintained across the 2 to 3 years of the follow-up study.

Attention-Deficit/Hyperactivity Disorder

Children with ADHD show deficiencies in the mechanisms that govern (1) sustained attention and effort, (2) inhibitory controls, and (3) the modulation of arousal levels to meet situational demands. DuPaul and colleagues (2012) described a process for working with children who have ADHD in schools. Shillingford, Lambie, and Walter (2007) also presented a way to use cognitive strategies with school children who have ADHD.

Ronen (1992), in a dated but nonetheless relevant essay, discusses cognitive therapy with children and its suitability for children's needs and ability levels. She lists the most frequent behavior problems of children (from most common to least common): loss of temper, hyperactivity, fears, restlessness, sleep disorders, enuresis, food intake, nail biting, tics, and stuttering. Her review of the literature revealed that children with behavior problems such as hyperactivity, impulsivity, and aggression tend to (1) generate fewer alternative solutions to interpersonal problems, (2) focus on ends or goals rather than on the intermediate steps toward obtaining them, (3) see fewer consequences associated with their behavior, (4) fail to recognize causes of others' behavior, and (5) be less sensitive to interpersonal conflict. Ronen then outlines some successful applications of CBT, such as self-assessment, self-instruction, self-reinforcement, and self-punishment. Cognitive treatments require children's active participation in learning to identify irrational thoughts, initiate internal dialogues, halt automatic thinking, change automatic thoughts to mediated ones, and use CBT to change unwanted behavior. Ronen responds to the question of whether children have developed sufficient cognitive skills to benefit from a cognitive approach by citing the similarity in difficulty between early childhood tasks and understanding CBT; she compares changing one's behavior with learning to ride a bicycle, use computers, or read and write. Ronen identifies three keys to such learning: (1) the knowledge of how to do it, (2) the desire to learn and practice, and (3) time to practice. Basically, our position is that good counselors should be able to teach children and adolescents almost any CBT skill that can be broken down into mediating steps that they understand and find meaningful to the events in their everyday lives.

Health Problems

Power and DeRosa (2012) outlined a CBT approach to intervening with health problems. They suggested a case conceptualization that included understanding and strengthening systems and system interconnections, identifying children's problems and resources to solve problems, analyzing problems and strengths, implementing interventions and evaluation effectiveness. The range of interventions they describe are adapted for educational settings.

Drug Use

Waldron and Kaminer (2004) reviewed the effectiveness of CBT for adolescent drug abuse. They noted that family therapy led to rapid improvement, but after 6 to 12 months of individual or group treatment, CBT was as effective. The protocols for CBT with adolescents with substance abuse include motivational interviewing, self-monitoring, contingency contracting, and refusal skills as well as coping, communication, and problem-solving skills.

Forman (2006) explained that a CBT substance abuse prevention approach focuses on developing coping skills that can offset risk factors and serve as buffers to substances abuse. The skills are self-management, decision making, problem-solving, communication, assertiveness, and anxiety and anger management skills as well as cognitive skills. The effective programs use interactive skills training. She cautioned schools to use only evidence-based substance abuse prevention programs.

Case Study*

ID of Problem

Derek is a 15-year-old boy in a residential treatment program. He was referred to the program by the Department of Juvenile Justice and Delinquency Prevention due to anger and aggression issues and his inability to function appropriately at home or in an alternative school. Derek consistently challenges authority and is often unwilling to take responsibility for his actions.

Academic

Prior to transitioning to the residential program, Derek was a student at an alternative school. He has difficulty completing classroom assignments without significant assistance and/or extensive explanation, and was often teased for being slow.

Family

Derek is the second of three children. His mother is recently disabled, and his father works in a factory. The family struggles to make ends meet. Derek's uncles and grandparents are alcoholics and share their substances with Derek and his siblings.

Social

Derek has a few friends in his neighborhood, but has difficulty making new friends. He has been accused of teasing and physically assaulting other children and has difficulty with regular social interactions.

Transcript

COUNSELOR: Hi Derek. What would you like to talk about today?

DEREK: You should have been here this morning, I got in trouble again. I'm on level one because of something stupid!! These people are always picking on me, and I don't get it. I didn't even do anything that bad!

COUNSELOR: You feel you're being treated unfairly.

DEREK: Yeah, I got my level dropped because I went outside to take a time-out because I was really angry, and I needed a break.

COUNSELOR: You went out to take a time-out?

DEREK: Yeah, I was really angry, and I needed to get away. People always telling us to using our "coping skills," and I do that by taking walks. They said they dropped my level because I didn't ask for permission to take a walk. That's dumb! They're just trying to make it hard—don't want me to get mad, don't want me to take a walk to cool off.

---

* The case of Derek was contributed by Tasha Hicks.

COUNSELOR:	You walked off without permission and got punished. You were angry before, and now you're even angrier.
DEREK:	Yeah, but…. it's not fair. I never get what I want.
COUNSELOR:	Derek, if I were watching a video of this incident, what would I see?
DEREK:	You'd see that dumb Tom pushing me outside my door and me getting ready to pop him. Then, hey, like we talked about it. I took a deep breath and then walked out the door at the end of the hall. Then that director person comes running out the door, yelling "Come back here, come back here, you know the rule," and I just kept on walking, thinking nobody can make me.
COUNSELOR:	That helps me understand how it happened. You said you were thinking nobody can make me—what other thoughts were going on in your head?
DEREK:	I keep getting in trouble. I can never stay on level, and I'm always going to be a bad kid. I can never be better because I keep doing stupid stuff. Man, I don't know why I even try.
COUNSELOR:	You think you're a failure and that people are out to get you. Then you are angry and do something to get in trouble—is that how it goes?
DEREK:	Pretty much.
COUNSELOR:	OK. Derek, what else could be going on?
DEREK:	What do you mean by that dumb question?
COUNSELOR:	I mean it sounds to me like you just put yourself in this box that has big FAILURE labels all over it.
DEREK:	Well so, yeah, but it's because everyone also tells me that.
COUNSELOR:	Anything else?
DEREK:	I don't have lots of friends and the guys at school tease me all the time about being slow.
COUNSELOR:	What else?
DEREK:	My mom and dad, they tell me they love me, but they never want to do anything with me; it's like they're ashamed of me or something.
COUNSELOR:	Okay, let's put all those things on a list—here's some paper. I'll help you remember, and you can write them down in that first column.
DEREK:	Here you go—
COUNSELOR:	Now there are three things there on that list. Which one of them is most important to your being a failure?
DEREK:	Those guys that tease me.
COUNSELOR:	So let me ask you some questions about that. I'm wondering if you ever tease anyone.
DEREK:	Yeah, my little brother—that's fun to see him get red in the face and push out his chest and then start crying—all I have to do is call him girly or stupid or something dumb.
COUNSELOR:	And that means he's a failure because you tease him?
DEREK:	Huh? No way—he's real smart and lots of fun to play basketball with and he likes the same video games—we play them lots.
COUNSELOR:	So teasing doesn't make him a failure, but it does make you one.

DEREK: Well, maybe not just teasing, maybe all those other things too.

COUNSELOR: Derek, I wonder if you'd like to let me help you figure out all those things and what's going on inside you that keeps you angry and feeling like a failure. Maybe we can look at what you are saying to yourself, go down this list and even make another one if you want or do some other things together to try to figure this out so maybe you can stay on the level you want to be on.

DEREK: Yeah let's do that. I feel better when I have privileges, like when I'm on a higher level. It's hard to keep up, but it feels good, and I want to stay on a good level.

COUNSELOR: Sounds to me like you tried really hard today when Tom pushed you so you got that right but then the second part didn't work out so well.

DEREK: Um … Well. I guess you could see it that way—like I got part one right but need to work on part two.

COUNSELOR: That's what it sounds like to me too—so maybe instead of being a failure, you are being a …

DEREK: like someone who is training for something like a race—like you can't do it all at once but you learn to get stronger and all.

COUNSELOR: Exactly—now let's see how we can help you more in that training.

DEREK: Sure.

COUNSELOR: OK, what else on this list can we talk about …

Cognitive-behavioral counseling helps people connect their thoughts, emotions, and behaviors. They identify their beliefs that maintain the distorted thinking that interferes with their lives. Derek thinks of himself as a failure and finds many things in his environment to keep that belief in place. Like many disruptive adolescents, he thinks he is treated unfairly and that people are always interfering with his goals. Furthermore, he is convinced all his future goals will be obstructed in the same way. The counselor has begun to help him connect his thoughts, feelings, and actions and to ask him to think of one particular instance (the teasing) in an alternative way. As their sessions continue, the counselor will use more interventions to help Derek challenge his distortions, self-monitor, and develop the skills he will need to get along better in his world.

Cognitive-Behavioral Play Therapy

Counselors realize that some children do not have the experiences or cognitive skills of an adult. For example, a preoperational child has limitations in seeing a situation from another point of view. Those perceptions can be modified with repeated experiences. Children may not attach meaning or beliefs to situations, and thus may be limited in developing coping behaviors. These concepts guide cognitive therapy for children and adolescents:

- Thoughts influence responses.
- Interpretations of events are based on beliefs.
- Children who have problems have errors in logic and may make assumptions that are incorrect.

Cognitive-behavioral play therapy incorporates cognitive and behavioral therapies through play using play activities to help the child solve problems. Knell (2011) explained that cognitive-behavioral play therapy provides structured, goal-directed activities, allowing the child to engage in an unstructured, spontaneous way. This therapy uses techniques chosen to relieve symptoms of distress by modifying the cognitive errors that accompany them.

The therapy is brief, directive, and problem oriented. In cognitive-behavioral play therapy, the therapeutic relationship is educational and collaborative. Knell (2009) explains that counselors see the child's words as basic data, and, rather than assuming unconscious meaning, the counselor uses focused questions to reveal the child's thoughts. A positive relationship is based on rapport and trust, with play activities being a means of communication. Play techniques, as well as verbal and nonverbal communication, are used to help children change their behavior and participate in the therapy. The active intervention involves the child and the counselor working together to establish goals. Both choose play materials and activities. The counselor focuses on the child's thoughts, feelings, fantasies, and environment.

During cognitive-behavioral play therapy, the child works through stages of introduction and orientation, assessment, middle, and termination phases. The introduction allows counselor and child to identify each other, and the orientation outlines the process of counseling. Assessment may occur by asking "What goes through your mind when __?" (Shapiro et al., 2006). During the middle stage, the therapy is focused on increasing the child's self-control and sense of accomplishment as well as learning different responses to situations.

Through play activities, such as using puppets to model, and cognitive strategies like disputing irrational beliefs and making positive statements about self, children can learn about counseling indirectly (Knell, 2009). The child learns new skills with the counselor's instruction. The counselor uses praise and interpretation to help the child learn new behaviors and increase understanding of his or her thoughts. The counselor also provides strategies for developing more adaptive thoughts and behaviors. The behavioral techniques used by the counselor may include systematic desensitization, contingency management, self-monitoring, and activity scheduling. Cognitive techniques include recording thoughts, cognitive change strategies, coping self-statements, and bibliotherapy. To accomplish the educative process, counselors use techniques such as modeling, role-playing, and using behavioral contingencies (Knell, 2011).

The counselor also emphasizes the issues of control, mastery, and responsibility for the client's own behavior change. Knell (2009) believes that combining cognitive and behavioral interventions increases the potency of the intervention. The change proceeds first in calming the child through the counselor's empathy and acceptance. Relaxation techniques and verbal approval also are appropriate. In the second stage, children are given opportunities to experience and test the thoughts that are associated with their emotions. Next, the children examine their distortions and learn to discern rational and irrational ideas to shift their perceptions. The counselor uses modeling tailored to the needs of the children to demonstrate adaptive coping skills. Cognitive change and adaptive behaviors are communicated indirectly.

Knell and Dasari (2009) outlined a process of changing behaviors and thoughts of children who are anxious and afraid. They explained that overcoming fears involves gaining mastery over them. The child may learn to deal with the source of the anxiety and fear, to manage feelings associated with the fear, or to use specific coping skills to deal with the fear and anxiety. Treatment with this type of play therapy included providing accurate information to the child, teaching deep breathing and muscle relaxation, cognitive restructuring, exposure and relapse prevention.

The success of cognitive-behavioral play therapy has been discussed in work with children who have ADHD (Young & Bramham, 2012), anger and aggression problems (Sukhodolsky & Scahill, 2012; Wilde, 2001), social adjustment concerns (Maryam, Mona, & Akram, 2014), insomnia (Tikotzky & Sadeh, 2010), and who have anxiety (Compton et al., 2004; Kendall & Treadwell, 2007).

Friedberg (1996) has given some specific suggestions for using cognitive-behavioral games and workbooks with distressed children in schools. He states that the flexibility and creativity of incorporating games and workbooks can promote the counseling relationship and augment the traditional counseling process. Utay and Lampe (1995) present a cognitive-behavioral group counseling game designed to increase the social skills of children with learning disabilities. Their study supports the effectiveness of the cognitive-behavioral approach to play therapy.

DIVERSITY APPLICATIONS OF COGNITIVE-BEHAVIORAL THERAPY

Cognitive-behavioral therapy is respectful, focused on current concerns and appeals to groups of all ages and backgrounds (Seligman & Reichenberg, 2014). Cognitive counseling techniques are especially appealing to those cultures and to those individuals in all cultures who prefer strong, directive counseling and an active counselor who favors dispensing information and helping people think, feel, and behave better. The approaches are not obtrusive, do not dwell on the past or the unconscious, and are respectful to the person. Cognitive-behavioral practitioners have an array of techniques and methods that can be taught to people from cultures favoring education and training that will, in turn, lead to empowering clients to solve problems and resolve conflicts. Seligman and Reichenberg note this approach is particularly appropriate if a person's culture does not emphasize insight or self-expression. Beck's work has been translated into more than a dozen languages.

Cognitive behavior counseling methods include relaxation and stress-reduction techniques, assertiveness training, anxiety management, modeling, role-playing, and goal setting. The counseling interview offers a "safe" environment for the counselor to explain and demonstrate each technique before giving clients a choice of which methods they would like to try. Clients feel safe in experimenting with the new methods they have been taught before using them in real-life situations. As for any client from any culture, the cognitive-behavioral counselor will want to be sure that the client's belief system is examined in the bright light of reality to see which beliefs are truly rational and irrational. For example, for a minority client, the belief that "I can't get a job" could very well be a rational belief in situations where discrimination against certain groups is practiced (Fuertes, Bartolomeo, & Nichols, 2001).

Hays and Iwamasa (2006) have compiled essays on the assessment, practice, and supervision of culturally responsive CBT. Their book focuses on the use of CBT with specific groups of Native, Latino, Asian, and African American heritage and people of Arab and Orthodox Jewish backgrounds. Cognitive-behavioral counselors will find this resource helpful in understanding and adapting this approach in a culturally appropriate manner.

EVALUATION OF COGNITIVE-BEHAVIORAL THERAPY

Butler, Chapman, Forman, and Beck (2006) and Epp and Dobson (2010) write that with children and adolescents, CBT has been clinically demonstrated in randomized controlled trials to be an effective treatment for the following disorders and problems:

- Depression (among adolescents and depressive symptoms among children)
- Anxiety disorders
  o Separation anxiety
  o Avoidant disorder
  o Overanxious disorder
  o Obsessive-compulsive disorder
  o Phobias
  o Post-traumatic stress disorder
- Conduct disorder (oppositional defiant disorder)
- Distress due to medical procedures (mainly for cancer)
- Recurrent abdominal pain
- Physical complaints not explained by a medical condition (somatoform disorders)

Fall et al. (2010) declare that during the past 20 years, evidence has accumulated on the effectiveness of cognitive therapy across a range of mental disorders, particularly on the treatment of fear and anxiety, specific phobias, and problems in adjustment. This therapy obviously emphasizes goal setting, accountability, and well-documented results.

SUMMARY

Aaron Beck and his associates have developed and refined CBT, an approach which has grown due to its empirical base and demonstrated usefulness. Beck and Weishaar (2014) explained that the common denominators across all effective therapies are an understandable framework, the client's active participation in counseling, and reality testing the situation. CBT embodies those criteria. CBT practitioners believe that people's thoughts give meaning to the events in their lives. Cognitive biases cause distortions in thinking and the negative direction of some of those biases lead to mental health problems.

Cognitive-behavioral counselors believe that helping people make positive changes means allowing them to identify, evaluate, and modify their thoughts. Emotions are not ignored, but distorted thoughts are the focus of treatment. CBT is brief, structured, collaborative, and effective. Clients have specific plans for change and receive clear explanation of the counseling process. They also have opportunities to learn and practice skills. CBT has been deemed effective in the treatment of depression, anxiety, substance abuse, and other mental disorders (Carr, 2009).

Ronen (1998) cautioned counselors to use simple and specific instructions with young children. Play therapy (Knell, 2009, 2011), as well as art activities and drama or role-playing, may be used by CBT counselors working with children. Friedberg and Wilt (2010) explain how to use metaphors with youngsters. Friedberg and McClure (2002; 2015) and Mennuti, Christner, and Freeman (2012) have provided specifics about using cognitive-behavioral counseling with children and adolescents.

WEB SITES FOR COGNITIVE-BEHAVIORAL THERAPY

Internet addresses frequently change. To find the sites listed here, visit www.cengage .com/counseling/henderson for an updated list of Internet addresses and direct links to relevant sites.

American Institute for Cognitive Therapy

Schema Therapy

The Center for Cognitive Therapy

The Beck Institute for Cognitive Therapy and Research

The Academy of Cognitive Therapy

REFERENCES

Beck, A. (1976). *Cognitive therapy and emotional disorders*. New York: International Universities Press.

Beck, A. (1996). Beyond belief: A theory of modes, personality, and psychopathology. In P. Salkovskis (Ed.), *Frontiers of cognitive therapy* (pp. 1–25). New York: Guilford.

Beck, A. T. (2008). The evolution of the cognitive model of depression and its neurobiological correlates. *American Journal of Psychiatry, 165,* 969–977.

Beck, A. T., Freeman, A., & Davis, D. D. (2006). *Cognitive therapy of personality disorders* (2nd ed.). New York: Guilford Press.

Beck, A. T., & Haigh, E. A. P. (2014). Advances in cognitive theory and therapy: The generic cognitive model. *Annual Review of Clinical Psychology, 10*(1), 1–24. doi:10.1146/annurev-clinpsy-032813-153734

Beck, A. T., & Weishaar, M. E. (2014). Cognitive therapy. In R. J. Corsini & D. Wedding (Eds.), *Current psychotherapies* (10th ed., pp. 231–264). Belmont, CA: Thomson.

Beck, J. S. (2011). *Cognitive therapy: Basics and beyond* (2nd ed.). New York: Guilford Press.

Beck, J., Beck, A., & Jolly, J. (2001). *Manual for the Beck youth inventories of emotional and social impairment*. San Antonio, TX: Psychological Corporation.

Beck, J. S., Beck, A. T., Jolly, J. B., & Steer, R. A. (2005). *Beck youth inventories adolescents manual* (2nd ed.). San Antonio, TX: Harcourt Assessment.

Benjamin, C. L., Puleo, C. M., Settipani, C. A., Brodman, D. M., Edmunds, J. M., Cummings, C. M., et al. (2011). History of cognitive-behavioral therapy in youth. *Child and Adolescent Psychiatric Clinics of North America, 20*(2), 179–189. doi:10.1016/j.chc.2011.01.011

Blocher, J. B., Fujikawa, M., Sung, C., Jackson, D. C., & Jones, J. E. (2013). Computer-assisted cognitive behavioral therapy for children with epilepsy and anxiety: A pilot study. *Epilepsy & Behavior, 27*(1), 70–76. doi:10.1016/j.yebeh.2012.12.014

Brent, D., & Poling, K. (1997). *Cognitive therapy treatment manual for depressed and suicidal youth*. Pittsburgh, PA: University of Pittsburgh, Services for Teens at Risk.

Burns, D. D. (1985). *Intimate connections*. New York: Morrow.

Butler, A. C., Chapman, J. E., Forman, E. M., & Beck, A. T. (2006). The empirical status of cognitive-behavioral therapy: A review of meta-analyses. *Clinical Psychology Review, 26*, 17–31.

Carr, A. (2009). *What works with children, adolescents, and adults? A review of research on the effectiveness of psychotherapy*. New York: Routledge.

Christner, R. W., Friedberg, R. D., & Sharp, L. (2006). Working with angry and aggressive youth. In R. B. Mennuti, A. Freeman, & R. W. Christner (Eds.), *Cognitive-behavioral interventions in educational settings: A handbook for practice* (pp. 203–220). New York: Routledge.

Compton, S. N., March, J. S., Brent, D., Albano, A. M., Weersing, V. R., & Curry, J. (2004). Cognitive-behavioral psychotherapy for anxiety and depressive disorders in children and adolescents: An evidence-based medicine review. *Journal of the American Academy of Child and Adolescent Psychiatry, 43*, 930–959.

Creed, T. A., Reisweber, J., & Beck, A. T. (2011). *Cognitive therapy for adolescents in school settings*. New York: Guilford Press.

Cuiipers, P., Muñoz, R. F., Clarke, G. N., & Lewinsohn, P. M. (2009). Psych educational treatment and prevention of depression: The "coping with depression" course thirty years later. *Child Psychology Review, 29*, 449–458. doi:10.1016/j.cpr.2009.04.005

Deblinger, E., Mannarino, A. P., Cohen, J. A., Runyon, M. K., & Steer, R. A. (2011). Trauma-focused cognitive behavioral therapy for children: impact of the trauma narrative and treatment length. *Depression & Anxiety (1091-4269), 28*(1), 67–75. doi:10.1002/da.20744

Donoghue, A. R., Wheeler, A. R., Prout, M. F., Wilson, H. W., & Reinecke, M. A. (2006). Understanding depression in children and adolescents: Cognitive-behavioral interventions. In R. B. Mennuti, A. Freeman, & R. W. Christner (Eds.), *Cognitive-behavioral interventions* (pp. 121–138). New York: Routledge.

DuPaul, G. J., Carson, K. M., Gormley, M. J., Junod, R. W., & Flammer-Rivera, L. M. (2012). Attention-deficit/hyperactivity disorder. In R. B. Mennuti, R. W. Christner, & A. Freeman (Eds.), *Cognitive-behavioral interventions in educational settings: A handbook for practice* (2nd ed., pp. 405–440). New York: Routledge.

Eckstein, D., & Gaynor, S. (2013). Combined individual cognitive behavior therapy and parent training for childhood depression: 2- to 3-year follow-up. *Child & Family Behavior Therapy, 35*(2), 132–143. doi:10.1080/07317107.2013.789362

Epp, A. M., & Dobson, K. S. (2010). The evidence base for cognitive-behavioral therapy. In K. S. Dobson (Ed.), *Handbook of cognitive-behavioral therapies* (pp. 39–73). New York: Guilford.

Fall, K. A., Holden, J. M., & Marquis, A. (2010). *Theoretical models of counseling and psychotherapy* (2nd ed.). New York: Brunner-Routledge.

Forman, S. G. (2006). Substance abuse prevention: School-based cognitive-behavioral approaches. In R. B. Mennuti, A. Freeman, & R. W. Christner (Eds.), *Cognitive-behavioral interventions in educational settings: A handbook for practice* (pp. 289–304). New York: Routledge.

Friedberg, R. D. (1996). Cognitive-behavioral games and workbooks: Tips for school counselors. *Elementary School Guidance & Counseling, 31*, 11–19.

Friedberg, R. D., & McClure, J. M. (2002). *Clinical practice of cognitive therapy with children and adolescents: The nuts and bolts*. New York: Guilford Press.

Friedberg, R. D., & McClure, J. M. (2015). *Clinical practice of cognitive therapy with children and adolescents: The nuts and bolts* (2nd ed.). New York: Guilford Press.

Friedberg, R. D., & Wilt, L. H. (2010). Metaphors and stories in cognitive behavioral therapy with children. *Journal of Rational-Emotive & Cognitive-Behavior Therapy, 28*(2), 100–113. doi:10.1007/s10942-009-0103-3

Fuertes, J., Bartolomeo, M., & Nichols, C. (2001). Future research directions in the study of counselor multicultural competency. *Journal of Multicultural Counseling & Development*, 29(1), 3–10.

Garland, A. F., Hawley, K. M., Brookman-Frazee, L., & Hurlburt, M. S. (2008). Identifying common elements of evidence-based psychosocial treatments for children's disruptive behavior problems. *Journal of the American Academy of Child & Adolescent Psychiatry*, 47(5), 505–514. doi:10.1097/CHI.0b013e31816765c2

Gibb, B. E., Beevers, C. G., & McGeary, J. E. (2013). Toward an integration of cognitive and genetic models of risk for depression. *Cognition and Emotion*, 27, 193–216.

Gilman, R., & Chard, K. M. (2007). Cognitive-behavioral and behavioral approaches. In H. T. Prout & D. T. Brown (Eds.), *Counseling and psychotherapy with children and adolescents: Theory and practice for school and clinical settings* (4th ed., pp. 241–278). Hoboken, NJ: Wiley.

Gosch, E. A., Flannery-Schroeder, E., & Brecher, R. J. (2012). School-based interventions for anxiety disorders. In R. B. Mennuti, R. W. Christner, & A. Freeman (Eds.), *Cognitive-behavioral interventions in educational settings: A handbook for practice* (2nd ed., pp. 117–160). New York: Routledge.

Hayden, E. P., & Mash, E. J. (2014). Child psychopathology: A developmental-systems perspective. In E. J. Mash & R. A. Barkley (Eds.), *Child psychopathology* (3rd ed., pp. 3–74). New York: Guilford Press.

Hays, P. A., & Iwamasa, G. Y. (2006). *Culturally responsive cognitive-behavioral therapy: Assessment, practice and supervision*. Washington, DC: American Psychological Association.

Kalodner, C. R. (2011). Cognitive-behavior theories. In D. Capuzzi & D. R. Gross (Eds.), *Counseling and psychotherapy: Theories and interventions* (5th ed., pp. 193–214). Alexandria, VA: American Counseling Association.

Kendall, P. C., & Hollon, S. D. (1979). Cognitive-behavioral interventions: Overview and current status. In P. C. Kendall & S. D. Hollon (Eds.), *Cognitive-behavioral interventions: Theory, research and procedures* (pp. 1–9). New York: Academic Press.

Kendall, P., Hudson, J., Choudhury, M., Webb, A., & Pimentel, S. (2005). Cognitive-behavioural treatment for childhood anxiety disorders. In E. Hibbs & P. Jensen (Eds.), *Psychosocial treatments for child and adolescent disorders: Empirically based strategies for clinical practice* (2nd ed., pp. 47–74). Washington, DC: American Psychological Association.

Kendall, P. C., & Treadwell, K. R. H. (2007). The role of self-statements as a mediator in treatment for youth with anxiety disorders. *Journal of Consulting and Clinical Psychology*, 75 (3), 380–389.

Khanna, M. S., & Kendall, P. C. (2010). Computer-assisted cognitive behavioral therapy for child anxiety: Results of a randomized clinical trial. *Journal of Consulting and Clinical Psychology*, 78(5), 737–745. doi:dx.doi.org/10.1037/a0019739

Knell, S. M. (2009). Cognitive-behavioral play therapy. In K. J. O'Connor & L. D. Braverman (Eds.), *Play therapy theory and practice: Comparing theories and techniques* (2nd ed., pp. 203–236). New York: Wiley.

Knell, S. M. (2011). Cognitive-behavioral play therapy. In C. E. Shaefer (Ed.), *Foundations of play therapy* (2nd ed.). Hoboken, NJ: John Wiley & Sons.

Knell, S. M., & Dasari, M. (2009). Cognitive-behavioral play therapy for children with anxiety and phobias. In H. G. Kaduson & C. E. Schaefer (Eds.), *Short-term play therapy for children* (2nd ed.). New York: Guilford Press.

Leahy, R. (1996). *Cognitive therapy: Basic principles and applications*. Northvale, NJ: Jason Aronson.

Lewinsohn, P. M., Clarke, G. N., Hops, H., & Andrews, J. (1990). Cognitive-behavioral group treatment of depression in adolescents. *Behavior Therapy*, 21, 385–401.

Lochman, J. E., Boxmeyer, C. L., Powell, N. P., Siddiquie, S., Stromeyer, S. L., & Kelly, M. (2012). Anger and aggression: School-based cognitive-behavioral interventions.

In R. B. Mennuti, R. W. Christner, & A. Freeman (Eds.), *Cognitive-behavioral interventions in educational settings: A handbook for practice* (2nd ed., pp. 305–338). New York: Routledge.

Lochman, J. E., Powell, N. P., Boxmeyer, C. L., & Jimenez-Camargo, L. (2011). Cognitive-behavioral therapy for externalizing disorders in children and adolescents. *Child and Adolescent Psychiatric Clinics of North America, 20,* 301–318.

Macdonald, G., Higgins, J., Ramchandani, P., Valentine, J., Bronger, L., Klein, P., & Taylor, M. (2012). Cognitive-behavioural interventions for children who have been sexually abused. *Cochrane Database of Systematic Reviews, 5(5),* CD001930. doi:10.1002/14651858.CD001930.pub3

Maryam, A. N., Mona, A. M., & Akram, M. (2014). Effectiveness of group play therapy through cognitive-behavioral method on social adjustment of children with behavioral disorder. *Kuwait Chapter of the Arabian Journal of Business and Management Review, 3(12),* 356.

Maultsby, M. (1976). *Rational self-analysis format.* Lexington, KY: Center for Rational Behavior Therapy and Training, University of Kentucky.

McLaughlin, C. L., & Christner, R. W. (2012). Depression. In R. B. Mennuti, R. W. Christner, & A. Freeman (Eds.), *Cognitive-behavioral interventions in educational settings: A handbook for practice* (2nd ed., pp. 215–238a). New York: Routledge.

Meichenbaum, D. (1977). *Cognitive behavior modification: An integrative approach.* New York: Plenum.

Meichenbaum, D. (1985). *Stress-inoculation training.* New York: Pergamon.

Mennuti, R. B., Christner, R. W., & Freeman, A. (Eds.). (2012). *Cognitive-behavioral interventions in educational settings: A handbook for practice* (2nd ed.). New York: Routledge.

National Registry of Evidence-based Programs and Practices (NREPP), a service of the Substance Abuse and Mental Health Services Administration (SAMHSA). (2014). Retrieved from http://www.nrepp.samhsa.gov/ViewIntervention.aspx?id=91

Power, T. J., & DeRosa, B. W. (2012). Children with chronic health conditions. In R. B. Mennuti, R. W. Christner, & A. Freeman (Eds.), *Cognitive-behavioral interventions* (2nd ed., pp. 531–552). New York: Routledge.

Reynolds, C. R., & Kamphaus, R. W. (2004). *Behavior assessment system for children* (2nd ed.). Circle Pines, MN: American Guidance Service.

Ronen, T. (1992). Cognitive therapy with children. *Child Psychiatry and Human Development, 23,* 19–30.

Ronen, T. (1998). Linking developmental and emotional elements into child and family cognitive-behavioural therapy. In P. Graham (Ed.), *Cognitive-behavioural therapy for children and families* (pp. 1–17). Cambridge, UK: Cambridge University Press.

Seligman, L., & Reichenberg, L. W. (2014). *Theories of counseling and psychotherapy: Systems, strategies, and skills* (4th ed.). Upper Saddle River, NJ: Pearson.

Shapiro, J. P., Friedberg, R. D., & Bardenstein, K. K. (2006). *Child and adolescent therapy: Science and art.* New York: Wiley.

Shillingford, M. A., Lambie, G. W., & Walter, S. M. (2007). An integrative, cognitive-behavioral, systemic approach to working with students diagnosed with attention deficit hyperactive disorder. *Professional School Counseling, 11(2),* 105–112.

Silverman, S., & DiGiuseppe, R. (2001). Cognitive-behavioral and emotional problems. *Journal of Rational-Emotive & Cognitive-Behavioral Therapy, 19,* 119–134.

Silverman, W. K., Ortiz, C. C., Viswesvaran, C., Burns, B. J., Kolko, D. J., Putman, F. W., et al. (2008). Evidence-based psychosocial treatments for children and adolescents exposed to traumatic events. *Journal of Clinical Child and Adolescent Psychology, 37,* 156–183.

Stein, C. C., Jayoux, L. H., Kataoka, S. H., Wond, M., Tu, W., Elliott, M. N., et al. (2003). A mental health intervention for school children exposed to violence. *Journal of American Medical Association, 290,* 603–611.

Sukhodolsky, D. G., Scahill, L., & Ebooks Corporation. (2012). *Cognitive-behavioral therapy for anger and aggression in children*. New York: Guilford Press.

Tikotzky, L., & Sadeh, A. (2010). The role of cognitive-behavioral therapy in behavioral childhood insomnia. *Sleep Medicine, 11*(7), 686–691. doi:10.1016/j.sleep.2009.11.017

Utay, J. M., & Lampe, R. E.(1995). Use of a group counseling game to enhance social skills of children with learning disabilities. *Journal of Specialists in Group Work, 20*, 114–121.

Waldron, H. B., & Kaminer, Y. (2004). On the learning curve: Cognitive-behavioral therapies for adolescent substance abuse. *Addiction, 99*, 93–105.

Watkins, C. E. (1983). Rational self-analysis for children. *Elementary School Guidance and Counseling, 17*, 304–306.

Wilde, J. (2001). Interventions for children with anger problems. *Journal of Rational-Emotive & Cognitive-Behavioral Therapy, 19*, 191–197.

Young, S., Bramham, J., & Ebooks Corporation. (2012). *Cognitive-behavioural therapy for ADHD in adolescents and adults: A psychological guide to practice*. Malden, MA; Chichester, West Sussex: Wiley-Blackwell.

Young, J., Klosko, J. S., & Weishaar, M. E. (2006). *Schema therapy*. New York: Guilford Press.

CHAPTER 14

Transactional Analysis

We do not grow absolutely, chronologically. We grow sometimes in one dimension, and not in another, unevenly. We grow partially. We are relative. We are mature in one realm, childish in another. The past, present, and future mingle and pull us backward, forward, or fix us in the present. We are made up of layers, cells, constellations.
—ANAÏS NIN

An unknown author once said we cannot not communicate. Messages, being received and given, are continuous parts of our lives. Proponents of transactional analysis (TA) have developed an analysis of communications that guide our lives. Even though TA practice is less common than it once was, this theory provides insights into life scripts, crossed transactions, and other means to understand the positions we choose in life. The theory offers several easy-to-learn concepts that may help children develop life communication skills. After reading this chapter, you should be able to:

▶ Outline the development of TA and Eric Berne
▶ Explain the theory of TA including its core concepts
▶ Discuss the counseling relationship and goals in TA
▶ Describe assessment, process, and techniques in TA
▶ Demonstrate some therapeutic techniques
▶ Clarify the effectiveness of TA

**ERIC BERNE
(1910–1970)**

Eric Lennard Bernstein was born May 10, 1910, in Montreal, Canada. His father was a general practitioner; his mother was a professional writer and editor; and he had a younger sister. Eric respected his father a great deal and was permitted to make house call rounds with him. He was 10 years old when his father died from tuberculosis, at which time his mother assumed responsibility for supporting the two children.

After receiving his medical degree from McGill University at the age of 25, Bernstein moved to the United States and began a psychiatric residency at Yale University. He became a U.S. citizen in 1938 and shortly thereafter changed his name to Eric Berne. After service with the armed forces from 1943 to 1946, he began working to earn the title of psychoanalyst. His first book, *The Mind in Action*, was published in 1947. That same year, Berne began analysis with Erik Erikson.

One of the major rejections of his life occurred when, in 1956, the Psychoanalytic Institute denied his application for membership and recommended that he continue through 4 more years of personal analysis and then reapply for the coveted title. This action greatly discouraged Berne, but at the same time motivated him, and he immediately began work on a new approach to psychotherapy.

Although Berne first published on the topic of the three ego states in his article "The Nature of Intuition" (1949), he formed the core of TA in 1954. At that time, Berne was involved in the psychoanalysis of a successful middle-aged lawyer he was treating by applying classic Freudian principles. During a session, the patient suddenly said, "I'm not a lawyer, I'm just a little boy," sparking Berne's idea that each of us contains a Child ego state accompanied by Parent and Adult ego states. After listening to his patients relating "games" for some 30 years, Berne decided to gather some of these into a catalog. Three years after its publication, *Games People Play* (1964) had been on the nonfiction best-seller list for 111 weeks—longer than any other book that decade. Some reviewers called the book psychiatric gimmickry, emphatically denying that it would ever be regarded as a contribution to psychological or psychiatric theory. Other reviewers found the book a real contribution to psychology and suggested that Berne had offered a thesaurus of social transactions with explanations and titles. In 1967, Berne attributed the book's success to the recognition factor—some of us recognize ourselves in it, whereas some of us recognize other people in the descriptions of winners and losers. The everyday language and categories he used came from his preferences.

Poker was Berne's favorite game because people play it to win. He had little patience with losers and believed that players should play to win if they were going to play. Berne believed losers spent a lot of time explaining why they lost. In the final years of his life, Berne shifted his emphasis from games to life scripts.

Berne published eight books and sixty-four articles in psychiatric and other periodicals; he also edited the *Transactional Analysis Bulletin*. In an article in the *New York Times* magazine in 1966, Berne renounced the therapeutic value of shock treatment, hypnosis, and medication in favor of his easy-to-understand approach to psychotherapy. TA is a social psychology that has applications to counseling, psychotherapy, education, and organizational development.

THE NATURE OF PEOPLE AND THEORY OF COUNSELING

The nature of people and the theory of counseling are covered together in this section because the TA theory of counseling is basically a statement describing the human personality.

Berne had a positive view of the nature of people. He believed children were born princes and princesses, but shortly thereafter their parents and the environment turned them into frogs. He believed that people had the potential to regain their royal status, providing they learned and applied the lessons of TA to their personal lives. Berne believed that the early childhood years were critical to personal development. During these early years, before children enter school, they form their basic life script and develop a sense of being either "OK" or "not OK." They also arrive at conclusions about other people's "OK-ness."

In Berne's view, life is very simple to live. However, people upset themselves to the point that they invent religions, pastimes, and games. These same people complain about how complicated life is, while persisting in making life even harder. Life is a series of decisions to be made and problems to be solved, and Berne believed that people have the rationality and freedom to make decisions and solve their own problems.

Seligman (2006) explained the developmental stages proposed by Berne as follows:

- Stage 1 occurs from birth to age 1. The child's ego state evolves with the early experiences, emotions, intuitions, inquisitiveness, and the capacity for joy and shame. All people are born with a *natural child* who is spontaneous, dependent, and lovable. The *adapted child* on the other hand is inhibited, well-behaved, socialized, conforming, and sometimes self-critical. *Free child* tendencies are spontaneity and intuitiveness like the natural child as well as playfulness and joy. The *little professor* portends the Adult ego state, which can be curious but also rigid and didactic.
- Stage 2 from ages 1 to 3 contains the development of the Adult and Parent ego states that continue to advance until about age 6. Social interactions, especially injunctions and restrictions on children's behavior, shape these states.
- Stage 3 from ages 3 to 6 continues the evolution of the ego states with messages from others and experiences shaping them.
- Stage 4 happens at age 6. The three major ego states have developed but will continue to grow.
- Stage 5 occurs between ages 6 and 12. Educational and interpersonal experiences contribute to changes in the ego states, especially the Adult ego state.
- Stage 6 encompasses ages 13 through 16 in which the Child ego state develops rapidly and may be revealed in rebellion and conflict.
- Stage 7, late adolescence, involves the time the Adult ego state may be able to provide balance between the three ego states, promoting a person's maturity and need fulfillment.
- Stage 8, adulthood, is the time when hopefully people have psychological maturity; they can function independently; make good decisions; have purpose and direction and a balance between Parent, Adult, and Child ego states.

Everything in TA emerges from the belief that the human personality has three separate ego states: Parent, Adult, and Child (PAC). These ego states are consistent patterns of feeling and experience with a related consistent pattern of behavior.

Prochaska and Norcross (2014) elaborate. People in their Child ego state sit, stand, speak, think, perceive, and feel as they did in childhood. Their behavior is impulsive, spontaneous, creative, and fun. The Child ego state is preserved intact from childhood, or, as Prochaska and Norcross explain, it is as if the person has a nonerasable inner tape from their lives at age 8 and younger that can be turned on at any time.

The Parent ego also comes from childhood and incorporates the behaviors and attitudes that mimic authority figures from childhood. The Parent ego includes the same type of recordings from childhood but can be modified as a person changes in life. The Adult ego includes the unfeeling, data-processing part of personality. This ego state develops gradually and emerges through the person's interactions with the environment.

Each of the ego states is healthy when used appropriately and the well-adapted personality switches easily from one state to another based on the needs of the current situation. Ego states form the structure of the personality but do not address the motivation of life which comes from the basic drive for survival and also from the psychological drives for recognition, structure, and excitement (Prochaska & Norcross, 2014). For those motivations, we move to the core concepts of TA.

CORE CONCEPTS

TA theory of human nature and human relationships derives from data collected through four types of analysis:

1. Structural analysis, in which an individual's personality is analyzed
2. TA, which is concerned with what people do and say to each other
3. Script analysis, which deals with the specific life dramas people compulsively enjoy
4. Game analysis, in which ulterior transactions leading to a payoff are analyzed

Structural Analysis

In explaining the TA view of human nature and the difficulties people encounter in their lives, the first step is to begin with the structural analysis of personality. Each individual's personality is divided into three separate and distinct sources of behavior, the three ego states: Parent, Adult, and Child (or P, A, and C). The ego states represent real people who now exist or once existed and had their own identities. Therefore, the conflicts among them often cause inconsistencies, as well as flexibility, in people.

The Parent, Adult, and Child ego states Berne proposed are not concepts like the superego, ego, and id of Freud, but rather phenomena based on actual realities. They each represent skeletomuscular and verbal patterns of behavior and feeling based on emotions and experiences perceived by people in their early years as discussed earlier. The Parent, Adult, and Child are all located in the conscious area of functioning and, as such, are readily available for use in our day-to-day living. In Freud's model, only the superego and ego are available to the conscious, with the id buried in the unconscious.

PARENT The Parent aspect of personality contains instructions, attitudes, and behaviors handed down mostly by parents and significant authority figures. It resembles a recording of all the admonitions, orders, punishments, encouragement, reinforcement, and caring experienced in the first years of life. The Parent ego state can take two different attitudes, depending on the situation: (1) *Nurturing Parent* manifests itself in nurturing or helping behavior, offering support, affirmation, and caring but can be overprotective and (2) *Critical Parent* provides rules, standards, control, and punishment; disapproves; and criticizes. The critical parent emerges from the rules, reprimands, praise, and rewards received from parents and other childhood caretakers (Seligman & Reichenberg, 2014; Harris, 1969). The Parent feels and behaves as the one who reared you did—both critical and nurturing. The Parent admonishes, "you should" or "you should not," "you can't win," "boys will be boys," or "a woman's place is in the home." The Parent uses words like *always*, *never*, and *should* and focuses on *you* and uses nonverbal signs like pointing, sighing, and a raised voice (Seligman & Reichenberg). The Parent, wanting to be in control and to be right, acts with superiority and authority, but the Parent is also responsible for giving love, nurturance, and respect to the Child in you. The Parent may give clear guidelines or mixed messages.

ADULT   The Adult ego state operates logically and unemotionally, providing objective information by using reality testing and a computer-like approach to life. Your Adult uses facts as a computer does to make decisions without emotion. The Adult values logic over emotion, processes information, solves problems, and integrates messages from the other ego states (Seligman & Reichenberg, 2014). The Adult says, "This is how this works" with mature, objective, logical, and rational thinking based on reality. The Adult ego state is not related to age but is straightforward. A child is also capable of dealing with reality by gathering facts and computing objectively. In fact, it is incumbent on the counselor to ensure that counseling sessions are conducted in an adult-to-adult format. Clients often work hard to shift communication to a parent-to-child format, where the counselor takes the parent role and tells the client what should be done. Counselors can deflect client attempts to shift the interview from adult to adult by using any of the counseling responses presented in this text. Active listening is effective, as is reality therapy and the other counseling responses, to return the interaction to adult–adult.

CHILD   All the childlike impulses common to everyone are in the Child state. The Child is an important part of personality because it contributes joy, creativity, spontaneity, intuition, pleasure, and enjoyment. The Child has two parts: (1) Adaptive Child emerges as a result of demands from significant authority figures and is marked by passivity; and (2) Natural or Free Child represents the impulsive, untrained, self-loving, pleasure-seeking part of the Child.

The Child part of us is an accumulation of impulses that come naturally to a young person and recorded internal events or responses to what is seen and heard. It has an element of immaturity but also deep feeling, affection, adaptation, expression, and fun. Figure 14-1 presents the ego states and their divisions in graphic form.

The well-adjusted person allows the situation to determine which ego state is in control during transactions, striking an even balance among the three. A common problem is allowing one ego state to assume predominant control. For example, the Constant Parent is seen as dictatorial or prejudiced; the Constant Adult is an analytical bore; and the Constant Child is immature or over-reactive. No age is implied by any of these states because even the young child has Adult and Parent states, and older adults can evince a Child response. In fact, whenever you are having fun or jumping up and down cheering at a ball game, you are in your Child ego state.

Transactional Analysis

The second type of analysis—the study of the transaction—is the heart of TA. The psychological motivation of giving and receiving strokes leads to the transactions, the exchange of strokes, which will be discussed more fully in a later section.

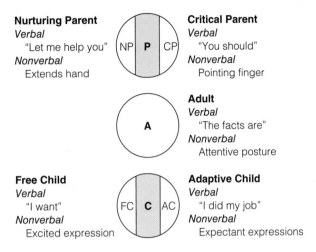

FIGURE 14-1   EGO STATES

Transaction is the basic unit of behaviors and occurs whenever a person acknowledges the presence of another person, either verbally or physically.

A *transaction* often is defined as a unit of human communication or as a stimulus–response connection between two people's ego states. TA defines three categories of transactions based on the source of the transactions, its target, and the replying ego state.

1. *Complementary transactions*, which Berne described as the natural communication of healthy human relationships, occur when a response comes from the ego state to which it was addressed. The target and replying ego state are the same. Complementary transactions lead to interactions that are clear, open, and rewarding because people say what they mean and can understand what others are saying. Disagreements are apparent and can be confronted (Seligman & Reichenberg, 2014).

    SUE: Billy, have you seen my bike?

    BILLY: Yes, it is in the backyard. (See Figure 14-2.)

2. *Crossed transactions* break communications. They occur when a response comes from an ego state *not* addressed. The target ego state and the replying state are not the same. In crossed transactions, people receive a response they

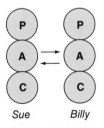

FIGURE 14-2   COMPLEMENTARY TRANSACTION

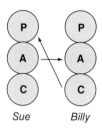

FIGURE 14-3   CROSSED TRANSACTION

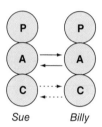

FIGURE 14-4   COVERT TRANSACTION

did not anticipate and they may feel ignored or misunderstood (Seligman & Reichenberg, 2014).

> **SUE:** Billy, would you help me find my bike?
>
> **BILLY:** Can't you see I'm watching my favorite program? (See Figure 14-3.)

3. *Covert*, or *ulterior*, *transactions* involve more than one ego state of each person and are basically dishonest. On the surface, the transaction looks and sounds like number 1 or 2, but the actual message sent is not spoken (Figure 14-4). Ulterior transactions cause problems because the overt communication does not match the covert communication so neither person knows what is in the mind of the other person. A continuing pattern of ulterior transactions leads to relationship difficulties. For example, the ulterior message being sent in number 1 could be on a social or overt level.

> **SUE:** Billy, why don't you help me find my bike so we can go riding?
>
> **BILLY:** Okay, it's a good day for a ride!
>
> Or the ulterior message could be on a psychological, covert, or ulterior level:
>
> **SUE:** I wish you would be my boyfriend.
>
> **BILLY:** I hope you like me better than the other boys.

Script Analysis

The nature of people can be further described by script analysis. A psychological script is a person's ongoing program for a life drama; it dictates where people are going with their lives and the paths that will lead there. The individual, consciously or unconsciously, acts compulsively according to that program. Scripts are shaped by both the strokes or positive messages and injunctions, disapproval, and prohibitions a child receives. As mentioned earlier, people are born basically "OK"; their difficulties come from bad scripts they learned during their childhood.

Berne (1961) developed the theory of scripts as part of TA theory from its inception. A life script is that life plan your Child selected in your early years, based mostly on messages you received from the Child in your parents. For example, at the request of her mother, a little girl takes it upon herself to save her alcoholic father, using the rescuer script. The same script may emerge once again later in life as she tries to save an alcoholic husband in an attempt to regain some of the payoffs from the original experience. The persecutor and victim scripts would also emerge in childhood and be revisited later in life.

Although the Parent and Adult of your mother and father may have told you sensible things such as "Be successful," the unspoken injunction from the Child in your parents may communicate the message "You can't make it" (Figure 14-5). Injunctions are prohibitions and negative commands usually delivered from the parent of the opposite sex. Injunctions are seldom discussed or verbalized aloud. Values we hold as guidelines for living may have come from injunctions. These injunctions determine how we think and feel about sex, work, money, marriage, family, play, and people. For example, "Do not waste your time and money."

The best way to learn about scripts is to examine ways we spend our time and how we relate (transactions) with others. Scripts have main themes, such as martyring, procrastinating, succeeding, failing, blaming, distracting, placating, and computing; scripts also have three basic types: winner, loser, and nonwinner. A small percentage of people seem to be natural winners; everything they touch turns to gold. Conversely, a slightly larger percentage of people seem to be natural losers; everything turns out badly for them. The majority, perhaps 80 or 85 percent, follow the nonwinners' script. Nonwinners are identified by a phrase they often use: "but at least …" (for example, "I went to school and made poor grades, *but at least* I did not flunk out.").

TA borrows heavily from fairy tales for its terminology and metaphors. For example, the Cinderella script is not an especially healthy plan because a prince or prize does not come to one who sits around waiting. Even martyrdom, as Cinderella did for her stepmother and stepsisters, does not help. The Santa Claus script is based on a similar myth. LeGuernic (2004) points out that many fairy tales, like the warm fuzzy story, provide children with different, positive relationship models and social roles that can lead to personal growth and autonomy. Because life scripts are formed in early childhood, selecting children's stories should be done with considerable care.

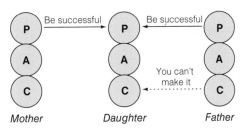

FIGURE 14-5　LIFE SCRIPT: INJUNCTIONS

In summary, Berne believed that scripts have five components: (1) directions from parents, (2) a corresponding personality development, (3) a confirming childhood decision about oneself and life, (4) a penchant for either success or failure, and (5) a pattern for behavior. Toth (2004) notes that script theories help teachers understand why students do what they do and how self-limiting behaviors such as fear of failure may be corrected.

Game Analysis

Unfortunately, most people, in following their scripts, learn how to use ulterior transactions; that is, they play games. A game is an ongoing series of complementary, ulterior transactions progressing to a well-defined, predictable outcome. Like every ulterior transaction, all games are basically dishonest, and they are by no means fun. One of the first games a child learns is, "Mine is better than yours." Its relatively benign outcome could range, in later years, to considerably more serious games. Three roles are played in games: persecutor, victim, and rescuer. There are no winners in these games; every player loses. *Games People Play* (Berne, 1964) offers a vastly entertaining, chilling overview of what might happen to a "not-OK" child.

Berne (1964) believed that the general advantages of a game are its stabilizing (homeostatic) functions. He defined *homeostasis* as the tendency of an individual to maintain internal psychological equilibrium by regulating his or her own internal processes. Change is difficult for people who automatically accept only what reinforces or confirms their personal prejudices, values, and views, and many people are not open to new data. Game playing functions to maintain homeostasis in one's life much like defense mechanisms do.

In reference to counseling, clients are ready to terminate counseling when their self-esteem is in order and they are able to exchange games for honest strokes from an "I'm OK, you're OK" view of human nature. In addition, fully functioning clients do confront and master the appropriate development tasks for age and stage. The ease with which children can understand TA concepts makes it a valuable approach for problem prevention.

In summary, games undermine the stability of relationships. Children's development, according to TA, is determined by the messages and responses they receive from significant people. Those messages may be strokes or injunctions and those become the basic motivation for interactions. The need for strokes often turns an honest transaction into a game, even negative strokes are better than no strokes which equates to being ignored (Seligman & Reichenberg, 2014). Game analysis deals with transactions between two people.

Life Positions

On the basis of the transactions and scripts, children develop life positions that summarize their concepts of self-worth and the worth of others. The four life positions are as follows:

1. "I'm OK, you're OK": This position of mentally healthy people (mature independence) enables them to possess realistic expectations, have good human relationships, and solve problems constructively. It is a "winner's" position,

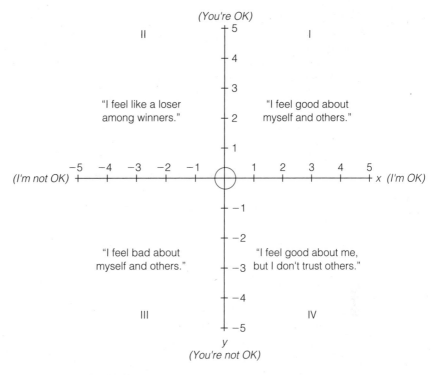

FIGURE 14-6 LIFE POSITIONS

defined as that of an authentic being. People feel good about themselves and about others. They focus on beneficial situations and have balanced ego states (Seligman, 2006). The extreme of this position is represented by +5 on both the *x*- and *y*-axes in Quadrant I of Figure 14-6. Marriages, business partnerships, and friendships work best when both people hold to the "I'm OK, you're OK" orientation to life.

2. "I'm not OK, you're OK": The universal position of childhood (total dependence) represents the position of those who feel powerless. Adults in this position often experience withdrawal and depression. They may feel guilty, powerless, and inferior even though they want appreciation and acceptance. They may always be following the rules in the hope of becoming accepted (Seligman & Reichenberg, 2014). The extremes of this position are represented by a −5 on the *x*-axis and +5 on the *y*-axis in Quadrant II of Figure 14-6. Those who like to parent their partners will choose one from the "I'm not OK, you're OK" orientation.

3. "I'm not OK, you're not OK": This is the most negative of the four positions. This life position is the arrival point of the child who cannot depend on parents for positive stroking (see discussion later in this chapter). Already not OK, the child perceives Mom and Dad as not OK too. Adults in this category are losers who go through a series of helpless, disappointing experiences and may

even become suicidal or homicidal, seeing no value in themselves or in others (Seligman, 2006). The extreme of this position is represented by a –5 on both the x- and y-axes in Quadrant III of Figure 14-6. Partners from this category are dangerous to your health and theirs.

4. "I'm OK, you're not OK": People who do not receive many positive strokes may be in this position. They have survived by stroking themselves (Seligman, 2006) and believe that they must rely only on themselves. They are angry, punitive, and have a sense of grandiosity and entitlement (Seligman, 2006). The individual feels victimized in this position. The brutalized, battered child ends up here. The position of the criminal and the psychopath is, "Whatever happens is someone else's fault." The extreme of this position is a +5 on the x-axis and a –5 on the y-axis in Quadrant IV of Figure 14-6. If you would like to be with a blamer, potential criminal, or sociopath, here is your person.

COUNSELING RELATIONSHIP

Practitioners have a flexible role in TA. They are collaborators who share responsibility with their clients for the treatment. In addition, TA is the ideal system for those who view the counseling process as teaching. As conveyed in this chapter, TA abounds with terms, diagrams, and models. Clients are taught the TA vocabulary so they can become proficient in identifying ego states, transactions, and scripts. The counselor's role includes teaching and providing a nurturing, supportive environment in which clients feel free to lift or eliminate restricting injunctions, attempt new behaviors, rewrite scripts, and move toward the "I'm OK, you're OK" life position. Counselors maintain the Adult ego state throughout sessions (Harris & Brockbank, 2011). Cooperation between counselor and client is a large part of the TA process in which children are expected to be open, responsible, and willing to take chances to make positive changes (Seligman & Reichenberg, 2014). Contracts are used to clarify the treatment process and delineate the roles of the counselor and the child.

Guy (2003) and Poda (2003) write that TA with children and adolescents promotes the developmental assistance needed to foster a healthy balance between attachment and autonomy, while providing these clients with a reassuring awareness of their potential.

Goals

Berne (1964) identified the goal of TA as autonomy, the autonomy of awareness, spontaneity, and intimacy. TA counselors want people to get to the "I'm OK; you're OK" position, balance their ego states, and use their time well.

Seligman and Reichenberg (2014) outline the goal of treatment is to uncover a picture of these components for each person: the balance of ego states, the nature of transactions with others, their games and rackets, the person's basic position and the person's life script. Clarkson (1993) and Stewart and Joines (2012) also articulate the goals and processes of therapy.

Games Clients Play

Among the many games Berne identified, the following is a list of those especially to be avoided in the counseling interview:

1. *"Why don't you; Yes, but ..."* The counselor's Adult is tricked into working for the client's Child as the Parent when the counselor gives advice.

   COUNSELOR: Why don't you ask your teacher to give you some extra help with math?

   CLIENT: Yes, but what if she says she doesn't have time?

The payoff comes to the client in spreading bad feelings, as in the misery-loves-company game: "I am not okay, and you aren't either because you can't help me solve my problem."

Summerton (2000) writes that Berne began his study of game analysis with the "Why don't you; Yes, but ..." game. The overt communication appears to be adult to adult, but the covert communication is actually a one-upmanship move by the Child ego state trying to hook the Parent ego state of the "helper" into giving advice on what the "helpee" needs to do to solve a particular problem. However, in the game, the advice is always rejected as inadequate in an attempt to make the "helper" feel bad for not having the wisdom to be helpful.

Woods (2000) distinguishes between the act of recognizing and confronting game playing and true game analysis. Recognition and confrontation of game playing is done to end the games. True game-playing analysis is done to explore how the client uses games as a defense and how games often communicate unconscious messages. Woods believes that people internalize the scenario of an early interpersonal relationship and unconsciously use it later as a template for further interpersonal interactions. One example is given of a client's father who always had a "Yes, but" statement for every self-assertive "I should" statement the client would make. In adulthood, the client projected his father's role onto others by rejecting all feedback, suggestions, and advice in the "Why don't you; Yes, but" game.

2. *"I'm only trying to help you."* Counselors sometimes play this game with their clients. The message to the client is, "You are not okay, and I know what is good for you." The payoff is for the counselor, who holds the faulty belief that "If I straighten my client out, then maybe I can get my own life in order." A truly helpful counselor offers help when it is requested, but believes that help can be accepted or rejected. When help fails or is rejected, the helpful counselor does not respond derogatorily, "Well, I was only trying to help you."

3. *Courtroom.* The courtroom game puts the counselor in the position of judge and jury if two clients can manipulate the counselor into placing blame. The payoff is bad feelings for all—persecutor, victim, and rescuer—because the rescuer (counselor) usually ends up being victimized by the other two players.

4. *Kick me and NIGY.* Counselors may find that some clients enjoy playing "kick me" with the counselor, just as they do with their bosses, colleagues, and spouses. They seem to enjoy being victimized and work at getting themselves rejected. They even work at getting themselves terminated from counseling before any gains have been made. Kick-me players manipulate others into playing NIGY (now I've got you) when they react to the bids for negative attention the

kick-me players make. The NIGY game is played by itself if a person tries to trap others in a double bind: damned if you do and damned if you don't.

MOTHER: Johnny, do you love me?

JOHNNY: Yes, I do.

MOTHER: How many times have I told you not to talk with your mouth full!

5. *Gossiping.* Gossiping refers to talking about people who are not present. In a counseling interview, the counselor may wish to have clients role-play dialogue between themselves and a missing person. For example, a student complaining about a teacher could role-play a conversation between the two of them, with the student playing the role of the teacher and then responding as the student would in the classroom. The technique uses an empty chair to represent the missing person. Role-playing and role-reversal methods have a way of limiting gossip while creating greater awareness of the problem situations and proper assignment of responsibility for the problem.

6. *Wooden leg.* The wooden-leg game is a display of the inadequacy pattern described in the chapter on individual psychology. Clients playing wooden-leg games work to increase their disabilities as a way of avoiding responsibility for taking care of themselves. These clients are experts at making people give up on them. Children are adept at convincing parents and teachers that they cannot handle certain chores and school subjects. Paradoxical strategies, which are at times effective with these clients, focus on harnessing their rebellion into productive activity. The counselor might say, for example, "Frank, you've got me convinced that you really can't make it." The rebellious client, Frank, often rises to the occasion to show that the counselor is a total idiot and begins to succeed in the face of the prediction that he could not. For clients who are really defeated and not rebellious, we recommend large doses of unconditional encouragement. Counselors of welfare and rehabilitation clients often find themselves in the wooden-leg game. The payoff goes to the clients, who justify not getting better, or even getting worse, as a way of increasing their benefits.

7. *If it weren't for you.* Related to the wooden leg, this game is another way of avoiding the assumption of responsibility for life and its unsolved problems. The client says, for example, "If it weren't for you and your good cooking, I could lose 10 pounds." The counselor may want to examine with the client the payoffs of being overweight and even develop a rationale of how being fat may be the preferred and "best" lifestyle for the client.

8. *Red Cross.* Red Cross happens when a person (the persecutor) pushes you (the victim) off a dock into deep water and then rescues you. This puts you (the victim) in debt to the rescuer. In this case, all three roles in the game are played by two people, with the persecutor and rescuer role played by the same person. Red Cross happens when people get other people in trouble and then "jump in" to "rescue" them from peril.

The Pursuit of Strokes

Human beings need recognition; to obtain it, they exchange what Berne called *strokes.* A stroke is any act implying recognition of another person's presence. In acknowledging the presence of another person, people give a stroke, which can be either positive or negative; which usually is obvious, except in the case of ulterior transactions. Young children receive positive or negative physical strokes when they are cuddled or spanked, whereas adults obtain primarily symbolic strokes in conversations or transactions with others. Positive strokes, such as compliments, handshakes, open affection, or uninterrupted listening, are the most desirable, but negative strokes, such as hatred or disagreement, are better than no recognition at all. A middle ground is maintenance strokes, which keep transactions going by giving recognition to the speaker but neither positive nor negative feedback. All these strokes can be either conditional or unconditional—that is, given as a result of some specific action or given just for being yourself. Unconditional regard—"I like you"—has more positive stroke value than conditional acceptance—"I like you when you are nice to me" (Figure 14-7).

The pattern of giving and receiving strokes an individual uses most is determined by the person's life position, as explained in the section on life positions. How people view themselves and others controls their ability to give and receive conditional and unconditional positive and negative strokes. People engage in transactions to exchange strokes. According to Berne (1964), people have an inherent psychological hunger for stimulation through human interactions and stroking, and any act implying recognition of another's presence is a means of satisfying these hungers. Failure to fulfill these needs may cause a failure to thrive in infants and feelings of abandonment and "not-OK-ness" in both children and adults. Satisfied hunger yields feelings of "OK-ness" and release of creative energy. Awareness of psychological hungers and the satisfaction of them are important.

Negative strokes, such as lack of attention, shin kicking, and hatred, send "You're not OK" messages. Diminishing, humiliating, and ridiculing strokes all treat people as though they are insignificant.

Positive strokes usually are complementary transactions. They may be verbal expressions of affection and appreciation, or they may give compliments or positive feedback; they may be physical, such as a touch, or they may be silent gestures or looks. Listening is one of the finest strokes one person can give another. All yield

	CONDITIONAL	UNCONDITIONAL
POSITIVE	2-Positive for doing something	1-Positive for being you
NEGATIVE	3-Negative for doing something	4-Negative for being you

FIGURE 14-7   TYPES OF STROKES

reinforcement to the "I'm OK, you're OK" position. Maintenance strokes, although lacking meaningful content, at least serve to give recognition and keep communication open.

STRUCTURING TIME   People have six options for structuring their time in pursuit of strokes:

1. *Withdrawing*—time alone in which no transaction takes place. It involves few risks, and no stroking occurs.
2. *Rituals*—involve prescribed social transactions such as "Hello," "Have a nice day," and "How are you?" These transactions are fairly impersonal.
3. *Pastimes*—provide mutually acceptable stroking. Pastimes are a means of self-expression but often involve only superficial transactions or conversations. Examples are conversations about baseball, automobiles, shopping, or other safe topics of conversation.
4. *Activities*—time is structured around some task or career. Activities are a way to deal with external reality and may involve more in-depth interaction with others.
5. *Games*—the need for strokes is met in dishonest or phony ways. Intense stroking often is received, but it may be unpleasant. Games are considered destructive transactions.
6. *Intimacy*—provides unconditional stroking. It is free of games, exploitation, and phony communication.

Obviously, some of these ways of structuring time are healthy and some are unhealthy, depending on the time and energy given to each. One of the goals of TA therapy is to help people learn productive ways of structuring their time.

Withdrawing may be the Adult's decision to relax or be alone, the Parent's way of coping with conflict, or the Child's adaptation for protection from pain or conflict. It is fairly harmless unless it happens all the time or when a person needs to pay attention. Withdrawing into fantasy may allow one to experience good stroking when the present setting does not appear to hold any.

A ritual is a socially programmed use of time in which everybody agrees to do the same thing. Brief encounters, worship rituals, greeting rituals, party rituals, and bedroom rituals may allow maintenance strokes without commitment or involvement. The outcome is predictable and pleasant, but most people need more intense stroking.

Pastimes are, as they imply, ways to pass time. They are superficial exchanges without involvement that people use to size up one another. Conversations concerning relative gas mileage, the weather, sports teams, or potty training may yield minimal stroking at the maintenance level but allow one to decide whether to risk a more intimate relationship.

Doing work or activities with others is time spent dealing with the realities of the world. It is getting something done that one may want to do, need to do, or have to do. Activities allow for positive strokes befitting a winner.

Berne (1964) defined games as an ongoing series of complementary, ulterior transactions progressing to a well-defined, predictable outcome. A person who sends an ulterior message to another person, for some hidden purpose, is playing a game. The Adult is unaware that the Child or Parent has a secret reason for playing or wanting to play. Harris (1969) believes all games derive from the Child's "mine is better than yours" attempt to ease the "not-OK" feeling; that is, to feel superior while the other feels put down. Games are differentiated from rituals and pastimes in two ways: (1) their ulterior quality and (2) the payoff. Games also are a way of passing time for people who cannot bear the stroking starvation of withdrawal, and yet whose "not-OK" position makes the ultimate form of relatedness—intimacy— impossible (Berne, 1964; Harris, 1969).

Intimacy is a deep human encounter stemming from genuine caring. Steiner (1974) views intimacy as the way of structuring time so there are no withdrawals, no rituals, no games, no pastimes, and no work. Conditions favorable for intimacy include a commitment to the "I'm OK, you're OK" position and a satisfying of psychological hungers through positive strokes. The traditional view of how people structure their time to meet their needs for emotional space between themselves and others has been one-dimensional, with intimacy and self-definition on opposite ends of the same continuum. The healthy position is viewed as holding the middle ground between the two extremes of total withdrawal from people versus being totally enmeshed in intimate relationships.

Kaplan (2001), taking issue with the traditional view, suggests that the needs for self-definition (withdrawal) and intimacy exist on different dimensions, with their own continuums of high and low needs for each dimension. This two-dimensional model, plotted on x- and y-axes, permits us to examine four lifestyles: (1) high needs for self-definition and intimacy, (2) high needs for intimacy and low needs for self-definition, (3) low needs for both self-definition and intimacy, and (4) high needs for self-definition and low needs for intimacy. The four-dimensional scale permits expansion of the two-scale model of high need for attachment versus fear of attachment to need for and fear of individuation and need for and fear of attachment. In other words, needs for intimacy and withdrawal are not opposite ends of the same continuum on the need to affiliate with people.

Rackets

Some people find themselves involved in what is known in TA theory as a "stamp-collecting enterprise"; they store bad feelings until they have enough to cash in for some psychological prize. The bad-feelings racket, or stamp collecting, works in much the same way that the former supermarket stamp-collecting enterprise once worked. People save brown stamps for all the bad things others have caused them to suffer and gold stamps for all the favors others owe them. Gray stamps refer to lowered self-esteem, red stamps symbolize anger, blue stamps mean depression, and white stamps connote purity (James & Jongeward, 1971). The filled-up, bad-feelings stamp books may be cashed in for such things as a free divorce, custody of children, nervous breakdown, blowup, drunken binge, bout of depression, tantrum, runaway attempt, or love affair. Good-feelings stamps are used to justify playtime, relaxation, and breaks from work. Stamp collecting is a racket learned from parents. The collector uses the stamps as excuses for behavior and feelings, and the suppliers may not even be aware they are giving them out. "I'm OK, you're OK" people do not need stamps because they need no excuses for their behavior, which is honest, open, and ethical.

COUNSELING METHOD

TA practitioners teach the principles of TA to participants and then let them use these principles to analyze and improve their own behavior. TA concepts have been taught to people of all ages and ability levels, from the very young to the very old and from mentally retarded children to gifted children. Pierini (2014) identifies the critical points of working with children as a TA therapist include tuning in to the logic of the child state, using imagination and creativity, and operating from a nurturing Parent ego state. The following TA points are most useful in counseling children and adolescents:

1. Definition and explanation of ego states
2. Analysis of transactions between ego states
3. Positive and negative stroking (or "warm fuzzies" and "cold pricklies")
4. I'm OK, you're OK
5. Games and rackets
6. Scripts

In simple terms, the primary goal in TA is to help the person achieve the "I'm OK, you're OK" life position. Various methods and techniques can accomplish this aim. Because children can easily learn and understand the terms and concepts of TA, the approach has become popular in helping school-age children.

The "I'm OK, you're OK" life position is one the child chooses to take. The other three positions more or less evolve of themselves; the child feels no sense of free choice in the matter. According to Harris (1969), the first three positions are based on feelings, and the fourth position—"I'm OK, you're OK"—is based on thought, faith, and initiation of action. The first three have to do with "why"; the fourth has to do with "why not." No one drifts into a new position; it is a decision a person makes. Figure 14-6 provides a guide to plotting a person's progress in moving from one quadrant to another, providing each step on the number axis is defined in operational terms. The x-axis refers to gains and losses in self-esteem; the y-axis indicates the same for relationships with others.

Process

Clarkson (1993), Stewart and Joines (2012), and Woollams and Brown (1979) talk about these stages of TA: motivation, awareness, the treatment contract, de-confusing the child, redecision, relearning, and termination. Counselors gather information about clients to explore early family backgrounds and people, strokes received, focus in their lives, and their social and cultural environment (Massey, 1995). Counselors are trying to have a picture of these facets of the client:

- The balance of ego states
- The nature of the person's transactions
- Their games and rackets
- The person's basic position
- The person's life script

Analyzing and understanding that information allows clients to become more aware of their patterns and origins, freeing them to change patterns and find healthier ways of relating (Prochaska & Norcross, 2014; Seligman & Reichenberg, 2014).

Techniques

Ideally, the role of a transactional analyst is teacher. TA concepts have been taught successfully to children, preadolescents, and adolescents (see Alvyn Freed's books *TA for Tots: And Other Prinzes* [1973/1998] and *TA for Teens and Other Important People* [1992] and Alvyn and Margaret Freed's book *TA for Kids: And Grown Ups Too* [1971/1998]).

A three-step process is effective in teaching TA to any child. First, explain the principle by using a story, a poster, puppets, or other age-appropriate methods. Second, ask the children to "read" back what they understand of the TA principle (correcting them as they go along). Third, ask the children to give examples of the principle from their own experience ("What positive strokes have you received today?") or to identify examples of the principle from the explanation ("'You must always go to bed early' comes from which ego state?").

We recommend that counselors begin teaching the PAC model by showing children that all of us have these three parts that tell us what to do in certain situations. For example, our *Parent* tells us what we should do, our *Adult* tells us how to figure things out, and our *Child* tells us what to do for fun.

Once children have been taught how to speak the language of TA, the counselor can help them analyze their own transactions and see how their behavior affects others and vice versa. Children learn to identify the source of the reasoning that goes into their decisions; that is, they learn how to use their Adult in dealing with the demands of their Parent and Child.

Children can then be taught about the differences between the nurturing and critical parts of the Parent part of their personality. The Critical Parent sounds a lot like our real parents, because it tells us the right thing to do. The Nurturing Parent tells us that we are all right and takes care of us in a loving way.

The Adult is compared with a computer. It helps us think for ourselves, solve problems, and learn new things. The Adult can be contaminated by the Child. For example, when you are studying for a test using your Adult, your Child might say, "Take time out for a snack and watch some TV."

Sometimes the Child part of our personality is divided into three parts: the adapted child, the little professor, and the free child. The adapted child is the part of you that might be the rebel who refuses to do what people in charge like parents and teachers want us to do. The adapted child seems to come alive at about age 2 and enjoys a rebirth during the adolescent years. However, the adapted child reaction is a natural reaction to any person, such as a peer or friend, who acts too bossy. The little professor is that part of the child that does the creative and clever planning to help the Child get what he or she wants. The little professor does the daydreaming that stimulates the make-believe games that often lead to future careers and hobbies. The free (or natural) child is the part of the child that engages in spontaneous fun. When we are playing in a fun game, we are in our natural child. The free child is also free to feel and express any emotion and feeling that may arise, including the negative feelings of hate and anger. Our free child does the playing, has the fun, and is often impulsive. However, it also needs to be monitored by our Adult and Parent to keep our behavior within the limits of responsible behavior.

The key to understanding PAC is to know which part of our personality is in charge at any particular moment and whether that is the appropriate one for the situation. We know which ego state is in charge by how we talk, how we act, how others react to us, and how we feel. The Parent says things such as "Shame on you," "That's stupid," or "I love you very much and you are pretty sharp." The Adult says things such as "I can figure it out," "I'm going to do my homework," and "The answer is 64." The Child says things such as "Cool," "I want," and "That sucks!"

After they understand how the PAC model works, children are ready to learn how positive and negative strokes are transacted between people. Positive strokes are identified as warm fuzzies (symbolized with soft balls of wool yarn) that include pats on the back, hugs, compliments, and handshakes that make you feel warm and fuzzy all over when you get them. Strokes can be earned by doing good work, but the best strokes are the freebies you get just for being you. Negative strokes are taught by using hard, spiny plastic objects called cold pricklies that are not fun to hold in your hand. Cold pricklies are criticisms, punishments, and insults, as well as name calling, hitting, and kicking you might get from somebody.

Children are taught they were born as Prinzes (prince or princess), and later on, when they get some cold pricklies, they may begin to think they have turned into Frozzes (girl and boy frogs). If we get too many cold pricklies about how we are "not OK" and everybody else is, we develop an "I'm not OK and you're OK" attitude, which could lead to developing and following a loser life script. The only cure for the "I'm not OK" position is to receive an abundance of unconditional, positive strokes and love from our parents and plenty of positive strokes (warm fuzzies) from our friends.

Stamp collecting is taught as a racket in which we save up incidents that hurt our feelings or made us angry and then trade these stamps in later for a guilt-free tantrum or blowup. As mentioned earlier, sometimes people use different colors to label the different bad feelings they collect, such as red for anger and blue for fear. However, brown stamps are now used to symbolize all bad feelings. The Adult has the task of acting rationally on these bad feelings to prevent them from being stored and saved for a later irrational act. These brown stamps can be saved or thrown away. In fact, our Adult can refuse to let us even print them.

These brown stamps can be avoided if you track them down. Children are taught to act as soon as they begin to feel uncomfortable because someone annoys them or hurts their feelings. The tracking down of brown stamps takes 30 seconds and consists of answering the following seven questions:

1. How do I hurt?—anger, fear or pain?
2. Which part of me hurts—Parent, Adult, or Child? (usually Child)
3. Who did it?
4. With what part? —Parent, Adult, or Child?
5. Why did he or she do it?
6. What can I do now?
7. What can I do differently next time?

Children also learn about the three types of transactions: complementary, crossed, and double (or hidden). Complementary transactions are parallel transactions where the arrows between your PAC and the other person's PAC do not cross. For example, the Adult question, "What was our math assignment?" is answered by the Adult response, "Page 104."

The transaction becomes crossed when the response to the Adult question comes from the Critical Parent: "You should have paid more attention in class." Another example of a crossed transaction might come from the Free Child, "Forget math, let's go shoot some hoops." Crossed transactions often lead to arguments, fights, and other bad feeling activities. Double transactions have a hidden, unspoken meaning. For example, the Adult might appear to be saying to another Adult, "Let's play some ball." The Hidden Child-to-Child message might be, "Let's not do that math assignment for tomorrow."

Children are taught that TA games are not the same as fun games. TA games are played to get strokes, but they are crooked ways of getting them because the transactions are not open and honest. As mentioned earlier, the first game children play is "mine is better than yours." Children play this game in an attempt to get rewarded with strokes when they do not believe they get strokes just for being themselves. "Tattletale" often becomes the next game, when children realize they can get strokes from people in charge by telling on their siblings or classmates. Both of these games are indications that children need to be reassured they are all right. Caretakers can also give strokes when children are trying to earn them by doing the right things and are not trying to earn them at the expense of others.

Rackets are identified as activities that can lead to games. Rackets are ways of trying to control others by making them responsible for the bad feelings you have that never seem to go away. For example, a person-in-charge might use to get children to do what they want is: "You really make me worried and nervous when you leave the house and go off with your friends," or "You know I have this heart condition and how upset I get when you don't make A's and B's."

Children recognize scripts as what they are going to be when they grow up, but they are not written in stone. Scripts can be changed (and often are) as we find out what we like to do and what we can do well. People can move from a loser's or nonwinner's script to a winner's script by being persistent in the pursuit of realistic, challenging goals that fall within their interest and ability levels. For children, the task involves moving from a failure identity to a success identity of "I am lovable and capable"—lovable because I have people in my life who care about me and whom I care about, and capable because I can do things such as succeed in school and other activities. In short, "I am OK."

Finally, children are taught about making and keeping contracts to make changes in their daily behavior. People do well when they keep their promises and hold to their contracts with friends and others. People who have difficulty in making and keeping their commitments to others get themselves in trouble. The way out of trouble is to commit to helpful behaviors they can and will do.

Probably the most important concept to remember when dealing with children is that everyone grows up feeling "not OK." Children function on the basis of the "OK-ness" they see in their parents. If Mommy frequently responds to the child with *her* "not-OK" Child, the stage is set for the establishment of the "I'm not OK, you're not OK" position. One of the best ways for youngsters to develop strong

Adult ego states is to observe their parents use their Adults in handling inappropriate responses from the demanding Parent or Child.

As mentioned earlier, the goal of TA counseling with children is to help them learn to control their responses with their Adult, thereby achieving the "I'm OK, you're OK" life position. However, strengthening a child's Adult causes his or her family role to shift. The child becomes less active in playing the destructive games that dominate many families. Other family members' roles of necessity also shift. For this reason, the child's parents must be included in the counseling process to achieve lasting results.

Children can learn all about warm fuzzies and cold pricklies, but because of the tremendous influence of their parents, it is next to impossible, without effective intervention, for them to reverse a "loser" life script if their parents have given it to them. Everything parents do and say to children tells them they are "OK" or "not OK," depending on what life position the parents themselves occupy. Positive stroking and respect are two things everyone needs to build a winner's script. The child needs positive strokes, both conditional ("We'll have some ice cream after you put away your toys.") and unconditional ("I love you no matter what."). Children come to see themselves as "OK" because their parents treat them that way. As a positive stroke, respect is hard to beat. The conclusion a child reaches is this: "If my OK parents think I'm OK, then I really must be OK."

Another useful TA principle for both teachers and parents is to teach "do" and *not* "don't." Parents' and other adults' attempts to teach appropriate behavior by catching children in *inappropriate* behavior baffle children. Because Mommy is "OK," a child thinks, "It must be all my fault, and I must be not OK."

A slightly different aspect of the same idea is that children who are counseled and taught to "do more" or "do better" must also know *what* to do. The Parent in everyone admonishes us to "do better"; the Adult supplies the "do *what* better."

As children and their families become more acquainted with the whys of their relationships, they learn to avoid undesirable ways of structuring time. Again, the goal of TA is to help the individual learn to lead a full, game-free life, and everyone has that choice. The usefulness of the PAC model is in creating awareness of how the Parent, Adult, and Child function in the decision-making process.

As mentioned earlier, several techniques can teach TA to children. The concepts of positive and negative stroking have been taught with smiling and frowning faces, as well as with fuzzy yarn balls and sharp, prickly plastic objects to connote warm fuzzies and cold pricklies, respectively. The following warm fuzzy, cold prickly fairy tale (Steiner, 1975) was written for the Child in everyone.

There once existed a town where people shared their warm fuzzies without fear of running out of their supply of fuzzies. One day a wicked witch appeared and planted the idea that people should hoard their fuzzies in case there happened to be a shortage of fuzzies. When the townspeople did this, their backbones began to shrivel up. The witch cured the shriveling backbones by giving everybody a bag of cold pricklies to share. The sharing of cold pricklies continued until a good witch arrived and put the townspeople back on the right track—sharing their warm fuzzies.

Posters can be made with representations of the various ideas of TA (stroking, ego states, "I'm OK, you're OK," lists of games with appropriate illustrations, lists of scripting phrases, and so on). Puppets, dolls, and make-believe stories can be successful with younger children who cannot yet read.

Counselors can teach new stroking patterns to children who are having interpersonal conflicts. They first need to analyze the other person's behavior. What response does parent, teacher, or friend give to the child's positive or negative strokes? What strokes does the other person like? Teach children new ways of stroking from among the following categories:

1. Self-strokes: doing nice things for yourself
2. Physical strokes: hugs, kisses, pats, back rubs, handshakes, "high fives" (be sure to distinguish between good and bad touching)
3. Silent strokes: winks, nods, waves, smiles
4. Verbal strokes: "I like you," "Good job," "Thanks"
5. Rewards or privileges: letting younger siblings go with you, playing with them, doing something for your parents

Young children (up to 7 years) may not be able to symbolize stroking and ego states as well as older children; thus, less technical language may be necessary. Young children can understand "warm fuzzy" if a stroke feels good and "cold prickly" if it feels bad after someone says or does something to them. They may need permission to ask for a warm fuzzy instead of manipulating for a cold prickly when they feel bad. Likewise, small children can understand "my bossy part," "my thinking part," "my angry part," or "my happy part" rather than the ego states, which they sometime confuse with actual people.

Ego-grams are bar graphs showing children "how much" of each ego state they use (Figure 14-8). An ego-gram can indicate what changes might be made. A child

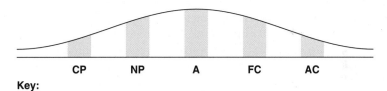

Key:

P The Parent refers to a person's values, beliefs, and morals.

   CP The Critical Parent finds fault, directs, orders, sets limits, makes rules, and enforces one's value system. Too much CP results in dictatorial or bossy behavior.

   NP The Nurturing Parent is empathic and promotes growth. The NP is warm and kind, but too much NP becomes smothering, and children will not be able to learn how to take care of themselves.

A The Adult acts like a computer. It takes in, stores, retrieves, and processes information. The A is a storehouse of facts and helps you think when you solve problems, but too much Adult is boring.

C The Child can be fun, expressive, and spontaneous, and sometimes it can be compliant and a follower of rules.

   FC The Free Child is the fun and spontaneous part of the child. When you cheer at a ballgame, you are in the Free Child part of your personality. However, too much FC might mean that you have lost control of yourself.

   AC The Adapting Child is the conforming, easy-to-get-along-with part of your personality. Too much AC results in guilt feelings, depression, other bad feelings, and robotlike behavior.

FIGURE 14-8 I EGO-GRAM

who wants to make a change can work on strengthening low ego states by practicing appropriate behaviors. Counselors can also help determine whether the child thinks the ego-gram differs in various situations—at home, at school, playing with friends.

Once children understand ego states, they can learn to distinguish complementary, crossed, and ulterior transactions. If they bring in a situation that illustrates one of these, have them diagram it. In the case of crossed or ulterior transactions, encourage children to use their Adult to figure out ways to obtain a more successful result.

Some other methods for teaching the various TA techniques are as follows:

1. Talk about the feelings and behaviors that go with each ego state. Have children identify their own and others' ego states by relating the ego states to what children say about their experiences.

   CHILD: My brother always tells me what to do. He's not my father.

   COUNSELOR: You feel rebellious when your brother acts like a bossy parent.

As children become aware of their ego states and can discriminate between them, their Adult can gain control of which ego state is expressed and give them permission to replace destructive ideas with constructive ones.

2. The OK Corral diagram is useful in helping children identify how they feel and think about themselves and other people. Children are able to discuss what "OK-ness" and "not-OK-ness" mean to them in terms of specific behaviors.

3. Games intrigue children. Once they have the concept, they can readily pick up on games in themselves and others and describe them. Any time children describe a pattern of games or recognize that "this always happens to me," the counselor can introduce the concept of games as a way of getting negative strokes to replace the positive strokes children think they cannot get. For example, "You seem to mess up a lot. How do you manage that?" "What does this mean about you?" "How did it feel after it happened?" "What do you really want? How could you get it better?" "What 'bad' (scary) thing does this game prevent?" Children can also identify the three game roles of persecutor, rescuer, and victim and learn to stay out of them. The persecutor role can be demonstrated by having the child try to "put someone down" by pressing straight down on his or her shoulders. Putting people down this way is difficult unless they lean over or bend their knees. You can demonstrate the rescuer role by trying to pick up a limp person (of about the same size). Holding up a person who does not want to stand is also difficult. The victim role is demonstrated in relation to the other two by the partner's "giving in," lying down, and staying limp.

4. Racket feelings can be discussed in terms of stamp collecting. Children can usually identify the bad feelings they save up and the prize they get. Hypothetical situations such as the following create bad feelings: "Did you ever have a rotten day? Your mom yells at you at breakfast, your teacher catches you talking, the other guys play keep-away with your hat, and you drop your books in the mud when your dog jumps on you because he's so glad to see you home. All day long you have felt mistreated and hurt, and that is the last straw. So you pick a fight with your little sister." Talk about how cashing in stamps feels and how getting dumped on feels. As small people, children are often the target

when stamps are cashed in. Awareness can help children stop collecting stamps (child abuse is the worst form of stamp cashing) by learning to talk about bad feelings with someone they can trust and by asking for and receiving the positive strokes they need.

5. For counselors working with script issues, useful questions for figuring out a child's script include many of the same questions used in the Adlerian lifestyle interview:

What are the "hurt" points in your family? (G)

Who is in your family? (BP)

What are the people in your family like? (BP)

Has anyone else ever lived with you? (BP)

What were they like? (BP)

Who is boss in your family? (PI, P)

What is your mother's (or father's) favorite saying? (PI, CI)

Describe yourself in three words. (BP, D)

What words would other people in your family use to describe you? (PI, CI, BP)

What bad feeling do you have a lot of the time? (R)

What good feeling do you have a lot of the time? (BP)

Who is your mother's favorite? (PI, CI)

Who is your father's favorite? (PI, CI)

The preceding questions are coded to fit parts of the life script:

BP—Basic life position regarding how I feel about myself and others

PI—Parental injunction (message from parent's Child): "Don't do as I do"

CI—Counter injunction (message from parent's Parent): "Do at least try"

G—Games (getting strokes at others' expense)

R—Racket (bad feelings)

D—Decision (how I have chosen to live my life)

P—Program (how to obey injunctions)

6. At some time during their lives, most people have kept a diary or journal in which they have recorded their innermost feelings, thoughts, and other events. Children and adolescents respond well to a homework assignment of keeping a diary. The diary provides the counselor and client with a record of feelings, thoughts, and life script to be explored. Keeping a journal or diary may also provide the child with a feeling of closeness to the counselor between sessions.

7. What *not* to do: The counselor who is not in a position to protect a child from negative consequences should not interfere with script behavior that still serves a purpose in the family. Do not ask children to give up their games or rackets before they learn more appropriate ways to get strokes. Do not decide for children what they "should" do. Do not encourage children to play TA counselor with people who have power over them and may not appreciate their comments.

However, scripts are not written in stone and can be modified or rewritten to help children and adults find better ways to meet their needs. All the preceding exercises can be used in group and family counseling, as well as in individual counseling. Role-playing and acting-out games are effective group techniques. Families in TA counseling come to recognize where their transactions become crossed, how and when scripting occurs, and how stroking behavior can change family feelings.

Morena (2014) and Poda (2011) talk about ways to work with childhood trauma and TA. Chiesa (2012, 2014) outlines using sand trays to uncover scripts, and Berardo (2012, 2014) recommends metaphors and writing as ways to understand adolescent scripts. Also, Evans (2014) connects the digital communication system to ego states and work with adolescents.

Case Studies

Transcript I

Jimmy, age 5, is being seen by the school counselor because he has recently begun fighting with other children in his kindergarten class.

COUNSELOR: Jimmy, remember when I came to your class and read the story about the warm fuzzies and the cold pricklies? [He nods.] Well, everybody, kids and grown-ups, needs to get some of these to live. Sometimes people do things to get cold pricklies like slaps or frowns, or being yelled at. Would you like to find out how to give yourself and other people nice warm fuzzies like smiles and hugs and pats on the back, and get them back from others?

JIMMY: Yes. Everybody doesn't like me now.

COUNSELOR: What do you do to get hugs and smiles from your mommy?

JIMMY: I don't do anything, she just gives them to me. Or sometimes I hug her first or say "I love you."

COUNSELOR: Sometimes mommies are busy. What do you do to get her attention then?

JIMMY: Well, I get a hug from Grandma. But if I can't get one, I make my little sister yell. Then somebody comes to see what's happening.

COUNSELOR: If you can't get a warm fuzzy, you get them to give you a cold prickly?

JIMMY: Yeah.

COUNSELOR: What do kids in your class have to do to get a smile?

JIMMY: The teacher smiles if you stay quiet when we go to the lunchroom, but I am usually talking to my friend.

COUNSELOR: If you can't get a smile or other warm fuzzy when you want one, is that what you do to get attention?

JIMMY: I make one of the other kids yell too by stepping on feet.

COUNSELOR: Sometimes getting yelled at is better than nothing, huh?

JIMMY:	Yeah.
COUNSELOR:	Do you think any of your teachers would give you a warm fuzzy?
JIMMY:	Mrs. Granite has a nice face and smiles lots kid's talk for often.
COUNSELOR:	So when you feel bad inside and need a warm fuzzy, you could get one from Mrs. Granite?
JIMMY:	Yeah, like when I miss my mommy. I could tell Mrs. Granite that and ask her to talk to me and give me a smile.
COUNSELOR:	That sounds like a good plan, Jimmy. And if you feel bad, or sad, or lonely, or angry, and need to talk about it, you can come here and talk to me about it.
JIMMY:	Okay.
COUNSELOR:	[gives Jimmy a hug] I give warm fuzzies too.
	Counselor feedback to Jimmy's teacher should include talking about giving Jimmy some strokes when he is being good and not making a bid for attention in the form of negative feedback.

Transcript II

The child in this interview is a 10-year-old boy.

COUNSELOR:	Christopher, you've read the Freed's book about stroking. Can you explain to me what they mean by strokes?
CHRISTOPHER:	Stroking is when somebody does something that makes you feel either good or not so good.
COUNSELOR:	I think that's a very good definition. Can you give me some examples of a positive stroke?
CHRISTOPHER:	Patting somebody on the back and saying "good job!", or helping them, or saying something nice.
COUNSELOR:	Like what?
CHRISTOPHER:	"You really helped me today."
COUNSELOR:	Can you think of a positive stroke you've given someone today?
CHRISTOPHER:	Not really.
COUNSELOR:	How about when I came in, and you looked up and smiled?
CHRISTOPHER:	I guess. I smiled at most everybody in the class today.
COUNSELOR:	You have to remember that they don't have to be words; just a smile is a positive stroke. Can you think of any negative strokes you've given anyone today?
CHRISTOPHER:	No.
COUNSELOR:	That's good. Of course, the same holds true for negative strokes; if, without realizing it, you looked at someone and gave them a frown or something that could be a negative stroke that you didn't realize you gave.
CHRISTOPHER:	I don't see why I would have given any, even by accident. There wasn't any reason to give any.
COUNSELOR:	Well, good. Can you think of any positive strokes anyone gave you today?
CHRISTOPHER:	When I got 100 on our test today, Mrs. Kincaid said that that was very good.

COUNSELOR:	I'm glad. Any negative strokes?
CHRISTOPHER:	No.
COUNSELOR:	Well, I told you your hands and face were dirty and I didn't like you coming around like that, right? You think you've got the idea about how positive and negative strokes work?
CHRISTOPHER:	Yes.
COUNSELOR:	How would you use stroking?
CHRISTOPHER:	Well, whenever I thought somebody did a good job on something, I could tell them.
COUNSELOR:	You know, there's such a thing as giving strokes that are not asked for, strokes that you just offer freely. Can you give an example of one of those, maybe?
CHRISTOPHER:	Just saying something nice when they don't even really need it … well, they do need it. Just saying it, but just saying it even if they haven't done anything.
COUNSELOR:	How about a more specific example?
CHRISTOPHER:	Well, if you meet somebody, you can say, "I like your shoes," or "Your hair looks nice," or something like that.
COUNSELOR:	Yes, those would be nice to hear. Can you tell me how you might use nonverbal positive strokes?
CHRISTOPHER:	By patting somebody, or smiling at them, or giving them a hug.
COUNSELOR:	How do you think you would feel if you started giving more positive strokes and getting more positive strokes?
CHRISTOPHER:	All covered over with strokes!

DIVERSITY APPLICATIONS OF TRANSACTIONAL ANALYSIS

Eric Berne believed that the concepts used in TA were universal. That is, all people possess Parent, Adult, and Child functions in their personality, and all people transact their business with others through communicating from each of the three ego states. The user-friendly nature of TA is an advantage for transcending cultural barriers. Cultures and individuals within all cultures who prefer a direct, straightforward, educational approach to personal development over a healing approach to mental illness will find TA comfortable. TA practitioners offer the opportunity to learn new skills in both group and individual settings. Considerable thought is required to analyze transactions and communication patterns between people. Analysis of scripts, games, and rackets puts a premium on cognitive processes. However, the focus on feelings is not disregarded, especially in dealing with the giving and receiving of positive and negative strokes.

In using TA across cultures, there is little variation in the method. Clients will learn the basic terminology and make contracts. TA has been used successfully in several different cultures. Mazzetti (1997) recommends TA for treating antisocial behavior by children of immigrant families in Italy. Robinson (1998) describes a TA program for treating seriously disturbed clients in a small, residential therapeutic community in England. Guimaraes (1997) uses TA to teach student doctors to communicate and work more effectively with patients from lower socioeconomic levels in Brazil. Beslija (1997) reports success with TA in working with the psychological problems of refugees from the former Yugoslavia.

EVALUATION OF TRANSACTIONAL ANALYSIS

Considerable work and progress toward counseling goals can be done in 10 group sessions, giving TA some advantage points for brief treatment and a goal-attainment focus. Setting goals may involve writing a new life script to replace the old script, which was not helping clients meet their needs. In fact, old ineffective scripts are generally written out and destroyed in a "public" burning during a group session. Rewriting one's life script also involves reviewing the messages one received from one's father and mother about such topics as education, work, fun, religion, marriage, family, sex, money, politics, love, and power. Messages that do not work for you are discarded in favor of those values that do work for you in your present life.

TA is viewed by some as being a versatile and integrative approach to counseling (Nabrady, 2005). TA practitioners use a variety of interventions that belong uniquely to the TA approach. Some examples include script analysis, group feedback on how one's communication style impacts others, structuring one's time, and clarification/evaluation of personal values. Hargaden and Sills (2002) refer to TA as a relational approach in much the same way the Rogers's person-centered counseling is described. Our view is that all counseling approaches need a significant relational component for interventions to be effective. TA practiced in groups does have a relationship focus, offering clients the opportunity to see themselves as others see them, which may result in clients altering their behavior to improve their relationships.

Some therapists have attached themselves to TA and identified themselves as transactional psychoanalysts (Novellino, 2005; Woods, 2005). Steiner and Novellino (2005) debate the merits of such a union. Novellino, supporting an integration of TA and psychoanalysis, practices transactional psychoanalysis that includes the standard psychoanalytic practice of analyzing transference, countertransference, and unconscious phenomena. Steiner, a veteran TA practitioner, makes the stronger case for TA being a radical departure from psychoanalysis as Berne intended it to be. Fowlie and Sills (2011) provide a useful explanation of relational TA. Widdowson (2010) provides a comprehensive, useful history of TA with its various transformations as well as the incorporation of the approach into other forms of counseling.

TA is a self-help psychology—people can be helped by reading about it because the concepts are easy to understand. In fact Stewart and Joines (2012) proclaim their book a self-help manual of TA approaches. People do not feel threatened by TA. It deals with observable behavior, the present, and the conscious area of functioning. The TA focus is on how people can change whatever they want to change; these changes often happen immediately as people learn how to communicate more effectively and develop contracts for behavior change.

SUMMARY

The practitioners of TA work to improve relationship and communication skills between individuals and within groups of various types. For example, Adams (2008) used TA to help a person make peace with his or her past. TA training is useful in conducting group guidance classes or group counseling sessions with students in the 5- to 17-year-old range. However, the language and concepts are easily understood. The focus on positive, helpful transactions and ways to increase and maintain those behaviors provides hope and momentum. The TA focus is on re-education rather than healing and, as such, is not based on the assumption that people are sick and need to be healed. Participants in TA groups appreciate their roles as learners over that of being patients and have a laboratory for analyzing and practicing transactions. TA instruction helps people to become aware of what they do and how this affects other people in their families and in their circles of friends and acquaintances. This information supports decisions to make changes in behavior.

WEB SITES FOR TRANSACTIONAL ANALYSIS

Internet addresses frequently change. To find the sites listed here, visit www.cengage .com/counseling/henderson for an updated list of Internet addresses and direct links to relevant sites.

International Transactional Analysis Association (ITAA) home page

USA Transactional Analysis Association

REFERENCES

Adams, S. A. (2008). Using transactional analysis and mental imagery to help shame-based identity adults make peace with their past. *Adultspan Journal, 7*, 2–12.

Berardo, C. (2012). The little red car: Metaphor as a tool for working with teenagers. *Transactional Analysis Journal, 42*(3), 220–227. doi:10.1177/036215371204200308

Berardo, C. (2014). Alice in writerland: Writing as a therapeutic tool and a way to understand adolescent needs. *Transactional Analysis Journal, 44*(2), 142–152. doi:10.1177/0362153714541950

Berne, E. (1947). *The mind in action.* New York: Simon & Schuster.

Berne, E. (1949). The nature of intuition. *Psychiatric Quarterly, 23*, 203–226.

Berne, E. (1961). *Transactional analysis in psychotherapy.* New York: Grove.

Berne, E. (1964). *Games people play.* New York: Grove.

Beslija, A. (1997). Psychotherapy with refugees from Bosnia-Herzegovina. *Transactional Analysis Journal, 27*, 49–54.

Chiesa, C. (2012). Scripts in the sand: Sandplay in transactional analysis psychotherapy with children. *Transactional Analysis Journal, 42*(4), 285–293. doi:10.1177/036215371204200407

Chiesa, C. (2014). On the seashore of an endless world, children play: Using transactional analysis in play therapy with children. *Transactional Analysis Journal, 44*(2), 128–141. doi:10.1177/0362153714539916

Clarkson, J. (1993). *Transactional analysis psychotherapy: An integrated approach*. New York: Routledge.

Evans, S. (2014). The challenge and potential of the digital age: Young people and the internet. *Transactional Analysis Journal, 44* (2), 153–166. doi:10.1177/0362153714545312

Fowlie, H., Sills, C., & Ebooks Corporation. (2011). *Relational transactional analysis: Principles in practice*. London: Karnac.

Freed, A. (1992). *TA for teens and other important people* (Rev. ed.). Rolling Hills Estates, CA: Jalmar.

Freed, A. (1998). *TA for tots: And other prinzes*. Rolling Hills Estates, CA: Jalmar. (Original work published 1973.)

Freed, A., & Freed, M. (1998). *TA for kids: And grown ups too*. Rolling Hills Estates, CA: Jalmar. (Original work published 1971.)

Guimaraes, B. (1997). Medical omnipotence and transactional analysis: A pedagogical proposal. *Transactional Analysis Journal, 27,* 272–277.

Guy, R. (2003). A theoretical-educational approach of developing positive self-esteem in children by implementing the theories of transactional analysis in the context of the family. *Dissertation-Abstracts, 64*(4-A), 1138.

Hargaden, H., & Sills, C. (2002). *Transactional Analysis: A relational approach*. Philadelphia, PA: Brunner-Routledge.

Harris, M., & Brockbank, A. (2011). *An integrative approach to therapy and supervision: A practical guide for counselors and psychotherapists*. Philadelphia, PA: Jessica Kingsley.

Harris, T. (1969). *I'm OK—You're OK*. New York: Harper & Row.

James, M., & Jongeward, D. (1971). *Born to win*. Reading, MA: Addison-Wesley.

Kaplan, K. (2001). TILT and structural pathology. *Transactional Analysis Journal Internet, 4,* 1–15.

LeGuernic, A. (2004). Fairy tales and psychological life plans. *Transactional Analysis Journal, 34,* 216–222.

Massey, R. F. (1995). Theory for treating individuals from a transactional analytic/systems perspective. *Transactional Analysis Journal, 25,* 271–284.

Mazzetti, M. (1997). A transactional analysis approach to adjustment problems of adolescents from immigrant families. *Transactional Analysis Journal, 27,* 220–227.

Morena, S. (2014). Children and their monsters: Childhood trauma and transactional analysis. *Transactional Analysis Journal, 44*(2), 118–127. doi:10.1177/0362153714539915

Nabrady, M. (2005). Emotion theories and transactional analysis emotion theory: A comparison. *Transactional Analysis Journal, 35,* 68–77.

Novellino, M. (2005). Transactional psychoanalysis: Epistemological foundations. *Transactional Analysis Journal, 35,* 157–172.

Pierini, A. (2014). Being a transactional analysis child therapist: How working with children is different. *Transactional Analysis Journal, 44*(2), 103–117. doi:10.1177/0362153714538937

Poda, D. (2003). A letter to parents about child therapy. *Transactional Analysis Journal, 33,* 89–93.

Poda, D. M. (2011). On receiving the Eric Berne memorial award for work with children. *Transactional Analysis Journal, 41,* 9–10.

Prochaska, J. O., & Norcross, J. C. (2014). *Systems of psychotherapy: A transtheoretical analysis* (8th ed.). Stamford, CT: Cengage Learning.

Robinson, J. (1998). Reparenting in a therapeutic community. *Transactional Analysis Journal, 28,* 88–94.

Seligman, L. (2006). *Theories of counseling and psychotherapy: Systems, strategies, and skills* (2nd ed.). Upper Saddle River, NJ: Pearson.

Seligman, L., & Reichenberg, L. W. (2014). *Theories of counseling and psychotherapy: Systems, strategies, and skills* (4th ed.). Upper Saddle River, NJ: Pearson.

Steiner, C. (1974). *Scripts people live*. New York: Grove.

Steiner, C. (1975). *Readings in radical psychiatry*. New York: Grove.

Steiner, C., & Novellino, M. (2005). TAJ theoretical diversity: A debate about transactional analysis and psychoanalysis. *Transactional Analysis Journal, 35*, 110–118.

Stewart, I., & Joines, V. (2012). *TA today: An introduction to transactional analysis* (2nd ed.). Chapel Hill, NC: Vann Joines and Southeast Institute.

Summerton, O. (2000). The development of game analysis. *Transactional Analysis Journal, 30*, 207–218.

Toth, M. (2004). Dealing with fear of failure: Working with script concepts in the classroom. *Transactional Analysis Journal, 34*, 209–215.

Widdowson, M., & Ebooks Corporation. (2010). *Transactional analysis: 100 key points and techniques*. New York; London: Routledge.

Woods, K. (2000). The defensive function of the game scenario. *Transactional Analysis Journal, 30*, 94–97.

Woods, K. (2005). Correlations between psychoanalysis and transactional analysis. *Transactional Analysis Journal, 35*, 205–210.

Woollams, S., & Brown, M. (1979). *T.A.: The total handbook of transactional analysis*. Upper Saddle River, NJ: Prentice Hall.

CHAPTER 15

Family Counseling

Perhaps the greatest social service that can be rendered by anybody to this country and to mankind is to bring up a family.
—GEORGE BERNARD SHAW

Until the 1930s, mental health treatment focused on the individual because therapists believed the person was the problem. The other theories we have discussed in this book started with this individual-based approach. Many of the supporters of those theories worked with families, but they concentrated on relieving the symptoms in the individual members in the family. Family counseling is an intervention in which members in a family identify and change problematic, maladaptive, repetitive relationship patterns and self-defeating belief systems (Goldenberg, Goldenberg, & Pelavin, 2014). This approach to treatment considers the identified patient (the person in the family that is exhibiting or is considered to be the problem) is having trouble as a result of the transactions within the family or community.

After reading this chapter, you should be able to:

▸ Outline the development of family counseling
▸ Explain the system's focus on family relationships
▸ Discuss the counseling relationship and goals in family counseling
▸ Describe the differences between healthy and unhealthy family systems
▸ Discuss some therapeutic techniques in family counseling
▸ Outline family counseling approaches to play therapy
▸ Clarify the effectiveness of family counseling

BACKGROUND The defining historical events in the family counseling field occurred in the 1950s when a number of researchers who were working independently began to look at schizophrenia as an area where family influences might be connected to the development of psychotic symptoms. Those efforts of Bateson's Palo Alto, California, group, Lidz's project at Yale, and Bowen and Wynn at the Institute

463

of Mental Health led to research discoveries of the therapeutic value of seeing family members together (Goldenberg et al., 2014).

Bateson, Jackson, Haley, and Weakland (1956) wrote a seminal paper about the "double-bind" hypothesis, their explanation of communication patterns that involved a consistent, contradictory message from the parent to the schizophrenic child. According to those researchers, the parent would put the child in a double bind by giving the child an either/or option and then responding negatively whichever way the child responded. The parent may say something like "Be more loving." If the child did not show affection, the parent scolded; but if the child did show warmth, the parent would ignore or demean the child (Fall, Holden, & Marquis, 2010). Thus, the child, who was compelled to respond, was doomed to fail. The conflicting messages caused the child to be confused and ultimately withdraw. Schizophrenia was therefore considered to be an interpersonal phenomenon, a consequence of the failure in a family's communication system (Goldenberg et al., 2014). These findings and those of Lidz, Gornelison, Fleck, and Terry (1957) and Bowen (1960) supported the systemic nature of symptoms and the impetus to further define systemic therapies.

HOW DOES FAMILY COUNSELING DIFFER FROM INDIVIDUAL COUNSELING?

The principal difference between family and individual counseling is that family counseling focuses on the family and its members' interactions and relations. Often, individual counseling tends to separate individuals and their problems from the family setting. Family counseling or family therapy, by contrast, almost always involves interventions to alter the way an entire family system operates. The family counseling and therapy label covers a wide variety of arrangements for the participants: It may be individual, couples, parent and child, or the entire family, including all who live in the home.

Common components of all types of family therapy include a brief duration, solution or crisis focus, action orientation, and attention to here-and-now interactions among family members as well as the ways the family creates, contributes to, and continues the problem. Therapists can work as coach, consultant, model, teacher, collaborator, or expert (Seligman & Reichenberg, 2014).

Carr (2014) conducted a thorough review of systemic interventions such as family therapy and parent training. He concluded the evidence from the research supports the effectiveness of systemic interventions either alone or as part of multimodal programs for sleep, feeding, and attachment problems in infancy; child abuse and neglect; conduct problems (including childhood behavioral difficulties, ADHD, delinquency, and drug abuse); emotional problems (including anxiety, depression, grief, bipolar disorder, and suicidality); eating disorders (including anorexia, bulimia, and obesity); and somatic problems (including enuresis, encopresis, recurrent abdominal pain, and poorly controlled asthma and diabetes). Diamond and Josephson (2005), in a 10-year review of family therapy, also found it to be effective in treating substance abuse and conduct disorders in children and adolescents. Parent management training, focused on teaching parents how to use positive reinforcement, was found to be effective in treating conduct disorders over a period of 14 years. Behavioral family therapy, similar to parent management training but including methods to reduce family factors such as stress in the parents' lives or the child's personality, also was found to be effective in reducing disruptive behavior in children and adolescents. Campbell and Palm (2004) concur about the benefits of parent education in helping parents understand how their behavior and child-rearing practices affect their children.

WHAT DEFINES A FAMILY?

Definitions of *family forms* range from the nuclear family unit of father, mother, and children to a single-parent family to blended (remarried or step) family. Other forms include multiple families living together; multigenerational families; and common law, communal, serial, polygamous, and cohabitation families. Families also are defined by their organizational structure, characterized by degrees of cohesiveness, love, loyalty, and purpose. High levels of shared values, interests, activities, and attention to the needs of its members serve to distinguish the functional family group from other organizational groups and teams.

Perhaps the most all-inclusive definition of family can be found in *Merriam-Webster's Collegiate Dictionary* (Mish, 2003), where *family* is defined as a group of people: "(1) bound together by philosophical, religious, or other convictions; (2) with a common ancestry; and (3) living together under the same roof" (p. 452). Another definition listed in Webster's defines *family* as "the basic bio social unit in society having as its nucleus two or more adults living together and cooperating in the care and rearing of their own or adopted children."

How Does General Systems Theory Relate to Families?

Understanding systems theory involves shifting attention from an individual to a social context. Two principles of general systems theory address the philosophical assumptions relative to family systems. First, systems are organized whole elements or units made up of several interdependent and interacting parts. The elements within the system are necessarily interdependent. The organized whole and interdependent parts are the philosophical core of systems theory (Fall et al., 2010).

System theorists believe that by understanding the interactive, interdependent relationships, counselors better understand the factors in the family functioning and that of each member of the family, as each person plays a part in influencing each other and the overall family atmosphere. The whole unit is greater than the sum of its parts, and change in any part affects all other parts. For example, any family member's graduation from high school or hospital admission has effects on all other family members. Thus, family therapists view the family as a system in which each member has a significant influence on all other members. It follows that they also believe that for significant positive change in an identified client, family members have to change the way they interact.

A second philosophical underpinning of systems thinking is that patterns in a system are circular instead of linear (Minuchin, 1984). An example of linear thinking is considering one person's maladjustment as being caused by something within that person. The concept of circular causality revolves around not only internal but also mutual influence. Yontef and Jacobs (2014) explain circular causality as a pattern. A causes B and B causes A. However an interaction begins, A triggers a response in B to which A reacts negatively with no awareness of a role in causing the negative reaction. Likewise, B triggers a harmful response by A without being aware of a role in the negative response. An example is a mother (A) who yells for her son (B) to clean up his room. He (B) shrugs and she (A) shouts about his lack of respect and on and on the interaction goes. This circular or reciprocal causality is a central concept in systems theory (Gladding, 2015).

Next, we consider a way to look at the causes of difficulties in families. A key difference between individual and family counseling is problem diagnosis. Family therapists use a circular causality diagnosis, whereas individual therapists tend to rely on linear causality. For example, a linear causality diagnosis might be as follows: Alice fails to turn in homework to her teacher and therefore earns a lower grade. A circular causality diagnosis might include how the teacher's reaction to Alice then influences how Alice reacts to her teacher, as well as to her parents. Mom nags Alice about not doing her homework; Alice, in turn, gets the attention, albeit negative, that she wants. The teacher sends home a failing note to Alice's parents, who, in turn, both start to nag Alice, who resists homework even more than before. In other words, a circular causality diagnosis involves the roles each family member plays. In fairness to the theories discussed in previous chapters, all have been effective in working with families.

A key point of interest to all family therapists is the balance families maintain between the several sets of bipolar extremes that characterize dysfunctional families. For example, families may struggle to find a healthy balance between too much involvement in each other's lives (*enmeshment*) and too much detachment from each other (*disengagement*). A family could be viewed as a canoe full of people heading into the current of a river. Some canoes are balanced and stable, but maintaining this balance requires each family member to assume an uncomfortable position; a shift by one person necessitates a shift by everyone else for the canoe to remain upright. Other families are paddling balanced canoes while sitting comfortably, allowing them to adapt to the changes all families face as they go through the stages of family development; still other canoes capsize, with family members hanging on to the side just trying to survive. Family therapists see their job as righting capsized canoes and making family members comfortable in their canoe-paddling roles. Staying with the canoe metaphor, family therapists see an obvious advantage in working with the whole crew as a group rather than focusing on the identified problem member of the family.

Shapiro, Friedberg, and Bardenstein (2006) summarized the differences in healthy and unhealthy families. Those authors explained that many of the differences link to a common theme. Dysfunctional families behave in an extreme position on some continuum, while healthy families achieve moderation or balance between opposite ways of functioning. The most common balancing acts are between enmeshment and disengagement, chaos and rigidity, and effective or ambiguous, complex or contradictory communication patterns. Healthy families do not have coalitions against each other, and the hierarchy of authority reflects the capabilities and needs of all family members. Gladding (2015) says that healthy families in almost all cultures adapt to change, set appropriate boundaries, build relationships by open communication, promote responsibility, show confidence in themselves and their children, and are optimistic about their future.

Counselors also need to consider the family life cycle. McGoldrick, Carter, and Garcia-Petro (2011) provide a six-stage model of an intact nuclear family with each

TABLE 15-1 MODELS OF FAMILY LIFE CYCLE

Haley Stages and Related Tasks	McGoldrick and Carter Stages and Tasks
Courtship—selecting a mate	Young adulthood—separating from family of origin
Marriage—making a formal commitment with lifelong expectations	Young couple—developing a partner relationship
Childbirth and dealing with the young—establishing a new nuclear family system	Families with children—establishing a new nuclear family
Middle marriage and child rearing—fulfilling the marriage and raising children	Families with adolescents—adjusting to adolescents' increased associations beyond the nuclear family
Parents' individuation from their adult children—transitioning to interdependent relationships	Families at midlife—adjusting to the departure of family members (children) and the arrival of new members (in-laws)
Retirement and old age—adjusting to end-of-life transitions	The family in later life—adjusting to retirement and old age
	Divorce, single parenting, and remarriage—marital transitions and/or contemporary characteristics of the family that influence the above stages

Adapted from Wagner (2008).

period having adjustments, tasks, and changes to be accomplished with the individual, family, and family members. Those stages are as follows:

- Single young adults leaving home
- New couple
- Families with young children
- Families with adolescents
- Families launching children and moving on
- Families in later life

The stages discussed by McGoldrick and Carter (2003) expanded the coverage to include families in divorce, single parenting, and remarriage. Hill (1986) collapses types of families into those with temporary or permanent single status. Those stages and related tasks as discussed by Wagner (2008) are summarized in Table 15-1.

Core Concepts

Appleton and Dykeman (2007) compiled family therapy terms critical to understanding the theories. Their summaries follow:

- *Centripetal and centrifugal:* terms from the field of physics used to describe relationship styles in families. Centripetal families look inward to the family as a source of joy and satisfaction. These families have rigid boundaries and agreeable familial interactions. Centrifugal families look outside for pleasure and satisfaction so family boundaries and interactions are minimal.
- *Cybernetics:* the study of processes that regulate systems, especially the control of information.

- *Family:* applies to two or more people who consider themselves family; usually share a residence and assume the responsibilities of family life.
- *Dyad:* a two-person system.
- *Marital dyad:* the relationship of husband and wife.
- *Nuclear family:* the nuclear family is the kinship group of caretakers and children.
- *Holon:* a term used to name whole units nested in larger whole units, such as a marital dyad in a nuclear family.
- *Family boundaries:* the explicit and implicit rules in a family system that govern how family members are expected to relate to one another and to people outside the family.
- *Family homeostasis:* a family system's tendency to maintain predictable patterns of interactions. When those processes are working, the family system is in equilibrium.
- *Family projection process:* this refers to the transmission of a problem in a couple to a child. This process allows the family to maintain an illusion of harmony but the transmission causes symptoms in the child. Often this child is the "identified patient" or the problem to be fixed.
- *Family system:* a social system built by repeated interaction of family members. The interactions include patterns of how, when, and to whom members relate.
- *Family therapist:* can be practiced as a specialty within a profession or as a stand-alone profession.
- *Family therapy:* an encompassing term for the therapeutic approaches that have the entire family as the unit of treatment. One can conduct family therapy using a variety of frameworks.
- *Feedback loop:* the process by which a system receives the information needed to correct itself. Self-correction is used to maintain a steady state (homeostasis) or to move toward a goal.
- *Triangulation:* the process of a third person or thing being added to a dyad to divert anxiety away from the relationship of the dyad (pp. 314–315).

Goldenberg and Goldenberg (2008) included some other fundamental concepts.

- *Family rules:* prescribed rules for the boundaries of permissible behavior. The rules may not be verbalized but are understood by all family members; the rules regulate and help stabilize the family system.
- *Family narratives and assumptions:* beliefs about the world shared by the family members. Some see the world as a friendly, orderly, predictable place in which they can function competently. Others see the world as threatening, unstable, and unpredictable, therefore, as dangerous. The family story links certain experiences into a sequence that justifies how and why they live as they do.
- *Pseudomutuality and pseudohostility:* the facade of togetherness that masks underlying conflict and the collusion of quarreling that is a superficial tactic for avoiding deeper issues.
- *Mystification:* an effort to obscure the real nature of family conflict by distorting experiences; contradicts one person's perceptions and, after repeated experiences, leads the person to question reality.
- *Scapegoating:* redirecting conflict by holding one person responsible for whatever goes wrong (pp. 415–417).

Now we will consider different approaches to providing family therapy.

SYSTEMS APPROACH TO FAMILY THERAPY

Family therapists may use a variety of approaches in counseling. Goldenberg et al. (2014) explain that family counselors would all agree on these principles:

1. People are products of their interactions and family relationships must be taken into account.
2. Problem behavior in a person comes from the context of relationships. Interventions to help the person are most effective when the faulty interaction patterns are changed.
3. Individual symptoms are maintained by the current family system transactions.
4. Conjoint sessions, with the family as the treatment unit and the focus on family interaction, are more effective in producing change than trying to uncover intrapsychic problems in individual sessions.
5. Assessing family subsystems and boundaries within the family and between the family and the external world provides clues about the family organization and susceptibility to change.
6. Traditional diagnostic labels based on individual psychopathology do not provide an understanding of family dysfunctions but rather tend to pathologize people.
7. The goals of family therapy are to change maladaptive or dysfunctional family patterns and/or to help people build alternative views about themselves to find new possibilities for the future (p. 389).

With those assumptions defined, a look at some major family theories can proceed.

Murray Bowen (1913–1990)

Family therapy roots reach back to the turn of the 20th century, beginning with Alfred Adler's parent groups and developing through various parent, family, and couple education groups within each decade until the 1950s, when family therapy as we know it today was born. Murray Bowen, an early theorist on family relationships, focused on how family members could maintain a healthy balance between being enmeshed and being disengaged. He believed each family member should develop an individual identity and independence separate from family identity, but also maintaining a sense of closeness and a feeling of togetherness with their families. The task for Bowen was to help people integrate the opposing forces of seeking independence from the family and maintaining a sense of family membership and closeness (Bowen, 1976, 1978).

Murray Bowen grew up in Waverly, Tennessee. He was the firstborn of five children in a cohesive and loving family. Bowen completed his bachelor's degree at the University of Tennessee in 1934 and his M.D. degree from the University of Tennessee Medical School in Memphis in 1937. He served in the army during World War II, and his war experiences influenced his decision to turn down a fellowship in surgery at the Mayo Clinic. Instead, he began psychiatric training at the Menninger Foundation in Topeka, Kansas, in 1946. He spent the next 8 years researching symbiotic relationships of mothers and their schizophrenic children at Menninger, where he developed the concepts of anxious and functional attachment involved in the mother–child relationship. From 1954 to 1959, Bowen served as the first director of the Family Division at the National Institute of Mental Health, where he broadened his research on family attachment to include fathers. In 1959, Bowen joined the Department of Psychiatry at Georgetown University Medical Center, where he directed family programs. He founded and directed the Georgetown Family Center in 1975, where he remained until his death. Among his many honors, he received the Distinguished Alumnus Award from the University of Tennessee in 1986.

Bowen saw the family as an emotional unit best understood as a multigenerational network. The healthy family has members who have learned to establish their own identities and to separate themselves from the family of origin. The dysfunctional family has no such differentiation of self, they are "stuck together." The counselor works as a coach to educate the family in a detached, objective, and neutral role. The goal of counseling is to help family members, especially the marital dyad, to move toward a better sense of self to reduce anxiety, increase differentiation of the self, and establish healthy boundaries between family members (Seligman & Reichenberg, 2014, p. 398). Genograms, the therapist's detachment, defining roles, and defusing emotions are the primary techniques of Bowenian family counseling (Fall et al., 2010).

Bowen used process questions designed to help family members shift from reacting emotionally about the negative aspects of other family members to thinking rationally about how they personally contribute to the family's dysfunction and what they can do to improve the situation. Bowen assumed the role of coach or educator, whose job was to create an environment in which the family can function at its best. To accomplish this, counselors need to be aware of the emotional processes working in the family while personally remaining neutral. Bowen focused on the following qualities: (1) relationship between the spouses, (2) differentiation of self, (3) triangles, (4) nuclear family emotional process, (5) family projection process, (6) multigenerational transmission process, (7) sibling position, (8) emotional cutoffs, and (9) emotional process in society.

The Spousal Relationship

Bowen and his followers gave attention to defining and clarifying the relationship between couples: How well do they move in and out of the various roles healthy couples play? Do they care for and nurture each other? Do they solve problems and make decisions well? Do they play well together? Do they work well together? Do they parent well together? Are they able to differentiate themselves as individuals apart from the couple? Do they enjoy time alone? Do they maintain individual relationships and friendships outside the marital dyad? Do they pursue individual goals, interests, and careers? Most important, how well do individuals handle differentiation within themselves and between other family members?

Differentiation of Self

Differentiation within oneself refers to the ability to separate feelings from thoughts. For example, in crises, does the person put rational thinking on hold and react emotionally to the situation? Lack of differentiation between individuals refers to the degree to which people absorb the thoughts and feelings of others or do the opposite by automatically reacting against these thoughts and feelings. Differentiation is our struggle to develop a sense of personal identity while still remaining a part of the family. This process is similar to being able to distinguish between thoughts and feelings. Bowen rated his patients' ability to differentiate on a scale of 0 to 100, with 0 being low. Those on the bottom end of the scale were regarded as undifferentiated, and their behavior, guided by their feelings, often left them with chronic anxiety resulting in relationship problems. Because they were undifferentiated from the family, their anxiety spilled over onto other family members. Highly differentiated people handle stress and anxiety better, because they are able to apply rational thought to the problem at hand. They are able to maintain a healthy balance between thinking and feeling. The high level of ego differentiation is a well-defined sense of self and low emotional reactivity. In contrast, a low level of ego differentiation refers to a poorly defined sense of self and high emotional reactivity (Appleton & Dykeman, 2007).

Bowen believed that marriage partners seek spouses with the same level of differentiation. Hence, the trait is passed down through several generations. Bowen, as noted earlier, believed that schizophrenia in children resulted from generations of undifferentiated individuals marrying each other. Thus, a primary goal for Bowen was to help people attain higher levels of differentiation from enmeshment in one's family. Differentiation enables people to enjoy meaningful relationships with family members while remaining autonomous and rational without falling back into unhealthy enmeshment with family patterns. Increased differentiation by one family member is likely to lead other family members to become more differentiated.

Self-differentiation was Bowen's principal goal of family therapy. He believed that progress toward self-differentiation had to be self-motivated rather than directed by the therapist. Serving in the role of educator and coach, the therapist's job was to move clients toward an intellectual processing of the couple's family system, rather than falling into the trap of responding to the emotional tone of the content brought to counseling. Also, Bowen observed that in providing too much "help," therapists could make the family situation worse. Bowen (1976) stated that "inappropriate helpfulness fosters helplessness."

Detriangulation of Self from the Family Emotional System

Triangulation, another important concept in Bowen's theory, refers to the practice of two family members bringing a third family member into conflictual situations (Appleton & Dykeman, 2007). Therapists attend to the extent a husband or wife involves one of their children in a problem situation that the two of them should handle. Another example of triangulation is involvement of a person outside the marital dyad, such as a lover, to fulfill unmet needs in the marriage. The chapter on transactional analysis discusses a form of triangulation in reference to games and the roles people play in them; for example, one family member may take the role of prosecutor, another the victim, and the third a rescuer. All three roles are needed to maintain the game, and a shift in role by any one of the three alters the roles of the other two. Many of these dysfunctional interactions are similar to dances, where it takes two people to keep the dance going and one to stop it. Bowen believed there was no such thing as a two-person system because a third party is always drawn in when there is increased anxiety. As mentioned previously, third parties can be from inside or outside the family and even can be the memory of a departed loved one. The shifting set of alliances and reactive behaviors that occur with third parties makes it more difficult to resolve the conflict between the original two parties.

Nuclear Family Emotional Process

The nuclear family emotional process refers to how the family system operates to handle anxiety and stress in times of crisis. Several symptoms are indicators of ways the system works. Emotional distance, when one family member avoids or gives the silent treatment to another, is an early symptom of family trouble. A second symptom could be transfer of a family problem to a child such as when a mother displaces her anxiety on the child by becoming worried and overly concerned about how the child is doing. A third symptom occurs when two family members become blamers, pointing their fingers at each other as the cause of the problem. Finally, a fourth symptom surfaces when one partner develops a disability or becomes dysfunctional. The second partner is forced to adapt to the dysfunctional partner by taking more control, making decisions, and handling responsibilities for the "dysfunctional" partner. Over time, the increased workload may be resented by the partner in charge as the dysfunctional partner becomes even more dependent and develops more symptoms. Such situations are generally headed toward major blowups.

Family Projection Process

The family projection process (FPP) refers to how parents pass good and bad things on to their children. The projection process follows three steps in the cases in which a parent is concerned about the child. First, the parent, fearing something is wrong, focuses on the child. Then the parent confirms the fear by interpreting the child's behavior in a way that supports the anxiety. Next, the parent begins treating the child as though something is really wrong. Thus the steps in this process include scanning, diagnosing, and then treating. The parents' perceptions affect the child's development who then grows to exhibit what has been feared (https://www.thebowencenter.org/pages/conceptfpp.html).

Multigenerational Transmission Process

Multigenerational transmission process refers to how a family passes its good and bad baggage from one generation to another. The bad baggage is the tendency of families to become less differentiated as this trait is handed down. Families become more vulnerable to stress, anxiety, and problems as they become less differentiated; this became the point where Bowen directed his method of family therapy for changing the way family members respond to each other in times of crisis.

Sibling Position

Bowen took the Adlerian position that birth order is a significant factor in how we develop our lifestyles. (See Chapter 11 for a detailed discussion of birth order traits.) Bowen held that birth order traits and behaviors carried to an extreme could lead to dysfunction in children. For example, a controlling firstborn may lead to a younger sibling's overly dependent behavior. As the younger child gets more service from the older child, dependence on the older child is increased, and developmental progress toward independence is blocked. Bowen also was concerned that trouble might arise when people of the same birth order married and each tried to maintain such respective birth order behaviors as leaders or followers.

Emotional Cutoff

As mentioned earlier, when a marriage partner's method for handling anxiety and stress is to distance himself or herself from others, problems do not get solved. Emotional cutoffs (sometimes referred to as pouting) are thought to be ways of dealing with unresolved attachment to parents. Whatever the cause, emotional distancing can achieve the ultimate distancing goal of divorce.

Emotional Process in Society

Bowen saw parallels in how family members react within the family and within society. Undifferentiated people typically react emotionally rather than rationally in times of conflict, stress, crisis, and general anxiety. They do this within the family and carry forth their emotionality when they react in society.

In teaching clients about family systems and the intergenerational transmission process, Bowen used genograms and questions to move his clients to the intellectual level in discussing how their own family system had been influenced by material and baggage inherited from prior generations of the family. The genogram, an elaboration of a family tree, maps family patterns and relationships. It provides a generational chart of the family including dates of marriages, births, and deaths; cultural and ethnic origins; socioeconomic status; work life; education; hobbies; religious affiliations; politics; and family relationships. In short, the genogram describes *who* makes up your family, *how* they got to be family (birth, marriage, adoption), *when* they arrived (birth date, birth order, marriage dates), *what* they did (work, hobbies), *what* they valued (religion, politics), and *when* they left the family (death, divorce, or separation) (Figure 15-1 and Figure 15-2).

Bowen (1980) included data from at least three generations in his genograms. He began by gathering as much information as he could (during the first interview) from the couple he was counseling. All family names and ages are listed on the genogram with the dates of significant life events. Notes explaining the significant events are added to the genogram. Completing the missing data can become a homework assignment for the couple to complete before the second session.

Thomas (1992) suggests the following questions that might be used in a genogram interview:

1. What were the ethnic/cultural, religious, and political values of the family members? How were these traditions passed on in the family?
2. Where did the family members live (city and state)? When, where, and why did they move?
3. How did people get along in the family? Who was close to whom? Did anyone not speak to another family member? What happened in these cases?

4. Which family members were very successful at what they did?
5. Which family members used alcohol or drugs, were arrested, had mental problems, committed suicide, or had other serious problems?
6. What illnesses are found in the family? How did family members cope with them?

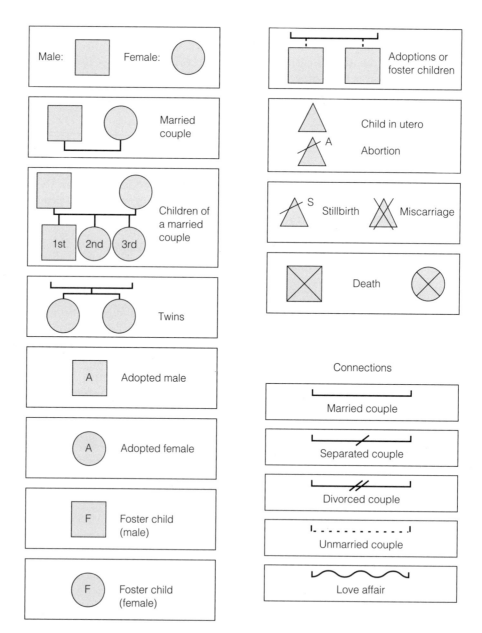

FIGURE 15-1   GENOGRAM KEY

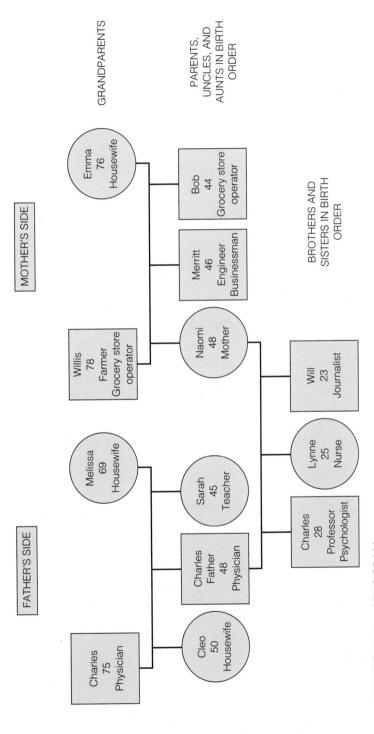

FATHER'S SIDE

MOTHER'S SIDE

GRANDPARENTS

PARENTS, UNCLES, AND AUNTS IN BIRTH ORDER

BROTHERS AND SISTERS IN BIRTH ORDER

Charles
75
Physician

Melissa
69
Housewife

Willis
78
Farmer
Grocery store operator

Emma
76
Housewife

Cleo
50
Housewife

Charles
Father
48
Physician

Sarah
45
Teacher

Naomi
48
Mother

Merritt
46
Engineer
Businessman

Bob
44
Grocery store operator

Charles
28
Professor
Psychologist

Lynne
25
Nurse

Will
23
Journalist

FIGURE 15-2   GENOGRAM

7. Can you tell me any special life events that happened—positive, neutral, and negative?
8. Tell me about the stories that have been passed down through the generations of your family.
9. Tell me about the family themes that seem to repeat in your family. If your family had a motto, what would it be?
10. If you were an elder in the family, what advice would you give to a younger member of the family?

Thomas (1992) offers the following ten questions to aid the family counselor in writing a genogram analysis:

1. *Health:* How healthy were the family members? What were the most common health problems? What was done to prevent or treat these health problems?
2. *Structure:* What types of family structures were repeated in the genogram (single parent, nuclear, extended, blended)?
3. *Themes:* What family themes have been carried through the generations?
4. *Occupations:* Which occupations occur most frequently in your family?
5. *Stages:* What stages in the life cycle have been easier for your family to handle? What stages have been the most difficult?
6. *Events:* Which life events have affected family functions throughout generations of your family?
7. *Triangles:* Where are the triangles present in the genogram? Which relationships are close, distant, conflicted, or fused? Where are the emotional cutoffs?
8. *Patterns:* What patterns are repeated, such as educational or work success, religious commitment, political activity, alcohol or drug use, or other behaviors?
9. *Size:* How large are the families in the genogram? Which families stand out as larger or smaller than the genogram norm? What stresses might have occurred due to the family size or family imbalance?
10. *Contract:* What values and behaviors passed on to you by your family have worked so well for you that you plan to keep them and even pass them on to your children? What family values and behaviors have not worked well for you, and what do you plan to do with them? Are there some family patterns that bother you? If so, what could you do to change them?

Gladding (2015) admonishes counselors to look for repetitive patterns, coincidences, and the impact of change and untimely life cycle transitions in the genogram.

Emotional Systems of the Family

Understanding family emotional systems and how they work is also central to Bowen's theory. Once again, failure to achieve differentiation between family members results in unhealthy family relationships that recycle from one generation to the next unless some helpful intervention interrupts the cycle. Bowen might well have envisioned himself as a cycle breaker, which is not a bad role for a counselor to take. In fact, Bowen often assumed the role of educator in teaching people about family emotional systems.

Modeling Differentiation

Bowen favored modeling for teaching differentiation to his patients. He did this by using "I" statements and taking ownership of his own thoughts, feelings, and behaviors; for example, he'd say, "I think the best thing for me to do is to confront my colleague about his behavior, but thinking about doing it gives me an uneasy feeling." In addition to owning one's thoughts and feelings, this statement lends some help for separating feelings and thoughts.

STRUCTURAL FAMILY THERAPY

Structural family therapy is closely related to Bowen's family systems theory. Structural family therapists also operate on the assumption that the individual client should be treated within the context of the family system. The therapist does not see the client as a sufficient source of information about the problems brought to counseling or as the only source of causes of the problem. Changes resulting from individual counseling are not stable enough to stand against the pressures a dysfunctional family brings to bear. Therefore, the overall goal of structural family therapists is to alter the family structure to empower the dysfunctional family to move toward functional ways of conducting or transacting family business and family communications.

In structural family therapy, the family involves the arrangements or patterns that govern the transactions of the members. The arrangements form a whole—the structure of the family. The well-functioning family has an underlying organizational structure that has fluid, flexible responses to changes in the family. The family provides mutual support and allows autonomy of its individual members. Symptoms arise when family structures are inflexible. Therefore, the dysfunctional family has not made appropriate structural adjustments to family changes. The counselor's role is both supportive and challenging—being for the family and against the sickness in the system. The therapist is an active and authoritative change agent. The basic goal of therapy is restructuring the family's system of rules so that interactions become more flexible (Fall et al., 2010).

Structural family therapy also is based on the assumption that families are evolving, hierarchical organizations with rules and behavioral patterns for interacting across and within the family subsystems. Wagner (2008) explained that family interactions occur within the context of subsystems such as spouses, parents, and siblings. A family member can belong to more than one subsystem. Some cultures include subsystems for extended family members. Minuchin (1974) defined subsystems by the differences in boundaries, the rules a family uses to dictate who and how members interact. Minuchin noted that families get into trouble when their members become either overly enmeshed in each other's business or totally disengaged (Appleton & Dykeman, 2007). Family members should feel a sense of belonging to the family that does not destroy their sense of being unique individuals within and outside the family context. In other words, functional families are characterized by each member's success in finding the healthy balance between belonging to a family and maintaining a separate identity.

One way to find the balance between family and individual identity is to define and clarify the boundaries between the subsystems. Each subsystem contains its own subject matter that is private and should remain within that subsystem. Spouses have matters they need to discuss that do not belong in the context of the parent–child and child–child subsystems. Such topics might include their sex life, financial concerns, and interpersonal conflicts. Dysfunctional families often discuss and play out these topics in an open family forum. Boundaries between subsystems range from rigid to diffuse. Private subject matter from one subsystem that leaks out to other subsystems indicates diffuse, poorly established boundaries. Diffuse boundaries can lead to family members becoming overly enmeshed in the private business of other family members; rigid boundaries allow too little interaction between family members, resulting in disengagement from the family. Once again, the secret to developing functional families is finding the right boundary balance between too rigid and too diffuse; boundaries need to be clearly defined. For example, parents need to provide enough love and support—but also enough room—for children to develop independence. A parent–child subsystem and a sibling subsystem also have communications and subject matter that belong to and are unique to those subsystems. Families who understand and respect differences between healthy and unhealthy subsystem boundaries and rules function successfully; families who do not understand and respect these differences find themselves in a dysfunctional state of conflict, either disengaged from or enmeshed in the family business.

Structural family therapy is directed toward changing the family organizational structure as a way of resolving the presenting problem or changing a family member's behavioral patterns. For example, in a particular session, Dad might be asked to give up being in charge of the children's homework assignments. The structural therapist actively directs the session and participates as a family member. The therapist may even take over the family ruler role as a way of sidetracking the dominant family member.

Salvador Minuchin's Contributions to Structural Family Therapy

Salvador Minuchin is considered the founder of structural family therapy as it is currently practiced. He was born in 1921 to Russian Jewish parents in a small town in Argentina. As a university student, he joined a Zionist organization and was arrested for taking part in a protest against Juan Perón in 1943. After spending 3 months in jail, Minuchin was expelled from the university and then studied in Uruguay for a time. He completed his medical degree in Argentina before taking a residency in child psychiatry and an 18-month tour of duty as a doctor in the 1948 Israeli war. Minuchin came to the United States with the intention of working with Bruno Bettelheim in Chicago's Orthogenic School; however, he met Nathan Ackerman in New York and eventually decided to work in Ackerman's child-development center. Minuchin worked with African and Asian immigrant children in Israel for 3 years before returning to New York and receiving more analytic training and becoming director of family research at the Wiltwyck School for Boys.

Noticing that some families produced several delinquent children, Minuchin concluded that families must be making a significant contribution to the problem. Therefore, he began to develop an approach for working with families who did not have the verbal skills for traditional psychotherapy, instead focusing on the nonverbal communication, a standard practice in individual, group, and family therapy.

Much of what Minuchin learned about families was by observation through a one-way glass and in collaboration with his colleagues at the school. In a method similar to the Adlerian method for working with families, Minuchin and his colleagues developed a three-step approach: Two counselors met with the entire family; then one counselor met with the parents, and the other with the children. The process culminated in a final stage in which everyone gathered to share information and plans for change. Further observation and study led to a language for describing family structure and a system of interventions designed to change unhelpful and even harmful patterns of family organization. Minuchin wrote *Families of the Slums* (1967) based on his experiences at Wiltwyck.

Minuchin's next project was transforming the Philadelphia Child Guidance Clinic into a model family therapy center. He had a flair for the dramatic and was highly critical of seminar case presentations that did not meet his standards. As a practicing family therapist, he set the family scene, assigned roles, started and stopped the action, and took a leading or supporting role himself.

Working with Jay Haley, Minuchin developed the clinic's family orientation and the Institute for Family Counseling, which was designed to train paraprofessionals. Perhaps his most notable accomplishment during this period was the treatment he developed for psychosomatic families, particularly those of anorexics. He wrote *Families and Family Therapy* (1974) during his 10 years as director of the clinic. After stepping down as director, Minuchin served as head of the training center until 1981. Minuchin continued family research with "normal" families and wrote several plays and a book for the lay public, *Family Kaleidoscope* (1984).

Minuchin has been praised for rescuing family therapy from intellectuality and mystery. His pragmatic approach contributed both to understanding how families function and to productive interventions for correcting malfunctions in them. Minuchin worked with children and families written off by the psychiatric community as unsuitable for treatment. His achievements are rooted in his philosophy of putting clients first and in his total commitment to their cases.

Once Minuchin diagnosed a flaw in the family system, he appeared willing to go to any length to bring about a needed change. His techniques ranged from gentle persuasion to outright provocation and confrontation. He viewed psychosomatic illness as a symptom brought on and maintained by the family and successfully treated eating disorders, asthma, and uncontrolled diabetes. He said that observers of his work would notice his attempts at getting the family transactions into the therapy room, his movement between participation and observation as a way to unbalance the current family system and his responses to family members' intruding into each other's space (Appleton & Dykeman, 2007).

Minuchin described traditional psychotherapy as a magnifying glass and structural family therapy as a zoom lens that can focus on the entire family or zoom in for a close-up of any family member. The structural therapist works with the family belief system to effect behavior changes between people. Rule changes may be the immediate goal as the family explores three questions: (1) How do family members relate to one another? (2) Who is allied with whom against whom? and (3) What is the nature of the parental dyad? The idea is to change the immediate context of the family situation and thereby change the family members' positions. The cognitive dissonance principle operates much the same way.

For example, Minuchin (1978) described the case of a 12-year-old girl with psychosomatically triggered asthma. She had a history of heavy medication, missed school, and several trips to the emergency department. During the first family interview, the counselor directed the family's attention to the eldest sister's weight problem, and the family's concern then shifted to the newly identified patient. The result for the asthmatic was fewer symptoms, less medication, and no lost school time.

Minuchin referred to the preceding case as the foundation of family therapy. The family structure had changed from two parents protectively concerned with one child's asthma to two parents concerned with one child's asthma and one child's obesity. The asthmatic child's position in the family changed, and that changed her experience.

As with all counseling approaches, the counselor's first step is to establish a trusting relationship with the family. Minuchin recommended three ways to establish trust: (1) *tracking*, or demonstrating interest in the family by asking a series of questions about the topics they bring up; (2) *mimicry*, or adapting the counselor's communication style to fit the family's; and (3) *support*, which includes the first two ways, plus acceptance of the problem as presented by the client. Minuchin's style was to get the family to talk briefly until he identified a central theme of concern and the leading and supporting roles in it. At this point, he operated like a play director or group dynamics consultant in determining the roles being played, what was interrupting the flow, what was silencing communication, and what diverting maneuvers were blocking family interaction.

Next, the counselor examines boundaries or family rules, which define (1) who participates in what and how, (2) areas of responsibility, (3) decision making, and (4) privacy. When rules have been broken, the family works on them with the help of "stage directions." The counselor may ask a family member to observe the family interaction but not to interfere. Minuchin paced the family by adopting their mood and tempo and gradually changing it as the interview proceeded. He asked questions in the enactive mode; that is, not "Why doesn't your mother talk to you?" but "See if you can get your mother to talk to you." The counselor might assign tasks related to the manipulation of space, such as asking a child to move his chair so he cannot see his mother's signals or asking a husband to sit next to his wife and hold her hand when she is anxious. Assigned tasks can dramatize family transactions and suggest change.

In summary, Minuchin's approach to structural family therapy was both active and directive. The first task is to shift the family focus from the identified client to the therapist, which allows the identified client to begin the process of rejoining the family as a regular family member. The shift in focus to the therapist occurs when the therapist joins the family and becomes part of the family system. When treatment is complete, the therapist moves outside the family structure and leaves the family intact and connected without the loss of individual family member identities (see Figure 15-3).

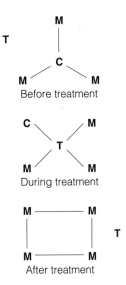

Key M – Family member
     C – Identified client
     T – Therapist

FIGURE 15-3   STAGES OF STRUCTURAL FAMILY THERAPY

STRATEGIC FAMILY THERAPY

Following the popularity of structural family therapy in the 1970s, strategic family therapy dominated the 1980s, led by Milton Erickson, Jay Haley, and Cloé Madanes. Strategic family therapy considers the family a system that has power relations and rules of operation. The power struggle does not involve who controls but who defines the relationship. Healthy families have appropriate, forthright ways of dealing with conflict and struggles. Functional families have clear rules and a balance of stability and flexibility. Symptoms are considered as attempts to control a relationship if one or both participants deny the issue of control or exhibit dysfunctional behavior in the attempt of controlling. The therapist is active and directive and takes charge of the power struggles, becoming the temporary family leader. The goal is to change the system, changing the behavior patterns that maintain the problem (Fall et al., 2010).

Therefore, strategic family therapy is based on the assumption that family member behavior, which is ongoing and repetitive, can be understood only in the family context. The family's ineffective problem solving develops and maintains symptoms. The counselor's role is to design a strategy for solving the presenting problem. Haley (1973) defines *strategic family therapy* as any therapy in which the therapist initiates what happens in therapy and designs a plan for solving each problem. It is characterized by its brief duration, generally no more than 10 sessions. The therapist takes on a very high activity level by giving specific directives for behavioral change that are carried out as homework assignments. The treatment process includes the six steps of introducing the process, clarifying the problem, identifying behaviors that maintain the problem, setting goals, creating and using interventions, and ending therapy (Seligman & Reichenberg, 2014). Many of the therapists' directives are paradoxical interventions and solution-focused brief counseling methods.

Paradoxical Interventions

One of the most controversial yet powerful techniques in strategic family therapy involves using paradox (Gladding, 2015). Paradoxical interventions harness the strong resistance clients have to change and to taking directives from the therapist. Rather than working against the client's resistance, the therapist uses it to bring about the changes in behavior needed to correct the problem and repair the family system. Therapists prescribe the symptom, giving the family members permission to do what they are already doing. The client is in the double-bind position of either obeying the therapist, which the client does not want to do, or stopping the problematic, "uncontrollable" behavior. The client soon discovers that the behavior is controllable and stops the undesirable behavior.

Paradox can take the forms of reframing, restraining, prescribing, and redefining. Restraining means the therapist tells the family they cannot do anything except what they are doing, setting up a situation for the family to prove otherwise. Prescribing involves therapists telling family members to act out the problem behavior (Gladding, 2015). For example, the counselor tells an insomniac to see how long the person can go without sleep, maybe even enter a stay-awake contest or go for the world's record, or tells a tantrum-throwing child to have more tantrums and the child's parents to provide a private room for the tantrums. Redefining allows the therapist to provide positive connotations to the symptom or trouble. The idea is that symptoms mean something to the people who are exhibiting them whether the meaning is logical or not. An example would be a counselor telling a family that the child who suddenly does not want to go to school is really trying to keep her parents together by keeping their attention on the child's problems (Gladding).

In another paradoxical intervention, the counselor takes a "one-down" position, encouraging the client not to do too much too soon. Clients often play the wooden-leg game which highlights the client's disabilities and the reasons why the client cannot function properly. In the one-down position, the counselor emphasizes all that the client is already doing despite problems and suggests that the client must have great inner strength even to show up for counseling.

Clients who handicap themselves through anticipatory anxiety over activities such as making speeches, taking tests, or meeting new people are directed to practice all the symptoms they fear, such as blushing, speaking in a trembling voice, stuttering, passing out, or completely failing the test. They often tell test-anxious people to take practice tests and fail each one. Appleton and Dykeman (2007) explained that therapists' directives are used to facilitate change and make things happen; to keep the therapists' influence and to provoke family reactions.

Although strategic or brief therapy is directed toward symptom removal, counselors distinguish between first-and second-order changes. First-order change occurs when the symptom is temporarily removed, only to reappear later because the family system has not been changed. Haley (1976) points out that the behaviors of family members do not occur in isolation. Rather, family behaviors occur in a sequence in which one member's behavior is both the result of and the catalyst for other members' behaviors. Fixing the symptom while failing to fix the system does not fix the family. First-order change is typical for dysfunctional families who work hard to maintain the status quo.

Second-order change occurs when the symptom *and* the system are repaired and the need for the symptom does not reappear. For example, Mom and Dad quarrel, the children start a fight, Mom and Dad stop their quarrel to deal with their children, and a period of family peace is achieved. Until Mom and Dad find a better way to resolve conflicts, the sequence repeats frequently and the peace is only temporary. Healthy families with an adaptive facility for repairing the family system when it is broken engage in second-order change.

Contributions of Milton Erickson, Jay Haley, and Cloé Madanes to Strategic Family Therapy

Jay Haley, director of the Family Therapy Institute of Washington, DC, described Milton Erickson as his mentor and major source of ideas about therapy. Since Erickson's death in 1980, Haley perhaps has been his best interpreter. Haley also worked closely with Salvador Minuchin at the Philadelphia Child Guidance Clinic. Haley worked with Cloé Madanes, including founding the Family Therapy Institute together.

To strategic family therapists, the term *strategic* refers to the development of a specific strategy, planned in advance by the therapist, to resolve the presenting problem as quickly and efficiently as possible. Erickson promoted the idea that insight, awareness, and emotional release are not necessary for change. Rather, people need to solve their immediate problems and eliminate bothersome symptoms to move ahead with their lives. Followers of Erickson's approach do not have the client's personal growth and development as a primary therapeutic goal. Problem solving through minimal intervention is the key goal for the strategic group. It is important to note that strategic interventions often foster changes in the family structure when structural interventions fail.

Erickson's approach incorporated three principles in addition to discounting the importance of achieving insight: (1) the therapist uses the client's reality rather than attempting to fit the client to the views of others in the world such as parents or colleagues, or even to those of the therapist; (2) both the therapist and client play active roles in the action-oriented process; and (3) minimal change must occur in one or more areas of the client's life for change in the family system to result. In family therapy practice, the therapist works to construct strategies to implement the needed changes.

The process of strategic family therapy is based on family member communication patterns. Haley realized that the family system functionality could be assessed by the communications among family members and their alliances. Neither insight nor generational information is needed in this approach. The process includes the counselor identifying solvable problems, setting goals, and then designing interventions focused on those goals. The therapist then examines the response to the intervention and the outcome of therapy. Problem solving is direct, concrete, and quick. In fact, Haley considered his greatest contribution was the practice of specific skills, ideas, and techniques (Haley & Reicheport-Haley, 2007).

As an example of this process, Haley (1976) combined a strategic and structural approach to treat a young boy's fear of dogs. A problem of family dynamics was that the boy was close to his mother but disengaged from his father. Haley's first step was to get father and son to interact by having them talk about the dangers of dogs in the neighborhood. When the mother tried to interrupt, Haley neutralized her by explaining that this was Dad's area of expertise. The second step was to get a dog into the home to help in three areas: (1) to continue the father–son interaction, (2) to achieve systematic desensitization of the dog phobia, and (3) to stimulate change in the family dynamics. Haley accomplished Step 2 by asking the boy to pick out a dog that was afraid and to work with his father on teaching the dog not to be afraid.

Dysfunctional symptoms in a family system might be evidenced in several ways. Intensive criticism between children and parents in families highly resistant to change could result in anything from suicidal depression to refusal to attend school. Strategic family counselors often fix both problems by prescribing more criticism and putting the family in the double bind of having to choose between obeying the counselor or disobeying by doing the "right" thing of stopping the criticism. Family resistance against counseling and the counselor is harnessed to work for the good of the family as they refuse to criticize each other.

A final example of strategic family therapy is the use of metaphor in bringing about rapid change. Parents bring an 8-year-old girl to family counseling with the problem that she is spoiled, stubborn, argumentative, and whiny. Although the parents obviously view this behavior as bad, their daughter does not. The counselor asks her age, and the child says she is 8. The counselor looks incredulously at the mother and father, shakes his head, and says to the parents, "This can't be, for this girl is 8, and this behavior you described is the behavior of a 6-year-old." With a puzzled look, the counselor asks the girl how old she was on her last birthday and how old she will be on her next birthday. The counselor notes that the behavior she is exhibiting during the session is that of an 8-year-old, and he asks the parents to keep a log of the child's behavior for 1 week. The direct challenge of age appeals to children's desire to look their age or older.

In summary, the job of the strategic family therapist is fourfold. First, the hierarchical structure of the family must be identified. "Who is in charge of whom and what?" and "What role does each family member play?" are the critical questions to be answered. Confusion about who is in charge and about role identity is characteristic of dysfunctional families. Second, the sequence of behaviors that causes and maintains the problem symptom needs to be identified. For example, what is the presenting problem, and what family conditions create and maintain the problem? Third, the therapist develops an intervention plan to serve as a directive for how family members are to change certain behaviors. Fourth, the therapist and family evaluate the plan's effectiveness in removing the symptom and repairing the family system. Haley (1976) distinguishes between advice and directives. Giving advice is telling people what they ought to do, what job to take, or what person to marry. Giving a directive is like assigning behavior homework or writing a behavior prescription designed to alter family interaction sequences.

Haley (1976) describes four stages of a typical first interview applying strategic therapy:

1. Stage 1, the *social stage*, accomplishes three tasks: building rapport, observing family communication patterns and alliances, and forming tentative hypotheses about how the family functions.

2. In Stage 2, the *problem stage*, the main task is obtaining a clear statement of the problem that meets with each family member's agreement. Haley suggests involving reluctant participants first in the problem discussion and the identified client last, a procedure followed in most family therapies to bring everybody into the discussion without focusing on the identified client as the scapegoat for the family's dysfunction.

3. Stage 3, the *interaction stage*, accomplishes two tasks: Everybody should discuss the problem, and everybody should interact with all other family members. During Stage 3, the therapist does not become personally involved in the family interaction because the family interaction patterns require full attention. The therapist directs the family to discuss their disagreements and to role-play or act out a typical family problem such as deciding who does what family chores. We prefer to observe how a typical family meeting might operate, even if the family is not accustomed to holding them. All these interactions provide valuable information about problem sequences, communication patterns, and the lines of authority in the family hierarchy.

4. In Stage 4, *goal setting*, the obvious task is to define the goal for therapy in concise, observable, behavioral terms. For example, in a family that does not discuss family conflicts, an acceptable goal might be weekly 30-minute family meetings to clear the air of conflicts. The therapist could add a paradoxical directive encouraging the family not to resolve any of the conflicts during the meetings. Again, complete clarity and agreement on the goals are necessary if the family is to have ownership in the therapy process and the resulting cooperation and commitment to make therapy work. Todd (2000) describes a similar, successful adaptation of strategic family therapy as it was applied to a parent-education class for rearing challenging teens.

Selekman (2010) uses what he refers to as reversal questions to tap adolescents' wisdom about what their parents can do differently to gain their cooperation on the conflicts that frequently occur between parents and teenagers, including following family rules, doing homework, maintaining good grades, and completing chores. Reversal questions, by putting teenagers in the expert role, help build the relationship between counselor and client. Examples of reversal questions include:

> Do you have any advice for your parents about how they can get you to do those things they always ask you about school and grades?

> What do you think your parents could do to reduce the number of arguments between you?

> What is the first thing your parents could do differently that would help all of you get along better?

Selekman's (2010) book contains other approaches to helping families discover their strengths and creative solutions to their concerns.

THE COMMUNICATIONS APPROACH TO FAMILY THERAPY

Our discussions of systems, structural, and strategic approaches to family therapy have highlighted several commonalities and overlap between methods, as well as specific differences. Perhaps the common thread that unites the field of family therapy is the focus on how family members communicate. Communication is the heart of the two methods presented next in our discussion: John Gottman's behavioral family therapy and Virginia Satir's conjoint family therapy.

John Gottman's Behavioral Interview Method

John Gottman earned three degrees with a mathematics focus before he turned to psychophysiology and clinical psychology. He has studied marriage stability and divorce prediction by following newly married couples. Through analysis of observations of married couples, he has created formulas to predict which couples will have successful relationships and which will divorce. Relationships that have a ratio of positive to negative interactions of 5 to 1 will succeed (Gladding, 2015). In his best-known book *The Seven Principles of Making Marriage Work* (Gottman & Silver, 1999), he outlines the guidelines he has discovered.

In Gottman's (1979, 1990) system, the therapist functions more as an educator than as a healer, as is true for most of the practitioners of the theories and systems presented in this book. Family therapists following a communications approach to family therapy naturally hold the view that accurate communication is the key to solving family problems. All families are faced with problems; however, some families solve more of their problems than other families do. Families that are good at problem solving have several traits in common. They communicate in an open and honest manner rather than relying on phony or manipulative roles when trying to meet needs or resolve family crises. In addition, these family members match the intent and impact of their communication. For example, a wife might want more cooperation from her husband on household chores. She stated her request in clear terms and listened empathically to her husband's response about his needs; the intent of her communication achieved the desired impact. Had she been sarcastic, the impact of her message might have resulted in less cooperation from her husband. Dysfunctional families have low success rates in matching the impact with the intent of their communications.

Gottman built his approach around matching the intent and impact of communication (Gottman, 1979, 1994; Gottman, Notarius, Gonzo, & Markman, 1976). He designed his behavioral interviewing method to teach people about what they are doing that is not working and to help them correct the situation by learning how to get the impact they want from their communication.

In Stage I, how a couple or family made the decision to seek therapy is explored. The therapist also determines the level of commitment to therapy and who, if anyone, might be a reluctant client. The dynamics give the therapist an opportunity to view the family interaction pattern firsthand. Areas of family or couple agreement and disagreement surface during this stage.

In Stage II, the goals each person has for therapy, some of the fears they have about coming to therapy, and fears about what could go wrong are identified.

The therapist asks clients what their situation would be like if all their goals were attained; that is, how would they be behaving differently, and how would an observer know they had met their goals? More specifically, what would their typical day be like if they achieved their goals? Couples in counseling often state their goals (for treatment) in terms of what they want for each other; a better focus would be the goals the couple wants for the partnership. The therapist can facilitate goal setting by presenting each client with a list of possible goals—improve communication, have more fun, do more things together, become more of a team, become better parents, end fighting, manage finances better, improve lovemaking, cooperate more on household jobs—and instructing them to select just one goal each. The clients then elaborate on their choices and explain why the goal is important to them. The second task in Stage II is to identify any fears or inhibitions the couple might have about counseling. A good introduction to the subject is asking the couple the worst possible thing that could happen from counseling. The therapist can use this opportunity to explain how treatment is conducted and the roles of the therapist and clients. If the couple is having a problem with finances, for example, the therapist's role is not to solve the money problem per se; rather, the therapist focuses on the couple's communications. Better and more effective communication should provide the means to solve problems more efficiently, including handling finances better.

In Stage III, the counselor asks the couple to articulate their perceptions of their marital issues or problems. Again, the couple completes a checklist of several marital issues and rates each issue for its severity on a scale of 0 to 10, with 10 being most severe. The typical list of issues approximates the goals list used in Stage II—for example, house and yard chores, fighting, finances, sex, in-laws, communication, cooperation, parenting, time together, and addictions. Again, the couple's discussion of their marital issues affords the therapist another opportunity to observe the couple's communication pattern.

In Stage IV, the therapist asks the couple to select one issue to discuss, just as they might try to resolve it at home, and then observes the free interaction to note whether the intent of each communication attempt is getting the desired impact.

In Stage V, a play-by-play analysis of the couple's interaction focuses on miscommunications in which the intent of the speaker's message did not get the desired impact. In fact, the miscommunication often gets an effect opposite the intended meaning. The intent might be to get a partner to help out around the house more, but the result is that the other partner is helping even less than before. After pointing out the differences between intent and impact for a series of communications, the therapist might ask one partner to assume the role of a play director to describe how the other partner could have responded better to the statement just made. Then the couple compares the desired response with the one actually made. As in reality therapy, the couple can decide whether what they are doing is getting the desired response, and they can stop or change what they are doing. The receiver of the message can validate the impact of the sender's message, and the sender then analyzes the receiver's return message for intent and impact. Step V might require the therapist to lecture on the intent and impact equation: *Good communication occurs when intent equals impact.* The therapist explains that choice of words, nonverbal communications, and the sender's and receiver's value filters can distort the intent of the message and lead to an undesired impact. Restating and clarifying the sender's message before reacting often can help. In other words, the couple may have to pass the message back and forth before the receiver understands it the way it was intended. Even with a clear message, the sender may not get the intended impact of the message and need to alter it to get the desired response. The receiving partner can help by stating how he or she wishes to be approached on the presenting issue.

In Stage VI, the therapist concludes the session by negotiating a contract with the couple on what goal(s) they will try to achieve and the method of treatment they will use. The clients' job is to decide on the objective, and the therapist's job is to supply the process. Again, as is true with most counseling approaches, the principal goal is to teach people a communication process that enables them to solve more of their own problems.

Virginia Satir's Conjoint Family Therapy

When Virginia Satir (1916–1988) was 5 years old, she decided to become a detective to help children figure out parents. She was not sure what she would be looking for, but even at that age she knew that more strange things were going on in families than met the eye. More than half a century later, after working with thousands of families, Satir reported that she still found a lot of puzzles in families.

Satir viewed family life as an iceberg. Most people are aware of only one-tenth of what is happening in the family—the tenth that they can see and hear. Like the ship that depends on the captain's awareness of the total iceberg, the family must depend on the total awareness of the family structure to survive. Satir referred to the hidden 90 percent as the family's needs, motives, and communication patterns. In four books, *Conjoint Family Therapy* (1967), *Peoplemaking* (1972), *Helping Families to Change* (Satir, Stachowiak, & Taschman, 1975), and *Step by Step* (Satir & Baldwin, 1983), Satir shared some of the answers she found to some family puzzles. According to Satir, she embellished some of the early concepts in *Conjoint Family Therapy* as a result of her work with the Gestalt concepts presented by Fritz Perls and the body-awareness work of Bernard Gunther.

Virginia Satir earned excellent qualifications as a parent detective: formal academic training in psychological social work at the University of Chicago and work as a teacher, consultant, and practitioner in psychiatric clinics, mental hospitals, family service centers, growth centers, and private practice. In 1959, she joined with two psychiatrists to form the initial staff of the Mental Research Institute in Palo Alto, California. She also served as the first director of training at the Easlen Institute in Big Sur, California, and lectured around the world. She was a visiting professor to at least 10 universities and a consultant to the Veterans Administration and several other agencies and schools.

Satir cited several contributors to the development of her system—including Harry Stack Sullivan's interpersonal theory of the 1920s (an individual's behavior is influenced by his or her interaction with another); the growth of group therapy, also during the 1920s, the major contributors of which were J. L. Moreno and S. R. Slavson; and Gregory Bateson and Murray Bowen, who looked at families to discover why individuals became "schizophrenic."

Satir had a positive view of human nature. After studying 12,000 families in depth, she was convinced that, at any time, whatever people are doing represents the best they are aware of and the best they can do. She believed that people are rational and have the freedom and ability to make choices in their lives. Although Satir viewed people as basically free, she considered the extent of their knowledge as the biggest limitation on personal freedom. People can learn what they do not know and change their ways of interacting with others. People can also make themselves healthier by freeing themselves from the past. Like Maslow, Satir believed that people are geared toward surviving, growing, and developing close relationships with others. Although some behaviors may be labeled psychotic, sick, or bad, Satir saw these behaviors as attempts to reach out for help.

Satir also saw families as balanced, rule-governed systems that are the context for growth and development. In healthy families, members recognize their own feelings, communicate congruently, accept others, and see differences as opportunities to learn and explore instead of threats. Congruence to Satir was using words that accurately match personal feelings; incongruence is communication when the nonverbal and verbal messages do not match (Appleton & Dykeman, 2007). Unhealthy families are people who are not free to grow and develop. Dysfunction comes from the interchange of low self-esteem, incongruent communication, poor system operations, and faulty family rules. The counselor, in Satir's model, is a facilitator, resource, observer, detective, and model of communication, warmth, and empathy. The goals of therapy are to help family members better understand themselves and increase their ability to communicate congruently, to build respect for each family member, and to view differences as opportunities to grow (Fall et al., 2010).

Self-esteem plays a prominent role in Satir's system. She believed that self-esteem and effective communication beget one another. Conversely, low self-esteem and dysfunctional communication are also correlated. Satir saw self-esteem—the degree to which people accept both their good and their bad points—as the basic human drive. Self-esteem is a changing variable that fluctuates within a healthy range, depending on the amount of stress one is experiencing. It is related to one's participation in the family interaction. When individual family members experience stress, their ability to communicate openly, give and receive feedback, and solve problems depends on the collective self-esteem of the family. Family members may try to block communication to protect their own self-esteem when they are under stress or in crises. Family members with low self-esteem are likely to create disturbances to make the others feel as bad as they do. For example, parents guilty of child abuse often have low self-esteem and may unconsciously internalize their feelings; for example, they may think, "One way to punish myself for my wasteful ways is to punish that same behavior in one of my children."

Satir (1967) held that children are the third angle of the family triangle. As such, their position may be intolerable, similar to the persecutor-victim-rescuer triangle described in transactional analysis (see Chapter 14). Parents in conflict consider any direction the child turns as a turn for or against one of the parents. Given this state of affairs, Satir wrote that children who seem to side with one parent run the risk of seeming not to love the other parent. Because children need both parents, making such a choice inevitably hurts them. Both parents have interlocking roles to play in the process of educating children emotionally, and the failure of one angle of the family triangle (one parent) disturbs the entire system; frequently, the result is disturbed children.

A further complication in the triangle is that the child has already established an identity with the same-sex parent, and the hurt of taking sides is further compounded by the stunted or stifled psychosexual development that may occur. Children need the opposite-sex parent to admire, respect, and love, and they need the same-sex parent as a good role model. When the parents are divided, arguing and fighting, children cannot achieve these identity and interpersonal goals. In a family with no parental coalition—that is, cooperation between father and mother to fulfill their respective roles as man and woman and husband and wife—the child may need counseling to fulfill unsatisfied wishes. Satir conceptualized this child as the *identified client*, even though the entire family is counseled.

Satir viewed mature people as those who are fully in charge of their feelings and who make choices based on accurate perceptions of themselves and others. The mature person takes full responsibility for choices that have been made. In summary, Satir regarded mature people as (1) being in touch with their feelings, (2) communicating clearly and effectively, and (3) accepting differences in others as a chance to learn.

Satir's theory of counseling is built on communication rules. She believed that four components in a family situation are subject to change and correction: the members' feelings of self-worth, the family's communication abilities, the system, and the rules of the family. The rules are the way things are accomplished in the family. Rules are the most difficult component to uncover during therapy sessions because they usually are not verbalized or are consciously known to all members of the family. Satir wanted all members of a family to understand the rules that govern their emotional interchanges, including (1) freedom to comment, (2) freedom to express what one is seeing or hearing, (3) freedom to agree or disapprove, and (4) freedom to ask questions when one does not understand. The family unit becomes dysfunctional when members do not understand the unwritten rules. Satir told families who were having problems with a member that families have no bad members who cause pain, only bad rules. She believed that what goes on at a given moment is the natural consequence of the experience of one's own life; consequently, anything can change. However, Satir believed that change is not a "have to," but rather one possibility among several choices. She believed in practitioners taking risks, controlling the counseling process, and leaving the outcome to the family. They must be able to put clients in touch with themselves at a feeling level. The counselor assumes the role of teacher to re-educate the family to new ways of thinking, feeling, and communicating.

Communication, the most important factor in Satir's system, is the main determinant of the kinds of relationships people have with one another and of how people adjust to their environment, as well as being the tie that binds the family together. When a family is operating smoothly, communication among family members is open, authentic, assertive, and received. Conversely, when a family system is in trouble, communication is blocked or distorted in a futile attempt to ward off anxiety and tension.

Fear of rejection is the common source of anxiety. As a result of fearing rejection, a person resorts to one response pattern or to a combination of patterns to communicate with others. These universal response roles are the placater, the blamer, the computer, the distractor, and the leveler. The last response, leveling, helps people develop healthy personalities; the other four responses hide real feelings for fear of rejection. In such situations, people feel and react to the threat of rejection, do not want to reveal "weakness," and attempt to conceal it. Satir (1971) agreed with Gestalt theory on nonverbal behavior: The body expresses your whole integration. Each response pattern is accompanied by a unique body posture and nonverbal behaviors, and each has its own way of dealing or not dealing with the context (or subject matter of the situation), the needs of the other family members, and the personal or self needs of the person playing the particular role.

PLACATER   Placaters pacify so others do not get angry. Their motto is "peace at any price." They talk in ingratiating ways to try to please, or they apologize. They never disagree and even take on the air of a "yes person." They have low self-esteem. They cannot negotiate solutions of mutual benefit because the process is too threatening. In other words, placaters negate self in the interest of serving others and staying within the context of the situation. Nonverbal behaviors of the placater send the message that "Whatever you want is okay with me; I am just here to make you happy."

BLAMER   Blamers are the faultfinders, directors, and bosses. They also do not feel good about themselves. They may feel lonely and unsuccessful and attempt to compensate by trying to coerce others into obeying them so they can feel that they amount to something. Blaming also is a good way to create distance and prevent others from getting too close. The blamers are good guilt inducers; for example, they may say, "After all I have done for you, how could you do this to me?" Blamers negate others while focusing on the context of the situation and on themselves. Nonverbal behaviors from the blamer send the message that "You never do anything right. What is the matter with you?"

COMPUTER   Computers are calm and accurate, show no feelings, and speak like a recording. They pretend there is no conflict when there is. Computers are the super-reasonable people. Their bodies reflect their rigid personalities. They negate the context of the situation and others to concentrate on getting what they want. They cover up their vulnerability with big words to establish self-worth. Nonverbal behaviors from the "computer" send messages that "I am cool, calm, and collected." They also may take the position of "See it my way" at the expense of others and the context of the situation.

DISTRACTOR   Distractors make completely irrelevant statements. They change the subject and never respond honestly. Their strong point is evading the issue. They may even resort to withdrawing from the situation to avoid a crisis or conflict. Distractors negate all three elements of reality: self, others, and the context of the situation. Nonverbal behaviors from distractors send messages that "Maybe if I do this long enough the problem will really go away." Distracting, doing and saying irrelevant things, withdrawing from family interaction, or a combination of these behaviors function to prevent the family from discussing painful, unresolved issues that should be faced in open and honest discussion.

LEVELER   Levelers communicate their honest thoughts and feelings in a straightfor-ward manner that addresses self, others, and the context of the situation (Figure 15-4). Their verbal messages and nonverbal body posture are consistent. Leveling occurs when all aspects of communication are congruent: body, vocal tone, context, and facial expression. Levelers do not cover up or put other people down in the name of being open and honest. They are not phonies. Levelers tell the truth about what they are thinking, feeling, and doing, and they allow others to do the same. Their relation-ships are free and honest, with few threats to self-esteem. The leveling response is the truthful message for a particular person at a given time. It is direct and to the point, with no hidden agenda. There is openness and a feeling of trust in interactions with

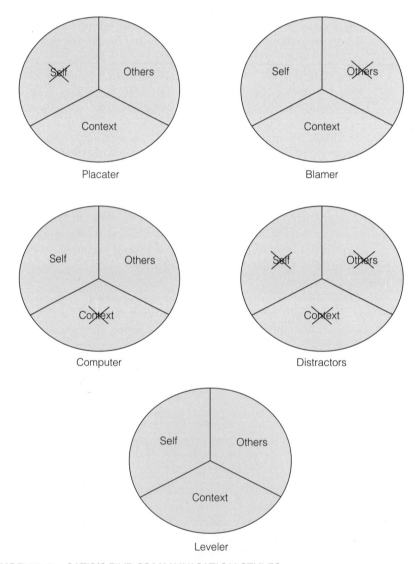

FIGURE 15-4   SATIR'S FIVE COMMUNICATION STYLES

a person who is leveling. This response allows people to live as complete persons in touch with their behavior, thinking, and feelings. The message of the leveler is consistent. If a leveler says, "I like you," the voice is warm and the eye contact and body speak the same message. If the leveler is angry, the voice is harsh, the face is tight, and the words are clear: "I am angry about what you have done!"

Being a leveler allows a person to have integrity, commitment, honesty, intimacy, competency, creativity, and the ability to solve real problems.

Satir pointed out that every person she has seen with a behavior or coping problem was a member of a family in which all significant communication was on a double level—that is, phony or hidden (Satir et al., 1975). If people learn to recognize harmful communication patterns and level with their family members, then the family has a chance to make its members' lives better and to solve problems more efficiently. Satir divided all families into two types: nurturing and troubled. Each type has varying degrees. Her main objective for her clients was recognition of their type, and then change from either troubled to nurturing or from nurturing to more nurturing. The nurturing family helps its members develop feelings of self-worth, whereas the troubled family diminishes these feelings. According to Satir (1972), aliveness, honesty, genuineness, and love mark nurturing families. These families have the following characteristics:

1. People are listened to and interested in listening to others.
2. People are not afraid to take risks because the family understands that mistakes are bound to happen when taking risks.
3. People's bodies are graceful and their facial expressions are relaxed.
4. People look at one another and not through one another or at the floor.
5. The children are friendly and open, and the rest of the family treats them as people.
6. People seem comfortable about touching one another and showing their affection.
7. People show love by talking and listening with concern and by being straightforward and real with one another.
8. Family members feel free to tell one another how they feel and what they think.
9. Anything can be discussed—fears, anger, hurt, criticism, joys, achievements.
10. Family members plan, but if something does not work out, they can adjust.
11. Human life and feelings are more important than anything else.
12. Parents see themselves as leaders and not as bosses. They acknowledge to their children their poor judgment, as well as their good judgment, and their hurt, anger, or disappointment, as well as their joy. Their behavior matches their teaching.
13. When nurturing, parents need to correct their children. They rely on listening, touching, understanding, and careful timing and are aware of children's feelings and their natural wish to learn.
14. Nurturing parents understand that children learn only when they are valued, so they do not respond in a way that makes the child feel devalued.

Counseling Method   The counseling method of conjoint family therapy involves the entire family and is based on communication, interaction, and general information. The approach Satir taught to families was both physical and emotional.

Satir's goals for family counseling were to establish the proper environment and to assist family members in clarifying what they want or hope for themselves and for the family. She wanted them to explore the present state of the family, including who plays which roles. She sought to build each member's self-esteem. Satir also worked to help families operationalize their definitions of words such as *respect* and *love*. For example, she asked clients, "What would be happening that would let us know you were getting the respect and love you desire?" or "What must be done for you to make you feel respected and loved?" Satir also used reframing to turn negatives into positives, thus allowing clients to view difficult situations in a better light and see possibilities for cooperation, conflict resolution, and change.

Satir led the family in role-playing both family situations and each other's actions and reactions to the happenings in a typical day. She used some Gestalt techniques of "sculpting" a family argument or interaction; she believed that the body is often a more honest reflection than the verbal message. Satir used videotape replay to teach communication, and her role-play dramas used various props such as ropes and stepladders, to demonstrate and analyze the types of family interactions. She staged these dramas to help family members learn how to level with each other, express their emotions, and use honest, direct language. Satir examined the family history by drawing family trees to look at how past and immediate family styles are passed on from parent to child. She used ropes to demonstrate the complicated process of communication between parents and children.

Even with a multitude of techniques, Satir proposed no formula for therapy because therapy involves human feelings and the ability to respond on a human level. Satir viewed the family as a "people-making factory" in which people are made by a process that is crude at best and destructive at worst.

In an example of Satir's method of family therapy, a 40-year-old woman sits in a fetal position on the floor, hiding behind a sofa. Her husband, sitting in a chair, points an accusing finger at her from across the room. One daughter, with arms outstretched, tries to make peace. Two children sit with their backs to the group, and a fourth child rubs his mother's back. Satir breaks the silent role-play, rests her hand on the father's shoulder, and asks how he feels right now. She has asked the family to act out silently how each feels during a family argument. This sculpting method is excellent in creating awareness of personal feelings, as well as awareness of the feelings of other family members.

Including children is imperative for family counseling success in Satir's system. Satir advocated inclusion of all the children, not just the child who has a problem, because all are part of the family homeostasis—a process by which the family balances forces within itself to achieve unity and working order. Satir operated from the assumption that all members feel dysfunction within the family in some way. Therefore, the counselor works with all members of the family to help them redefine their relationships. Family members have their own perceptions of what is going on in the family, and each member's input is vital in building a functional family. The counselor works with the family's interpersonal relationships to discover how the members interact so they can strengthen their bonding.

Satir suggested meeting with the marital pair before bringing in the children. She made the couple aware of themselves as individuals, as well as mates and parents. She also suggested preparing the parents in the initial interview for bringing the children into the counseling sessions. After the parents agreed that the children's role in family counseling was important, the children were included.

The counselor should begin by recognizing all the children and repeating their names, ages, and birth order to let the children know they are being heard. The counselor also sets rules for the sessions; for example, no one may destroy property within the room, no one may speak for anyone else, all must speak so they can be heard, and everyone must enable others to be heard. When the ground rules have been established, in-depth discussion can begin.

Children need to know that the counselor will treat them as people with perceptions and feelings. The counselor should demonstrate individuality by speaking to each child separately, differentiating each child, and restating and summarizing what each child says. Counselors need to convey their sincerity by honoring all questions from each child and demonstrating that questions are not troublemaking and illegitimate, and that all family members should ask questions about what they do not know or are unsure about. Counselors who convey their expectations of the children increase the likelihood that the children will rise to meet them. Children listen, are interested, and contribute to the discussions.

The counselor must ask the children their ideas about why they are in counseling and then repeat what each child says to make sure the child's meaning is understood. The counselor may proceed by asking the children where they got their ideas about why they are there, who told them, and what was said. From this exchange, the counselor can gain insight into communication within the family. The counselor encourages the children to talk about themselves and their feelings in relation to each family member. The counselor also helps the children express frustration and anger and has the children ask their family members for answers to any questions they may have. The counselor may use confronting questions to provoke thought in the child. As the counseling sessions advance, questions concerning family rules and roles arise. After establishing good rapport and a comfortable atmosphere, the counselor may begin to bring out underlying feelings and confront people concerning the family's dysfunction. The basis for further probing and confronting must be established between counselor and parent; counselor and child; parent and child; and counselor, parent, and child in the initial interviews. From the initial interviews, the counselor must gain the child's confidence to move forward.

The counselor wants to see each child's place in the family unit. In the beginning, to build the children's self-esteem, the counselor focuses on them—not ignoring the parents, but having the parents respond intermittently. Counselors help children understand their parents as parents and people and themselves as children and people (Johnsen, Sundet, & Torsteinsson, 2004).

Satir's approach to family counseling focused on three key ingredients:

1. Increase the self-esteem of all family members by facilitating their understanding of the family system and teaching them to implement changes toward open systems and nurturing attitudes and behaviors.
2. Help family members better understand and analyze their encounters with each other and learn the leveling response so that they can improve and open communication patterns.

3. Use experiential learning techniques in the counseling setting to help the family understand present interactions and encourage family members to take personal responsibility for their own actions and feelings.

Family therapists use a variety of techniques to assist the family in self-discovery. Satir's method was designed to help family members discover what patterns do not work and how to better understand and express their feelings in an open, level manner. Rather than have them rehash past hurts, Satir had the family analyze its "systems" in a present interaction in the counseling setting. Among the many ways to accomplish this analysis are the following: enacting a situation, simulating a decision, constructing a family structure, role-playing, and games.

Satir's games, which are used for counselor training, as well as for family therapy, are based on her definition of a *growth model*, which assumes that an individual's behavior changes as a process that is represented by transactions with other people. People function fully when they are removed from the maladaptive system or when the system is changed to promote growth. This model differs greatly from the *sick model*, which proposes that a client's thinking, values, and attitudes are wrong and therefore must be changed, and from the *medical model*, which purports that the cause of the problem is an illness located in the patient.

Satir developed games to deal with the family's behavior when family members operate within these three models. All family members are present during the family counseling process, including the games.

Simulated Family Game   In the simulated family game, various family members simulate each other's behavior; for example, the son plays the mother. The therapist may also ask family members to pretend that they are a different family. After this enactment, the counselor and family members discuss how they differ from or identify with the roles.

Systems Games   Systems games are based on either open or closed family systems; learning and insight can be obtained from both family types. Satir believed that emotional and behavioral disturbances result directly from a member being caught in a closed family system. The closed system does not allow an individual the right to honest self-expression. The family views differences as dangerous, and the overriding "rule" is to have the same values, feelings, and opinions. In the open-system family, honest expression and differences are received as natural occurrences, and open negotiation resolves such differences by "compromising," "agreeing to disagree," "taking turns," or finding win–win solutions.

One set of games entails having family members take roles revolving around the five interactional patterns of behavior discussed earlier: (1) the placater, (2) the blamer, (3) the distractor, (4) the computer, and (5) the leveler. Various games have been constructed from these interactional patterns, including:

1. *Rescue game:* Behaviors 1, 2, 3, and 4 are played. Who plays each role is variable, but each member must remain in this role throughout the session.
2. *Coalition game:* Behaviors 1 and 2 are played. Two people always disagree and gang up on a third person.

3. *Lethal game:* Behavior 1 is used. Everyone agrees.
4. *Growth vitality game:* Each person includes himself or herself and others by honest expression and by permitting others to express themselves (leveling).

These techniques can be broadened beyond the initial family triad by incorporating all family members into a prescribed family situation and assigning various roles to each member. These sessions are vital for younger children who have been ruled by the adage "Children should be seen but not heard." The games aid families in understanding the nature of their own family system. They also allow family members to experience new interactional patterns through identification of their current behavior and insight into possible alternatives. By using the growth vitality game and the leveling role, families can experience movement from a pathological system of interaction to a growth-producing one.

Communication Games   Communication games are aimed at establishing communication skills. Satir believed that an insincere or phony message is almost impossible to deliver if the communicator has skin contact, steady eye contact, or both forms of contact with the listener. One communication game involves having two members sit back to back while they talk. Then they are turned around and instructed to stare into each other's eyes without talking or touching. Satir (1967) reported that this type of interaction leads to many insights concerning the assumptions that each makes about the other's thoughts and feelings. Next, the participants continue to stare and then touch each other without talking. This process continues in steps until each partner is talking, touching, and "eyeballing" the other. Assuming these positions, they are asked to disagree, which Satir found was nearly impossible. People either enjoy the effort or are forced to pull back physically and divert their eyes to get angry.

The counselor's role is an important part of these games. Throughout and after each session, the counselor intervenes and discusses each member's responses, feelings, and reactions to himself or herself and to other family members.

In Satir's approach to family counseling, the counselor is a facilitator who gives total commitment and attention to the process and the interactions. The counselor does not take charge and must be careful not to manipulate the participants' reactions and verbalizations. By careful and sensitive attention to each family member's interactions, transactions, and responses (or lack of responses), the counselor can intervene at certain points to ask whether the messages are clear and correct and how a particular person is feeling. Each person thus has a chance to interact or make corrections. For example, the counselor might interrupt the dialogue when one person makes a statement about how another feels or thinks by asking the second person if the statement is accurate and how he or she feels at that moment.

In summary, the counselor intervenes to assist leveling and taking responsibility for one's own actions and feelings. The counselor also intervenes to give quieter family members permission to talk and be heard. Analyzing a present interaction in the counseling setting should help family members understand past hurts and problems. Understanding what patterns produced the trouble also helps family members. With experience in openness and leveling, family members can change their communication style and growth can occur. The family then is better able to continue the discussions, come to new insights, and implement appropriate changes.

Case Study

People's ability to assume other roles in the family group situation supports the idea that people can change their response roles and families can change their ways of interacting and solving problems. Family members need to learn to share both positive and negative feedback in ways that do not hurt or belittle others. Following is a family role-play transcript in which the leveling response is omitted:

DON: [Father/husband, blaming] Why isn't our dinner ready?

SANDY: [Mother/wife, blaming] What are you yelling about? You've got as much time as I have.

BILL: [Son, blaming] Aw, shut up. You two are always yelling. I don't want any dinner, anyway.

DON: [Blaming] You keep your trap shut. I'm the one who makes the rules around here *because* I'm the one who pays the bills.

SANDY: [Blaming] Says who? Besides, young man, keep your nose out of this.

DON: [Placating] Maybe you'd like to go out to dinner for a change?

SANDY: [Computer] According to the last issue of *Woman's Day*, they say eating out is cheaper than cooking the same things at home.

DON: [Placating] Whatever you would like to do, dear.

BILL: [Placating] You always have good ideas, Mother.

SANDY: [Computer] That's right. I have a list of the restaurants offering specials this week.

Perhaps one good leveling response by any of the family members could have helped these short exchanges. Perhaps Sandy could have said that she needed a rest from a long, hard day and would like to have dinner out. Don could have made a statement rather than asking a phony question. Perhaps a leveling remark by Don might have informed Sandy that he was wondering what she wanted to do about dinner. Bill could have changed his remark to "I really worry when we argue and fight in this family, and I would like this to stop." The counselor's job is to rehearse these leveling responses until the problem is solved in the role-playing setting, and then make plans to try the leveling response in real life.

In a second family session with the counselor present, the Frazier family is seated clockwise around the counselor: Jody, 43-year-old wife/mother; Frank, 11-year-old son; Larry, 44-year-old husband/father; Joyce, 14-year-old daughter; and Kathy, 16-year-old daughter.

KATHY: Mom, just say yes or no. Am I going to be allowed to go out on weekdays or not?

JODY: Why don't you do what you want? You always do anyway.

COUNSELOR: [To Kathy] How does this make you feel?

KATHY: Angry. I'd like to be able to do what the rest of the kids are doing, but I know Mom and Dad don't approve.

COUNSELOR: That sounds funny because I heard your mom say it was up to you. [To Jody] Is that what you said? Maybe it was the expression on your face and the way you spoke your message to Kathy that made her think you didn't really mean "Do what you want to do."

KATHY: Yes, her stern face said "no."

COUNSELOR: What did she do with her face to tip you off?

KATHY: Well, she squinted her eyes and wrinkled up her nose.

COUNSELOR: It's hard to read your mom's mind, but I am guessing that she thinks nobody listens to her very much. We can check this with her later. But I'm wondering if you have ever felt this way.

KATHY: Sometimes.

COUNSELOR: [To Jody] Do you ever have this feeling?

JODY: I think maybe we've hit on something new.

COUNSELOR: Do you think no one listens to you?

JODY: I have a rough day just keeping house for this family. Larry comes home from work too tired to talk, and all I ever talk to the children about are their fights and arguments. I have to handle all the family problems.

LARRY: Well, my job is all I can handle.

JODY: See, no one listens to my side of the story.

COUNSELOR: [To Larry] Were you aware of what Jody was saying when she said that? What did it feel like, Larry?

LARRY: It irritates me that everybody thinks it's my fault that things don't go better in our family.

COUNSELOR: Hold it one minute. Frank is doing something over here.

LARRY: [To Frank] Settle down over there and shape up.

COUNSELOR: Let's take some time out and find out what's going on with Frank. I haven't been paying much attention to Frank and Joyce. [To Frank] How did you feel about what was going on over here?

FRANK: Well, I, uh …

JOYCE: [Blaming Frank] You weren't even paying attention.

KATHY: Frank, if you move over here with me, we can get along better.

JODY: [To Larry] Can't you do anything to make him mind me? It's all your fault he acts like he does.

COUNSELOR: [To Kathy and Larry] An interesting thing happened before Frank started acting up. I was wondering, Kathy, how you felt when your father said to your mother, "It's all my fault that things don't go better in our family."

In this short segment, the counselor attempts to look at present communication patterns and the feelings these patterns conceal. After achieving awareness of the communication blocks, the family can begin to practice leveling as an alternative way of communicating.

Virginia Satir's method could fit well into a systems, structural, or communications approach for counseling families. She focused on developing better family communication by making family members aware of how others in the family react to their communication styles. Satir saw improved communication skills as leading to better family conflict resolution and problem solving.

PLAY THERAPY WITH FAMILIES

Play therapy has the advantage of helping children communicate their story to the therapist. Engaging the family in play therapy activities offers a rich observational field for evaluating the family system in action. A principal therapeutic effect from play therapy is the opportunity to help children move from dysfunctional enmeshment with a parent to functional individualization. Likewise, overly rigid family boundaries might be relaxed to allow for a healthy sense of family cohesion. Similar breakthroughs in family therapy with children have been reported for storytelling, art therapy, and outdoor adventure programs.

Ray, Bratton, Rhine, and Jones (2001) completed a meta-analysis of published play therapy outcomes. Play therapy had an overall effect size of 0.80 that dropped to 0.73 when parents were not involved. Other studies have similar results (Bratton, Ray, Rhine, & Jones, 2005; LeBlanc & Ritchie, 2001). In addition, Bratton and Holt (2009) listed research support for caregivers as effective therapeutic change agents (Becker-Weidman, 2006; Eyberg, Nelson, & Boggs, 2008; Landreth & Bratton, 2006; Lender & Lindaman, 2007; Lieberman & Van Horn, 2005, 2008; Weir et al., 2013).

Some models for promoting play therapy with families are discussed in the following section.

Dynamic Family Play Therapy

Harvey (2006) has explained dynamic family play therapy that is based on the developmental concepts of attachment and attunement. Harvey explained that the treatment builds the positive feeling, motivation, and creative variables of play in order to engage the family in problem solving. Family members learn to engage in play episodes using movement, drama, storytelling, and artistic expressions as they address their concerns. The counselor's goal is to help the family develop and use creativity to be better able to adapt to the current situation with more flexibility and emotional responsiveness. The idea is that creativity is activated when people play and that creativity allows problem solving and emotional closeness.

Dynamic play therapy developed from expressive art therapies of dance, drama, and art. Those expressive means are used by counselors to induce metaphors for emotional experiences. The counselor identifies and uses the dramatic themes that emerge. As family members engage in creative play moments, the counselor guides them into initiating interactive play in which metaphors emerge. The metaphors help them experience a mutual catharsis, understanding, and sense of mastery in their experiences with each other. Harvey identifies themes and images that often occur as anger, loss, death, grief, fear, protection, and hope as well as events of change, leaving, and transition.

By helping family members engage in play, counselors help families develop or restart their own natural play with each other. Over the progression of therapy, painful and conflicting issues emerge through play. Counselors can guide family members to generate the naturally creative playful spirit that will produce trust and affiliation. Then counselors can focus on the content of play to help family members reconstruct their relationships. Attuned communication occurs when parents follow the child's play and play flow is created when a parent recognizes the child's play initiatives and responds.

Dynamic play therapy evolves by having the family develop mutual play and then using the play to communicate and resolve emotional issues while the family members experience the pleasure and restoration of play. To accomplish this, the counselor teaches the family to appreciate the metaphoric qualities of play, to develop attuned play, to be able to use expressive flow with each other, to have parents respond to children's emotions, and to use metaphors to find family meaning for difficult events. Each stage requires evaluation, games, addressing the core scene, and using ritual and termination.

The counselor begins by issuing directive activities such as tug-of-war, scribble war, or follow the leader. The counselor remains alert to avoidance, interference, and resistance. The family members' actions evolve into more elaborate and flexible interactions, and eventually they develop their own unique style of play episodes (Harvey, 2006). In his study of the changes in problem behavior outcomes after dynamic family play therapy, Harvey (2008) concluded that positive changes in child behavior were reported and that the treatment can be a flexible medium for children and parent(s) to use interactive play in creatively adapting to stress together. Stagniti (2014) also presents a manual that outlines how parents learn to play with their children.

Filial Therapy

Bernard and Louise Guerney developed filial therapy, a play therapy method in which the parents are directly involved. Filial therapy is based on the principles of child-centered therapy. Guerney (1997) believed that adjustment problems experienced by children were caused by parents' failing to learn how to understand their children. She defined these problems as learning problems and thought that teaching parents to conduct child-centered play sessions might overcome parental shortcomings. Parents are so important to their children that she felt acceptance from them would be extremely meaningful for their children.

Filial therapy uses play as a way of helping parents and children communicate, work through problems, and strengthen their relationships (VanFleet, 2009). Filial therapy is a psychoeducational intervention that provides both knowledge and skills to parents. It is process oriented so that counselors create an empathic, accepting, and child-focused environment focused on relationships. Filial therapy empowers children, parents, and families by engaging parents in the partnership of play with children (VanFleet, 2011). The goals of filial therapy are to reduce the children's problem behaviors, to help parents gain the skills of the child-centered play therapists use when relating to their children, and to improve the parent–child relationship.

In filial therapy, the counselor trains and supervises parents or caregivers to carry out unstructured play sessions with children. After they have learned, become competent, and confident, parents hold play sessions at home with the counselor monitoring the child's play, parents' skills, and therapy progress (VanFleet, 2009).

The intervention proceeds by using learning theory and behavioral therapy for the parent training principles. Counselors complete the following steps:

1. Introduce parents to methods for conducting client-centered play therapy.
2. Consider the other demands of parents' lives, and assure them they are expected to practice these skills only in the play sessions.
3. Model the behaviors as complete tasks by coaching parent interactions.
4. Reduce each task to small, separate components and practice each component.
5. Reassemble the complete tasks and role-play without children.
6. Encourage parents to conduct sessions observed by the counselor or held at home and reported to the counselor.
7. Gradually increase the length of the sessions and have home play weekly.

As in child-centered play therapy, the child is encouraged to express his or her needs, thoughts, and feelings. Optimally, during the process, children and parents perceive each other in a more positive light as they learn how to play and talk together more effectively.

Parents learn four basic skills in filial therapy. They practice structuring, empathic listening, child-centered imaginary play, and limit-setting. Structuring helps parents begin and end the sessions so that children understand these times are different from their regular interactions. Empathic listening allows parents to recognize, accept, and understand their children's feelings. Child-centered imaginary play involves caretakers playing out roles assigned and directed by the child. Limit-setting helps parents establish authority when needed. Within those boundaries, children have a chance to correct their behaviors with rules enforced by the parents if children do not self-correct. Limit-setting in filial therapy is a three-step skill. The parent states the rule for the child and redirects the play in a general way—"you may not hit me with the block." The parent then gives a warning if the child breaks the same rule again—"remember you may not hit me with those—if you do it again, our play time will end today." Finally, if the child breaks the rule a third time, the parent enforces the consequence. Parents also develop the skill of interpreting play themes by learning to recognize and understand patterns of play (VanFleet, 2005, 2009).

Bratton et al. (2005) reported the effectiveness of play therapy was enhanced if parents participated, particularly as they do in filial therapy. VanFleet, Ryan, and Smith (2005) likewise concluded that filial therapy studies have consistently indicated improvements in child behaviors and problems, parent empathy and acceptance, parent skills, parent stress, and satisfaction with family life. Grskovic and Goetze (2008) taught German mothers and their children filial therapy and found an increase in acceptance, empathy, positive attention, and education competence for mothers and decreased rating of children's behavioral disruptions. Filial therapy has been used with a wide range of child and family concerns such as anxiety, conduct disorders, depression, trauma, anger, grief and loss, and others (VanFleet, 2011). Generally, the positive outcomes of filial therapy include improvements in child behavior and presenting problems, greater parent acceptance and empathy, parent skill levels improve, parent stress levels decrease, and more satisfaction with family life (VanFleet et al., 2005).

TheraplayBundy-Myrow and Booth (2009) describe Theraplay as an "engaging, playful, relationship-focused treatment method that is modeled on the healthy, attuned interaction between parents and their children" (p. 315). The approach is intense, short-term methods with the goal of building attachment, self-regulation, self-esteem, trust, and joyful engagement as parents learn to continue the health-promoting interactions. Booth and Jernberg (2010) explains that in Theraplay no toys or props are used and no questions are asked. Focusing on health, the play counselor structures the sessions to meet the needs of the child and to enhance the parent–child attachment.

Booth and Jernberg (2010) observed normal parent–child interactions and categorized them into four main dimensions: structure, engagement, nurture, and challenge. Descriptions of those dimensions and related techniques follow (Bundy-Myrow & Booth, 2009; Munns, 2010).

Structure refers to situations in which the parents give clear directions, rules, and boundaries, thus making the child's world safe and predictable. In Theraplay, this occurs in distinct parts. Throughout the play interaction structure occurs by the therapist or parent leading the activities. The adults clearly state safety rules. Finally structure is provided through games that have a clear beginning, middle, and end. The child learns to follow rules and directions. Games like "Mother May I" or "Simon Says" are examples of structuring activities.

Engagement means connecting with another person in an intimate way with mutual enjoyment. Engagement builds empathy with one another. The adult meets the child with enthusiasm but also knows how to modulate excitement so the child does not escalate inappropriately. Imitation games such as mirroring and clapping patterns are examples of engagement activities.

Nurture stands as the most important dimension of Theraplay. Children need care, comfort, affection, and security that their basic needs will be met. Nurturing is the key to secure attachment so that children learn regulate themselves and parents learn how to comfort their child and meet security needs. In Theraplay, children are nurtured in every session. They may be given food, soothed when they have scratches or other "boo-boos," and comforted by having lotion smoothed on their hands.

Challenge allows the child to take mild, age-appropriate risks. Children learn to master activities that are stressful, to explore and to promote feelings of competence when they are challenged. Activities may be done cooperatively. The tasks must be within the range of the child's abilities so the child does not fail. Some challenging activities that might be used include catching bubbles, balloon tennis, and feather blowing.

In the first three sessions of Theraplay, parents observe through a one-way mirror or from the corner of the playroom. In the remaining sessions, parents participate with the child under the guidance of the counselor. Sessions are usually 30 minutes of play and 30 minutes of debriefing and parent counseling.

Theraplay has been used with children who are impulsive (Booth & Jernberg, 2010), aggressive (Eyles, Boada, & Munns, 2009), as well as those who are withdrawn (Manery, 2000; Wettig, Coleman, & Geider, 2011). It has also been successful with foster and adopted children (Lindaman & Lender, 2009; Miller-Mroz, Lender,

Rubin, & Lindaman, 2010). This structured, relationship-based, short-term play therapy with parents and children has a growing amount of evidence to support its effectiveness. These and other approaches to family play therapy have promising potential for children and their caretakers.

DIVERSITY APPLICATIONS OF FAMILY COUNSELING

Sue and Sue (2012) point out that many different cultures are represented in the United States and that counselors are finding people from many various cultures coming to their offices for family counseling. Therefore, in addition to understanding psychopathology, counselors need to familiarize themselves with the customs, styles, symbols, and standards of behavior of these diverse groups. Family counselors are not expected to become experts on all cultures but rather to be open to understanding the uniqueness of every family they counsel, how that family's behavior matches its culture, and how it adapts to U.S. culture (Weitan & Lloyd, 2003). Goldenberg and Goldenberg (2012) explained that family counselors must be culturally sensitive, but they must not blindly adopt a stereotypic view that all members of a particular group are alike.

Some guidelines for working with culturally diverse families have been compiled. Bean, Perry, and Bedell (2002) outline competence for non—African American family therapists working with African American families. Kim, Bean, and Harper (2004) provide guidelines for working with Asian American families and Beitin and Allen (2005) do the same for Arab American families. Filial therapy is an effective treatment with Latino families (Garza & Watts, 2010).

The Center for Family Studies at the University of Miami School of Medicine has concentrated research on Latino and African American families. The center identified Brief Strategic Family Therapy as a family-based approach for Cuban immigrants and Structural Ecosystems Therapy for Hispanic and African American adolescents (Muir, Schwartz, & Szapocznik, 2004). Shapiro et al. (2006) stated that brief strategic family therapy provides a culturally sensitive intervention for Hispanic young people who are abusing drugs and exhibiting conduct disorder. The intervention produced more reduction in conduct problems than an unstructured group model.

McGoldrick, Giordano, and Pearce (2005) have more guidelines for providing family therapy across ethnic groups. These authors explained that effective family counseling with culturally diverse families demands sensitivity, experience, acceptance, ingenuity, specificity, and intervention by the therapist.

Gladding (2015) suggests the counselor who wants one approach to working with culturally diverse families will be disappointed. He offers some helpful guidelines. One is to determine whether the family's problems are mainly internal or external. Counselors should also gauge the family's degree of acculturation before selecting an intervention. Counselors will want to explore the family's commitment to problem resolution as well as explore what has previously been tried to solve the concern. Generally culturally skilled family therapists are aware and sensitive to their own cultural heritage, comfortable with the differences between them and their clients, sensitive to family circumstances, and knowledgeable about their own attitudes, beliefs, and feelings (Sue & Sue, 2013).

EVALUATION OF FAMILY COUNSELING

As noted in the opening paragraphs of this chapter, Carr (2014) reviewed studies of family therapy and found evidence of effectiveness with a range of behavioral and relationship problems.

Shadish and Baldwin (2003) reviewed 20 meta-analytic reviews of family interventions and concluded that outcome research indicates abundant evidence for the effectiveness of systemic therapy. Gladding (2015) summarized findings on research on family therapy. He noted that family interventions are more effective than no treatment and that improvement rates are similar to improvement rates in individual counseling. He also noted that different kinds of family therapy tend to produce similar results and that brief therapy of 20 sessions or less is as effective as long-term therapy.

Goldenberg and Goldenberg (2012) identified factors in family counseling sessions that lead to change. One is the alliance between the family and a caring, competent counselor who understands the problem. Another factor relates to cognitive changes in the family that lead to greater awareness, understanding, and a shared sense of purpose. Behavioral changes of staying engaged with other family members and having feelings validated by the family also lead to better outcomes in family counseling. Strengthening family relations, promoting constructive dialogue, and enhancing disclosure are the other mechanisms that stimulate change in families. Counselors who are aware of, create, and monitor those conditions will have a greater likelihood of successful family therapy.

SUMMARY

Systems theory emphasizes family interactions and reciprocal influence. Table 15-2 includes an overview of selected theorists' views of the family, of healthy and unhealthy families, the goal of counseling and concepts particular to the theory. Although this chapter focuses on differences between the schools and proponents of the various family therapies, similarities do exist. First, all agree that families are like engines with interdependent parts. When one part malfunctions, the total engine is adversely affected; that is, one malfunction may cause other parts to break down as well. For lasting behavioral change, therefore, the entire family may need to change. Second (to change the analogy), the family is like a canoe floating downstream; that is, maintaining its balance only because one member is leaning way out over the right side and two other members are tilted slightly to the left. In other words, the canoe is balanced, but uncomfortably so. The goal of family therapy is to relieve the pain by finding a more comfortable balance without upsetting the canoe. Families often say, "Stabilize us, but do not change anything." Third, to bring about successful change, the counselor may need to tip the canoe; however, the counselor's job is to ensure that the emergency process is a safe one. Fourth, all family therapy approaches borrow heavily from the material discussed in the previous chapters, as well as from sources outside this book. Once again, as with other theories, eclectic and integrative themes continue in the current literature on family therapy.

TABLE 15-2 COMPARISON OF VIEWPOINTS IN FAMILY COUNSELING

Model	View of Family	Healthy Family	Unhealthy Family	Goals of Counseling	Major Concepts
Family systems therapy—Bowen	Family is an emotional unit	Emotional detachment, separate identities	Marital dyad have no differentiation; self and spouse are "stuck together"	To move toward a better level of separation to reduce anxiety and reduce symptoms	Genograms, differentiation of self, multigenerational transmission
Structural—Minuchin	Family members relate by certain arrangements or the structure of the family	Has an underlying organizational structure that supports fluid and flexible responses	Inflexible structures cause dysfunction	Restructuring the family system of rules to be more flexible	Boundaries, subsystems, enmeshment, and disengagement
Strategic—Haley and Madanes	Family is a system of power relations	Have developed a suitable way to deal with conflict/control struggles	Symptoms are an attempt to control a relationship	Change the system by altering behavior patterns	Complementary communication patterns, paradox
Communication—Satir	Families are balanced, rule-governed systems with basics of communication and self-esteem; they provide a place to grow	Members know their own feelings; communicate congruently; accept that others are different and differences as opportunities	The freedom to grow and develop has been blocked by low self-esteem, incongruent communication, poor functioning, and rules	Growth in self-understanding and communication, increased respect for family members, members see individual differences as chances to learn	Self-esteem, clear communication

Adapted from Fall, Holden, and Marquis (2010) and Goldenberg and Goldenberg (2008).

INTRODUCTION TO FAMILY COUNSELING

To gain a more in-depth understanding of the concepts in this chapter, visit www
.cengage.com/counseling/henderson to view a short clip of an actual therapist–client
session demonstrating family counseling.

WEB SITES FOR FAMILY COUNSELING

Internet addresses frequently change. To find the sites listed here, visit www
.cengage.com/counseling/henderson for an updated list of Internet addresses and
direct links to relevant sites.

American Association for Marriage and Family Therapy (AAMFT)

International Association of Marriage and Family Counselors (IAMFC)

National Council on Family Relations

REFERENCES

Appleton, V. E., & Dykeman, C. (2007). Family therapy. In D. Capuzzi & D. R. Gross (Eds.),
Counseling and psychotherapy: Theories and interventions (4th ed., pp. 313–337). Upper
Saddle River, NJ: Merrill.

Bateson, G., Jackson, D. D., Haley, J., & Weakland, J. (1956). Towards a theory of schizophrenia. *Behavioral Science, 1*, 251–264.

Bean, R. A., Perry, B. J., & Bedell, T. M. (2002). Developing culturally competent marriage and family therapists: Treatment guidelines for non-African-American therapists
working with African-American families. *Journal of Marital and Family Therapy, 28*,
153–161.

Becker-Weidman, A. (2006) Treatment for children with reactive attachment disorder: Dyadic
developmental psychotherapy. *Child and Adolescent Social Work, 23*(2), 147–171.

Beitin, B. K., & Allen, K. R. (2005). Resilience in Arab American couples after September 11,
2001: A systems perspective. *Journal of Marital and Family Therapy, 31*, 251–267.

Booth, P., & Jernberg, A. (2010). *Theraplay: Helping parents and children build better relationships through attachment-based play* (3rd ed.). San Francisco, CA: Jossey-Bass.

Bowen, M. (1960). A family concept of schizophrenia. In D. D. Jackson (Ed.), *The etiology of
schizophrenia.* New York: Basic Books.

Bowen, M. (1976). Theory in the practice of psychotherapy. In P. J. Guerin, Jr. (Ed.), *Family
therapy: Theory and practice* (pp. 42–89). New York: Gardner.

Bowen, M. (1978). *Family therapy in clinical practice.* New York: Aronson.

Bowen, M. (1980). Preface. In E. A. Carter & M. Goldrick (Eds.), *A framework for family
therapy* (p. xiii). New York: Gardner.

Bratton, S., & Holt, K. (July 2009). Mining Report: Involving Caregivers as Therapeutic Agents
in Their Children's Therapy: Empirically Supported Play Therapy Models. Retrieved from
http://www.a4pt.org/

Bratton, S. C., Ray, D., Rhine, T., & Jones, L. (2005). The efficacy of play therapy with children: A meta-analytic review of treatment outcomes. *Professional Psychology: Research and Practice, 36,* 376–390.

Bundy-Murow, S., & Booth, P. B. (2009). Theraplay: Supporting attachment relationships. In K. J. O'Connor & L. D. Braverman (Eds.), *Play therapy theory and practice* (2nd ed., pp. 315–366). Hoboken, NJ: Wiley and Sons.

Campbell, D., & Palm, G. (2004). *Group parent education.* Thousand Oaks, CA: Sage.

Carr, A. (2014). The evidence base for family therapy and systemic interventions for child-focused problems. *Journal of Family Therapy, 36*(2), 107–157. doi:10.1111/1467-6427

Diamond, G., & Josephson, A. (2005). Family-based treatment research: A 10-year update. *Journal of the American Academy of Child & Adolescent Psychiatry, 44,* 872–888.

Eyberg, S., Nelson, M., & Boggs, S. (2008). Evidence-based treatments for child and adolescent disruptive behavior disorders. *Journal of Clinical Child and Adolescent Psychology, 37,* 213–235.

Eyles, S., Boada, M., & Munns, C. (2009). Theraplay with overtly and passively resistant children. In E. Munns (Ed.), *Applications of family and group Theraplay* (pp. 45–55). Northvale, NJ: Aronson.

Fall, K. A., Holden, J. M., & Marquis, A. (2010). *Theoretical models of counseling and psychotherapy* (2nd ed.). New York: Brunner-Routledge.

Garza, Y., & Watts, R. (2010). Filial therapy and Hispanic values: Common ground for culturally sensitive helping. *Journal of Counseling and Development, 88,* 108–113.

Gladding, S. T. (2015). *Family therapy: History, theory, and practice* (6th ed.). Upper Saddle River, NJ: Merrill.

Goldenberg, I., & Goldenberg, H. (2008). Family therapy. In R. J. Corsini & D. Wedding (Eds.), *Current psychotherapies* (8th ed., pp. 402–436). Belmont, CA: Thomas.

Goldenberg, H., & Goldenberg, I. (2012). *Family therapy: An overview.* Belmont, CA: Cengage.

Goldenberg, I., Goldenberg, H., & Pelavin, E. G. (2014). Family therapy. In D. Wedding & R. J. Corsini (Eds.), *Current psychotherapies* (10th ed., pp. 372–410). Belmont, CA: Thomson.

Gottman, J. (1979). *Marital interaction: Experimental investigations.* New York: Academic Press.

Gottman, J. (1990). Finding the laws of close personal relationships. *Methods of Family Research, 1,* 249–263.

Gottman, J. (1994). *What predicts divorce?* Hillsdale, NJ: Lawrence Erlbaum.

Gottman, J., Notarius, C., Gonzo, J., & Markman, H. (1976). *A couple's guide to communication.* Champaign, IL: Research Press.

Gottman, J., & Silver, N. (1999). *The seven principles of making marriage work.* New York: Three Rivers Press.

Grskovic, J. A., & Goetze, H. (2008). Short-term filial therapy with German mothers: Findings from a controlled study. *International Journal of Play Therapy, 17,* 39–51.

Guerney, L. (1997). Filial therapy. In K. O'Connor & L. M. Braverman (Eds.), *Play therapy theory and practice: A comparative presentation* (pp. 131–159). New York: Wiley.

Haley, J. (1973). *Uncommon therapy.* New York: Norton.

Haley, J. (1976). *Problem-solving therapy.* New York: Harper & Row.

Haley, J., & Reicheport-Haley, M. (2007). *Directive family therapy.* Binghamton, NY: Haworth Press.

Harvey, S. (2006). Dynamic play therapy. In C. E. Schaefer & H. G. Kaduson (Eds.), *Contemporary play therapy: Theory, research and practice* (pp. 55–81). New York: Guilford.

Harvey, S. (2008). An initial look at the outcomes for dynamic play therapy. *International Journal of Play Therapy, 17*, 86–101.

Hill, R. (1986). Life cycle stages for types of single parent families: Of family development theory. *Family Relations, 35*(1), 19–29.

Johnsen, A., Sundet, R., & Torsteinsson, V. (2004). *Self in relationship: Perspectives on family therapy from developmental psychology.* London: Karnac.

Kim, E. Y. K., Bean, R. A., & Harper, J. M. (2004). Do general treatment guidelines for Asian American families have applications to specific ethnic groups? The case of culturally-competent therapy with Korean Americans. *Journal of Marital and Family Therapy, 30*, 359–372.

Landreth, G. L., & Bratton, S. C. (2006). *Child parent relationship therapy (CPRT): A ten-session filial therapy model.* New York: Routledge.

LeBlanc, M., & Ritchie, M. (2001). A meta-analysis of play therapy outcomes. *Counseling Psychology Quarterly, 12*(2), 149–163.

Lender, D., & Lindaman, S. (2007). Research supporting the effectiveness of theraplay and Marschak interaction method (MIM). *Theraplay Institute Research Overview.* Retrieved from http://www.theraplay.org/

Lidz, T., Gornelison, A., Fleck, S., & Terry, D. (1957). The intrafamilial environment of schizophrenic patients. II. Marital schism and marital skew. *American Journal of Psychiatry, 114*, 241–248.

Lieberman, A., & Van Horn, P. (2005). *Don't hit my mommy: A manual for child-parent psychotherapy with young witnesses of family violence.* Washington, DC: Zero to Three Press.

Lieberman, A., & Van Horn, P. (2008). *Psychotherapy with infants and young children: Repairing the effects of stress and trauma on early attachment.* New York: Guilford Press.

Lindaman, S., & Lender, D. (2009). Theraplay with adopted children. In E. Munns (Ed.), *Applications of family and group Theraplay.* Northvale, NJ: Aronson.

Manery, G. (2000). Dual family Theraplay with withdrawn children in a cross-cultural content. In E. Munns (Ed.), *Theraplay: Innovations in attachment enhancing play therapy* (pp. 151–194). Northvale, NJ: Aronson.

McGoldrick, M., & Carter, B. (2003). The family life cycle. In F. Walsh (Ed.), *Normal family processes: Growing diversity and complexity* (3rd ed.). New York: Guilford Press.

McGoldrick, M., Carter, B., & Garcia-Petro, N. (2011). *The expanded family life cycle: Individual, family, and social perspectives* (4th ed.). Upper Saddle River, NJ: Pearson.

McGoldrick, M., Giordano, J., & Pearce, J. K. (2005). *Ethnicity and family therapy* (3rd ed.). New York: Guilford Press.

Miller-Mroz, J., Lender, D., Rubin, P., & Lindaman, S. (2010). Theraplay for children who are adopted or in foster care. In P. Booth & A. Jernberg (Eds.), *Theraplay: Helping parents and children build better relationships through attachment-based play* (3rd ed., pp. 405–493). San Francisco, CA: Jossey-Bass.

Minuchin, S. (1967). *Families of the slums.* New York: Basic Books.

Minuchin, S. (1974). *Families and family therapy.* Cambridge, MA: Harvard University Press.

Minuchin, S. (1978). *Psychosomatic families.* Cambridge, MA: Harvard University Press.

Minuchin, S. (1984). *Family kaleidoscope.* Cambridge, MA: Harvard University Press.

Mish, F. C. (Ed.). (2003). *Merriam-Webster's Collegiate Dictionary* (11th ed.). Springfield, MA: Merriam-Webster.

Muir, J. A., Schwartz, S. J., & Szapocznik, J. (2004). A program of research with Hispanic and African American families: Three decades of intervention development and testing influenced by the changing cultural context of Miami. *Journal of Marital and Family Therapy, 30*, 285–303.

Munns, E. (2010). Theraplay: Attachment-enhancing play therapy. In C. Schaefer (Ed.), *Foundations of play therapy* (2nd ed., pp. 275–296). Hoboken, NJ: Wiley and Sons.

Ray, D., Bratton, S., Rhine, T., & Jones, L. (2001). The effectiveness of play therapy: Responding to the critics. *International Journal of Play Therapy, 10*(1), 85–108.

Satir, V. (1967). *Conjoint family therapy: A guide to theory and technique* (Rev. ed.). Palo Alto, CA: Science and Behavior Books.

Satir, V. (1971, January). Conjoint family therapy. In G. Gazda (Ed.), *Proceedings of a symposium on family counseling and therapy* (pp. 1–14). Athens, GA: University of Georgia.

Satir, V. (1972). *People making*. Palo Alto, CA: Science and Behavior Books.

Satir, V., & Baldwin, M. (1983). *Step by step*. Palo Alto, CA: Science and Behavior Books.

Satir, V., Stachowiak, J., & Taschman, H. (1975). *Helping families to change*. New York: Tiffany.

Selekman, M. (2010). *Collaborative brief therapy with children*. New York: Guilford Press.

Seligman, L., & Reichenberg, L. W. (2014). *Theories of counseling and psychotherapy: Systems, strategies and skills* (4th ed.). Upper Saddle River, NJ: Pearson.

Shapiro, J. P., Friedberg, R. D., & Bardenstein, K. K. (2006). *Child and adolescent therapy: Science and art*. Hoboken, NJ: Wiley.

Stagniti, K. (2014). The parent learn to play program. In E. Prendiville & J. Howard (Eds.), *Play therapy today: Contemporary practice with individuals, groups and carers* (pp. 149–162). Abingdon, Oxon: Taylor and Francis.

Sue, D., & Sue, D. (2012). *Counseling the culturally different: Theory and practice* (6th ed.). New York: Wiley.

Thomas, M. (1992). *An introduction to marital and family therapy*. New York: Prentice Hall.

Todd, T. (2000). Solution-focused strategic parenting of challenging teens: A class for parents. *Family Relations, 49*, 165–168.

VanFleet, R. (2005). *Filial therapy: Strengthening parent-child relationships through play* (2nd ed.). Sarasota, FL: Professional Resource Press.

VanFleet, R. (2009). Filial therapy. In K. J. O'Connor & L. D. Braverman (Eds.), *Play therapy: Theory and practice* (2nd ed., pp. 163–201). Hoboken, NJ: Wiley and Sons.

VanFleet, R. (2011). Filial therapy. In C. E. Schaefer (Ed.), *Foundations of play therapy* (2nd ed., pp. 153–170). Hoboken, NJ: Wiley and Sons.

VanFleet, R., Ryan, S. D., & Smith, S. K. (2005). Filial Therapy: A critical review. In L. Reddy, T. Files-Hall, & C. E. Schaefer (Eds.), *Empirically-based play interventions for children* (pp. 241–264). Washington, DC: American Psychological Association.

Wagner, W. G. (2008). *Counseling, psychology, and children* (2nd ed.). Upper Saddle River, NJ: Merrill.

Weiten, W., & Lloyd, M. (2003). *Psychology applied to modern life: Adjustment in the 21st century* (7th ed.). Belmont, CA: Wadsworth/Thomson Learning.

Weir, K. N., Lee, S., Canosa, P., Rodrigues, N., McWilliams, M., & Parker, L. (2013). Whole Family Theraplay: Integrating Family Systems Theory and Theraplay to Treat Adoptive Families. Adoption Quarterly, 16(3–4), 175–200.

Wettig, H. G., Coleman, A. R., & Geider, F. J. (2011). Evaluating the effectiveness of Theraplay in treating shy, socially withdrawn children. *International Journal of Play Therapy*, *20*(1), 26–37.

Yontef, G., & Jacobs, J. (2014). Gestalt therapy. In D. Wedding & R. Corsini (Eds.), *Current psychotherapies* (10th ed., pp. 299–338). Belmont, CA: Brooks/Cole.

CHAPTER 16

Consultation and Collaboration

You must be the change you wish to see in the world.
—MAHATMA GANDHI

Counselors may expand their opportunities to improve children's lives by engaging in cooperative relationships with other adults. The processes of consultation and collaboration provide ways to build those types of working relationships. These related kinds of interactions allow counselors to serve children indirectly.

After reading this chapter, you should be able to:

▸ Define consultation and collaboration
▸ Discuss models of consultation
▸ Talk about roles of consultants
▸ Explain collaboration
▸ Outline ways to build teams
▸ Describe assessment types and instruments

Brown, Pryzwansky, and Schulte (2011) explained that consultation and collaboration have these common characteristics:

▸ Problem-solving processes
▸ Communication
▸ Clarity of roles
▸ Relationships built on respect and trust
▸ Using specialized information to achieve goals
▸ Sharing resources
▸ Stimulating change or improvement

For purposes of our discussion, we use the following parameters to differentiate consultation and collaboration. Consultation is considered as a method of sharing expertise. Collaboration is used as a term for an interactive relationship of conferring and collective problem solving. Team collaboration refers to a group that works together for the good of the whole in which each person contributes a specific effort to a plan of action. The following more specialized definitions, models, and examples will allow counselors to determine ways to incorporate each of these methods in working with children. That discussion is followed by examples of some specific consultation interventions.

CONSULTATION

Consultation is a process in which the consultant (counselor) works with the consultee (parent, teacher, or other adult) with the goal of bringing about a positive change in the client (child). Kurpius and Fuqua (1993) summarize consultation as follows: "In general, consultants help consultees to think of their immediate problem as part of the larger system, and not only to understand how problems are solved but also to understand how they were developed, maintained, or avoided" (p. 598).

Brown et al. (2011) offer a definition for consultation that identifies it as a voluntary problem-solving process aimed at helping consultees develop attitudes and skills that will allow them to work more effectively with a client, which can be an individual, group, or organization. According to these authors, the twofold goals of consultation are enhanced services and improved functioning.

Dougherty (2013) and Keys, Green, Lockhart, and Luongo (2003) further report that human service professionals may be asked to consult with adults who work and live with children, and the young people are ultimately the beneficiaries of the services. They suggest that consultants work with principals to discuss the concerns of students. Consultants may be asked to consult about a particular school program, or they may be involved in organization development. Consultants also work with teachers to enhance professional skills in areas such as effective parenting, enhancing children's self-concepts, choosing instructional materials, or conflict resolution. Although they do not engage parents as frequently as might be expected or as may prove beneficial, consultants may meet with parents to help them understand more about children's growth and development or behavior. Dougherty suggests that the range of roles in which a consultant may practice include that of advocate, expert, trainer/educator, collaborator, fact finder, process specialist, or other less common roles.

According to Glosoff and Koprowicz (1990), consultation directed primarily toward children typically involves the following:

- Conducting professional development workshops and discussions with teachers and other school personnel on subjects such as substance abuse or child abuse
- Assisting teachers in working with individual students or groups of students
- Providing relevant materials and resources to teachers, especially relating to classroom guidance curriculum
- Helping to identify and develop programs for students with special needs

- Participating in school committees that address substance abuse, human growth and development, school climate, and other guidance-related areas
- Designing and conducting parent education classes
- Interpreting student information, such as results of standardized tests, for students and team members
- Consulting regularly with other specialists such as social workers, psychologists, and other representatives from community agencies

Brown and Trusty (2005) suggest that consultation might be considered an information function or a problem-solving function that focuses on children's immediate needs and is not often a stand-alone activity when working in the child's interest.

Models of Consultation

MENTAL HEALTH CONSULTATION   Mental health consultation focuses on primary prevention and involves helping professionals and nonprofessionals. Caplan and Caplan (1999) explain mental health consultation as a "process of interaction between two professionals—the consultant, who is a specialist, and the consultee, who invokes the consultant's help in a current work problem that he believes is within the consultant's area of specialized competence" (p. 11). In this model, the consultant, considered an expert, diagnoses a problem and provides a solution. However, the consultant has no responsibility for carrying out the changes that have been recommended. Caplan thought that communities devoted to the well-being of people were positioned to prevent mental illness, ease future distress, and build wellness capacity in the community as well mitigate the need for direct mental health services (Albee & Fryer, 2003). Consultation provided the means for supporting those prevention possibilities.

The model proposed by Caplan and Caplan (1999) consists of four ways of approaching the consultation relationship.

1. In *client-centered case consultation*, the consultant helps the consultee with a client. The consultant assesses the problem and recommends a plan for the consultee to implement. The consultant's responsibilities include performing an accurate diagnosis and suggesting an effective intervention that focuses on the client.
2. In *consultee-centered case consultation*, the consultant helps the consultee gain the knowledge, skills, self-confidence, and/or objectivity needed to work with a particular client. By focusing on the consultee's behavior and attitude, the consultant facilitates change.
3. A consultant using *program-centered administrative consultation* focuses on the area of planning and administration such as the development of a program or the improvement of an existing project. The consultant collects information about the organization and suggests solutions with the goal of prescribing an effective course of action.
4. Finally, *consultee-centered administrative consultation* focuses on remedying difficulties among consultees that interfere with their abilities to perform their work. These problems may be the individual difficulties noted in consultee-

centered case consultation or may be the result of poor leadership, authority difficulties, communication blocks, and other group problems. Table 16.1 provides a comparison of these four types of consultation.

Across the different types of mental health consultation, consultants consider these fundamental assumptions. Both characteristics of the consultee and the environment must be considered. Consultee's beliefs, feelings, and attitudes impact behavior. Furthermore problems do not reside completely within the client but also at several levels within and outside of the organization. Other assumptions rest on the idea that technical expertise must be incorporated into intervention design. That belief recognizes that the norms, roles, language, and body of knowledge of the profession combine for the unique aspects of the context of the consultation. Furthermore, the responsibility for action belongs to the consultee. That practice promotes learning and generalization to other situations for the consultee. Caplan and Caplan (1999) explain that mental health consultation provides a supplement to other problem-solving mechanisms within an organization and that consultee attitudes and affect cannot be addressed directly—that would upset the working relationship in many ways (Brown et al., 2011). Sandoval (2014) has compiled an excellent volume about the application of consultee-centered consultation in schools.

Knotek and Sandoval (2003) pointed to a new definition of consultee-centered consultation that identifies the goals as a joint development of new ways to see the work problem. The process includes orderly reflection, generating hypothesis, and exchanging information. The relationship between consultant and consultee is supportive and equal. The goal of the relationship is changing the consultee's understanding of the situation. The consultant helps the consultee think differently by using a range of techniques (Caplan & Caplan-Moskovich, 2004), with dialogue being used to explore the consultee's view of the problem, introduce alternative viewpoints or new information, or reframing the problem to a solution focus. Nonetheless, the consultee is free to accept or reject the consultant's ideas (Brown et al., 2011).

Another modification of mental health consultation is the ecological approach in which the consultant sees the client system as the source of difficulties between the individual's ability and the demands of the environment (Gutkin, 2009, 2012). This approach involves three premises. The first assumption is that each setting has finite resources for maintaining and developing itself. Next, the model posits that in an adaptive environment the members have a variety of competencies. Therefore, the goal of intervention is to activate and develop resources. The ecological perspective focuses on consultation that cultivates opportunities to build competencies for self-development (Dougherty, 2013).

BEHAVIORAL AND COGNITIVE-BEHAVIORAL CONSULTATION   For school or mental health counselors interested in a more structured model of consultation, behavioral consultation may be appealing. This approach to consultation requires a deep understanding of behavioral theory and practice, especially Bandura's social learning theory (Bandura, 1977). The foundation of behavioral consultation is that behavior is observable and can be modified through the use of learning principles.

TABLE 16-1 MENTAL HEALTH CONSULTATION

	Client-centered Case Consultation	Consultee-centered Case Consultation	Program-centered Administrative Consultation	Consultee-centered Administrative Consultation
Focus	Client-centered case consultation focuses on developing a plan that will help a specific client.	Consultee-centered case consultation focuses on improvement of the consultee's professional functioning in relation to specific cases.	Program-centered administrative consultation focuses on improvement of programs or policies.	Consultee-centered administrative consultation focuses on improvement of consultee's professional functioning in relation to specific programs or policies.
Goal	To advise the consultee regarding client treatment.	To educate consultee using his or her problems with the client as a lever.	To help develop a new program or policy or improve an existing one.	To help consultee improve problem-solving skills in dealing with current organizational problems.
Example	School psychologist called in to diagnose a student's reading problem.	School counselor asks for help in dealing with students' drug-related problems.	Nursing home director requests help in developing staff orientation program.	Police chief asks for help in developing ongoing program to deal with interpersonal problems between veteran and new officers.
Consultant's Role and Responsibilities	Usually meets with consultee's client to help diagnose problem. Is responsible for assessing problem and prescribing course of action.	Never, or rarely, meets with consultee's client. Must be able to recognize source of consultee's difficulties and deal with them indirectly.	Meets with groups and individuals in an attempt to accurately assess problems. Is responsible for correctly assessing problem and providing a plan for administrative action.	Meets with groups and individuals in an attempt to help them develop their problem-solving skills. Must be able to recognize source of organizational difficulty and serve as catalyst for action by administrators.

From Brown, D., Pryzwansky, W. B., & Schulte A. C. (2006). *Psychological consultation: Introduction to theory practice* (6th ed., p. 32). Boston, MA: Allyn and Bacon. Copyright 2006 by Allyn and Bacon. Reprinted with permission.

Kratochwill, Elliott, and Callan-Stoiber (2002) outlined behavioral consultation and therapy as the application of systems theory and principles of learning a problem-solving process. The consultant gathers information from the consultee and then defines the problem in concrete, behavioral terms, as well as identifying the environmental conditions that maintain it. The consultant tries to help the consultee solve the problem by changing either the client's or consultee's behavior or the system in which the client and the consultee exist. Dougherty (2013) and Scott, Royal, and Kissinger (2015) detail the sequence of behavioral consultation as follows:

1. *Problem identification:* After a detailed analysis is performed, the problem is formulated in succinct, behavioral terms.
2. *Problem analysis:* A functional analysis of the problem is studied within its framework; antecedents and consequences are identified as well as task demands (cognitive, time, educational, and others).
3. *Selection of a target behavior:* The focus of the consultation is chosen.
4. *Behavior objectives:* Specific goals of the intervention are generated.
5. *Plan design and implementation:* A behavioral plan is developed and applied.
6. *Evaluation of the behavioral change program:* Measurement of behavioral outcomes in relation to goals established occurs.

The guiding principles of this model are the scientific perspective of using evidence-based practices, an orientation to the present, and the use of behavior change processes of operant conditioning—reinforcement, punishment, and shaping of behavior. Interventions begin with the agreement of consultant and consultee on a behavioral objective with one of three broad goals—reducing inappropriate behavior, increasing appropriate behavior, or eliminating an identified behavior. Consultant and consultee collaborate to change behavior. Intervention strategies, such as those described by social learning theory and cognitivebehavioral theory, also can be applied in the consultative setting to address either the antecedent or the consequence of the identified behavior. The choice of the intervention would be based on the one best suited to the knowledge, skills, and goals of the consultee (Scott et al., 2015).

MacLeod, Jones, Somers, and Havey (2001) have investigated the effectiveness of school-based behavioral consultation. Their findings support the importance of consultant skills and the quality of consultation in generating successful outcomes. Wagner (2008) identified behavioral consultation as one of the two most common methods to work with parents. The consultant promotes behavior change by closely examining the environmental antecedents and consequences of the child's actions. Parents learn to observe and monitor the behaviors also and then apply behavioral techniques to modify the actions. Operant conditioning, which includes the use of positive reinforcement, punishment, and extinction, is the technique parents are taught. Danforth (1998) provided a Behavior Management Flow Chart, which gives parents a step-by-step decision-making process to respond to their child's behavior.

Brown, Pryzwansky, and Schulte (2006) have developed general interview guidelines for behavioral noncrisis and crisis consulting. The consultant in a noncrisis situation (developmental interview) focuses on the following tasks:

1. Establishing clear general objectives
2. Reaching agreement with the consultee in the relationship between general objectives and more specific ones
3. Generating clearly defined, prioritized performance objectives with the consultee
4. Deciding how accomplishment of performance objectives will be assessed and recorded
5. Deciding on follow-up meetings

In a crisis or problem-centered interview, the outline focuses on the following tasks:

1. Identifying and describing problematic behavior(s) by collecting data from several sources concerning the nature of the problem
2. Determining the conditions under which these behaviors occur, their antecedents, and their consequences; the consultant and consultee analyze either the setting or interpersonal factors that contribute to the problem or the client's skill deficits
3. Deciding on assessment procedures; the consultant and consultee design a plan to deal with the problem by identifying objectives, selecting behavioral interventions, considering barriers to overcome, and evaluating progress
4. Scheduling future meetings (Brown et al., 2006, pp. 52–53)

MacLeod et al. (2001) conclude that intervention planning was positively correlated to student outcome. A step-by-step plan, adhering to the treatment plan, and the comparison of baseline and treatment data all related to student behavioral change.

Consultants who use the cognitive-behavioral consultation approach also rely on collaboration and shared problem solving. Those consultants believe that both internal and external factors influence behavior. Antecedents to behavior may be complicated by cognitive, environmental, biological, and cultural factors. They concur that behavior has a purpose but caution that a person may not immediately know that actual purpose.

In cognitive-behavioral consultation, the consultee identifies the problem behavior or the absence of an expected behavior. The problem identification moves into a detailed description of observable, measurable behavior. A functional behavioral assessment involves identifying the cognitive, emotional, and contextual data that might be used to help select appropriate interventions. Scatter plots might be used for tracing behavior as well as personal interviews and other means of compiling a complete picture of the behavior. Chosen intervention should be simple and nonintrusive and closely monitored for effectiveness. Observing and assessing the impact of the intervention focuses on the accuracy and efficacy of the treatment (Scott et al., 2015).

SOLUTION-FOCUSED CONSULTEE-CENTERED CONSULTATION   The models presented earlier are based on a philosophy known as modernist. That knowledge base assumes that reality is a knowable, objective reality. Those philosophers contend that only the scientific method of research identifies and verifies new knowledge. In addition, they presume that human behavior can be measured and quantified in meaningful ways. Cause-and-effect relationships exist and are discoverable through appropriate research methods. Accordingly, the context in which people exist are considered either neutral or unimportant.

On the other hand, social constructivism, a postmodern philosophy, is based on the premise that a person cannot be separated from context, people must be studied in their environments. These theorists repudiate the idea that cause-and-effect relationships can be inferred and that the only legitimate source of knowledge about a person is the subjective frame of reference of that individual. Finally, these thinkers propose that the acquisition of knowledge occurs through social interaction.

This approach to consultation borrows significantly from the work of Steve de Shazer (1985) and his wife Insoo Kim Berg that was discussed in Chapter 10. In this approach to consultation, consultant works to understand how or what the consultee identifies as the problem and potential solution. Using brief solution-focused interventions, such as finding exceptions, the miracle question, scaling questions, and understanding the clients' stories based on their perceptions, the consultant structures the process mirroring the therapeutic one.

During the first session, the consultant helps the consultee reframe the problem in manageable ways. The strengths of the consultee are identified and the consultant may distinguish themselves as coaches or facilitators of the problem-solving process. Problem identification begins with the question "what can I do for you today?" which quickly moves to forming a goal as well as scaling the problem. Solution-finding starts when the problem is identified and continues as consultant and consultee consider what has been tried and how that action has worked previously—exceptions to the problem help the dyad build a way to another outcome to the problem. Kahn (2000) presents a case study of this model used with a teacher in a middle school.

PROCESS CONSULTATION   Edward Schein (1999) has proposed a model of consultation he labels *process consultation*. He considers this approach to consultation as a skill. He emphasizes the interest in how things happen between people rather than what is actually done. More specifically, he defines process consultation as a "set of activities on the part of the consultant which help the (consultee) to perceive, understand, and act upon process events which occur in the (consultee's) environment" (Schein, 1988, p. 11).

This type of consultation focuses on the ways problems are solved and on the system in which the problems occur. The consultant and consultee examine six different areas: (1) communication patterns, (2) group member roles, (3) group problem solving and decision making, (4) group norms and growth, (5) leadership and authority, and (6) intergroup cooperation and competition. The consultant may operate as a catalyst in helping the consultee find a solution or as a facilitator who aids the consultee through a problem-solving process (Dougherty, 2013).

Harrison (2004) explains three strategic goals of process consultation. The first is to encourage a situation in which the client will ask for help. The next is to diagnose or create a situation so that information will surface and people understand better what is happening. The third goal is to build a team or create an environment in which the client will take responsibility for the problem and the solution. To accomplish these broad goals, Schein (1999) outlines these principles that can guide any consultation approach:

1. Constantly try to be helpful.
2. Stay in touch with reality by being alert to what is going on with you, with the situation, and in the consultee and client system.
3. Remain open to information and monitor your own ignorance particularly around racial, ethnic, and gender differences.
4. Remember that everything done is an intervention.
5. The client owns the problem and the solution.
6. Go with the sense of flow that emerges from the process.
7. Timing is critical in everything but particularly in shifting focus or method.
8. Find and build on existing motivation and cultural strengths.
9. Errors are inevitable.
10. When in doubt, share the problem (summarized in Harrison, 2004, pp. 228–232).

CROSS-CULTURAL CONSULTATION   Sheridan (2000) and Sheridan, Eagle, and Doll (2006) identified considerations of multiculturalism to the behavioral consultation process. They recommend particular attention to the awareness and sensitivity of the consultant, that is, the ability to consider various perspectives and procedures and to include those qualities into the process. They also discuss factors that may enhance the multicultural consultative relationship such as trust, acknowledgment of diversity, avoiding technical jargon, and considering the effect of interpreters. Although specific to behavioral consultation, their suggestions are also applicable to other models.

Ingraham (2007, 2008) offers a summary of her ideas of multicultural consultation. She emphasizes methods for supporting consultee and client success that a consultant should consider using. Consultants should value multiple perspectives and create emotional safety and support. That support should be balanced between new learning and interventions based on principles of mastery. Systems that support learning and development should be part of a consultant's strategy. Those strategies would include cross-cultural learning, bridging methods matched to the consultee's style, building confidence and self-efficacy, and working to increase knowledge, skill, and objectivity. For the consultant's development, Ingraham suggests continuing to learn, engaging in professional development, seeking feedback, and finding cultural teachers.

Brown et al. (2006) caution that cross-cultural consultation has many complexities. They emphasize that the cultural beliefs of the consultee influence verbal and nonverbal communication, the consultation model, the hierarchy in the relationship, and the nature of the intervention. They recommend asking the following questions or making these statements before making decisions about the consulting process:

- *To help determine the hierarchy:* I'm used to people calling me by my first name, but some people prefer something more formal. What do you prefer?
- *To assess who should be involved:* Based on the situation, what people other than you and me should be included in the consulting process?
- *To determine what leads to use:* Some people are uneasy talking about their emotions. We can focus only on behavior. Which is your preference?
- *Allowing the right not to participate:* Any time our discussion makes you uncomfortable, just tell me that you would rather not answer (p. 168).

Consulting Process

Brown et al. (2011) clarify that consultation is a process devoted to a consultant and consultee working to change a problem situation. That problem solving moves through the typical steps of assessment, problem identification, strategy, implementation, and evaluation. Dougherty (2013) suggests four stages. Following is a summary of the sequence, tasks, and goals of the consulting process and the steps suggested by those authors.

The first step is *pre-entry.* Consultants look at themselves to see whether they are right for the task and what services they can provide. Consultants may consider these questions: As a consultant, how do I view humans? Am I more attracted to some than others? How do I listen and respond to leaders at the top of the organization as compared with workers at the bottom? What do I think and feel when consultees disagree with me and confront me or my ideas? What about my espoused theories versus my theories-in-use (Kurpius, Fuqua, & Rozecki, 1993, p. 601)? Dougherty states that effective consultants must possess a personal and professional growth orientation, knowledge of consultation, and human behavior and consultation skills. How do you rate yourself on those requirements?

The second step is *entry, problem exploration, and contracting.* During the initial contact, the consultant needs to learn about the presenting problem, the people involved, what interventions have been tried, and the expectations of the person or organization seeking consultative services. At this point, the consultant must decide whether he or she can be helpful and establish a contract. Kurpius et al. (1993) recommended for any work other than individual consultation a written contract describing the purposes, objectives, ground rules, expectations, resources needed, and timelines for consultation; individual consultation, such as between a counselor and a classroom teacher or another helping professional, should have a brief written agreement, even if it is only a memorandum of understanding. Dougherty (2013) summarizes these steps of the entry stage as exploring the needs of the organization, contracting, then physically and psychologically entering the system.

The third step is *information gathering, problem confirmation, and goal setting.* Kurpius et al. (1993) encourage consultants to spend enough time gathering valid and reliable data, both qualitative and quantitative, to ensure delivery of high-quality services. Accurate data are important for defining the problem and attributing ownership—all essential steps to establishing the problem as a goal to be reached. Without agreement about the ownership of the problem (the teacher, parent, child, other child, or adult), interventions the consultant suggests are ineffective because no one takes responsibility for implementing the plan. According to Dougherty (2013), the diagnosis stage includes gathering information, defining the problem, setting goals, and generating possible interventions.

Wagner (2000) has identified four processes that consultants use in their conversations to promote change. They help externalize the problem so the person sees the difficulty in a different way. The consultant also allows the consultee to gain a larger, more detached view of the problem. According to Wagner, that process allows a paradigm shift, where there is recognition of the complex patterns between the focus and features of the situation, as well as the possibilities of change. Finally, Wagner remarks that the process of consultation encourages consultees to engage in self-reflection, recognizing their own roles, and avoiding the dynamics of blame.

In the fourth step, *solution searching and intervention selection*, consultants must avoid seeing all problems in the light of their favorite paradigm or counseling theory. Pointing out that human service organizations tend to see human factors as causing most problems and that industry and business most often see their problems as coming from structural causes, Kurpius et al. (1993) suggest that consultants carefully consider both the human and structural factors (the school or other systems in the child's life) as possible causes of the problem and areas for intervention. Therefore, this implementation stage includes choosing an intervention, developing and implementing the plan, and then evaluating the success of the intervention (Dougherty, 2013).

As noted earlier, Kahn (2000) proposes a model of Solution-Focused Consultation that shifts the consultation emphasis to solutions and strengths. The model rests on the assumptions of a future orientation and the helper being seen as a facilitator or coach, among other roles. Little time is spent exploring the problem before a goal is set. The goal is stated in positive language. The helper and the helpee explore exceptions to the problem, choose the best solutions, and create a plan to implement these solutions. The helper also encourages trying something different to change the problem. Kahn encourages school counselors to consider her propositions.

The fifth step is *evaluation*. As with any counseling task, evaluation ensures professional effectiveness. Kurpius et al. (1993) suggest asking certain questions to evaluate the outcomes of consulting services. For example, have the consulting goals been achieved and to what degree? How well have interventions worked? Were there unexpected outcomes, and have they been addressed effectively? Evaluation should give the consultant information about how each step in the process worked. Outcomes may include the changes in the client or in the system in which the client exists. Dougherty (2013) concludes that three ways to evaluate a plan's outcome are individual goal-attainment measures, standardized outcome assessment devices, and consumer satisfaction surveys. Sladeczek, Elliott, Kratochwill, Robertson-Mjaanes, and Stoiber (2001) use goal-attainment scaling not only to evaluate but also to facilitate a behavioral consultation case. Hughes, Hasbrouck, Serdahl, Heidgerken, and McHaney (2001) have tested another instrument, the Consultant Evaluation Rating Form (CERF), used to assess the effectiveness of the consultant.

During the sixth step, *termination*, when the consultant and consultee agree that the process should be terminated, the consultant should review with the consultee each step in the process, describing what was successful or unsuccessful. If the work was successful, this review process provides an opportunity for clarification, recognition of successes, and reflection on how the process brought about improvements. If the consultation process was unsuccessful, the session helps all members understand the reasons for the failure. Brown et al. (2006) provide several instruments that can be used to assess all aspects of the consultation process.

Consultant Roles

Young and Basham (2010) explained that the complexity of consultation involves many different roles. They summarized the different ways consultants may work as these:

Expert: The consultant has a specialized expertise and is expected to share that knowledge or skill set.

Advisor: Consultants can use their objective assessment of the problem to guide the consultee.

Researcher: The consultant gathers facts, collects data for evaluation, for decision making, or for developing awareness of trends.

Program evaluator: Consultants may be asked to document program outcomes or make recommendations about program implementation.

Teacher/trainer/educator: The consultant may provide and present instructional materials for new information or skills for the consultee.

Advocate: The consultant stands up for the rights of a person or group.

Process specialist: Consultants may also focus on the interactive process rather than the problem content. This type of consulting highlights the relationship dynamics of the group.

Collaborator: The consultant and consultee work together to identify and solve the problem.

Combinations

Myrick (2011) has explained a model of consultation that may also serve as framework for the processes of collaborating and teamwork. His systematic facilitative approach for practice involves the following steps:

1. Identify the problem clearly after careful discussion and listening.
2. Continue to clarify the situation by determining:
   a. The emotional and value components
   b. The specific behaviors involved
   c. The expectations of the people involved
   d. What has been done previously
   e. The strengths of the people, systems, or both
   f. The resources available
3. Determine the desired goal or outcome in specific (preferably behavioral) terms.
4. Gather any needed information for further clarity.
5. Develop a plan of action and determine the responsibilities for implementing it.
6. Evaluate and revise as needed and discuss the next steps.

Persi (1997) proposes a set of questions to encourage discussion in a consulting relationship. His questions mirror Myrick's consultation model. These questions are:

1. How have these problems affected you?
2. What has worked well for you with these problems?
3. What has not worked?
4. What type of support do you need?
5. Is there anything I can do for you?
6. Have we left anything out?
7. May I come back for a follow-up visit? (p. 347)

The tasks of consultation that Kurpius et al. (1993) describe are, in summary, assessing one's own competency, collecting data, defining the problem, setting a goal, selecting interventions, evaluating results, and terminating the relationship—all activities with which counselors are familiar. To ensure high-quality consultative services, however, counselors inexperienced in consulting should work with a colleague or seek supervision as they begin their consultative work, and all counselor-consultants should periodically evaluate the effectiveness of their professional services.

Consultation Interventions

Consulting can help counselors reach more children by teaching adults (parents, teachers, and other significant people in the children's lives) to behave in more helpful ways. Thus providing indirect services to children through consultation can be an important part of the counselor's role.

Counselors can work with parents and teachers in several ways. They can help adults learn to observe their children and look for good behavior. Practitioners can help teachers and parents understand their children and their motivations. Counselors can provide parent and teacher training that includes skills for building strong connections to their children. One example of a prevention program aimed at parents is PMHP, the Primary Mental Health Project (Johnson, Pedro-Carroll, & Demanchick, 2005). This program shows ways professionals may offer adults suggestions and recommendations for helping their child.

Guli (2005) defines parent consultation as interactions between a professional and a parent while others consider it a structured, problem-solving, collaborative relationship. The same type of interactions occurs with teachers. Other authors (Holcomb-McCoy & Bryan, 2010) identified conjoint behavioral consultation, Adlerian consultation, and values-based consultation as the models most used with adults working with children.

Conjoint behavioral consultation incorporates school and home resources to help the child. Parents, teachers, and consultants work cooperatively to address the needs of the child. This team works through a problem-solving process, use behavioral assessment techniques and interventions, and evaluate outcomes based on behavioral analysis. Sheridan et al. (2006) found positive results with 125 diverse students, as did Auster, Feeney-Kettler, and Kratochwill (2006) with students with anxiety.

Adlerian parent consultation assumes that behavior is goal directed and that change happens when the person recognizes that capacity. The concept of goals of misbehavior predominates and parents learn encouragement, respect, faith in the child, and belief in the consultant (White, Mullis, Early, & Brigman, 1995). This model includes these stages:

- developing a relationship with parents,
- identifying the problem, and
- exploring and formulating a plan.

Dinkmeyer and Carlson (2006) provide specific consultation procedures to help adults implement these and other Adlerian interventions with children.

Values-based parent consultation involves caring and compassion, diversity, self-determination, health, and social justice. This approach moves through six steps to implement consultation and prevention programs in schools.

Consultants create partnership, clarify values, identify and merge strengths of different partners, define the problem collaboratively. They develop a prevention program together and monitor the outcomes (Nelson, Amio, Prilleltensky, & Nickels, 2000).

An example of a prevention program aimed at parents is the STAR Parenting Program (Fox & Fox, 1992). Parents in the STAR program learn to respond to their child's misbehavior in a thoughtful rather than an emotional way (Nicholson, Anderson, Fox, & Brenner, 2002). Parents learn to:

S—**stop,** rather than responding immediately;

T—**think;** focusing on their own feelings and getting control of the emotions;

A—**ask** themselves—do you have a realistic expectation for your child?

R—**respond** by acting in a planful manner to their child's misbehavior.

Bartholomew, Knight, Chatham, and Simpson (2000) have compiled a manual for leading groups focused on learning and practicing parenting skills. This comprehensive and easy-to-use guide could easily be adopted for any setting in which consulting with parents would be appropriate. These are only a few of the ways consulting would be appropriate for teachers, parents, and other adults who work with children. Holcomb-McCoy and Bryan (2010) recommend a consulting approach that combines empowerment and advocacy to connect and collaborate to help children.

Next are techniques counselors may wish to try in their consultative efforts with the adults in the child's world. Each child's uniqueness and specific needs must be considered before one selects any counseling or consulting procedure.

ROLE SHIFT   Simply changing one's own behavior may elicit a behavioral change in another person. Adults who change their responses to children's behaviors may cease to reinforce them or present children with an unexpected response that causes change.

Consultants might want to ask adults to list *everything* they have tried with the child that has been effective and ineffective. The consultant then asks them to commit themselves to dropping those ineffective techniques with this child. The list should be kept as a reminder of what not to do with the child, as well as what responses work.

When the child has behaved inappropriately, adults can stop and ask themselves, "What response does this child expect?" Does the child expect the adult to be shocked, outraged, or angry? For instance, Glen reacted to his mother's scolding by drawing grotesque pictures of her and placing them around the house. He took great delight in watching her reactions when she found the pictures. Glen's mother decided that Glen enjoyed her outrage. The next time she found a picture, she calmly commented to him, "I must have really made you angry when I scolded you for you to draw me like this." She left the picture up and went on with her work. Glen quietly removed his pictures later that day. This technique appears to work best when the child expects to get attention, elicit shock (as with curse words or dirty language), cause frustration or anger, or get revenge.

LISTING OF BEHAVIORS   Another technique is listing behaviors. For instance, Mr. Jones told the counselor that Sherry was a crybaby who cried at *everything* that did not go her way. The counselor asked Mr. Jones to keep an exact count of the times that Sherry cried during the next week. The next week Mr. Jones admitted that, according to his count, Sherry had cried only three times that week—once when she fell, once when she was told to go to bed, and once when she was refused a request. Mr. Jones began to change his perception of Sherry as a crybaby.

Listing the number of times a behavior occurs also can provide a baseline count to determine whether an intervention has reduced an inappropriate behavior or increased an appropriate one.

LOGICAL CONSEQUENCES   Proponents of Adler's individual psychology advocate allowing children to experience the natural or logical consequences of their behavior, rather than punishment, as the preferred form of discipline. They suggest that adults who punish children become authority figures and lose the friendship of the child. They also point out that natural or logical consequences are reality oriented and teach the child the rules of society, whereas punishment may teach unwanted lessons such as "power is authority." Obviously, adults cannot allow children to experience the consequences of all their behaviors; for example, children cannot learn that busy streets are dangerous by playing in them. However, a thoughtful adult can find ways for children to see the consequences of inappropriate behavior. When Peter colors on the walls instead of on paper, for instance, he is responsible for using the sponge and cleanser to remove the coloring. The natural consequence of being late is to miss an event or a meal. The logical consequence of damaging someone's property is to earn enough money to replace it. The logical consequence of behaving inappropriately in a group is usually rejection by the group or isolation. Discipline with logical consequences quickly teaches children the order and rules of society.

COLLABORATION

Dougherty (2013) refers to collaboration as an increasingly necessary competency of helping professionals. He suggests it has grown as a way to allow the people involved to assume more ownership in the problem-solving process, especially in the implementation of the interventions (Finello, 2011).

Friend and Cook (2012) explain that collaboration involves voluntarily working together in shared decision making toward a shared goal. They note this definition conveys how the process occurs—as a partnership. These authors identify defining characteristics of collaboration to clarify their definition. First, they emphasize that collaboration is voluntary. Collaboration requires parity among participants. That is, each participant has a voice equal to any other participant, and all contributions are valued equitably. The parties involved in collaboration base their work on mutual goals, and they share responsibility for the process and the outcomes. They also share their resources and decision making. Curtis and Stollar (2002) defined collaboration as two or more people planning, problem solving, and achieving desired outcomes. The collaborative process involves shared goals, two-way communication, and joint activity (Dougherty, 2013).

Harrison (2004) explains that the goals of collaboration are centered on the relationship and the treatment. The primary goal focuses on developing a working relationship with all the members of the collaborative effort. The second goal refers to the treatment, arriving at the best possible solution for the client. People involved in collaborations need to be effective, cooperative decision makers. They build upon each other's capacity for achieving the goals (Conoley & Conoley, 2010). They focus on the key elements of result and the connection between the purpose of collaboration and its goals (Gibbons & Silberglitt, 2008). In fact, collaboration can provide social support to the people involved by helping them feel more productive as well as having more tools (Conoley & Conoley, 2010).

Collaboration among school professionals is a necessity. Collaborative relationships in schools include work with administrators (Paisley & Milsom, 2007; Ysseldyke, Burns, & Rosenfeld, 2009) who, for example, may request help implementing a school-wide program, or incorporating a primary prevention program or in working with particular children. Relationships with teachers may involve direct service such as an inclusion model in which school counselors and teachers provide direct services together in the classroom setting rather than pulling students out for services (Clark & Breman, 2009). Another example involves home-school collaboration, a partnership between school-based personnel and the family with the goal of enhancing student achievement (Epstein & Van Voorhis, 2010). This preventive, problem-solving approach incorporates both educators and families to support learners with opportunities for parent participation and shared goals of the collaboration (Esler, Godber, & Christenson, 2008).

Keys, Bemak, and Lockhart (1998) believe that a collaborative consultation model can result in a "more comprehensive and integrated program" to address the complex problems of youth and families (p. 123). They point to the increasing number of youths and families facing serious problems such as poverty, family instability, substance abuse, physical and sexual abuse, violence, and other societal issues, and conclude that new ways of helping require service integration through collaboration. According to these authors, "Collaborative consultation is a model that actively involves parents, educators, youths, and counselors as equal participants and experts in problem solving a specific issue ... it is the sharing and transferring of knowledge and information between and among all team members that enables the group to determine and carry out a more comprehensive plan" (p. 127). Their five stages of problem solving for collaborative consultation involve the following:

1. Coming together—establishing a commitment among all participants to collaborate on a certain issue
2. Defining a shared vision—sharing knowledge and information; building trust; and defining vision, goals, and objectives
3. Developing a strategic plan to accomplish goals and objectives
4. Taking action on the plan
5. Evaluating progress by determining if specific objectives are accomplished

The authors called for school and community mental health counselors to redefine their roles and to see themselves as a part of the broader community.

Some authors (Taylor & Adelman, 2000; Porter, Epp, & Bryant, 2000) suggest that collaborative efforts may involve nurturing relationships to increase resources, to enhance effectiveness, to decrease fragmentation, and to be cost-efficient. Their ideas of "school-community" collaboration include agencies; organizations that provide services and programs, such as health and human services, juvenile justice, and economic development; institutions that share facilities such as schools, parks, and libraries; and other entities such as young people, families, religious groups, civic groups, and businesses. Porter et al. (2000) argue that collaboration among school mental health professionals must occur and provide examples of collaborative programs that have been implemented successfully. Within the school, collaborators work with school administrators to collect and share data on school performance, to develop programs to overcome barriers, to design strategies for school problems, and to emphasize a healthy school climate. Collaborators work with teachers to improve classroom performance, to understand cultural learning styles, and to develop group skills and conflict resolution strategies.

Dougherty (2013) suggests guidelines to help in determining whether consultation or collaboration should be chosen. First, one should determine how the two services are viewed by the consumer. Next, consultants should reflect on their personal reactions to the two services and their comfort with the assumptions of each. Dougherty suggests that collaboration may be the method to choose if the parameters of consultation cannot be met. The consultant's skill level and the consultee's (or collaborator's) skill level also influence the decision. Fundamental to the choice are the nature of the problem, the context in which it occurs, and the skills of everyone involved.

Harrison (2004) lists prerequisites for collaborative efforts. First, the participants need to understand the language of each discipline that is involved. All team members should be trusted and respected. The shared responsibilities should be acknowledged. Cultural differences should be recognized and understood. Collaborators should create models, goals, and strategies that promote children and families. Open communication must be maintained. Finally, collaborators must accept that each professional will have different outcome orientations.

Some activities have been proposed by Dettmer, Knackendoffel, and Thurston (2012) to advance collaborative discussions and to build interactive formats. Three activities are as follows:

Jigsaw: The group decides on an issue and several subtopics. The large group divides into smaller groups. Each small group researches one of the subtopics and shares what is learned by teaching it to the others.

Compare-and-contrast: A small group identifies terms and phrases that represent different perspectives on an issue. The group's work is combined with all the work in the larger group to result in a broad list of ways of thinking about an issue.

Circle response: A small group sits in a circle. A leader begins by introducing or by repeating a topic. Moving clockwise, each person takes a turn responding to the issue or by saying "I pass." At the end of the time, the ideas are summarized and integrated into the larger group.

Collaborative efforts occur across settings. The efforts may be about individual, group, and system problems. Working together allow the talents, viewpoints, and focus of participants to combine in creating and implementing solutions. Often those efforts unfold in a team.

Teaming

Collaboration also can take place in specialized groups called teams that have a specific work purpose. Teams have shared goals and are interdependent. Gravois, Groff, and Rosenfeld (2009) explain that successful teams have similar characteristics. Teams manage their work of solving problems and evaluating solution as well as giving and receiving feedback (Barnett, Hawkins, & Lentz, 2011). They deal with conflict through an agreed upon mechanism (Finello, 2011) and have strong leadership qualities, commitment, and focus (Yetter, 2010). Team members are committed to building and maintaining constructive relationships among themselves. Effective teams have goals and identified roles. Each person on the team is aware of the focus of the team, the responsibilities of the members, and the plan for accomplishing the task of the team. Effective teams have members that value each other's input, define interventions explicitly, and are accountable for their outcomes (Kirst-Ashman & Hull, 2012).

Teams in schools include grade-level teams, school-based special needs teams, and referral teams (Brigman, Mullis, Webb, & White, 2005). Collaboration may occur in collaborative teams that assess students' progress (Gravois et al., 2009), intervention teams (Young & Gaughan, 2010), or multidisciplinary problem-solving groups (Burns, Wiley, & Viglietta, 2008). Some collaboration teams focus on helping the system (Kirst-Ashman & Hull, 2012). Student assistance, teacher support, and school-wide support (Adelman & Taylor, 2008) may be addressed in school collaboration which can be seen as a process of connecting schools, families, and communities (Taylor & Adelman, 2000). Counselors who are interested in developing team expertise in educational settings may find the monograph by Basham, Appleton, and Dykeman (2004) a road map for team building.

ASSESSMENT AS A CONSULTING AND COUNSELING INTERVENTION

In their attempts to understand children's developmental and other critical problems, counselors often use a variety of tools such as self-report surveys, interviews, tests, case histories, and behavioral observations. Counselors also need to be familiar with standardized tests, understand their results, and use them effectively in counseling and in consulting with other professionals. Some of the more commonly used assessment tools are discussed in the following section.

THE INTERVIEW Counselors usually are comfortable with interviewing their child clients and can obtain much information through this procedure. Counselors are adept not only in listening to what is being said but also in noting how it is said and the accompanying behaviors. Typically, the interviewer seeks to learn something about the child (name, age, family information) and the presenting problem. While interviewing the child, the counselor has an opportunity to observe whether the child makes good eye contact, is outgoing or shy, attentive or distracted, overactive or lethargic, talkative or reluctant to speak, confused or thinking clearly, anxious or depressed. Some counselors prefer structured interviews; others allow clients to reveal themselves at their own pace. Some counselors will use self-report surveys that ask children open-ended questions (my best friend ...; I like it when my mother ...). Counselors can learn much through observation of appearance, behaviors, affect, and verbal and nonverbal communications of children.

One interview, the Mental Status Examination (MSE), may be used to provide an inventory of the person's behavior. Hohenshil and Getz (2001) outline the following types of observations to be included:

General appearance, behavior, and attitude: Counselors note whether the child's appearance and dress are appropriate to the situation. Observations may also include posture, odd mannerisms, activity level, and facial expression. Whether the client is cooperative, sullen, assertive, impulsive, dependent, evasive, or friendly may also be noted.

Speech characteristics and thought process: Hohenshil and Getz (2001) note that speech indicates thought processes. Characteristics of verbal activity such as the pattern of speech, the amount of detail, the goal of speech, fragmented ideas, loosely connected phrases, and silences are included.

Emotional status and reactions: What the client says and how he or she behaves provide evidence of emotional status. The counselor observes facial expressions, whether he or she is flushed, and whether the affect is appropriate to the situation.

Content of thought: This involves a determination of whether the client's thought patterns are within normal limits. Delusional thinking, rigidly held false beliefs, and obsessions are examples of thoughts beyond the normal range.

Orientation and awareness: The counselor ascertains whether the client is oriented to time, place, and person. This is a critical element of a mental status examination and may be chosen to begin the interview. The counselor may ask the client the setting, his or her name, and the day, month, and year. This may need to be modified to the cognitive ability of the child.

Memory: The counselor may ask the person to talk about the previous day, a birthday, or some past life experience.

General intellectual functioning: A child may be asked to demonstrate an academic skill relevant to his or her grade level to assess general knowledge. Judgment and reasoning might include something like "What would you do if you saw a fire?" or "How are a cat and dog alike?"

Insight: The counselor tries to determine how much the client understands about the current problem situation.

MSE summary: The counselor summarizes the observations and may include recommendations for further assessment (Hohenshil & Getz, 2001, pp. 272–273).

Wagner (2008) outlined a six-stage model for an interview that uses puppets. To start, the counselor introduces the assessment to the child and family. Then the child chooses from a collection of puppets. Next, the child introduces the puppets; counselors may prompt this by saying something like "This character is ...." The practitioner then asks the child to tell a story using the puppets. The counselor then interviews the puppets in order to get more information on the clinically relevant information in the story. Finally, the counselor and child discuss the puppet experience, which may include the child's reasons for the story, possible connections to the child's life, and favorite characters in the tale.

Shapiro, Friedberg, and Bardenstein (2006) offered a set of assessment questions that are applicable to most situations when counselors are trying to understand the child's concerns.

- What is involved in the problem? Tell me specifically what this problem looks like please. What thoughts and feelings happen as a result?
- How often does the problem happen? How many times per day or week?
- When does it happen? In what situations does it not occur?
- When did it start? What was happening at that time?

And for adults, the additional ones below.

- What has the child said about the problem that might help us know his thoughts about it?
- What have you tried to solve or manage the problem? What has been the result of those efforts? (p. 16)
- What are the child's strengths? (talents, relationships, positive traits)
- What are the child's resources? (family, friends, school personnel)

CASE HISTORIES   A case history gives professionals complete biographical information about the child client. Interviewing the child and his or her parents and other family members and reviewing school records and the records of other professionals working with the child (doctors, speech therapists, special teachers, and others) provide data for the case history.

Behavior Observations and Rating Forms

BEHAVIORAL OBSERVATIONS   In certain cases, the counselor will need to observe children in their work and play situations to understand more about their functioning and their relationships with others. Personal observation can tell the counselor whether a child's behavior is appropriate, any circumstances that stimulated certain responses, and how others around the child respond. Counselors may use published checklists or develop their own methods for recording behavioral observations.

BEHAVIOR RATING SCALES, FORMS, CHECKLISTS   Counselors can obtain objective data about a child's behavior by using behavior rating instruments that allow a comparison of a child's behavior to appropriate norms. A variety of those instruments exists and many can be used by parents, teachers, and other caregivers, as well as the counselor. Some of those widely used scales are listed below:

Achenbach System of Empirically Based Assessment (ASEBA; Achenbach & Rescorla, 2001) has forms for teachers, parents, direct observation, and a semi-structured clinical interview format.

The Behavior Assessment System for Children-2 (Reynolds & Kamphaus, 2002, 2004) has rating scales and self-report forms to assess both the behaviors and emotions of children and adolescents.

The Connors Third Edition (Connors, 2008) is used for screening children with disruptive behaviors and for tracking progress with these youngsters.

The Vineland Adaptive Behavior Scales-II (Sparrow, Cicchetti, & Balla, 2005) allows someone who is familiar with the child's behavior in several settings to rate adaptive behavior or the child's ability to carry out daily activities.

Formal Psychological and Educational Tests

Children referred for learning and behavioral problems often take a battery of tests to help professionals understand more about their level of functioning. Psychologists working with the child usually decide the tests to be included in the battery.

INTELLIGENCE TESTS   Intelligence is a difficult concept to define, but most agree that it is related to a person's general mental ability and intellectual performance. Tests for children usually include some measure of knowledge, concept formation, and reasoning. Many tests tap both verbal and nonverbal abilities. Intelligence tests are popular but also controversial (Wicks-Nelson & Israel, 2013). Some of the more popular tests for measuring children's intelligence are:

Stanford-Binet Intelligence Scale, 5th edition (Roid, 2003)

Wechsler Intelligence Scale for Children–Fourth Edition (WISC-IV: Wechsler, 2003)

Wechsler Preschool and Primary Scale of Intelligence, Third Edition (WPPSI-III; Wechsler, 2002)

Wechsler Abbreviated Scale of Intelligence (WASI; Wechsler, 1999)

For a quick screening estimate of intelligence, the Otis-Lennon School Ability Test (OLSAT-8; Otis & Lennon, 2004) is available.

The Stanford-Binet and Wechsler scales must be administered individually by a trained professional; the OLSAT-8 can be administered in the classroom to groups in grades 1 through 12. The tests yield a numerical intelligence quotient, the IQ score, with 100 being the mean or average and a 15- to 16-point standard deviation to indicate how far above or below the mean the child scores.

A quick estimate of intelligence can be obtained with the Peabody Picture Vocabulary Test, Fourth Edition (PPVT-IV; Dunn & Dunn, 2006). Children respond by pointing to the picture that best describes the word read by the administrator. The test taps only one area of the child's ability, and therefore is not considered to be a measure of general intelligence.

A newer test of intelligence and achievement is the Kaufman Assessment Battery for Children, Second Edition (KABC-II; Kaufman & Kaufman, 2004a) and the Kaufman Brief Intelligence Test, Second Edition (KBIT-2; Kaufman & Kaufman, 2004b). The developers of the KABC and KBIT define *intelligence* in terms of a child's information-processing skills and problem-solving abilities. The test has been a helpful diagnostic tool for both normal and exceptional children. Individuals using either the PPVT-R or the KABC-II need training and supervision in the administration and interpretation of these instruments.

Children often are labeled or classified by intelligence test results, and extreme care is needed to avoid harming any child through the misuse of assessment measures. Hohenshil and Getz (2001) caution counselors in interpreting results for ethnic and cultural groups.

PROJECTIVE TECHNIQUES   Professionals sometimes ask children to respond to an unstructured stimulus, a picture, or a story to learn more about their thoughts and feelings. One projective technique, the Children's Apperception Test (CAT-A; Bellak & Bellak, 1949), uses animals as stimuli for children aged 3 to 10. An alternative form, the CAT-H (Bellak & Bellak, 1965), uses human figures. The administrator asks the children what they see when they are shown each card.

Trained professionals can use Draw-A-Person (DAP; Goodenough & Harris, 1963), the Kinetic Family Drawing (K-F-D; Burns & Kaufman, 1970), and the Kinetic House-Tree-Person Drawing (K-HTP; Burns, 1987) tests to learn more about the child's psychological functioning. They ask children to draw a person or their family on a blank sheet of paper, and these pictures reveal how children feel about themselves and the relationships among their family members.

The Tell-Me-A-Story (TEMAS; Constantino, Malgady, & Rogler, 1988) multicultural inventory for children between ages 5 and 13 has two sets of color pictures—one for European American children and another for Latino and African American young people. The children are asked to talk about what is happening in the pictures, what happened previously, and what will happen in the future. The stories are scored for cognitive, personality, and affective functions (Constantino, Malgady, & Rogler, 1988).

Projective tests are less commonly used than previously due to concerns about reliability and validity (Wicks-Nelson & Israel, 2013). Counselors do not ordinarily administer, score, or interpret projective instruments; however, counselors may need to be familiar with the tests to consult effectively with other professionals about their clients and families.

ACHIEVEMENT TESTS   Achievement tests are educational assessments that measure learning. These tests are standardized and well-normed. They are administered in a very structured, prescribed manner either in groups or individually. These instruments focus on the level of knowledge, skill, or accomplishment in a particular area—what the person currently knows or can do. A battery of achievement tests covers more than one academic area (reading, mathematics, language, and others).

Some of the more popular group-administered achievement tests used in kindergarten through grade 12 include these:

Iowa Test of Basic Skills, Form A (ITBS; Hoover, Hieronymus, Dunbar & Frisbee, 2001)

Stanford Achievement Test, Tenth Edition (Stanford-10; Harcourt Brace Educational Measurement, 2003)

TerraNova-2/CAT 6. (Seton Testing, 2005)

Some commonly used achievement tests that are administered individually are as follows:

Kaufman Test of Educational Achievement-Second Edition (KTES-II; Kaufman & Kaufman, 2005)

Peabody Individual Achievement Test-Revised (PIAT-R; Markwardt, 1998)

Wechsler Individual Achievement Test, Second Edition (WIAT-II; Wechsler, 2001)

Wide Range Achievement Test, Fourth Edition (WRAT4; Wilkinson & Robertson, 2006)

Woodcock-Johnson III Tests of Achievement (Woodcock, Mather, & McGrew, 2001)

The results of achievement tests can be used for placement of children or to determine educational areas of strengths and weaknesses.

APTITUDE TESTS   Aptitude tests are similar to achievement tests but are given to predict learning or behavior, for example, school or reading readiness. The Metropolitan Readiness Test, Sixth Edition (MRT-6; Nurss & McGauvran, 1995) measures children's school readiness in reading and mathematics. Other tests of general aptitude include:

Differential Aptitude Test, Fifth Edition (DAT; Bennett, Seashore, & Wesman, 1990)

O*Net Ability Profiler (U.S. Department of Labor, 2005)

Armed Services Vocational Aptitude Battery (ASVAB; United States Military Entrance Processing Command, 2005)

PERSONALITY TESTS   Objective personality tests allow counselors to understand the child's attitudes, characteristics, emotional, motivational, and interpersonal styles and needs. Some of these assessments focus on subsets of personality such as depression. A few of those instruments used with children are:

Beck Youth Inventories, Second Edition (BYI-II; Beck, Beck, & Jolly, 2005)

Children's Depression Inventory (CDI 2; Kovacs, 2010)

Multidimensional Anxiety Scale for Children (MASC 2; Marsh, n.d.)

Personality Inventory for Children-2 (PIC-2; Lachar & Gruber, 2001)

Personality Inventory for Youth (PIY; Lachar & Gruber, 1995)

Piers-Harris Children's Self-Concept Scale, Second Edition (Piers-Harris 2; Piers, Harris, &Herzberg, 2002)

OTHER TESTS   Counselors may want to administer other tests, surveys, or scales to learn more about a child's interests, values, study habits, social acceptance by peers, or the age appropriateness of their behaviors. Follow-up diagnostic testing in mathematics or reading may be helpful after the results of an initial intelligence or achievement test have been obtained. Special tests are available for children with exceptional conditions—children with learning disabilities, hearing or visual challenges, mental or emotional conditions, and others. The *Myers-Briggs*[1] Type *Indicator* (Myers, McCaulley, Quenk, & Hammer, 1998), a self-report instrument, may help students develop self-awareness and self-acceptance. Counselors select assessments according to the nature of the child's problem and the counseling objectives to be accomplished.

Before selecting any test for administration—and before accepting the results of any test—the user of assessment data should know whether the test is a good measure. At least two concepts give counselors an indication of the "goodness" of a particular instrument: validity and reliability. *Validity* is the extent to which a test measures what it is supposed to measure—intelligence, interests, achievement, or aptitude. A test that measures the child's current level of achievement in grade 2 is not a measure of the child's aptitude or intelligence; the test is valid only for measuring achievement. The *reliability* of a test indicates the consistency with which the test provides accurate measurements. Are the results of an intelligence test similar when the test is administered to the same child 2 days, 2 weeks, or 2 months apart? Correlation coefficients indicate the degree to which tests are valid and reliable. Counselors also need to know the type of population used in the process to determine the "normal" values. A test with normative data for children younger than 5 years is not appropriate for administration to a 6-year-old child. Complete information on validity and reliability, as well as a description of the norm group, can be found in the technical manuals that accompany tests, or the counselor can consult other references such as catalogs, journal reviews, *Tests in Print*, or *The Mental Measurement Yearbook*.

Counselors must be cautious in working in the area of assessment. Most are trained in interviewing, developing case histories, and behavioral observation. However, their training in assessment procedures varies, and counselors should administer and interpret only those tests for which they have received instruction. Practitioners who use assessment instruments must continue studying this area to keep current about new and revised instruments. Professionals can refer to their appropriate professional code of ethics to determine their roles in assessment and appraisal.

---

[1] Myers-Briggs Type Indicator is a trademark or registered trademark of the Myers-Briggs Type Indicator Trust in the United States and other countries.

SUMMARY

Consultation and collaboration are indirect ways to assist children in need. Helping techniques presented to significant people in children's lives through small groups, psychological education, outreach programs, and preventive education may reach children to whom a lone counselor's direct services would not be available. For our purposes, consultation refers to the one-to-one interaction between the counselor and a significant adult in the child's life or to a counselor-led group of significant adults, with the purpose of finding ways to assist children in functioning more effectively. Counselors will also have opportunities to work collaboratively with other health services and educational professionals, as well as other people who influence a child's life. In addition, the use of teamwork allows counselors to contribute to cooperative efforts on the behalf of young people. Another form of consultation and collaboration occurs when counselors use and/or interpret assessment instruments in their practice.

WEB SITES FOR CONSULTATION AND COLLABORATION

Internet addresses frequently change. To find the sites listed here, visit www.cengage .com/counseling/henderson for an updated list of Internet addresses and direct links to relevant sites.

Association for Supervision and Curriculum Development (ASCD)

Georgetown University Center for Child and Human Development

American Educational Research Association (AERA)

Association for Assessment and Research in Counseling and Education (AARC)

REFERENCES

Achenbach, T. M., & Rescorla, L. A. (2001). *Manual for the Achenbach system for empirically based assessment (ASEBA)*. Burlington, VT: University of Vermont, Research Center for Children, Youth, & Families.

Adelman, H. S., & Taylor, L. (2008). Best practices in the use of resource teams to enhance learning supports. In A. Thomas & J. Grimes (Eds.), *Best practices in school psychology* (5th ed., pp. 1689–1705). Bethesda, MD: National Association of School Psychologists.

Albee, G. W., & Fryer, D. M. (2003). Praxis: Toward a public health psychology. *Journal of Community & Applied Social Psychology, 13,* 71–75.

Auster, E. R., Feeney-Kettler, K. A., & Kratochwill, T. R. (2006). Conjoint behavioral consultation: Application to the school-based treatment of anxiety disorders. *Education and Treatment of Children, 29,* 243–256.

Bandura, A. (1977). *Social learning theory.* Englewood Cliffs, NJ: Prentice Hall.

Barnett, D., Hawkins, R., & Lentz, F. E., Jr. (2011). Intervention adherence for research and practice: Necessity or triage outcome? *Journal of Educational and Psychological Consultation, 21,* 175–190.

Bartholomew, N. G., Knight, D. K., Chatham, L. R., & Simpson, D. D. (2000). Partners in parenting. Retrieved from http://ibr.tcu.edu/manuals/partners-in-parenting-the-parenting-manual-2/

Beck, J. S., Beck, A. T., & Jolly, J. (2005). *Manual for the Beck youth inventories, second edition*. San Antonio, TX: Pearson.

Bellak, L., & Bellak, S. S. (1949). *Children's apperception test*. Larchmont, Lutz, FL: PAR.

Bellak, L., & Bellak, S. S. (1965). *Children's apperception test—human figures*. Lutz, FL: PAR.

Bennett, G. K., Seashore, H. G., & Wesman, A. G. (1990). *Manual for the differential aptitude test*. San Antonio, TX: Pearson.

Basham, A., Appleton, V., & Dykeman, C. (2004). Team building in educational settings. *Counseling and Human Development, 36*, 1–8.

Brigman, G., Mullis, R., Webb, L., & White, J. (2005). *School counselor consultation: Skills for working effectively with parents, teachers, and other school personnel*. Hoboken, NJ: Wiley.

Brown, D., Pryzwansky, W. B., & Schulte, A. C. (2006). *Psychological consultation and collaboration: Introduction to theory and practice* (6th ed.). Boston, MA: Pearson.

Brown, D., Pryzwansky, W. B., & Schulte, A. C. (2011). *Psychological consultation and collaboration: Introduction to theory and practice* (7th ed.). Boston, MA: Pearson.

Brown, D., & Trusty, J. (2005). *Designing and leading comprehensive school counseling programs: Promoting student competence and meeting student needs*. Belmont, CA: Brooks/Cole.

Burns, M. K., Wiley, H. I., & Viglietta, E. (2008). Best practices in implementing problem-solving teams. In A. Thomas & J. Grimes (Eds.), *Best practices in school psychology* (5th ed., pp. 1633–1644). Bethesda, MD: National Association of School Psychologists.

Burns, R. C. (1987). *Kinetic House-Tree-Person Drawings (K-HTP): An interpretative manual*. New York: Routledge.

Burns, R. C., & Kaufman, S. H. (1970). *Kinetic Family Drawings (K-F-D): An introduction to understanding children through kinetic drawing*. New York: Routledge.

Caplan, G., & Caplan, R. B. (1999). *Mental health consultation and collaboration*. San Francisco, CA: Jossey-Bass.

Caplan, G., & Caplan-Moskovich, R. B. (2004). Recent advances in mental health consultation. In N. M. Lambert, I. Hylander, & J. H. Sandoval (Eds.), *Consultee-centered consultation: Improving the quality of professional services in school and community organizations* (pp. 21–35). Mahwah, NJ: Erlbaum.

Clark, M. A., & Breman, J. C. (2009). School counselor inclusion: A collaborative model to provide academic and socio-emotional support in the classroom setting. *Journal of Counseling & Development, 87*, 6–11.

Connors, C. K. (2008). *Manual for the Connors' rating scales* (3rd ed.). North Tonawanda, NY: Multi-Health Systems.

Conoley, J. C., & Conoley, C. W. (2010). Why does collaboration work? Linking positive psychology and collaboration. *Journal of Educational and Psychological Consultation, 20*, 75–82.

Constantino, G., Malgady, R. G., & Rogler, L. H. (1988). *TEMAS (Tell-Me-A-Story)*. Los Angeles, CA: Western Psychological Services.

Curtis, M. J., & Stollar, S. A. (2002). Best practices in system-level change. In A. Thomas & J. Grimes (Eds.), *Best practices in school psychology* (4th ed., pp. 223–243). Washington, DC: National Association of School Psychologists.

Danforth, J. S. (1998). The behavior management flow chart: A component analysis of behavior management strategies. *Clinical Psychology Review, 18*, 229–257.

Dettmer, P. A., Knackendoffel, A. P., & Thurston, L. P. (2012). *Consultation, collaboration and teamwork for students with special needs* (7th ed.). Upper Saddle River, NJ: Pearson.

De Shazer, S. (1985). *Keys to solution in brief therapy*. New York: Norton.

Dinkmeyer, D., Jr., & Carlson, J. (2006). *Consultation: Creating school-based interventions* (3rd ed.). Philadelphia, PA: Brunner-Routledge.

Dougherty, A. M. (2013). *Psychological consultation and collaboration in school and community settings* (6th ed.). Belmont, CA: Brooks/Cole.

Dunn, L. M., & Dunn, L. M. (2006). PPVT-IV: *Peabody picture vocabulary test, fourth edition*. Bloomington, MN: Pearson Assessments.

Epstein, J. L., & Van Voorhis, F. L. (2010). School counselors' roles in developing partnerships with families and communities for student success. *Professional School Counseling, 14*, 1–14.

Esler, A. N., Godber, Y., & Christenson, S. L. (2008). Best practices in supporting home-school collaboration. In A. Thomas & J. Grimes (Eds.), *Best practices in school psychology* (5th ed., pp. 917–936). Bethesda, MD: National Association of School Psychologists.

Finello, K. M. (2011). Collaboration in the assessment and diagnosis of preschoolers: Challenges and opportunities. *Psychology in the Schools, 48*, 442–453.

Fox, R. A., & Fox, T. A. (1992). *Leader's guide: STAR parenting program.* Bellevue, WA: STAR Parenting.

Friend, M., & Cook, L. (2012). *Interactions: Collaboration skills for school professionals* (7th ed.). New York: Longman.

Gibbons, K. A., & Silberglitt, B. (2008). Best practices in evaluating psychoeducational services based on student outcome data. In A. Thomas & J. Grimes (Eds.), *Best practices in school psychology* (5th ed., pp. 2103–2116). Bethesda, MD: National Association of School Psychologists.

Glosoff, H., & Koprowicz, C. (1990). *Children achieving potential: An introduction to elementary school counseling and state-level policies.* Washington, DC: National Conference of State Legislatures and American Association for Counseling and Development.

Goodenough, D. B., & Harris, F. L. (1963). *The Goodenough Harris drawing test.* San Antonio, TX: PsychCorp.

Gravois, T. A., Groff, S., & Rosenfeld, S. (2009). Teams as value-added consultation services. In T. B. Gutkin & C. E. Reynolds (Eds.), *The handbook of school psychology* (4th ed., pp. 80–820). Hoboken, NJ: Wiley.

Guli, L. A. (2005). Evidence-based parent consultation with school-related outcomes. *School Psychology Quarterly, 20*, 455–472.

Gutkin, T. B. (2009). Ecological school psychology. In T. B. Gutkin & C. R. Reynolds (Eds.), *Handbook of school psychology* (4th ed., pp. 463–496). Hoboken, NJ: Wiley.

Gutkin, T. B. (2012). Ecological psychology: Replacing the medical model paradigm for school-based psychological and psychoeducational services. *Journal of Educational & Psychological Consultation, 22*(1–2), 1–20. doi:10.1080/10474412.2011.649652

Harrison, T. C. (2004). *Consultation for contemporary helping professionals.* Boston: Pearson.

Hohenshil, T. H., & Getz, H. (2001). Assessment, diagnosis, and treatment planning in counseling. In D. C. Locke, J. E. Myers, & E. I. Herr (Eds.), *The handbook of counseling* (pp. 269–285). Thousand Oaks, CA: Sage.

Holcomb-McCoy, C., & Bryan, J. (2010). Advocacy and empowerment in parent consultation: Implications for theory and practice. *Journal of Counseling and Development, 88*, 259–268.

Hoover, H. D., Hieronymus, A. N., Dunbar, S. B., & Frisbie, D. A. (2001). *Iowa Test of Basic Skills (ITBS).* Itasca, IL: Riverside Publishing.

Hughes, J. N., Hasbrouck, J. E., Serdahl, E., Heidgerken, A., & McHaney, L. (2001). Responsive systems consultation: A preliminary evaluation of implementation and outcomes. *Journal of Educational and Psychological Consultation, 12*, 179–201.

Ingraham, C. L. (2007). Focusing on consultees in multicultural consultation. In G. B. Esquivel, E. C. Lopez, & S. Nahari (Eds.), *Handbook of multicultural school psychology* (pp. 98–118). Mahwah, NJ: Erlbaum.

Ingraham, C. L. (2008). Studying multicultural aspects of consultation. In W. P. Erchul and S. M. Sheridan (Eds.), *Handbook of research in consultation* (pp. 269–291). New York: Erlbaum.

Johnson, D. B., Pedro-Carroll, J. L., & Demanchick, S. P. (2005). The Primary Mental Health Project: A play intervention for school-age children. In L. A. Reddy, T. M. Files-Hall, & C. E. Schaefer (Eds.), *Empirically based play interventions for children* (pp. 13–30). Washington, DC: American Psychological Association.

Kahn, B. B. (2000). A model of solution-focused consultation for school counselors. *Professional School Counseling, 3,* 248–254.

Kaufman, A. S., & Kaufman, N. L. (2004a). *KABC-II: Kaufman assessment battery for children* (2nd ed.). Bloomington, MN: Pearson Assessments.

Kaufman, A. S., & Kaufman, N. L. (2004b). *KBIT-2: Kaufman brief intelligence test* (2nd ed.). Bloomington, MN: Pearson Assessments.

Kaufman, A. S., & Kaufman, N. L. (2005). *KTEA-II: Kaufman test of educational achievement, second edition.* Bloomington, MN: Pearson Assessments.

Keys, S. G., Bemak, F., & Lockhart, E. J. (1998). Transforming school counseling to serve the mental health needs of at-risk youth. *Journal of Counseling and Development, 76,* 381–388.

Kirst-Ashman, K. K., & Hull, G. H., Jr. (2012). *Generalist practice with organizations and communities* (5th ed.). Belmont, CA: Brooks/Cole.

Knotek, S. E., & Sandoval, J. (2003). Current research in consultee-centered consultation. *Journal of Educational and Psychological Consultation, 4,* 243–250.

Kovacs, M. (2010). *CDI: Children's depression inventory 2.* San Antonio, TX: Pearson.

Kratochwill, T. R., Elliott, S. N., & Callan-Stoiber, K. (2002). Best practices in school-based problem-solving consultation. In A. Thomas & J. Grimes (Eds.), *Best practices in school psychology* (4th ed., pp. 438–608). Washington, DC: National Association of School Psychologists.

Kurpius, D., & Fuqua, D. (1993). Fundamental issues in defining consultation. *Journal of Counseling and Development, 70,* 598–600.

Kurpius, D., Fuqua, D., & Rozecki, T. (1993). The consulting process: A multidimensional approach. *Journal of Counseling and Development, 7,* 601–606.

Lachar, D., & Gruber, C. P. (1995). *Manual for the personality inventory for youth.* Los Angeles, CA: Western Psychological Services.

Lachar, D., & Gruber, C. P. (2001). *Manual for the personality inventory for children, second edition.* Los Angeles, CA: Western Psychological Services.

MacLeod, I. R., Jones, K. M., Somers, C. L., & Havey, J. M. (2001). An evaluation of the effectiveness of school-based behavioral consultation. *Journal of Educational and Psychological Consultation, 12,* 203–216.

Markwardt, F. C., Jr. (1998). *Peabody individual achievement test* (Rev. ed.). Bloomington, MN: Pearson Assessments.

Marsh, J. S. (n.d.). *MASC: Multidimensional anxiety scale for children 2.* North Tonawanda, NY: Multi-Health Systems.

Myers, I. B., McCaulley, M. H., Quenk, N. L., & Hammer, A. L. (1998). *MBTI Manual: A guide to the development and use of the Myers-Briggs Type Indicator* (3rd ed.). Palo Alto, CA: Consulting Psychologists Press.

Myrick, R. D. (2011). *Developmental guidance and counseling: A practical approach* (5th ed.). Minneapolis, MN: Educational Media.

Nelson, G., Amio, J. L., Prilleltensky, I., & Nickels, P. (2000). Partnerships for implementing school and community prevention programs. *Journal of Educational and Psychological Consultation, 11,* 121–145.

Nicholson, B., Anderson, M., Fox, R., & Brenner, V. (2002). One family at a time: A prevention program for at-risk parents. *Journal of Counseling and Development, 80,* 362–371.

Nurss, J., & McGauvran, M. (1995). *Metropolitan readiness tests, sixth edition (MRT6)*. San Antonio, TX: Psychological Press.

Otis, A. S., & Lennon, R. T. (2004). *Manual for the Otis-Lennon School Ability Test, eighth edition (OLSAT-8)*. Bloomington, MN: Pearson Assessment.

Paisley, P. O., & Milsom, A. (2007). Group work as an essential contribution to transforming school counseling. *Journal of Specialists in Group Work, 32*, 9–17.

Persi, J. (1997). When emotionally troubled teachers refer emotionally troubled students. *The School Counselor, 44*, 344–352.

Piers, E. V., Harris, D. B., & Herzberg, D. S. (2002). *Piers-Harris children's self-concept scale, second edition*. Los Angeles, CA: Western Psychological Press.

Porter, G., Epp, L., & Bryant, S. (2000). Collaboration among school mental health professionals: A necessity, not a luxury. *Professional School Counseling, 3*, 315–322.

Reynolds, C. R., & Kamphaus, R. W. (2002). *A clinician's guide to the behavior assessment system for children*. New York: Guilford.

Reynolds, C. R., & Kamphaus, R. W. (2004). *Manual for the behavior assessment system for children* (2nd ed.). Bloomington, MN: Pearson Assessments.

Roid, G. H. (2003). *Stanford-Binet intelligence scales, fifth edition*. Itasca, IL: Riverside.

Sandoval, J. (2014). *An introduction to consultee-centered consultation in the schools: A step-by-step guide to the process and skills*. New York: Routledge.

Schein, E. (1988). *Process consultation: Vol. 1. Its role in organization development* (2nd ed.). Reading, MA: Addison-Wesley.

Schein, E. (1999). *Process consultation revisited: Building the helping relationship*. Menlo Part, CA: Addison-Wesley.

Scott, D. A., Royal, C. W., & Kissinger, D. B. (2015). *Counselor as consultant*. Thousand Oaks, CA: Sage Publishing.

Shapiro, J. P., Friedberg, R. D., & Bardenstein, K. K. (2006). *Child and adolescent therapy: Science and art*. Hoboken, NJ: Wiley.

Sheridan, S. M. (2000). Considerations of multiculturalism and diversity in behavior consultation with parents and teachers. *School Psychology Review, 29*, 344–353.

Sheridan, S. M., Eagle, J. W., & Doll, B. (2006). An examination of the efficacy of conjoint behavioral consultation with diverse clients. *School Psychology Review, 41*, 23–46.

Sladeczek, I. E., Elliott, S. N., Kratochwill, T. R., Robertson-Mjaanes, S., & Stoiber, K. C. (2001). Application of goal attainment scaling to a conjoint behavioral consultation case. *Journal of Educational and Psychological Consultation, 12*, 45–58.

Sparrow, S. S., Cicchetti, D. V., & Balla, D. A. (2005). *Vineland adaptive behavior scales, second edition (Vineland-II)*. Bloomington, MN: Pearson Assessments.

Stanford Achievement Test-Tenth Edition (Standford 10). (2003). Bloomington, MN: Pearson Assessment.

Taylor, L., & Adelman, H. S. (2000). Connecting schools, families, and communities. *Professional School Counseling, 3*, 298–307.

TerraNova 2/CAT 6. (2005). Front Royal, VA: Seton Testing Company.

United States Department of Labor. (2005). *O*NET work importance profiler*. Retrieved from http://www.onetcenter.org.

United States Military Entrance Processing Command. (2005). *Armed Services Vocational Aptitude Battery (ASVAB)*. Retrieved from http://official-asvab.com/counselors.htm.

Wagner, P. (2000). Consultation: Developing a comprehensive approach to service delivery. *Educational Psychology in Practice, 16*, 9–18.

Wagner, W. G. (2008). *Counseling, psychology, and children*. Upper Saddle River, NJ: Pearson.

Wechsler, D. (1999). *Manual for the Wechsler abbreviated scale of intelligence*. San Antonio, TX: Pearson.

Wechsler, D. (2001). *Manual for the Wechsler individual achievement test* (2nd ed.). San Antonio, TX: Pearson.

Wechsler, D. (2002). *Manual for the Wechsler preschool and primary school scale of intelligence* (3rd ed.). San Antonio, TX: Pearson.

Wechsler, D. (2003). *Manual for the Wechsler intelligence scale for children* (4th ed.). San Antonio, TX: Pearson.

White, J., Mullis, F., Early, B., & Brigman, G. (1995). *Consultation in schools: The counselor's role*. Portland, ME: Weston Walch.

Wicks-Nelson, R., & Israel, A. C. (2013). *Behavior disorders of childhood* (8th ed.). Upper Saddle River, NJ: Pearson.

Wilkinson, G. S., & Robertson, G. J. (2006). *Manual for the wide range achievement test, fourth edition*. Lutz, FL: Psychological Assessment Resources.

Woodcock, R., Mather, N., & McGrew, K. (2001). *Woodcock-Johnson III tests of achievement*. Itasca, IL: Riverside.

Yetter, G. (2010). Assessing the acceptability of problem-solving procedures by school teams: Preliminary development of the pre-referral intervention team inventory. *Journal of Educational and Psychological Consultation, 20*, 139–168.

Young, H. L., & Gaughan, E. (2010). A multiple method longitudinal investigation of pre-referral intervention team functioning: Four years in rural schools. *Journal of Educational and Psychological Consultation, 20*, 106–138.

Young, M. A., & Basham, A. (2010). Consultation and supervision. In B. T. Erford (Ed.), *Orientation to the counseling profession: Advocacy, ethics, and essential professional foundations* (pp. 193–213). Upper Saddle River, NJ: Merrill.

Ysseldyke, J. E., Burns, M., & Rosenfield, S. (2009). Blueprints on the future of training and practice in school psychology. What do they say about educational and psychological consultation? *Journal of Educational and Psychological Consultation, 19*, 177–196.

PART III

COUNSELING WITH CHILDREN: SPECIAL TOPICS

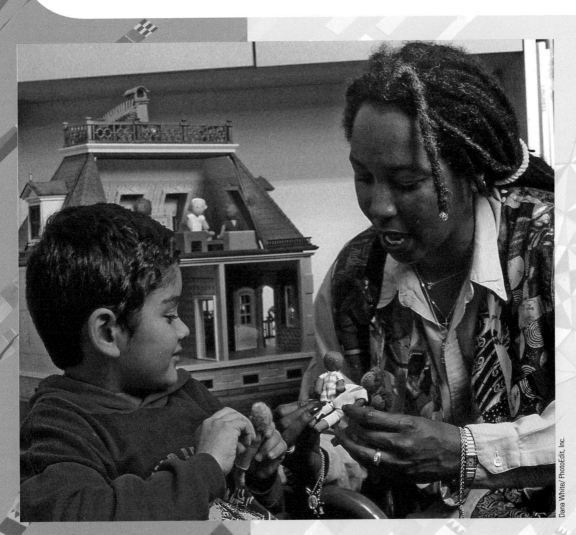

Dana White/ PhotoEdit, Inc.

CHAPTER 17

Play Therapy

You can discover more about a person in an hour of play than in a year of conversation.
—PLATO

Rather than Freud's "talking cure" as a descriptor of therapy, Kaduson, Cangelosi, and Schaefer (1997) proposed "playing cure" as more appropriate to describe therapy with children. In fact, Brown and Vaughan (2009) states that play is as necessary as oxygen for the well-being of human beings. Play is "the child's natural medium of self expression" according to Virginia Axline (1947, p. 9) in her classic book *Play Therapy: The Inner Dynamics of Childhood.*

The Association for Play Therapy (2014) explains the importance of play. Play is the opposite of work. It has no purpose other than itself. Play is an enjoyable activity, freely chosen, and unconstrained. Play lifts spirits and brightens outlooks. Play evokes self-expression, self-knowledge, self-actualization, and self-efficacy. Play eases stress and boredom, connects us to people, stimulates creative thinking, encourages exploration, moderates emotions, and boosts ego (Landreth, 2012). Play provides a context to practice skills and roles needed for life. Play is fun, a way to learn and grow. Webb (2007) noted that in spite of the differences in theory and treatment approach, play therapists all agree on the unique meaning of play to children.

After reading this chapter, you should be able to:

▶ Outline the history of play therapy
▶ Define and explain the goals of play therapy
▶ List the advantages and diversity applications of play therapy
▶ Demonstrate the skills of play therapy
▶ Discuss some play therapy strategies

INTRODUCTION

Heidemann and Hewitt (2010) explain that play skills are life skills, social skills used throughout life. These authors dub play "the main event" in children's lives. While playing children learn to communicate and explore. They learn things like the language of emotions, their own feelings as well as their likes and dislikes. Children think during play using mental pictures, curiosity, and problem-solving in their pretend land. In addition, during play children organize themselves and plan. Schaefer (2011) notes the corresponding therapeutic powers of play in eight categories: communication, emotional regulation, relationship enhancement, moral judgment, stress management, ego boosting, preparation for life, and self-actualization. Each of these will be discussed in a later section.

Schaefer (1993) has identified other common characteristics of play. He stated that play is pleasurable and, therefore, intrinsically motivating. During play the child is often engrossed in it and more concerned with the play itself than with the end result. Play is not literal—it has a make-believe quality. Play is flexible. It has the power to enhance normal development and alleviate abnormal behavior. The child feels comfortable when playing. Play is a natural way for children to express themselves, to act out sensitive material, to gain security, and to increase their self-confidence. Another significant attribute of play is that it is free from evaluation and judgment by adults so that children are safe to make mistakes (Sweeney, 2001).

Landreth (2012) explains that play is children's symbolic language and provides a way for them to express their experiences and emotions in a natural, self-healing process. "A child's play is his talk and toys are his words," proposed Ginott (1994, p. 33), who believed that in manipulating toys, children can show more adequately than through words how they feel about themselves and people and events in life. Play is the child's language (Landreth, 2012). Bettelheim (1987, p. 35) said that "play is the royal road to the child's conscious and unconscious world; if we want to understand his inner world and help him with it, we must learn to walk this road." Play therapy allows counseling a way to undertake that journey.

HISTORY OF PLAY THERAPY

Some people consider play therapy a relatively new phenomenon. However, the practice of using play as a medium for treatment has roots from 1799, according to Carmichael (2006). Most trace the early work in play therapy to Sigmund Freud, Hermine Hug-Hellmuth, Anna Freud, Melanie Klein, and Margaret Lowenfeld. Their contributions are outlined in the following section.

Sigmund Freud (1909) wrote about his work with Little Hans, thus introducing the idea of play in the practice of therapy. Freud wrote that play serves the purposes of promoting freer expression, fulfilling wishes, and mastering traumatic events. Children work through catastrophic events by reenacting the crisis, gaining a sense of power over it. Children may relive repressed memories by bringing them to consciousness and appropriately releasing the previously subjugated emotions. Abreaction refers to this reliving and mastery of the traumatic experience. It is different than catharsis which refers only to the release of emotion. (Erwin, 2001). Freud connected play to abreaction.

Hermine Hug-Hellmuth (1921) was the first therapist to use play with children. She did not create a method of play therapy but used play as the basis of analysis. She also identified three things that make children different clients than adults: the child does not come willingly, the child is suffering from present rather than past experiences, and the child does not want to give up being difficult (Carmichael, 2006; Landreth, 2012).

Anna Freud (1926) played games, recorded dreams and stories, and created toys to encourage children to participate in treatment and to reveal their secrets to her. Anna Freud emphasized building a relationship with children by playing with them before interpreting their motivations. She used fantasies and dreams and interpretation in her therapy with children (Carmichael, 2006; Landreth, 2012).

Melanie Klein (1932) used play as a way to uncover children's motivations. She explained that children, through the use of play and drawings, projected their feelings and that therapists could understand children's unconscious lives by considering their nonverbal behavior. Klein encouraged children to express their fantasies, anxieties, and defenses and then she interpreted those play activities. She attempted to relieve children of disabling guilt by having them transfer to the therapist the aggressive feelings they could not express to their parents.

A contemporary of Klein and Anna Freud, Margaret Lowenfeld (1935, 1991) believed play therapy allowed children to work through and master emotions and cognitions. She focused on the child's ability to make sense of the world. She used the *world technique* and *mosaic test* as concrete ways to see how children reason. In the world technique, children have the opportunity to create an imaginary world in which they can express whatever they want. The worlds may be realistic or fantastic, peaceful or aggressive, orderly or chaotic (Lowenfeld, 1939). Hug-Hellmuth, Klein, Anna Freud, and Lowenfeld paved the way for contemporary play therapy.

Other people have also influenced the history of play therapy. Release therapy (Levy, 1938) was used to reenact a traumatic incident, and active play therapy (Solomon, 1938) provides a way to redirect acting-out behavior into more socially appropriate behavior. Moustakas (1959) patterned structured play therapy after release therapy. Rank (1936), Allen (1942), and Taft (1933) explained the importance of the relationship with the child as a curative factor. Bixler (1949) wrote "Limits Are Therapy," an article focused on the idea that properly set limits allow children to develop a sense of security and trust. Most importantly, Virginia Axline (1969), a student and colleague of Carl Rogers, developed child-centered play therapy based on eight principles that continue to guide the practice of play therapy and counseling children.

1. A counselor is genuinely interested in the child and develops a warm, friendly relationship as quickly as possible.
2. The counselor accepts the child exactly as he or she is and does not wish the child were different.
3. The therapist establishes a feeling of safety and permissiveness so the child feels free to explore and express.
4. The practitioner is alert to the child's feelings and gently reflects those feelings back to the child so that he or she can develop self-understanding.
5. The counselor believes in the child's capacity to be responsible and to solve problems and allows the child to do so.

6. The therapist trusts the child's inner direction and allows the child to lead.
7. The therapist allows the gradual nature of the treatment to unfold and does not hurry.
8. The counselor sets up on the limits that are necessary to anchor the session in reality and to help the child accept responsibility (Landreth, 2012, p. 80).

Table 17-1 contains a brief summary of these historical events in the history of play therapy.

DEFINING PLAY THERAPY

Play therapy is a helping interaction between a trained adult and a child in order to relieve the child's distress. It is a structured, theoretically based approach to therapy. Play therapy uses the normal communicative and learning processes of children in a way that allows the therapist to help children address and hopefully resolve their problems (Axline, 1947; Carmichael, 2006; Landreth, 2012; O'Connor & Schaefer, 1994). The benefits of play therapy include children learning to communicate, express feelings, change behavior, develop skills, and master a variety of relationship skills. With play children have a safe psychological distance from their problems and a way to express their thoughts and feelings. The emphasis should not be placed on the word *play*, but on the word *therapy* (Carmichael, 2006).

Play therapists choose play therapy techniques to help children express what is troubling them when they lack the words to express their thoughts and feelings (Gil, 1991). In summary, the Association for Play Therapy defines play therapy as "the systematic use of a theoretical model to establish an interpersonal process wherein trained play therapists use the therapeutic powers of play to help clients prevent or resolve psychosocial difficulties and achieve optimal growth and development" (http://www.a4pt.org/?page=PTMakesADifference).

TABLE 17-1 HISTORY OF PLAY THERAPY

H. Hug-Hellmuth (1921)	First used play directly in sessions with children
Melanie Klein (1932)	Incorporated play into treatment to encourage expression of fantasies, anxieties, and defenses, which she then interpreted
Anna Freud (1926)	Used play as a way to build a child's attachment to the therapist and to gain access into the child's unconscious
Margaret Lowenfeld (1935)	Saw play as a way for children to work on and master their thoughts and feelings; world technique and mosaic test used as indicators of how children reason
David Levy (1938)	Release play therapy, structured play for children who had suffered a specific stress; children reenact the experience
Jesse Taft (1933) Frederick Allen (1942)	Relationship therapy built on work of Otto Rank (1936) that stressed the development of the counselor–client relationship as the curative component in therapy
Virginia Axline (1947)	Applied client-centered therapy principles, such as the belief in a person's capacity to grow, to children

Goals of Play Therapy

Webb (2007) explained that as well as working for symptom relief, play therapists attempt to remove barriers to children's development and future growth. Therefore, goals of therapy are twofold—lessened symptoms and enhanced development. Carmichael (2006) and Pedro-Carroll and Reddy (2005) included goals of providing children with skills and experiences to help overcome behavioral difficulties, adjustment problems, trauma, or deficits in emotional or social skills. Kottman (2009) included building a sense of competence by allowing children to do things for themselves and make decisions in the play relationship. Kottman listed the typical goals of play therapy:

- Boost self-acceptance, self-confidence, and self-reliance
- Facilitate learning about self and others
- Explore and express feelings
- Encourage ability to make good decisions
- Arrange opportunities to practice control and responsibility
- Explore alternative views of problems and relationships
- Learn and practice problem-solving and relationship skills
- Increase feeling vocabulary and emotional concepts (p. 540)

The positive relationship that develops between therapist and child during play therapy sessions provides a corrective emotional experience necessary for healing (Moustakas, 1997). Play therapy may also be used to promote cognitive development and provide insight about and resolution of inner conflicts or dysfunctional thinking in the child (Drewes & Schaefer, 2010).

The theory from which the play therapist works would also dictate more specific goals. LaBauve, Watts, and Kottman (2001) provided an overview of approaches to play therapy that included their goals. Adlerian play therapy focuses on the reduction of discouragement, increase of social interest, the recognition of strengths, and improvement of behavior. Cognitive-behavioral play therapy goals are to shift thinking from irrational to rational. Gestalt play therapy attempts to restore the child to a pattern of growth. The chapters on counseling theories in this book provide further descriptions of the process and goals of play therapy.

Therapeutic Advantages of Play Therapy

Schaefer (1993) and Schaefer and Drewes (2009) outlined 14 therapeutic powers of play and the beneficial outcome of each, which Kottman (2011) and Sweeney (2001) interpreted. They are as follows:

1. **Overcoming resistance:** Play draws children into a working alliance with the counselor since many children do not make the choice to enter counseling.
2. **Communication:** Play provides a natural medium of self-expression. Counselors convey their respect by being willing to "speak" in the child's language. Watching the child's activity and choices provides the counselor with a quick and smooth understanding.
3. **Competence:** Play satisfies the need to explore and master, thereby building self-esteem. Counselors build confidence by pointing out that the child is working hard and making progress.

4. **Creative thinking:** Problem-solving skills are encouraged so that innovative solutions to dilemmas can occur. Play provides opportunities for creativity and imaginative solutions.
5. **Catharsis:** Children can release strong emotions they have had difficulty confronting. The sense of relief can be an experience that leads to growth for the child.
6. **Abreaction:** In play, children can process and adjust to difficulties by symbolically reliving them with appropriate emotional expression. Play gives children a place to reenact and gain a sense of mastery over the negative experience.
7. **Role-play:** Children can practice new behaviors and develop empathy for others.
8. **Fantasy:** Children use their imagination to make sense of painful reality. They can also experiment with the possibility of changing their lives, a process that instills hope.
9. **Metaphoric teaching:** Children gain insight by facing their conflicts and fears through the metaphors generated in play. Stories, play, and artwork can be used to look at situations differently.
10. **Attachment formation:** Children develop a bond with the counselor and learn to increase their connections with others.
11. **Relationship enhancement:** Play enhances the positive therapeutic relationship, allowing children to move toward self-actualization and grow closer to others. The children begin to believe they are worthy of love and positive attention.
12. **Positive emotion:** Children enjoy playing. They can laugh and have a good time in an accepting place.
13. **Mastering developmental fears:** Repeated play activities help reduce anxiety and fear. By working with toys, art supplies, and other play media, children can recognize their skills for coping with fear and for taking care of themselves.
14. **Game play:** Games help children socialize and develop ego strength. They have opportunities to expand their interaction skills.

Carmichael (2006) and Reddy, Files-Hall, and Schaefer (2005) explained that play therapy is the treatment of choice in mental health, school, agency, developmental, hospital, residential, and recreational settings, with clients of all ages. Reddy et al. summarized that play therapy research supports the effectiveness of play therapy with children experiencing a wide variety of social, emotional, behavioral, and learning problems. Play therapy helps children:

- Become more responsible for behaviors and develop more successful strategies.
- Develop new and creative solutions to problems.
- Develop respect and acceptance of self and others.
- Learn to experience and express emotion.
- Cultivate empathy and respect for thoughts and feelings of others.
- Learn new social skills and relational skills with family.
- Develop self-efficacy and thus a better assuredness about their abilities (https://a4pt.site-ym.com/?PTMakesADifference).

Henniger (1995) proposed that play could serve as an antidote to childhood stress, and Albon (1996) recognized that play allows children to expose and explore troublesome emotions. Fall (1999) investigated child-centered interventions in the school setting with children with poor coping skills and had positive results during the six sessions of play therapy. Bratton and Ray (2000) summarized further support in their review of the case study research in this field. They summarized 82 studies and presented the effectiveness of play therapy with several specific issues and populations.

Diversity Applications of Play Therapy

One valuable benefit of play therapy is that it is applicable within and across many groups. The play counselor who is careful to understand the traditions of a particular culture or ethnic group will be able to provide culturally sensitive interventions (Chang, Ritter, & Hays, 2005; Gil & Drewes, 2005). As outlined in a previous chapter, counselors need to consider several variables to understand the child's world. The degree of acculturation of the child and family, in-groups and out-groups, age, gender, religion, spirituality and philosophy, and communication patterns all impact perceptions and customs the child brings to the play therapy setting. Language boundaries are obvious differences as are the limits of roles, status, inclusion, race, tribe, family, identity, self-concept, time, and individualism (Chang et al., 2005; Kottman, 2011).

Drewes (2005) admonishes counselors who are play therapists to become more culturally sensitive and improve their knowledge about cultures and the ways play and therapy are viewed. Play therapists should expand the understanding of cultures and increase their flexibility in working with a variety of issues. She stresses the need to consider these factors that greatly impact work with culturally diverse clients:

1. The importance of family
2. Issues of privacy, trust, and beliefs
3. English as a second language
4. Culturally related syndromes
5. Personal space, eye contact, and nonverbal expressions

Carmichael (2006) reminded play therapists that knowing about a child's culture helps build relationships with the parents and child. She suggested counselors may expand their offer of confidentiality to the extended family or other caretakers. She also pointed out that consulting with other healers in the community helps clients and counselors. Finding bridges between present and future time orientations may also be a need in counseling diverse clients. Carmichael recommended play therapy interventions across a continuum from nondirective to directive to meet the needs of diverse children.

Some authors have described play materials for particular groups such as Japanese (Ji, Ramirez, & Kranz, 2008), Chinese (Kao & Landreth, 2001), and Korean children (Kim & Nahm, 2008). The selection of toy materials should always be guided by sensitivity to cultural issues and the need to include materials and toys that show respect for cultural groups. Hinman (2003) and Gil and Drewes (2005) have extensive lists of culture-specific possibilities.

O'Connor (2009) cautioned play therapists to be aware of problems that may interfere. He began by emphasizing the obvious difficulty of discussing ethnic groups as having particular characteristics. The generalizations that are identified may not apply to specific children or parents. In addition, some of the basic assumptions of play therapy may conflict with the values of some cultures. One conflict is that play is similar across cultures. Another problem is the play therapists often encourage children to express feelings as a step toward problem solving and conflict resolution; but some cultures avoid direct expression of emotions and handle conflict indirectly. In addition, the interpretation of nonverbal communications by the child or by the therapist may be compromised. O'Connor noted that most play therapy practiced in the United States is unstructured, not goal oriented, and based on a causal relationship. Parents may be troubled and find it incomprehensible that playing with a child will help resolve problems. Another conflict emerges when therapists expect the parents and child to voluntarily disclose problems to the therapist, a practice that is inconsistent with the values and customs of some cultural groups. One last conflict occurs when the linear and logical problem solving valued by Western groups is uncomfortable with the more intuitive and holistic approach of some other groups.

Kottman (2011) and Glover (2001) provided the following specifics for working with children from multicultural populations:

1. Respect the historical, psychological, sociological, and political aspects of the child's culture. The counselor may gather information about and gain experience of the culture. Play materials should be chosen to express respect for cultural differences. Carmichael (2006) provided these guidelines: check images and dolls to be sure ethnic diversity is represented; do not use objects that are sacred to a group in a profane manner; and avoid stereotypes in selecting toys.
2. Investigate the role of play in diverse populations in order to avoid comments or interpretations that may violate the cultural standards. Stock the playroom with toys appropriate for the self-expression of a child in that particular group.
3. Become familiar with the values, beliefs, customs, and traditions of a child's culture, paying particular attention to language differences, roles, and acculturation.
4. Seek a match between the child's cultural background and the appropriate techniques to us with the child in play therapy.
5. Recognize the ongoing process of becoming culturally competent.
6. Examine the appropriateness of the philosophical basis of the play therapy theory to determine whether there is a mismatch with cultural values.
7. Be aware of your own personal cultural biases, values, beliefs, and attitudes.
8. Interact with multicultural populations and consult with healers in the community.

As well as working with children, play therapy counselors will want to include parents in the treatment. The counselor may ask parents about their background, such as their traditions, celebrations, and religion. Gonzalez-Mena (2012) provides one way of understanding a home environment. That author explained two opposing goals of parenting styles—individualism versus connectedness. Parents who value individualism will work to help the child develop autonomy and self-help skills. The parent may encourage the idea of passion, making choices, and expression of feelings. Independence, self-assurance, competence, and a sense of specialness may be emphasized with this type of parenting. Parenting to maintain connections emphasizes interdependence as the greatest value. Parents may promote peace and harmony among family members rather than independence and autonomy because humility and humbleness are valued. Worthiness is connected to fitting in, belonging, and putting others first. Counselors working with children from diverse cultures will want to seek out other helpful explanations.

The counselor who uses play therapy must begin by considering personal characteristics that may indicate the child's and the counselor's suitability for that type of intervention. Then, by considering the varying theoretical approaches to play therapy, the counselor can construct an understanding of that process. Awareness of the stages of play therapy, criteria for the selection of play materials, and examples of play therapy techniques will contribute to a foundation for integrating play into counseling practices.

Children Appropriate for Play Therapy

Kottman (2009) identifies most play therapy clients as children younger than 12 years of age as the theory of choice. Older children and adults may also benefit from participation (Demanchick, Cochran, & Cochran, 2003). They suggest that counselors ask the children whether they would rather sit and talk or play with toys, especially with older elementary children, preadolescents, and young teens. Older children may be interested in working with craft supplies, carpentry tools, office supplies and equipment, and more complex games or games created for intervention purposes (Kottman).

Anderson and Richards (1995) directed counselors to begin by assessing the following capabilities of the potential client:

1. The ability to tolerate/build/use a relationship with an adult
2. The ability to tolerate/accept a protective environment
3. The capacity to learn new ways of coping
4. The potential to gain new insight and the motivation to try
5. The attention span and cognitive organization to participate

Those authors also admonish counselors to consider whether play therapy is an effective way to address this particular child's concern and whether conditions in the child's environment will impede the play therapy process. A limited ability in the five things mentioned in the list or a negative answer to the other considerations would imply that play therapy would not be the appropriate choice for that child.

The Play Therapist

Kottman (2011), Landreth (2012), and Schaefer (2011) stress that counselors cannot learn play therapy by reading a book or attending a workshop. Play therapy requires the counselor to think differently in order to communicate through play and toys. Concentrated training and practice are needed to master the knowledge and skills needed. The Association for Play Therapy, the Canadian Association for Child and Play Therapy, and Play Therapy International all have certification standards for education and clinical experience.

Cattanach (2008) commented on various ways to be a play therapist. Whatever theoretical choice a counselor makes, keeping the child safe in the play therapy process is the top priority. She emphasized that the counselor is responsible for the process and should have appropriate training and continuing supervision. The play therapist needs to understand the developmental processes of the child and needs to learn to play in ways to stimulate the child's participation. The counselor's style of interacting depends on the children who are clients, as well as the personality and skills of the counselor and the level of his or her training.

Landreth (2012) identified the principles that guide a client-centered play therapist and seem applicable across several theoretical approaches. The guidelines include the therapist being interested in the child as well as being warm, caring, and accepting. The therapist creates an environment of safety and allows the child opportunities to express freely. Landreth emphasized the play therapist is an adult who "intently observes, empathically listens, and encouragingly recognizes not only the child's play but also the child's wants, needs, and feelings" (p. 97). The therapist trusts the child's inner directions and respects the child's capacity to act responsibly. The counselor is objective and flexible, unwilling to judge, tolerant of ambiguity, and willing to follow the child. Patience and courage are also required.

Some (Kottman, 2011; Landreth, 2012; Schaefer & Greenberg, 1997) identify the personal characteristics and personality of the counselor as key elements in the play therapy process. According to these authors, the effective play therapist will most likely be a person who has the following qualities:

a. Appreciation of children, treating them with a respectful, kind manner
b. A sense of humor and willingness to laugh at self
c. Playful and fun-loving attitude
d. Self-confidence and self-reliance
e. Openness and honesty
f. Accepting
g. Willingness to use play and metaphors as communication tools
h. Flexibility and ability to deal with ambiguity
i. Comfort with children and experience interacting with them
j. Ability to set limits and maintain personal boundaries
k. Self-aware

Ray (2010) notes the knowledge base needed for play therapists. She says these counselors need to know child development theories, both the historical and the current understanding of how children change, particularly important are the history and role of play in child development. Information about common drugs prescribed for children, educational practices, parenting methods, and current research on childhood and mental health issues must be mastered by play therapists. Counselors should also be familiar with the diagnostic criteria, symptoms, prognosis, and current research on childhood disorders. Finally, play therapists need the knowledge to critically analyze and synthesize the literature and research on working with children. Ray (2011) acknowledges the fundamental skills of play therapists as silence, focus, organization, and strong conceptualization of the complexities of the child client.

Anderson and Richards (1995) recommended counselors who are considering the use of play therapy ask themselves these questions:

1. Do I have the necessary skills? Is supervision or consultation available if I need it?
2. Is my office suitable (such as do I have adequate space, treatment duration, and funding issues) for effectively treating this child?
3. If I need to work with other professionals with this case, do I have the skills and knowledge needed?
4. Are my energy or stress levels adequate for me to commit to working with this child?

Kottman (2009) recommended that if play therapists can answer yes to the above questions, they are ready to begin counseling the child.

Play Stages

Nash and Schaefer (2011) identify three main stages to play therapy. Early session focus on *rapport building* with the child and counselor building a working relationship. The therapist is learning about the child and the child is learning about the play space and process of counseling. These sessions are often supportive, allowing the child time to feel safe and become comfortable. The second stage is *working through* the time in which therapeutic change evolves. During this time the therapist selects and applies the theory and techniques designed to create for the child an environment for resolving problems. Play themes often become evident, allowing the counselor to see the child's inner world. Nash and Schaefer explain the themes reappear across sessions. They suggest common themes are aggression, attachment, competition, control, cooperation, traumatic events, death/grief/loss, fears, repairing something that is broken, gender, good versus evil, identity, limits, mastery, need for approval, power, problem solving, regression, reenactment, school, sexuality, rules, transitions, vulnerability, and win/lose circumstances. The use of the themes will be determined based on the theoretical approach (p. 9). The final stage of play therapy is *termination*, in which the child takes ownership of the changes and further improvements.

Orton (1997) presented an integrated approach to the therapeutic play process that moves through five stages: (1) relationship, (2) release, (3) re-creation, (4) re-experiencing, and (5) resolving. Through this process, a strong relationship is built in which the child feels accepted and understood. The child uses play to release feelings and to ease tension through cathartic release. As the relationship grows, the child begins to explore significant events or relationships that trigger uncomfortable thoughts and feelings. Children begin to understand the links between past events and to connect that knowledge with current thoughts, behaviors, and feelings. The final stage is reached when children are able to act on the understanding and to experiment with various solutions.

Theories of Play Therapy

Many of the theories discussed earlier in this book include descriptions of play therapy that are directly related to the theories presented. Some other practices of play therapy are briefly outlined in the following section.

ECOSYSTEMIC PLAY THERAPY   O'Connor (2011) explained a model of ecosystemic play therapy that he described as a hybrid approach that integrates biology, several theories of psychotherapy (psychoanalysis, child-centered, and cognitive-behavioral), and developmental concepts. The child's interactions and experiences in the world as well as the internal, symbolic world of the child are emphasized in this type of play therapy. Based on the biological term *ecosystem*, which means the total environment that influences the subject being studied (Carmichael, 2006), the therapy model contains a comprehensive model of case conceptualization and intervention. O'Connor and Ammen (1997) expanded this description and provided a workbook for counselors to use in implementing this type of play therapy.

One key element of the theory is the ecosystemic worldview, the perspective that community and environment form nested systems in which an individual exists. The basic unit of the model, however, is the individual rather than the system. The counselor considers all the systems when conceptualizing the child's problem and the treatment plan. The goal of the intervention is to help children have their needs met without interfering with the ability of other people to get their needs met. The strategies that are used are aimed at altering the problem, the child's view of the problem, and the child's response to the problem. The ultimate goal is to help the child change beliefs that are causing difficulties (Carmichael, 2006). O'Connor (2009) further explained working on complementary levels of experience/behavior and cognitive/emotional to help the child. As the child becomes reflective about his or her behavior in the relationship systems, he or she may choose alternative ways of behaving. Symbolic play facilitates this reflective process.

The counselor assists in the process by providing interventions that allow children to (1) recognize their own needs, (2) identify potential resources for meeting those needs, (3) develop strategies for activating the resources, (4) tolerate frustration, and (5) value and accept gratitude when they are successful. Children must learn to recognize the needs of others and to balance those needs against their own. O'Connor (2000) explains the fundamental goal of ecosystemic play therapy includes maximizing the child's ability to meet needs in ways that do not interfere with the ability of others to get their needs met (p. 347). Appropriate developmental functioning is emphasized.

O'Connor (2009) explained that children will progress through steps in this therapy. The first is an introduction and exploration in which the relationship is established. One of the differences in this approach is that from the outset, the therapist presents a potential treatment contract focusing on the needs of the child, emphasizing concrete improvements to the child's quality of life (O'Connor, 2011). During the next stage, tentative acceptance, children have accepted the process and seem to be cooperative, but they are anxious. Once the children begin to resist the therapy, the next stage, negative reaction, has begun. The reactions may be overt or may be very mild and difficult to detect. After at least one difficult session, children move into the fourth phase—growing and trusting. In this phase, active problem solving is initiated. The final phase is termination, which includes a review of the therapy, the problems faced, and the strategies used (O'Connor & Ammen, 1997).

In ecosystemic play therapy, the most important goal is to help the children resume a normal life, having their needs met without infringing on others. Specific treatment objects are developed after extensive assessments. Counselors are active and directive and use structuring, challenging, intruding, and nurturing to engage and maintain "an optimal level of arousal so that learning and change can occur" (O'Connor, 2009, p. 407). Working with parents is stressed (O'Connor, 2011) and may include exchanging information, consulting about management strategies or parenting skills, and problem solving.

GROUP PLAY THERAPY   Children age 2 to 12 with similar problems or experiences affecting their behavior may benefit from a play therapy group. Using play in group counseling is similar to using it with individuals; the previously mentioned theoretical approaches will guide a counselor in those decisions.

Sweeney (2011) identified many advantages to using group play therapy. Children will have experiences that help them learn to function well, explore their actions, develop tolerance, and find joy in working with others. Groups provide opportunities for vicarious learning, self-growth, and self-exploration. The group play may decrease a child's tendency to be repetitious or to retreat to fantasy play. In addition, the group offers a forum for practicing behaviors and strategies in a safe place. Trice-Black, Bailey, and Riechel (2013) outline ways to deliver play therapy groups in schools.

The goals of group play therapy suggested by Corey, Corey, Callahan, and Russell (2014) regardless of theoretical approach include the following:

- Trust for self and others
- Self-knowledge
- Recognition of commonality of members' needs
- Acceptance of self and others
- Concern and compassion for others
- Discovery of alternative ways to cope
- Increased self-direction, interdependence, and responsibility for self and others
- Awareness of choices
- Planning
- Building social skills
- Enhanced sensitivity
- Learning how to challenge with care, concern, honesty, and directness
- Clarity of values

O'Connor (1991) stated that the children selected for group play therapy should display a range of functioning both to avoid competition for attention and to provide models. He suggested no more than six children per adult in the group, and no more than 10 children in a group with two adults. Children should be within a 3-year age span among members, come from a similar socioeconomic status and ethnic background, and have no more than 15 IQ points separating them. The advisability of mixing boys and girls in one group depends on the age of the members, the type of group, and the group goals. The length and frequency of group play therapy correlates with the group purpose.

The setting for group play therapy requires adequate size as well as floor and equipment that are sturdy and easy to clean. Play materials are chosen to allow expression and engage children's interests.

The therapist serves as a facilitator of the process, working to instill hope, to promote altruism and universality, to develop social skills and adaptive behavior and catharsis. The counselor must have a high tolerance for messiness and noise and must be willing to handle chaos. The therapist must keep responses balanced among group members being intentional about using the child's name in any response to avoid other group members' confusion. The group play therapist must be an expert limit setter (Sweeney, 2011).

Group play therapy has been successful with a number of child populations. A few of those group are trauma victims (Hansen, 2006; Shen, 2010); those who have been sexually abused (Gallo-Lopez, 2006; Jones, 2002); some with anger issues (Badau & Esquivel, 2005; Fischetti, 2010); with social skills problems (Blundon & Schaefer, 2006), and children with divorcing parents (Ludlow & Williams, 2006) as well as homeless children (Baggerly, 2004). Paone and colleagues (2008) found significant positive effects on moral reasoning after group activity therapy with at-risk high school students. Group play therapy has also been effective with children with diverse backgrounds. Baggerly and Parker worked with African American boys; Hopkins, Huici, and Bermudez (2005) with Hispanic clients; and Kao (2005) with Asian children.

Nisivoccia and Lynn (2007) outlined group work with children who have been exposed to violence. The goals of the group were to give the young people opportunities to have a corrective emotional experience and to increase social skills. The content of the groups incorporates expressing feelings, talking about isolation and shame, discussing who was responsible for the violence, and learning conflict resolution. The authors discussed the activities they used to move through the group stages with the children who had witnessed a violent incident. Schuurman and DeCristofaro (2007) provided similar specifics for group play therapy with children who have suffered the death of a parent.

PRESCRIPTIVE PLAY THERAPY   Gil and Shaw (2009) described prescriptive play therapy as a child-led, practitioner-informed way to select and apply a particular play therapy approach that research supports as being most effective for a specific symptom or problem. Schaefer (2001) explained that prescriptive play therapy "challenges the clinician to weave together a variety of play interventions into one comprehensive, tailor-made treatment program for a particular client" (p. 57). To do this, practitioners must have both a conceptual and practical knowledge base about the many theories of play therapy. That knowledge will allow the counselor to understand the child and the child's problems and then match the issue to a play therapy approach. Effective implementation of prescriptive play therapy means a counselor balances the recommendations from research with information from the child, taking the strengths, limitations, external factors, and readiness into account.

Schaefer (2011) notes that the therapist's role in prescriptive play therapy varies based on the chosen play approach. Counselors suited to this matching approach are open, flexible, and skilled in adapting treatment. Kaduson et al. (1997) outlined the responsibilities of counselors who use prescriptive play therapy:

- know every approach to play therapy, including the theory's philosophical foundations, constructs, and strategies
- have skill in applying the constructs and strategies
- understand the psychological and emotional issues related to childhood disorders

- be capable of identifying the short- and long-term needs of children with specific diagnoses to form treatment plans for those needs
- know the current outcome research in order to choose the most effective treatment for the specific problem

To find the best fit of child and treatment course, therapists have three considerations. First, they decide the relevant patient and treatment variables and characteristics. Next, they weigh the combination of client and treatment qualities that best predict and facilitate success. Finally, the counselor looks at the contributions of the client condition, treatment, therapeutic relationship, and match of treatment to client (Beutler, Consoli, & Lane, 2005). The goal is symptom relief so if the first choice of treatment is not successful, the prescriptive play therapist will use the same method to select an alternative. As Gil and Shaw (2009) explain, this is an approach to play therapy that is guided by the questions; "*What* treatment, by *whom*, is most effective for this individual with *that* specific problem and under *which* set of circumstances?" (p. 455).

Beyond the specific objective of symptom reduction, prescriptive play therapists work to help children improve their psychological health, increase their positive regard for themselves, be open to experience, and form successful interpersonal relationships.

Prescriptive play therapists use their assessment skills to isolate the problem to be addressed and then investigate the concern in the context of current research of the evidence-based practices successful in the treatment of the issue (Gil & Shaw, 2009).

Play Therapy with Children and Adults

Interventions combining family and play therapy have been used in prevention programs in elementary schools (Morrison & Bratton, 2010) and in helping parents identify children's strengths (Sheely-Moore & Bratton, 2010). Johnson (2000) discussed the use of play therapy to work with a child who had attention difficulties. Those authors coached parents in relationship-building techniques with a successful outcome for both the child and the parents.

Some authors have successfully used play therapy to build teacher–child relationships (Helker, Schottelkorb, & Ray, 2007; Helker & Ray, 2008; Ray, Henson, Schottelkorb, Brown, & Muro, 2008). One article summarized research on the use of play therapy in elementary schools and contained practical information on developing a program (Landreth, Ray, & Bratton, 2009).

Gladding (1993) encourages families to play, but in a manner that is fair, tolerant, and trusting. His admonition was to set up cooperative play environments where everyone shares and wins. Rotter and Bush (2000) also emphasize the importance of families playing together in therapy. Several theorists have provided models for promoting that type of play therapy with families. Our chapter on family counseling outlines two approaches to helping families and children play together.

PARENT–CHILD INTERACTION THERAPY   Parent–child interaction therapy (PCIT) model was developed to treat children who were showing behavioral problems such as resistance and aggression—behaviors that are part of the diagnostic conditions for conduct disorder (CD) and oppositional defiant disorder (ODD) (Herschell & McNeil, 2005). In treating these behaviors, PCIT focuses on the parent–child relationship and is based on developmental psychology and social learning theory. Those fields of knowledge have established a link between parent–child relationships, parenting styles, and the behavior of children. In fact, Herschell and McNeil asserted that programs with an emphasis comparable with PCIT are "currently considered the treatment of choice for child conduct problems" (p. 174).

PCIT is based on the ideas that when parents use controlling or coercive ways to deal with behavior, they reinforce inappropriate, noncompliant behavior. Thus PCIT helps parents establish and maintain a secure, nurturing relationship while maintaining consistent, appropriate discipline (Kottman, 2011).

PCIT takes place once a week in a 1-hour therapy session. The duration of treatment is from 10 to 14 weeks (Herschell & McNeil, 2005). Herschell and McNeil describe the two stages that make up the actual process of PCIT, which centers on teaching parents effective ways to interact with their child. Counselors use coaching for at least 30 minutes of each session. The therapist gives immediate feedback to the parent during play sessions with the child by using a one-way mirror and a bug in the ear or with "in-room" coaching (Herschell & McNeil, p. 180). Before beginning each stage, parents receive a didactic session in which they not only have a lesson but also participate in role-plays. Counselors model the skills that parents will then display in an interaction with their child.

In the initial stage of PCIT, termed *child-directed interaction*, parents are coached to ignore the negative and disruptive behaviors of their child and to concentrate on the positive, suitable behaviors that their child presents. Parents learn about strategic attention and selective ignoring (McNeil, Bahl, & Herschell, 2009). In the second stage of *parent-directed interaction*, parents are coached on methods to gain and maintain the compliance of their child, such as learning to give understandable commands and to set up house rules (Herschell & McNeil, 2005). Parents also commit to interact and play with their child every day for 5 to 10 minutes outside the play therapy room. That interaction is an essential portion of PCIT (Herschell & McNeil). Ongoing assessments are also a vital portion of this therapy. Several instruments have been designed to measure PCIT goals, outcomes, and treatment progress according to these ongoing assessments. Brestan, Jacobs, Rayfield, and Eyberg (1999) have documented the psychometric soundness of the Therapy Attitude Inventory, an instrument developed specifically for PCIT to evaluate the satisfaction of parents after the course of therapy.

The second phase, which lasts between 7 and 10 sessions, is the parent-directed interaction focused on the skills for parents to become authoritative. Those skills include these in the acronym BE DIRECT:

Be specific and clear so children know what is expected

Every request should be stated positively

Developmentally appropriate commands ensure the child is capable of doing what is asked

Individual demands are more effective than multiple requests

Respectful and polite requests encourage reciprocal responses

Essential commands help parents remember to assess whether what they are asking is trivial or necessary

Choices help children build independence and problem-solving skills

Tone of voice that is neutral and calm, parents relaxed and in control

After parents learn these skills, they receive more information on establishing house rules, managing difficult behavior in public, and recognizing the need for booster sessions of training. Parents will hopefully generalize and transfer the learned skills (Kottman, 2011).

The effectiveness of PCIT has been documented with measurable changes in children's behavior noted; specifically, the decline of disruptive behavior and the increase of compliant behavior have occurred across treatment. PCIT gains have also generalized to school behavior (Boggs et al., 2004; Eisenstadt, Eyberg, McNeil, Newcomb, & Funderbunk, 1993; Gallagher, 2003; Hood & Eyberg, 2003; McNeil, Capage, Bahl, & Blanc, 1999; McNeil, Eyberg, Eisenstadt, Newcomb, & Funderbunk, 1991).

PCIT, although used primarily for disruptive behavioral disorders in children, is also being used for other childhood problems. Other studies (Chaffin et al., 2004) have focused on the use of PCIT for families in which physical abuse has occurred and in which the child welfare system was involved (Chaffin, Funderburk, Bard, Valle, & Gurwitch, 2011). In addition, Choate, Pincus, Eyberg, and Barlow (2005) have conducted a pilot study on the use of PCIT to treat separation anxiety disorder in children and reported a reduction in separation anxiety behaviors. Impressively, the gains children show during the treatment are maintained according to 1- and 2-year follow-up studies of PCIT (Eyberg et al., 2001). Furthermore, a recent comprehensive analysis of this type of therapy resulted in strong evidence for the efficacy of PCIT (Cooley, Veldorale-Griffin, Petren, & Mullis, 2014).

THERAPLAY   Is a treatment method modeled after the healthy parent–child bond, the kind of relationship between parents and children that fosters secure attachments and high self-esteem (Bundy-Myrow & Booth, 2009). Munns (2011) explains this intensive, short-term approach as a therapy in which parents are involved as observers and then as co-therapists. The goal of the therapy is to foster attachment, self-esteem, self-regulation, trust, and joyful engagement.

Jernberg (1979) distinguished Theraplay from other approaches by noting it is playful, requiring no toys and few props with the person using this approach avoiding questions and focusing on health. The adult structures the sessions, and physical contact is encouraged. The assumptions of Theraplay are that people are motivated toward relatedness and the parent–child interaction is the foundation for personality. Another premise is that the empathic, playful responsiveness of caregivers builds a strong sense of self as well as the capacity to understand and empathize with other people. Theraplay practitioners also believe that self-regulation in adults depends on early experiences of co-regulation with caregivers. Finally, these counselors assume that early, secure attachments lead to positive and hopeful people (Bundy-Myrow & Booth, 2009).

The agenda of Theraplay sessions is designed to meet the child's needs, encouraging regression and enhancing the parent–child attachment. Theraplay integrates the elements of structure, engagement, nurture, and challenge. The adult enforces structure by clearly stating safety rules. Engaging activities are unexpected, delightful, and stimulating. Nurturing activities calm and reassure children, while challenging activities are opportunities for the child to explore and master new experiences. The duration of Theraplay is usually eight to twelve sessions. During that time, the counselor explains the process, describes activities, and elaborates on the process for parents. The counselor also coaches parents and gives support and encouragement (Kottman, 2009).

Theraplay has been used in many settings and with many ages. This approach to play therapy has been chosen especially in situations where attachment issues are evident such as with stepchildren, foster and adopted children (Miller-Morz, Lender, Rubin, & Lindaman, 2010; Lindaman & Booth, 2010; Schlanger, 2010). It has been used with impulsive children (Booth & Jernberg, 2010) as well as aggressive young ones (Eyles, Boada, & Munns, 2009). Siu (2009) provides evidence of the growing body of research on this approach. Theraplay Institute has an Activities Flip Book, Group Activity Cards, and other resources for Theraplay activities.

EFFECTIVENESS

Reddy et al. (2005) edited a compilation of play therapy research in their useful book, *Empirically Based Play Interventions for Children*, a highly recommended reference for counselors working with children. Different studies have focused on the effectiveness of play therapy. Bratton, Ray, Rhine, and Jones (2005) have conducted meta-analyses of play therapy studies across several years. Their conclusions were that play therapy was effective for a variety of problems, populations, in numerous settings, and with a multitude of clinical orientations. Both of these analyses resulted in the findings that parental involvement and therapy duration of 35 to 45 sessions were common elements of effective play interventions. LeBlanc and Ritchie (2001) also found a strong average effect size of play therapy outcomes. Those studies suggest that play therapy can be considered as effective as talk therapy. The inclusion of parents as co-therapists or active participants increases those positive changes for children.

Play therapists may be concerned with identifying appropriate outcomes for interventions. Hendricks (2014) explained play as a medium for self-realization, a worthy outcome. Barnes (1991) suggested criteria for assessing progress toward goals of play therapy that continue to be applicable:

1. The child comes to the sessions looking more hopeful and relaxed.
2. The child appears to have increased confidence.
3. The child can summarize what has happened and what has been learned.
4. The child's interactions with parents appear more relaxed.
5. Play patterns, interactions, and/or body language have changed.
6. The child openly raises a problem or concern (Table 17-2).

These criteria could be used to help formulate outcomes for the goals of the play therapy, allowing counselors to document the effectiveness of play therapy for themselves, for their clients, and for other interested parties.

TABLE 17-2 PLAY THERAPY

Play therapy (regardless of the approach) would be treatment of choice	Certain approaches to play therapy have been useful in treating these children	Play therapy can be an effective intervention when combined with other interventions	Play therapy would not be the treatment of choice for these children
Adjustment Disorder	Attachment Disorder	Attention Deficit Hyperactivity Disorder	Severe Conduct Disorder
Post-traumatic Stress Disorder	(Theraplay & Thematic Play)	Autism Spectrum Disorder	Severe Attachment Disorder
Dissociative Disorder	Selective Mutism (Cognitive-Behavioral Play-Therapy & Client-Centered Play Therapy)	Separation Anxiety Disorder	Manifest Signs of Psychosis
Depressive Episodes	Moderate to Severe Behavior Problems (Filial Therapy, Adlerian Play Therapy, and Ecosystematic Play Therapy)	Mood disorders	
Specific Fears and Phobias		Learning Disabilities	
Aggressive, Acting-out Behavior		Mental Retardation Physical Handicaps	
Anxiety and Withdrawn Behavior			
Abuse and/or Neglect			
Divorce of Parents			
Family Violence and Other Family Problems			
Grief Issues			
Adoption and Foster Care-Related Issues			
Severe Trauma (e.g., earthquake, car wreck, war, or kidnapping)			
Hospitalization			
Chronic or Terminal Illness			

Source: Kottman, T. (2011). Play therapy: Basics and beyond. Alexandria, VA: American Counseling Association, pp. 18–21.
© ACA. Reprinted by permission. No further reproduction authorized without written permission of the American Counseling Association.

PLAY THERAPY MEDIA AND STRATEGIES

Play media includes the materials and props a counselor may use in the play therapy session. These tools can help capture children's interest and provide them with a way to express themselves. Carmichael (2006) provided some guidelines and suggested that the quality of therapy does not depend on the quality of the toys. She added that the more generic toys allow open interpretation by the child so counselors should not choose toys that are associated with specific, well-known characters. She also alerted counselors to cleanliness concerns and suggested that selected toys be sanitized or laundered regularly.

Landreth (2012) said that play media should be chosen based on the following criteria:

1. The toys are interesting.
2. They help the child show creativity.
3. The toys facilitate expressive and exploratory play.
4. They allow success and noncommittal play.
5. They encourage mastery for children.
6. The toys can take rough treatment without breaking.

Furthermore, the selected toys should help children with the following:

- build a positive relationship with the counselor and with any other children in group play therapy
- express a range of feelings
- explore/reenact situations
- test limits
- increase self-control
- build their understanding of self and others
- improve their self-image (Kottman, 2009, p. 127)

The material should be selected carefully rather than merely accumulated (Landreth, 2012). Different therapy approaches have different philosophies of toy selection, but toys should always be sturdy and safe. Kottman (2011) provided a general list of play media to have available. Therapists should have family/nurturing toys, scary toys, aggressive toys, expressive toys, and pretend/fantasy toys. VanFleet, Sywulak, and Sniscak (2010) suggested the following specific examples for each of some other toy categories:

Creative expression toys: dress-up clothes, hats, scarves, fabric pieces; masks; play money; watercolor paints, markers, crayons (8 colors); drawing paper, easel; blackboard or whiteboard, colored chalk or markers, eraser; small sandbox/container with miniature toys; sandbox and sand pencils; paints and brushes, white and colored paper; tape, paste, blunt scissors, Play-Doh® clay, pipe cleaners, popsicle sticks, hand puppets, costumes, newsprint, rags or old towels, hand puppets; mirror; magic wand; cars, trucks, school bus, train set; emergency vehicles; medical kit

Family/Nurturing toys: doll house and furniture, dolls, doll clothes and blanket, doll buggy, bendable doll family, rag doll, household items (iron, ironing board, play kitchen, two play dishes and cups, spoons), baby bottles, cars, airplane, farm animals and buildings, medical kit, Band-Aids®, school kit, play money, plastic fruit, purse, costume jewelry

Acting-out and aggressive-release toys: handcuffs, balls, dart gun and suction darts, dartboard, suction throwing darts, pounding bench and hammer, drum, blocks, toy soldiers (20 are enough) and military equipment, rubber knife, toy gun, masks, inflatable punching toy, aggressive hand puppet such as biting figure; foam bats or swimming "noodles"

Scary toys: snakes, rats, monster figures, sharks, dinosaurs, dragons, alligators, and animal puppets like a wolf, bear, or other predator

Communication toys: telephones including cell/mobile phones, megaphone, binoculars, walkie-talkies

Mastery toys: Plastic container with 1–2 cups water; measuring cups, play cooking utensils; bean bag toss game; jump rope, hula-hoop; ringtoss game; bowling pins; large checkers; deck of cards; building toys such as block or Legos; heavy cardboard bricks (Kottman, 2011, pp. 90–91; VanFleet et al., 2010, pp. 50–52).

Landreth (2012) listed items for a portable play bag to be used by a traveling play therapist in a school. Chang et al. (2005) found that multicultural dolls and puppets, markers, crayons, and Play-Doh in multicultural shades and toys with various environmental elements are important for children from diverse backgrounds. Gil (1991) emphasized the use of sunglasses in her work with abused children noting that children believe they are invisible when they put on sunglasses. She also noted the use of therapeutic stories in her therapy. Kottman (2009) included toys for older children such as craft supplies, carpentry tools, office supplies and equipment, and more sophisticated games.

Basic Skills of Play Therapy

VanFleet et al. (2010) state that whatever form of play therapy counselors practice, the process is relationship oriented and attuned to the child's feelings and needs. The counselor must be able to build a helpful relationship with the child, understand the child's problem, plan, and have time for spending with the child.

Kool and Lawver (2010), Kottman (2009, 2011) and Landreth et al. (2009) explain the basic verbal skills used by all play therapists. They talk about responding, pacing, tracking, restating, reflecting feelings, and returning responsibility to the child. The effective response should be succinct, tailored to the language ability and age of the child, and interactive. Longer answers may confuse children, make them lose interest, and imply the counselor does not understand. If the child is quiet and reserved, the counselor should slow down; if the child is talkative, the counselor matches that energy (Landreth et al.).

Kottman and Landreth and his colleagues also identified and explained the generic skills of play therapy. Counselors use tracking to reflect the child's nonverbal behavior and connect with the child by conveying that what the child is doing is important. In tracking, counselors describe what the child is doing with no interpretations and no assumptions. The counselor avoids labeling objects by keeping descriptions vague. Counselors use pronouns such as "this" or "it" and phrases such as "moving back and forth" or "looking up and down." An example of tracking would be the response "You are picking that up" as the counselor sees a child lift a doll off the shelf.

Restating content refers to paraphrasing what the child has said to convey concern and understanding. Again, the purpose is to build the therapeutic relationship. Counselors use their own words to relay the content, but choose vocabulary appropriate to the child's level of understanding. An illustration of restating occurs in the following interchange. A child says, "My mom likes for me to practice piano, but I hate it," and the counselor replies "Your mom and you have different ideas about playing the piano."

Counselors reflect children's feelings to deepen the therapy relationship and to help the child understand emotions, learn more about being with others, and expand their affective vocabulary. Counselors use phrases such as "You seem happy today" or "You're scared when the puppet yells." To help children learn responsibility, the counselor does not use the phrase "makes you feel" but rather "You feel. . . ." The counselor is alert to both surface, obvious emotions and the underlying deeper ones as well (Kottman, 2011).

Kottman (2009) and Landreth (2012) explain that the strategy of returning responsibility to the child builds self-reliance, self-confidence, and self-responsibility. The practice can also help with decision making, a sense of accomplishment, and feelings of mastery and control. Counselors allow children to take action ("I think you know how to close the play chest.") or to make decisions ("It can be whatever you want it to be."). The counselor can use a direct approach of returning responsibility by just telling the child to make the choice or a less direct approach by restating content, reflecting feelings, or tracking. Landreth said the rule of thumb is never do for children what they can do for themselves.

Facilitating creativity and spontaneity sends a message of being uniquely special. When children have freedom of expression, they develop confidence and flexibility in thinking (Landreth et al., 2009). An example would be responding "you can do whatever you want" when a child asks about using some play media. After the child does several things, the counselor could then acknowledge "you know lots of things you can make" as a statement to facilitate creativity.

Esteem building and encouraging is another example of helping children see themselves as capable. Landreth et al. (2009) gave examples of a child trying to open a bottle and trying several different things with the counselor saying "You're trying lots of ideas. You're not giving up." Another illustration would be a child struggling to do something and finding a solution. The therapist would respond "You got it" or "You figured it out."

Using the child's metaphor means that the counselor maintains the child's story without imposing the counselor's interpretation of the meaning. Kottman (2009) explains this as the counselor being careful to restrain and "avoid 'breaking' the metaphor by going outside the story to the 'real' world" (p. 133–134). Using a metaphor means the counselor tracks, restates content, reflects feelings, and returns responsibility to the child without imposing the counselor's meaning onto the child's story. Chesley, Gillett, and Wagner (2008) provided a valuable overview of using both verbal and nonverbal metaphors with children in play therapy.

Facilitating the relationship involves using relational responses that recognize the child's attempts to make contact with the counselor, relay the counselor's care for the child, and help the child learn appropriate communication patterns. The responses should include a reference to the child and to the counselor. An example would be the child dropping something, looking at the counselor, and saying nothing. A relational response would be "You're wondering what I'm thinking" (Landreth et al., 2009).

Finally, the skill of setting limits in the play area keeps the child safe, increases a sense of self-control, and enhances self-responsibility. Appropriate limits include those intended to (1) protect the child from hurting self or others, (2) keep the child from damaging the play setting, (3) maintain the toys and play media in the play setting, and (4) stay in the session for the scheduled amount of time. Kottman (2009) offered three steps for redirecting a child's misbehavior. First, state the limit in a nonjudgmental way ("It's against the rules to throw things that are sharp"), reflect the child's feelings and make guesses about the reason for the behavior ("You're mad at me and you want me to know you are the boss"). The third step involves asking the child for ideas about a better behavior choice ("I'll bet you can figure out something in the playroom you can throw"). If the child agrees, no further action is necessary; if not, the counselor arranges logical consequences that the child can enforce ("We need to think of what would be a consequence if you decide to throw that at me again. What do you think would be fair?"). Landreth (2012) suggested the A-C-T model of limit-setting that is different. The counselor does the following: (1) Acknowledges the feeling, (2) Communicates the limit, and (3) Targets an alternative. An example would go like this: "You are pleased with your clay creation." Then a short, concrete limit "but we don't take it out of the playroom" and an alternative "You could put it in that slot and it will be there the next time we meet."

Counselors who use these basic skills may find the following strategies helpful in conducting play therapy sessions based on the combination of the child's characteristics, problem(s), and needs, as well as the stage of the play therapy process.

Some common techniques and media useful in communicating with children are art, puppets, and sandplay. These are further explored as examples of play therapy techniques in the section below. Counselors and children engaging in play therapy have many other possibilities from which to choose. The books *101 Favorite Play Therapy Techniques, Volume III* (Kaduson & Schaefer, 2003), *Creative arts and play therapy for attachment problems* (Malchiodi & Crenshaw, 2014), *Integrating expressive Arts and Play Therapy with Children and Adolescents* (Green & Drewes, 2014), *Popular Culture in Counseling, Psychotherapy, and Play-based Interventions* (Rubin, 2008) and *Windows to our Children* (Oaklander, 1988), as well as many others, contain valuable examples of the use of storytelling, drama, poetry, games, and other techniques.

Hall, Kaduson, and Schaefer (2002) outline fifteen play therapy techniques useful for children with depression, anxiety, impulsivity, and distractibility. Play Therapy International (http://www.playtherapy.org/) is a valuable resource for play therapy information. That society provides a toolkit for play therapists that include these techniques: creative visualization, therapeutic storytelling, drama, puppets and masks, sand tray and sand world, art, drawing, music, and clay. Play counselors will choose activities in order to facilitate the child's growth; therefore, treatment choices should always be decided based on the counseling goals such as building a relationship, self-awareness, decision making, or others that are listed previously.

VISUALIZATION   Visualization may be used in many ways. For example, children and adolescents may find their engagement in an imaginary world without the barriers of their reality allows them to revise their thinking about problems, discover strengths they had not recognized, or adjust their expectations about other people. Counselors should be cautious in using visualizations because some agencies and schools forbid the use of imagery with children (Bradley, Gould, & Hendricks, 2004). In the following two stories, children are encouraged to determine some things valuable to them and to talk about how that discovery can help in their current situation. Oaklander (2006) provided two fantasy exercises that she used with adolescents. Her scripts follow.

The Pawn Shop: Imagine you are in a time machine that will take you back to the middle ages. You land safely and when you leave the time machine you are on a cobblestone street with shops of all kinds and people walking all around. You see an interesting store with unusual items in the window and you go in to what turns out to be a pawn shop. The owner greets you warmly and invites you to look around. He can tell you are from another time and offers to give you anything in the store you want. You look around and see beautiful stone, unusual boxes, instruments, jewelry, figurines and many other wonderful-looking things. Finally, you decide on something. Soon you have to leave and get back into your time machine and now you are here with me. Draw what you chose and anything else you want and then let's talk about it.

The Boat in a Storm: Imagine you are a boat or ship or yacht. You can be any kind of water vessel—a canoe, sailboat, ocean liner, submarine—anything you want. You are in a body of water—an ocean or lake or river—any kind of water. You are happily moving along when a terrible storm starts. The rain is pounding down, the wind howling, lightning and thunder roar—it is a massive, strong, angry storm. What happens to you? Draw me a picture of you—before the storm, during the storm and after the storm is over (pp. 115–116).

STORYTELLING   Storytelling is a way to explore emotions, and it can be used to help children and adolescents learn about themselves. The only limitation on topics is the imagination of the child or counselor (Bradley et al., 2004). In a previous chapter, we discussed the Mutual Storytelling technique described by Gardner (1979). The method has been used successfully with depressed and suicidal children between 9 and 14 years of age (Bradley, Hendricks, & Crews, 2009). The strategy proceeds with the counselor asking the child to tell a story with a beginning, middle, and end. Then the counselor retells the story with the same beginning but with more constructive problem solving and a more successful resolution. Specifically using a device to record the story, the counselor proceeds in this manner:

1. Invite the child to make a recording with you of a make-believe show. The child is the guest of honor.
2. Turn on the device and briefly introduce the "show." Ask the child to state name, age, school, and grade.
3. Ask the child to tell a story. If the child needs help getting started, ask about interests, hobbies, family, and other things related to life.

4. While the child tells the story, take notes on content and meanings.
5. After the story is finished, ask the child if there is a moral lesson in the tale. Also ask for more details.
6. Comment on the story, such as how exciting, unusual, interesting, or whatever it was.
7. Turn off the recorder and discuss the story with the child in order to get the information you need to prepare your own version of the story. Ask the child which figure in the story represented him or her and other significant people in his or her life. Ask about symbols and the feel of the setting or atmosphere of the story. Take into account the emotional reactions the child had when telling the story. Use the moral lesson to select the story's theme and figure out healthier resolutions or coping with the problems in the story.
8. Turn on the tape recorder and tell your version of the story, include the same characters, settings, and situation as the original story but revise it for a better resolution of the conflict, alternatives to problems, and indications that behavior can change. Emphasize healthier ways to cope.
9. Turn off the tape recorder and ask if the child would like to hear the complete story (Bradley et al., 2004, pp. 94–95; Kottman, 2011, 227–234).

DRAMA   Playacting increases concentration, develops creativity, and allows the actors to enhance their communication skills. Children can take a role unfamiliar to them, thus changing their perspectives and practicing new behaviors. Participants can "act" themselves, others, or some symbolic character (Bradley et al., 2004).

One group activity that could be used for teaching children and adolescents how we impact each other involves sculpturing. The group is divided in half—artists and clay. The directions are for the artists to mold their clay into sculptures. Children may not touch each other during the activity, but they may give directions to achieve their "sculpture." After the sculptures are complete and frozen, the group leader can take a tour of the exhibit, allowing each creator to explain the creation and its significance. After the tour, the participants change roles and the process is repeated (http://www.childdrama.com/lessons.html).

Another possible activity, by Watts and Garza (2008), outlined an expressive and reflective approach to helping children act "as if" they were who they want to be. First, children draw a picture of the person, asking reflective questions about the drawing, identifying behaviors to reach the goals, and then enacting those behaviors. Those practice sessions would incorporate art and drama. Rubin and Livesay (2006) talked about helping children identify superheroes as examples of the ideal person the children want to become. Young people could then act "as if" they were these heroes.

MUSIC   Most adolescents listen to music daily. Music eases feelings of depression, anxiety, loneliness, and grief and gives words to many of the important facets of life. In counseling, music can be used to increase emotional awareness, deepen understanding, reduce fears, and invite self-disclosure (Bradley et al., 2009). Counselors can ask clients to bring in songs that have strong personal meaning and listen to the music together. They can then talk about the feelings and thoughts the music generated and how the emotions and cognitions are connected to the client's current situation. Another possibility would be to ask the client to create a song or to find a song that has a useful message. Finally, Hadley and Steele (2014) provide resources and procedures for music performance, composition, and movement.

ART   Gladding (2011) noted that visual arts offer five benefits for counselors. One is the access to the unconscious. A second advantage is the symbolizing of emotions in tangible ways. A third benefit is that visual arts help people become more self-aware. Fourth, the visual arts are a nonthreatening method and are open to self-interpretation. Finally, they can easily be combined with other play methods. Orton (1997) stated that art helps establish a relationship, helps children express and resolve their conflicts, and promotes self-expression, problem solving, and confidence.

Naumburg (1966) and Kramer (1971) developed art therapy. Naumburg's psychoanalytic understanding included the interpretation of art as being a window to the unconscious, insight as being central to the process, and obtaining the client's interpretation of the symbols as crucial to therapy. Kramer focused on the healing power of the act of creating. She explained that process and product are ways of releasing conflict, re-experiencing and rechanneling it, and resolving it.

Art materials can include crayons, finger paint, felt-tip markers, paints, clay and Play-Doh, paper, scissors, paste, glue, and glitter. Gladding (2011) also suggested using published pictures and photography. Counselors might also keep an easel with paper, paint, and brushes available for children to use while talking.

For counselors to use the Magic Art technique, they need to have a range of colors of construction paper and assorted colors of liquid tempera paint with very small openings in the tops. The child is allowed to select a piece of paper and at least three colors of paint to make a magic picture. The counselor tells the children to draw lines, dots, or any figure they like. After the picture is finished, the child is asked to fold the paper lengthwise. The counselor says "magic picture, what will (child's name) draw today?" Then the child unfolds the paper to reveal the new "picture." The counselor asks the child to describe what he or she sees in the picture and is questioned about what makes it look like that (Walker, 1998). Another strategy for counselors is to use yarn to create drawings. Leben (1997) stated this alternative to paper-and-pencil drawing is more appealing to children with low self-esteem.

CLAY   Clay is an art medium that can be used in play therapy with activities connected to therapeutic goals. Children can roll clay into a ball and then smash it down. They could also squeeze the clay through their fingers with varying degrees of pressure. To use clay as an activity for self-awareness, children can create a personal mobile. They may use different amounts of clay to represent the value they place on decision points. Clay can also be used to help children clarify goals, build communication skills, and develop time management strategies.

Bratton, Taylor, and Akay (2014) discuss a group for preadolescent girls in which the participants were asked to imagine traveling to the future, a world with creatures never before seen. The girls shape the creatures they would like to be using clay. They then create a home where all their creatures can live together. This group activity built trust and acceptance among the girls.

PUPPETS   Axline (1964, 1969) suggested that puppets provide opportunities for children to play out their feelings, to reenact events that produced anxiety, and to try out new behaviors. Puppets also allow children to develop communication skills, overcome isolation, build self-esteem, release emotions, and make decisions (Jewel, 1989).

Children can use puppets to tell stories, play out their fantasies, and deal with their thoughts. The child can create a separate person who communicates things too difficult for the child to express directly. Finally, the puppet may be the target of the child's strong emotion, an object of displacement so that anger can be expressed in a healthy way (Bradley et al., 2004). Gil (1991) identified a benefit of puppet play as the child creating a story anonymously, using characters to enact hidden concerns. Puppet play is also an effective activity for large or small groups of children. Nims (2009) also used puppets to act out the miracle in a solution-focused session.

Puppets can be bought or handmade. Carter and Mason (1998) explained some practical guidelines for selecting puppets. Some of the guidelines are also useful in selecting dolls. Counselors should determine how they intend to use the puppets and should have a variety for the children's choice. The puppets should be chosen to represent a range of emotions such as aggression, friendship, and neutrality. Puppets should also be representative of family and cultural groups. Other categories for puppets are occupations, symbolic types (witch, pirate), and wild and tame animals. The collection of puppets should relate symbolically to the problems of children. James and Myer (1987) listed these other important selection considerations such as ease of manipulation, lack of universal symbolism, fit, soft and cuddly, and cleanable.

The final selection consideration is whether the puppet has a "personality" to which the counselor responds with an engaged imagination (Carter & Mason, 1998).

The counselor who plans to use puppets does not have to be a ventriloquist. Basic skills are developing a voice for the puppet's personality, keeping the puppet active enough to engage and hold the child's attention, and knowing when to talk to the child and when to talk to the puppet. To use puppets successfully, counselors must become transparent, real, and courageous. The puppet should look up and out. Only the lower jaw of the puppet should move. Counselors should practice creating emotional expressions and other "moves" in front of a mirror to achieve a realistic presentation (Carter & Mason, 1998).

Bromfield (1995) and Irwin (1991) discussed many uses of puppets in which the child is offered a selection of puppets and invited to tell a story using them as characters. The child chooses the puppets and creates the story as the counselor observes the child's coping skills in dealing with this experience. The child introduces the puppets as "characters" in the show and "enacts" the story. After the play, the counselor asks the puppets about the plot and themes of the story, extending the make-believe. For the final step, the child is invited to discuss the story and the experience with the counselor.

SAND   Kalff (2003) identified the counselor's role in sand play as being a respectful witness. Gil (1991) suggested that children enjoy the experience of touching, molding, and shaping sand as well as letting it run through their fingers. She concluded that some children feel nurtured, calmed, or soothed by sand play. Other children use sandplay to "make a world" as first discussed by Lowenfeld (1935/1991) as "the World Technique." Kalff stated that the child resolves conflicts and traumas by externalizing and developing a sense of mastery and control when using sand play. Hong (2011) believed that sand play provides immediate access to the personal inner world and initiates instinctual self-healing. Robson (2008) described eight sessions of sand play therapy with a bereaved child in which the young person learned to adapt to life after the loss.

The sand tray is a container with the general dimensions of 20 × 3 × 30 × 3 × 3 inches. Some counselors use two trays, one for dry sand and one for wet sand; others use only a dry tray. The interior of the tray is painted blue to simulate water.

Carmichael (2006) suggested a transparent plastic storage container with a blue top that can be placed under the tray to provide the blue color. Some dry materials that can be substituted for sand are cornmeal, dried beans or peas, rice, popcorn, and aquarium gravel. The child is offered a choice of miniatures in the following categories:

- Buildings: houses, schools, churches, castles
- People: domestic, military, fantasy, mythological
- Animals: domestic, wild, zoo, prehistoric, marine
- Vehicles: land, air, water, space, war machines
- Vegetation: trees, bushes, shrubs, plants, vegetables
- Structures: bridges, fences, gates, doorways, corrals
- Natural objects: shells, driftwood, stones, bones
- Symbolic objects: wishing well, treasure chests, jewelry.

Hutton (2004) reviewed the "world techniques" originated by Lowenfeld (1939), a method of sand play that has stood the test of time. Another process in sand play begins with an invitation to create a miniature world. The counselor provides unconditional positive regard, empathy, warmth, and genuineness. Allan and Berry (1987) described "the sand as the process, the sand tray as the medium, and the world as the product" (p. 301). The session should progress without adult interference with the counselor as an attentive observer in the process.

According to Allan and Berry (1987), three stages occur in sand play: chaos, struggle, and resolution. In the chaos stage, the child imposes no order on the toys or sand. During the struggle phase, battles are waged. At the beginning no winner emerges. As the sessions progress, the fighting may become more intense and organized and struggles may become more balanced. A hero emerges who wins the fight. The child who demonstrates resolution restores order and balance in the sand play. The toy figures are in place and completion and wholeness are apparent (Allan & Berry, 1987; Kalff, 2003).

Mulherin (2001) provided a case study using the sand tray with a mother and child. She discussed the processes of separation, individuation, rapprochement, and recovery that occurred during the stage of treatment. She provided pictures to illustrate how the child represented his emotional states. Vaz (2000) also presented pictures to chronicle the process of sand play. Vaz surveyed other therapists who use sand play. She concluded that most therapists consider the sand play process complete when the images used in the tray reflect the client's return to a more effective approach to life.

TECHNOLOGY   Technology presents another media for interacting with young people. Children use computers and other devices to communicate with each other; to produce homework, music, and videos; and to entertain themselves with games, social sites, and other online enticements. Apps for smartphones and tablets include programs for drawing, recording, identifying emotions, problem solving, and many other possibilities that could be incorporated into a counseling relationship.

Bradley et al. (2009) suggest a few ways to use technology in counseling children. Counselors can ask the young client to explain the profile on the person's social networking page, create a slide show that represents the person's life, create a Web page memorial or discuss video game characters. Brezinka (2014) outline the use of computer games to support therapy. In addition, counselors should continue to investigate the potential of using virtual reality sites for role-playing opportunities as well as problem-solving situations.

This brief overview of this play therapy toolkit serves as an example of the possibilities of play media. Counselors are encouraged to investigate others as well as to create their own ways of incorporating play materials into their counseling practice. The following case study illustrates one additional method.

Case Study[1]

Identification of the Problem

Amos is a sixth-grade student in a rural middle school. His teacher referred him to the school counselor because his grades had dropped since the beginning of the school year and he was frequently distracted in class.

Individual and Background Information

Academic

School records indicate that Amos's ability is in the average range. He received good grades in elementary school and teachers noted his positive disposition and quiet nature. End-of-grade tests indicate that his math skills are much stronger than his verbal skills.

Family

Amos lives with his mother and stepfather. He has an older half-brother who is in eighth grade at the same school and a younger brother in the third grade at a nearby elementary school. Although Amos has not told the counselor, she knows his older brother was in a serious accident during the past summer and has recently had an operation. The brother has not returned to school.

---

[1] The case of Amos was contributed by Margery Peskin.

Social

According to teachers' reports, Amos is well liked and easily forms friendships. He is involved with several school sports teams and clubs. He enjoys interacting with his classmates.

Counseling Method

After meeting with Amos initially to assess the problem, the counselor decided he might benefit from an alternative method of counseling rather than verbal interactions only. She decided to use a nondirected play therapy approach.

Transcript

COUNSELOR: Hi, Amos! How are you doing today?

AMOS: Fine.

COUNSELOR: Last time we met you mentioned you had a basketball game that night. How did it go?

AMOS: Okay.

COUNSELOR: How did you think the game went?

AMOS: Pretty good.

COUNSELOR: That sounds positive. Today I thought we could try something a little different than what we've been doing. I put some supplies on the table. You can see I've got colored paper, markers, crayons, glue, yarn, scissors, clay, and watercolors.

AMOS: I love clay. I work with clay at home all the time.

COUNSELOR: Great. It sounds like you've had some experience with some of these materials. Here's what I'd like you to do. Using any combination of the materials here, create something that shows me what you have been thinking about the most over the past few days. You can use just one kind of material or as many as you want. Also, I want you to understand that there is not a "right" or "wrong" way to do this; create anything you want. Remember that our relationship is confidential, so I'm not going to show what you've made to anyone else unless you ask me to. Any questions?

AMOS: No.

COUNSELOR: Okay.

After some time has passed:

AMOS: I'm done.

COUNSELOR: I wonder if you'd tell me what you've made.

AMOS: Well, the two clay figures are my parents. See, my mom has long blond hair, so this one has yellow string on the top, and my dad has short blond hair, so this one has a short yellow string. This rectangle of paper on the table is a hospital bed and this clay is my brother because he's been really sick and had an operation on his neck.

COUNSELOR: It must be hard that your brother is so sick. One thing I notice is that you're not in this scene.

AMOS: Well, I would have made myself, but there wasn't enough clay.

COUNSELOR: You're feeling left out.

AMOS:	Lots of time I think they have forgotten me.
COUNSELOR:	So it sounds like your parents are spending a lot of time with your brother in the hospital.
AMOS:	Yeah, they go there every afternoon so when I get home from school no one is at home.
COUNSELOR:	That must be pretty difficult because you are worried about your brother but feel lonely, too.
AMOS:	Yeah, sometimes.
COUNSELOR:	I'm wondering if you ever feel guilty because you wish your parents weren't spending so much time with your brother so they might have more time to spend with you.
AMOS:	Exactly. But I feel really bad about that.
COUNSELOR:	It sounds like there are a lot of different things for you to be worried about that might be making it hard to concentrate in school.
AMOS:	Usually I like school, but right now I'm sad all the time. I keep wondering if the doctors have found out anything about my brother, and then I wonder if my mom or dad will be home after school and then I feel bad because my brother needs them, too.
COUNSELOR:	You have lots of different things fighting for your attention. Maybe we can figure out some ways to help you relax a bit. Let's meet again on Wednesday to see what we can try.
AMOS:	That sounds good.

SUMMARY

Virginia Axline (1964) chronicled her work with Dibs, a child who found himself through play therapy. That classical work stands as a testimony to the power of play. Lowenfeld (1935/1991) and her staff at the Institute of Child Psychology in London recorded and classified the play of 229 children between the years of 1928 and 1934. Her book documents the classification of the children's play as bodily activity, repetition of experience, demonstration of fantasies, realization of the environment, and preparation for life. She concluded that play served four purposes for children:

1. Play is children's means for making contact with the environment in a way similar to the social aspect of work in an adult's life;
2. Play helps children bridge consciousness and emotional experience as conversation, introspection, philosophy, and religion do for adults;
3. Play represents to the child the overt expression of his emotional life as does art for an adult; and
4. Play serves the child as relaxation and amusement (Lowenfeld, 1935/1991, p. 232).

She argued that play is an essential function of moving from immaturity to emotional maturity. Counselors strive to enhance the development of children; play therapy is a significant way of influencing that growth. Carr (2009), in his careful review of the effectiveness of the processes of counseling, noted empirical support for play therapy treatments for children who have experienced parents separating, domestic violence, trauma, chronic illness, hospital stays, and conduct or developmental disorders. Gil (Sori & Schnur, 2014) captures the impact of play therapy as the healing power of an adult being inviting, engaging, and connecting to the child.

WEB SITES FOR PLAY THERAPY

Internet addresses frequently change. To find the sites listed here, visit www.cengage.com/counseling/henderson for an updated list of Internet addresses and direct links to relevant sites.

Association for Play Therapy, Inc.

Canadian Play Therapy Institute

Play Therapy International

REFERENCES

Albon, S. L. (1996). The therapeutic action of play. *Journal of American Academy of Child Adolescent Psychiatry, 35*(4), 545–547.

Allen, F. (1942). *Psychotherapy with children.* New York: Norton.

Allan, J., & Berry, P. (1987). Sandplay. *Elementary School Guidance & Counseling, 21,* 300–306.

Anderson, J., & Richards, N. (October, 1995). *Play therapy in the real world: Coping with managed care, challenging children, skeptical colleagues, time and space constraints.* Paper presented at the First Annual Conference of the Iowa Association of Play Therapy, Iowa City, IA.

Association for Play Therapy. (2014). Play therapy makes a difference. Retrieved from http://www.a4pt.org/?page=PTMakesADifference.

Axline, V. (1947). *Play therapy: The inner dynamics of childhood.* Boston: Houghton Mifflin.

Axline, V. (1964). *Dibs: In search of self.* Boston, MA: Houghton Mifflin.

Axline, V. (1969). *Play therapy.* New York: Ballantine.

Badau, K., & Esquivel, G. (2005). Group therapy for adolescents with anger problems. In L. Gallo-Lopez & C. Schaefer (Eds.), *Play therapy for adolescents* (pp. 239–266). Lanham, MD: Rowman & Littlefield.

Baggerly, J. (2004). The effects of child-centered group play therapy on self-concept, depression, and anxiety of children who are homeless. *International Journal of Play Therapy, 13,* 31–51.

Barnes, M. (1991). *The magic of play therapy: A workshop on specialized therapeutic skills with children.* Ontario, Canada: Mandala Therapeutic Services.

Bettelheim, B. (1987). The importance of play. *Atlantic Monthly, 3,* 35–46.

Beutler, L. E., Consoli, A. J., & Lane, G. (2005). Systematic treatment selection and prescriptive psychotherapy: An integrative eclectic approach. In J. C. Norcross & M. R. Goldfried (Eds.), *Handbook of Psychotherapy Integration* (2nd ed., pp. 121–143). New York: Oxford University Press.

Bixler, R. (1949). Limits are therapy. In M. Haworth (Ed.), *Child psychotherapy* (pp. 134–147). New York: Basic Books.

Blundon, J., & Schaefer, C. (2006). The use of group play therapy for children with social skills deficits. In H. Kaduson & C. Schaefer (Eds.), *Short-term play therapy for children* (2nd ed., pp. 336–376). New York: Guilford Press.

Boggs, S., Eyberg, S., Edwards, D., Rayfield, A., Jacobs, J., Bagner, D., & Hood, K. (2004). Outcomes of parent-child interaction therapy: A comparison of treatment completers and study dropouts one to three years later. *Child & Family Behavior Therapy, 26*(4), 1–22.

Booth, P., & Jernberg, A. (2010). *Theraplay: Helping parents and children build better relationships through attachment-based play.* San Francisco, CA: Jossey-Bass.

Bradley, L. J., Gould, L. J., & Hendricks, P. B. (2004). Using innovative techniques for counseling children and adolescents. In A. Vernon (Ed.), *Counseling children and adolescents* (3rd ed., pp. 75–110). Denver, CO: Love.

Bradley, L. J., Hendricks, P. B., & Crews, C. R. (2009). Expressive techniques: Counseling interventions for children and adolescents. In A. Vernon (Ed.), *Counseling children and adolescents* (3rd ed., pp. 75–122). Denver, CO: Love.

Bratton, S. C., & Ray, D. (2000). What the research shows about play therapy. *International Journal of Play Therapy, 9*(1), 47–88.

Bratton, S. C., Ray, D., Rhine, T., & Jones, L. (2005). The efficacy of play therapy with children: A meta-analytic review of treatment outcomes. *Professional Psychology: Research and Practice, 36,* 376–390.

Bratton, S. C., Taylor, D. D., & Akay, S. (2014). Integrating play and expressive art therapy into small group counseling with preadolescents: A humanistic approach. In E. Green & A. A. Drewes (Eds.), *Integrating expressive arts and play therapy with children and adolescent* (pp. 253–282). Hoboken, NJ: Wiley and Sons.

Brestan, E., Jacobs, J., Rayfield, A., & Eyberg, S. (1999). A consumer satisfaction measure for parent-child treatments and its relations for measures of child behavior change. *Behavior Therapy, 30,* 17–30.

Brezinka, V. (2014). Computer games supporting cognitive behaviour therapy in children. *Clinical Child Psychology and Psychiatry, 19*(1), 100–110. doi: 10.1177/1359104512468288

Bromfield, R. (1995). The use of puppets in play therapy. *Child & Adolescent Social Work Journal, 12*(6), 435.

Brown, S. L., & Vaughan, C. C. (2009). *Play: How it shapes the brain, opens the imagination, and invigorates the soul.* New York: Avery.

Bundy-Myrow, S., & Booth, P. B. (2009). Theraplay: Supporting attachment relationships. In K. J. O'Connor & L. D. Braverman (Eds.), *Play therapy theory and practice: Comparing theories and techniques* (2nd ed., pp. 315–366). Hoboken, NJ: Wiley.

Carmichael, K. D. (2006). *Play therapy: An introduction.* Upper Saddle River, NJ: Merrill.

Carr, A. (2009). *What works with children, adolescents and adults? A review of research on the effectiveness of psychotherapy.* New York: Routledge.

Carter, R. B., & Mason, P. S. (1998). The selection and use of puppets in counseling. *Professional School Counseling, 1*(5), 50–53.

Cattanach, A. (2008). *Play therapy with abused children.* London and Philadelphia: Jessica Kingsley.

Chaffin, M., Silovsky, J. F., Funderburk, B., Valle, L. A., Brestan, E. V., Balachova, T., Jackson, S., Lensgraf, J., & Bonner, B. (2004). Parent-child interaction therapy with physically abusive parents: Efficacy for reducing further abuse reports. *Journal of Consulting and Clinical Psychology, 72*(3), 500–510.

Chaffin, M., Funderburk, B., Bard, D., Valle, L. A., & Gurwitch, R. (2011). A motivation-PCIT package reduces child welfare recidivism in a randomized dismantling field trial. *Journal of Consulting and Clinical Psychology, 79*(1), 84–95.

Chang, C. Y., Ritter, K. B., & Hays, D. G. (2005). Multicultural trends and toys in play therapy. *International Journal of Play Therapy*, *14*, 69–85.

Chesley, G. L., Gillett, D. A., & Wagner, W. G. (2008). Verbal and nonverbal metaphor with children in counseling. *Journal of Counseling & Development*, *86*, 399–411.

Choate, M., Pincus, D., Eyberg, S., & Barlow, D. (2005). Parent-child interaction therapy for the treatment of separation anxiety disorder in young children: A pilot study. *Cognitive and Behavioral Practice*, *12*, 126–135.

Cooley, M. E., Veldorale-Griffin, A., Petren, R. E., & Mullis, A. K. (2014). Parent-child interaction therapy: A meta-analysis of child behavior outcomes and parent stress. *Journal of Family Social Work*, *17*(3), 191–208. doi:10.1080/10522158.2014.888696

Corey, G., Corey, M. S., Callahan, P., & Russell, J. M. (2014). *Group techniques* (4th ed.). Belmont, CA: Cengage.

Demanchick, S. P., Cochran, N., & Cochran, J. (2003). Person-centered play therapy with adults with developmental disabilities. *International Journal of Play Therapy*, *12*(1), 47–65.

Drewes, A. (2005). Suggestions and research on multicultural play therapy. In E. Gil & A. Drewes (Eds.), *Cultural issues in play therapy* (pp. 72–95). New York: Guilford.

Drewes, A. A., & Schaefer, C. E. (2010). *School-based play therapy*. Hoboken, NJ: John Wiley & Sons, Inc.

Eisenstadt, T., Eyberg, S., McNeil, C., Newcomb, K., & Funderbunk, B. (1993). Parent-child interaction therapy with behavior problem children: Relative effectiveness of two stages and overall treatment outcomes. *Journal of Clinical Child Psychology*, *22*(1), 42–51.

Erwin, E. (Ed.). (2001). *The Freud encyclopedia: Theory, therapy, and culture*. New York: Routledge.

Eyberg, S., Funderbunk, B., Hembree-Kigin, T., McNeil, C., Querido, J., & Hood, K. (2001). Parent-child interaction therapy with behavior problem children: One and two year maintenance of treatment effects in the family. *Child & Family Behavior Therapy*, *23*(4), 1–20.

Eyles, S., Boada, M., & Munns, C. (2009). Theraplay with overtly and passively resistant children. In E. Munns (Ed.), *Applications of family and group Theraplay* (pp. 45–55). Northvale, NJ: Aronson.

Fall, M. (1999). A play therapy intervention and its relationship to self-efficacy and learning behaviors. *Professional School Counseling*, *2*, 194–205.

Fischetti, B. (2010). Play therapy for anger management in the schools. In A. Drewes & C. Schaefer (Eds.), *School-based play therapy* (2nd ed., pp. 283–306). Hoboken, NJ: Wiley.

Freud, A. (1926). *Psychoanalytic treatment of children*. London: Imago Press.

Freud, S. (1909). *Analysis of a phobia in a five year old boy*. London: Hogarth Press.

Gallagher, N. (2003). Effects of parent-child interaction therapy on young children with disruptive behavior disorders. *Bridges: Practice-Based Research Synthesis*, *4*(1), 1–17.

Gallo-Lopez, L. (2006). A creative play therapy approach to the group treatment of young sexually abused children. In H. Kaduson & C. Schaefer (Eds.), *Short-term play therapy for children* (2nd ed., pp. 245–272). New York: Guilford Press.

Gardner, R. A. (1979). Mutual storytelling technique. In C. E. Schaefer (Ed.), *The therapeutic use of child's play* (pp. 313–321). New York: Jason Aronson.

Green, E., & Drewes, A. A. (2014). *Integrating expressive arts and play therapy with children and adolescents*. Hoboken, NJ: John Wiley and Sons.

Gil, E. (1991). *The healing power of play: Working with abused children*. New York: Guilford Press.

Gil, E., & Drewes, A. (Eds.). (2005). *Cultural issues in play therapy*. New York: Guilford.

Gil, E., & Shaw, J. A. (2009). Prescriptive play therapy. In K. J. O'Connor & L. D. Braverman (Eds.), *Play therapy theory and practice: Comparing theories and techniques* (2nd ed., pp. 451–488). Hoboken, NJ: Wiley.

Ginott, H. G. (1994). The nature of play: Quotation. In C. E. Schaefer & H. Kaduson (Eds.), *The quotable play therapist: 238 of the all-time best quotes on play and play therapy* (p. 33). Northvale, NJ: Jason Aronson.

Gladding, S. T. (1993). The therapeutic use of play in counseling: An overview. *Journal of Humanistic Education and Development, 31*, 106–115.

Gladding, S. T. (2011). *The creative arts in counseling*. Alexandria, VA: American Counseling Association.

Glover, C. J. (2001). Cultural considerations in play therapy. In G. L. Landreth (Ed.), *Innovations in play therapy: Issues, process, and special populations* (pp. 31–42). Philadelphia, PA: Brunner-Routledge.

Gonzalez-Mena, J. (2012). *Child, family and community* (6th ed.). Upper Saddle River, NJ: Pearson.

Hadley, S., & Steele, N. (2014). Music therapy. In E. Green & A. A. Drewes (Eds.), *Integrating expressive arts and play therapy with children and adolescents* (pp. 149–179). Hoboken, NJ: Wiley and Sons.

Hall, T. M., Kaduson, H., & Schaefer, C. E. (2002). Fifteen effective play therapy techniques. *Professional Psychology: Research and Practice, 33*(6), 515–522. doi:10.1037/0735-7028.33.6.515

Hansen, S. (2006). An expressive arts therapy model with groups for post-traumatic stress disorder. In L. Carey (Ed.), *Expressive and creative arts methods for trauma survivors* (pp. 73–91). London: Kingsley.

Heidemann, S., & Hewitt, D. (2010). *Play: The pathway from theory to practice*. St. Paul, MN: Redleaf Press.

Helker, W. P., & Ray, D. (2008). The impact child-teacher relationship training on teachers' and aides' use of relationship-building skills and the effect on student classroom behavior. *International Journal of Play Therapy, 18*, 70–83.

Helker, W. P., Schottelkorb, A. A., & Ray, D. (2007). Helping students and teachers CONNECT: An intervention model for school counselors. *Journal of Professional Counseling, Practice, Theory, & Research, 35*, 31–45.

Hendricks, T. S. (2014). Play as self-realization: Toward a general theory of play. *American Journal of Play, 6*(2), 190.

Henniger, M. L. (1995). Play: Antidote for childhood stress. *Early Child Development and Care, 105*, 7–12.

Herschell, A., & McNeil, C. (2005). Parent-child interaction therapy for children experiencing externalizing behavior problems. In L. A. Reddy, T. M. Files-Hall, & C. E. Schaefer (Eds.), *Empirically based play interventions for children* (pp. 169–190). Washington, DC: American Psychological Association.

Hinman, C. (2003). Multicultural considerations in the delivery of play therapy services. *International Journal of Play Therapy, 12*(2), 107–122. doi:10.1037/h0088881

Hong, G. (2011). *Sandplay therapy: Research and practice*. New York; London: Routledge.

Hood, K., & Eyberg, S. (2003). Outcomes of parent-child interaction therapy: Mothers' reports of maintenance three to six years after treatment. *Journal of Clinical Child and Adolescent Psychology, 32*(3), 419–429.

Hopkins, S., Huici, V., & Bermudez, D. (2005). Therapeutic play with Hispanic clients. In E. Gil & A. Drewes (Eds.), *Cultural issues in play therapy* (pp. 148–167). New York: Guilford Press.

Hug-Hellmuth, H. (1921). On the technique of child analysis. *International Journal of Psychoanalysis, 2,* 287.

Hutton, D. (2004). Margaret Lowenfeld's 'world technique.' *Clinical Child Psychology and Psychiatry, 9*(4), 605–612. doi:10.1177/1359104504046164

Irwin, E. C. (1991). The use of a puppet interview to understand children. In C. E. Schaefer, K. Gitlin, & A. Sandgrund (Eds.), *Play diagnosis and assessment* (pp. 617–642). New York: Wiley.

James, R. K., & Myer, R. (1987). Puppets: The elementary school counselors' right or left arm. *Elementary School Guidance and Counseling, 21,* 262–265.

Jernberg, A. (1979). *Theraplay: A new treatment using structured play for problem children and their families.* San Francisco, CA: Jossey-Bass.

Jewel, D. L. (1989). *Confronting child abuse through recreation.* Springfield, IL: Charles C. Thomas.

Ji, Y., Ramirez, S. Z., & Kranz, P. L. (2008). Physical settings and materials recommended for play therapy with Japanese children. *Journal of Instructional Psychology, 34,* 53–61.

Johnson, B. (2000). Parent training through play: Parent-child interaction therapy with a hyperactive child. *Family Journal, 8,* 180–187.

Jones, K. D. (2002). Group play therapy with sexually abused preschool children. *Journal for Specialists in Group Work, 27,* 377–389.

Kaduson, H. G., Cangelosi, D., & Schaefer, C. E. (1997). *The playing cure: Individualized play therapy for specific childhood problems.* Northvale, NJ: Jason Aronson.

Kaduson, H., & Schaefer, C. (Eds.). (2003). *101 favorite play therapy techniques, Volume III.* Northvale, NJ: Jason Aronson.

Kalff, D. M. (2003). *Sandplay: A psychotherapeutic approach to the psyche.* Cloverdale, CA: Temenos Press.

Kao, S. (2005). Play therapy with Asian children. In E. Gil & A. Drewes (Eds.), *Cultural issues in play therapy* (pp. 195–206). New York: Guilford Press.

Kao, S., & Landreth, G. (2001). Play therapy with Chinese children. In G. Landreth (Ed.), *Innovations in play therapy: Issues, process, and special populations* (pp. 43–49). Philadelphia, PA: Taylor & Francis.

Kim, Y., & Nahm, S. (2008). Cultural considerations in adapting and implementing play therapy. *International Journal of Play Therapy, 17,* 66–77.

Klein, M. (1932). *The psychoanalysis of children.* London: Hogarth Press.

Kool, R., & Lawver, T. (2010). Play therapy: Considerations and applications for the practitioner. *Psychiatry, 7*(10), 19.

Kottman, T. (2009). Play therapy. In A. Vernon (Ed.), *Counseling children and adolescents* (3rd ed., pp. 123–146). Denver, CO: Love.

Kottman, T. (2011). *Play therapy: Basics and beyond* (2nd ed.). Alexandria, VA: American Counseling Association.

Kramer, E. (1971). *Art as therapy with children.* New York: Schocken.

Landreth, G. L. (2012). *Play therapy: The art of the relationship* (3rd ed.). New York: Routledge.

Landreth, G. L., Ray, D. C., & Bratton, S. C. (2009). Play therapy in elementary schools. *Psychology in the Schools, 46,* 281–289.

LaBauve, B. J., Watts, R. E., & Kottman, T. (2001). Approaches to play therapy: A tabular overview. *TCA Journal, 29,* 104–113.

Leben, N. Y. (1997). The yarn drawing game. In H. Kaduson & C. Schaefer (Eds.), *101 favorite play therapy techniques* (pp. 61–63). Northvale, NJ: Jason Aronson.

Leblanc, M., & Ritchie, M. (2001). A meta-analysis of play therapy outcomes. *Counselling Psychology Quarterly, 14,* 149–164.

Levy, D. (1938). "Release Therapy" in young children. *Psychiatry*, *1*, 387–389.

Lindaman, S., & Booth, P. (2010). Theraplay for children with autism spectrum disorders. In P. Booth & A. Jernberg (Eds.), *Theraplay: Helping parents and children build better relationships through attachment-based play* (pp. 301–358). San Francisco, CA: Jossey-Bass.

Lowenfeld, M. (1935/1991). *Play in childhood*. London: MacKeith Press.

Lowenfeld, M. (1939). The world pictures of children: A method of recording and studying them. *British Journal of Medical Psychology*, *18*, 65–101.

Ludlow, W., & Williams, M. (2006). Short-term group play therapy for children whose parents are divorcing. In H. Kaduson & C. Schaefer (Eds.), *Short-term play therapy for children* (2nd ed., pp. 304–335). New York: Guilford Press.

Malchiodi, C. A., & Crenshaw, D. A. (2014). *Creative arts and play therapy for attachment problems*. New York: The Guilford Press.

McNeil, C., Bahl, A., & Herschell, A. (2009). Involving and empowering parents in short-term play therapy for disruptive children. In H. Kaduson & C. Schaefer (Eds.), *Short-term play therapy for children* (2nd ed., pp. 169–202). New York: Guilford Press.

McNeil, C., Capage, L., Bahl, A., & Blanc, H. (1999). Importance of early intervention for disruptive behavior problems: Comparison of treatment and waitlist-control groups. *Early Education & Development*, *10*(4), 445–454.

McNeil, C., Eyberg, S., Eisenstadt, T., Newcomb, K., & Funderbunk, B. (1991). Parent-child interaction therapy with behavior problem children: Generalization of treatment effects to the school setting. *Journal of Clinical Child Psychology*, *20*(2), 140–151.

Miller-Morz, J., Lender, D., Rubin, P., & Lindaman, S. (2010). Theraplay for children who are adopted or in foster care. In P. Booth & A. Jernberg (Eds.), *Theraplay: Helping parents and children build better relationships through attachment-based play* (pp. 405–493). San Francisco, CA: Jossey-Bass.

Morrison, M., & Bratton, S. (2010). An early mental health intervention for Head Start programs: The effectiveness of child-teacher relationship training (CTRT) on children's behavior problems. *Psychology in the Schools*, *47*, 1003–1017.

Moustakas, C. (1959). *Psychotherapy with children*. New York: Ballantine Books.

Moustakas, C. (1997). *Relationship play therapy*. Northvale, NJ: Jason Aronson.

Mulherin, M. A. (2001). The Masterson approach with play therapy: A parallel process between mother and child. *American Journal of Psychotherapy*, *55*, 251–272.

Munns, E. (2011). Integration of child-centered play therapy and theraplay. In A. A. Drewes., S. C. Bratton, & C. E. Schaefer (Eds.), *Integrative play therapy* (pp. 325–340). Hoboken, NJ: John Wiley & Sons.

Nash, J. B., & Schaefer, C. E. (2011). Play therapy: Basic concepts and practices. In C. E. Schaefer (Ed.), *Foundations of play therapy* (2nd ed., p. 9). Hoboken, NJ: John Wiley & Sons.

Naumburg, M. (1966). *Dynamically oriented art therapy*. New York: Grune & Stratton.

Nims, D. R. (2009). Integrating play therapy techniques into solution-focused brief therapy. *International Journal of Play Therapy*, *16*(1), 54–68. doi:10.1037/1555-6824.16.1.54

Nisivoccia, D., & Lynn, M. (2007). Helping forgotten victims: Using activity groups with children who witness violence. In N. B. Webb (Ed.), *Play therapy with children in crisis: Individual, group, and family treatment* (pp. 294–321). New York: Guilford Press.

Oaklander, V. (1988). *Windows to our children: A gestalt therapy approach to children and adolescents*. Highland, NY: The Center for Gestalt Development.

Oaklander, V. (2006). *Hidden treasure: A map to the child's inner self*. London: Karnac.

O'Connor, K. (2000). *The play therapy primer* (2nd ed.). New York: Wiley.

O'Connor, K. (2009). The ecosystemic model. In K. J. O'Connor & L. D. Braverman (Eds.), *Play therapy theory and practice* (2nd ed., pp. 367–450). Hoboken, NJ: Wiley.

O'Connor, K. (2011). Ecosystemic play therapy. In C. Schaefer (Ed.), *Foundations of play therapy* (2nd ed., pp. 253–273). Hoboken, NJ: John Wiley and Sons.

O'Connor, K. J., & Ammen, S. (1997). *Play therapy treatment planning and interventions: The ecosystemic model and workbook*. New York: Academic Press.

O'Connor, K., & Schaefer, C. (1994). *The handbook of play therapy, Volume II: Advances and innovations*. New York: Wiley.

Orton, G. L. (1997). *Strategies for counseling with children and their parents*. Pacific Grove, CA: Brooks/Cole.

Paone, T., Packman, J., Madduz, C., & Rothman, T. (2008). A school-based group activity therapy intervention with at-risk high school students as it relates to their moral reasoning. *International Journal of Play Therapy, 17*, 122–137.

Pedro-Carroll, J., & Reddy, L. (2005). A preventive play intervention to foster children's resilience in the aftermath of divorce. In L. Reddy, T. Files-Hall, & C. Schaefer (Eds.), *Empirically based play interventions for children* (pp. 51–75). Washington, DC: American Psychological Association.

Rank, O. (1936). *Will therapy*. New York: Knopf.

Ray, D. C. (2010). *Advanced play therapy: Essential conditions, knowledge, and skills for child practice*. New York: Brunner-Routledge.

Ray, D. (2011). *Advanced play therapy: The complete picture*. New York: Routledge Ltd.

Ray, D. C., Henson, R. K., Schottelkorb, A. A., Brown, A. G., & Muro, J. (2008). Effect of short- and long-term play therapy services on teacher-child relationship stress. *Psychology in the Schools, 45*, 994–1009.

Reddy, L., Files-Hall, T., & Schaefer, C. E. (Eds.). (2005). *Empirically based play interventions for children*. Washington, DC: American Psychological Association.

Robson, M. (2008). The driver whose heart was full of sand: Leigh's story – a play therapy case study of a bereaved child. *British Journal of Guidance & Counselling, 36*, 71–80.

Rotter, J. C., & Bush, M. V. (2000). Play and family therapy. *Family Journal, 8*, 172–177.

Rubin, L. C. (Ed.). (2008). *Popular culture in counseling, psychotherapy, and play-based interventions*. New York: Springer.

Rubin, L., & Livesay, H. (2006). Look, up in the sky! Using superheroes in play therapy. *International Journal of Play Therapy, 15*, 117–133.

Schaefer, C. (Ed.). (1993). *The therapeutic power of play*. Northvale, NJ: Jason Aronson.

Schaefer, C. (2001). Prescriptive play therapy [Abstract]. *International Journal of Play Therapy, 10*, 57–73.

Schaefer, C. E. (2011). Prescriptive play therapy. In C. E. Schaefer (Ed.), *Foundations of play therapy* (2nd ed., pp. 365–378). Hoboken, NJ: John Wiley & Sons.

Schaefer, C. E., & Drewes, A. A. (2009). The therapeutic powers of play and play therapy. In A. Drewes (Ed.), *Blending play therapy with cognitive behavioral therapy: Evidence-based and other effective treatments and techniques*. Hoboken, NJ: John Wiley & Sons.

Schaefer, C. E., & Greenberg, R. (1997). Measurement of playfulness: A neglected therapist variable. *International Journal of Play Therapy, 6*(2), 21–32.

Schlanger, R. (2010). *For the love of Melissa*. Bloomington, IN: Author House.

Schuurman, D. L., & DeCristofaro, J. (2007). After a parent's death: Group, family, and individual therapy to help children. In N. B. Webb (Ed.), *Play therapy with children in crisis: Individual, group, and family treatment* (pp. 173–196). New York: Guilford Press.

Sheely-Moore, A., & Bratton, S. (2010). A strengths-based parenting intervention with low-income African American families. *Professional School Counseling, 13*, 175–183.

Shen, Y-J. (2010). Trauma-focused group play therapy in the schools. In A. Drewes & C. Schaefer (Eds.), *School-based play therapy* (2nd ed., pp. 237–256). Hoboken, NJ: Wiley.

Siu, A. F. Y. (2009). Theraplay in the Chinese world: An intervention program for Hong Kong children with internalizing problems. *International Journal of Play Therapy, 18*, 1–12.

Solomon, J. (1938). Active play therapy. *American Journal of Orthopsychiatry, 8*, 479–498.

Sori, C. F., & Schnur, S. (2014). Trauma-focused integrated play therapy: An interview with Eliana Gil, part I. *The Family Journal, 22*(1), 113–118. doi:10.1177/1066480713505280

Sweeney, D. S. (2001). *Counseling children through the world of play*. Eugene, OR: Wipf & Stock Publishers.

Sweeney, D. (2011). Group play therapy. In C. Schaefer (Ed.), *Foundations of play therapy* (2nd ed., pp. 227–252). Hoboken, NJ: John Wiley and Sons.

Taft, J. (1933). *The dynamics of therapy in a controlled relationship*. New York: Macmillan.

Trice-Black, S., Bailey, C. L., & Riechel, M. E. K. (2013). Play therapy in school counseling. *Professional School Counseling, 16*(5), 303.

VanFleet, R., Sywulak, A. E., & Sniscak, C. C. (2010). *Child-centered play therapy*. New York: Guilford Press.

Vaz, K. M. (2000). When is a sand play psychotherapy process completed? *International Journal of Action Methods: Psychodrama, Skill Training, and Role Playing, 53*, 66–81.

Walker, R. (1998). Magic art. In H. Kaduson & C. Schaefer (Eds.), *101 favorite play therapy techniques* (pp. 61–63). Northvale, NJ: Jason Aronson.

Watts, R. E., & Garza, Y. (2008). Using children's drawings to facilitate the acting "as if" technique. *The Journal of Individual Psychology, 64*, 113–118.

Webb, N. B. (2007). Crisis intervention play therapy with children. In N. B. Webb (Ed.), *Play therapy with children in crisis* (3rd ed., pp. 45–72). New York: Guilford Press.

Group Counseling with Children

Good leadership consists of doing less and being more.
—JOHN HEIDER

Many counselors find that working with groups is more effective than individual counseling. Children and adults function as members of groups in their daily activities—in the classroom, the work setting, or their neighborhoods. Our beliefs about ourselves and about other people evolve from the feedback of significant people who are important to us—especially our family, friends, and peers. This chapter will help you understand some of the considerations for planning, implementing, and evaluating groups.

After reading this chapter, you should be able to:

▶ List reasons for conducting groups
▶ Define groups and group types
▶ Outline different theoretical group orientations
▶ Explain group leadership and planning skills
▶ Discuss group stages and processes
▶ Describe a group model for crisis response

RATIONALE

Psychologists such as Alfred Adler emphasized that people are social beings and groups around them significantly influence their development; therefore, group counseling contains a real-world orientation, what Corey, Corey, and Corey (2014) considered a "natural laboratory." For children who have difficulties forming or maintaining relationships, being included in group counseling provides opportunities to improve those relationship skills. In groups, young people can improve their awareness of their own and other people's values and priorities. They can develop an appreciation for different views. Most important, groups provide a place where children can unlearn inappropriate behaviors and replace them with new ways of relating. Small groups provide young people with interaction and feedback in a safe practice situation with their peers. Goodnough and Lee (2010) agree and state that children learn best when they learn from each other.

Some current societal influences increase the need for children to be engaged in groups counseling. Certainly, the rapid increase in the use of electronic devices such as smartphones and computers has switched much communication from face-to-face contact to other means. Families may be less stable with increased economic concerns and no job security. They may also be more transient with the extended family living in a distant location. All of these and other world conditions exacerbate the child's natural need to have a forum for discussing concerns and decisions.

Bergin and Klein (2009) explain that the interactive process of groups influences children in several ways. As group members express caring, acceptance, and support for each other, participants learn to trust and share. In addition, the group's reality and emphasis on conscious thought allow participants to explore and genuinely express their thoughts, feelings, and actions. Finally, Bergin and Klein point out that as group members show understanding to each other, they grow in tolerance and an accepting attitude. They encourage participation of all group members in helping each other make educated choices about their personal behaviors. Therefore, the overarching benefit of group counseling is the creation of opportunities for group members to learn about themselves and others and to have a place to make choices and plan for carrying out those decisions in a supportive group.

Meta-analysis refers to the process of compiling several research studies that focus on a specific construct and then applying statistical tests to determine the effect size associated with outcomes across those studies. Such studies on group counseling with children indicate support for the effectiveness of group counseling with young people (Durlak & Wells, 1997; Hoag & Burlingame, 1997; Whiston & Sexton, 1998). Durlak and Wells looked at 177 primary prevention programs designed to prevent behavioral and social problems with children and adolescents. Many of those were delivered in small groups with strong success rates; results were also expressed in other studies (Kulic, Horne, & Dagley, 2004). Hoag and Burlingame (1997) conducted a meta-analysis of group treatment for children and adolescents, with the most common issues being behavioral problems, social skills, and divorce adjustment. They found that group treatments produced significantly better effects than wait-list or placebo control group. Shechtman (2002) also reviewed studies of group work in schools and concluded group counseling was effective and approximately 70 percent of groups for children occurred in school settings. Whiston, WendiLee, Rahardja, and Eder (2011) found small group interventions were comparatively effective so school counselors could maximize time by using groups to address guidance topics and to assist with emotional and personal problems. Forsyth (2010) captures the rationale for providing group counseling for children in these words—"groups are scientifically, practically and clinically significant" (p. 27). Clearly these positive outcomes suggest that counselors will want to include groups in their practice.

Counselors who are prepared to conduct groups will have completed the coursework and a supervised practicum to help them develop skills in this area. This chapter presents an overview of working with children in groups, with suggestions for those who already possess the knowledge and skills to conduct groups or for those who intend to pursue further training.

DEFINITION OF GROUP

Gladding (2012) defines a group as "a collection of two or more individuals who meet in face-to-face interaction, interdependently, with the awareness that each belongs to the group and for the purpose of achieving mutually agreed-on goals" (p. 4). These characteristics allow members in groups to deal with their own concerns, as well as to help other participants develop.

Dye (2002) has identified assumptions basic to group work. One assumption maintains that social behavior is learned; therefore, new experiences can produce new understandings. A group forum presents an environment in which those new ways of seeing situations can occur. Another foundation is that people have reasons for their actions and groups may allow opportunities to express and alter those purposes. The elements of group counseling consist of expressed goals, membership criteria, roles of members and leader(s), counseling methods and techniques, and interactions among the participants.

Jacobs, Masson, Harvill, and Schimmel (2012) summarized the benefits of group counseling as the following:

- *Efficiency:* having more than one person at a time saves time and effort.
- *Experience of commonality:* group members can discover their thoughts, and feelings may be shared with other people who have similar concerns.
- *Variety of resources and viewpoints:* group members have a range of opinions and ideas to share with each other.
- *Sense of belonging:* members may identify with each other and feel a part of something bigger than themselves.
- *Skills practice:* groups provide a place for safe practice.
- *Feedback:* group members have opportunities to receive feedback from each other and from the group leader.
- *Vicarious learning:* the opportunities to hear other members addressing similar concerns allow a group participant to apply the lessons.
- *Real-life approximation:* group members learn ways of relating and coping they can use in everyday living.
- *Commitment:* motivation to change is stronger when made to more than one person (pp. 2–5).

Group members support each other in several ways. Expressing their thoughts and perceptions leads to honest interactions as well as using feedback. As members connect across similar problems, they help each other identify alternative solutions. They may also speak to inconsistencies noted in order to help another become more aware of conflicting stories or details. Group members support each other and offer encouragement to other participants. The group becomes a place to experiment with appropriate responses and to talk about concerns in a caring environment. More specifically, some of the universal therapeutic factors that help group member include the following:

- *Acceptance*: being supported by members and leaders
- *Universality*: realizing I am not the only one with the problem
- *Self-disclosure*: trusting leaders and members, so revealing self honestly
- *Insight*: gaining self-awareness
- *Interpersonal interaction*: learning from other members
- *Catharsis*: experiencing emotional release and feeling of relief afterward
- *Guidance*: receiving and providing information and suggestions for improvement
- *Vicarious learning*: learning from observing and listening when working with others
- *Altruism*: feeling of worthiness when helping others
- *Hope*: taking positive action and believing things will improve (Yalom & Leszca, 2005)

TYPES OF GROUPS

Groups function in many ways depending on the goal of the group process. The main goal of group work consists of promoting personal growth and resolving problems and conflicts. Groups create opportunities for children to increase knowledge and skills to help them make and accomplish their choices (Bergin & Klein, 2009). Explanations of some common types of groups allow a counselor to determine which might be most appropriate to the situation and population with which they are working. Even though these descriptions may appear to indicate clear distinctions across types of groups, considering the types along a continuum would be more accurate. Jacobs and Schimmel (2005) remind us that group leaders must be clear about the type and purpose of the group.

Psychoeducational groups, sometimes referred to as educational or guidance groups, emphasize using educational methods to deliver and use information as well as develop skills. Corey et al. (2014) remarked that psychoeducational groups are particularly effective with children and adolescents because the new knowledge group members gain leads to their growth. The groups may focus on such topics as attitudes, beliefs, working together, communicating, and building friendship skills. Corey et al. (2014) explained that psychoeducational groups focus on the development of cognitive, affective, and behavioral skills through the use of a structured procedure. The groups focus on a theme and attempt to give members a better awareness of a life problem and the tools to cope with it. Gerrity and DeLucia-Waack (2007) reviewed research and found significant support for the use of psychoeducational groups in schools.

Bergin and Klein (2009) suggest that psychoeducational groups may be planned to help children investigate their identity concerns, developmental transitions, academic matters, and career planning. According to Boutwell and Myrick (1992), the social interaction in the group helps the members gain a sense of well-being that can lead to preventing future problems. When young people encounter others in the group who are facing similar concerns, they have opportunities to master more than the targeted skills, as well as gain an understanding of different types of coping. Fall, Landreth, and Berg (2013) consolidate that growth into the realization that others have problems too and therefore, not feeling all alone.

Some psychoeducational groups occur as classroom guidance activities in schools. Furr (2000) provides a format for designing a psychoeducational group. This format includes stating the purpose, establishing goals, identifying objectives, determining content, choosing exercises, and conducting evaluation. The design she proposes contains three components: giving information, practicing skills, and talking about the process. Her outline and examples would help counselors plan and deliver these groups. Akos, Goodnough, and Milsom (2004) provide another useful resource in planning groups. These authors recommend that when planning groups, leaders consider the developmental level of group participants, multicultural issues, school climate, and the overall mission of the program. DeLucia-Waack (2006) has a comprehensive textbook on leading psychoeducational groups for children and adolescents with extensive lists of resources and planning documents.

Counseling groups are also growth oriented, preventive, and remedial. Each person's behavior and development is the focus as group members attempt to develop or change within the group and through the help of the group (Gladding, 2012). The members of counseling groups are generally normal people who are experiencing some stress in their lives. Topics may revolve around concerns with interpersonal relationships, social skills, study skills, values, problem solving, or making decisions. The groups may also be centered on problems and topic determined by the concerns of individual participants at the time of the meeting. Goals of counseling groups include the following:

- Helping members develop more positive attitudes and interpersonal skills
- Using the group to help change behavior
- Assisting the transfer of the skills learned in the group to the world outside the group (Corey et al., 2014)

Arman (2000) suggests that counseling groups help children reduce their sense of social isolation and negative emotions. The groups may also be designed for children who are facing transitions in their lives such as divorce of parents, a death, or school problems. Children with behavioral problems may also benefit from counseling groups. Orton (1997) lists the benefits of the group as trust, caring, understanding, and support. In groups, children can help not only themselves but also others. Counseling groups may be held in schools, institutions, or mental health agencies.

Group therapy deals with unconscious motivations with the goal of personality change for the group members. These groups are held for the remediation and treatment of people who are severely disturbed, are suffering from deep psychological problems, or are exhibiting socially deviant behavior. The depth and extent of the disturbance is significant, so the group goals involve rebuilding, alleviating symptoms, and creating a place to explore problems (Corey et al., 2014). Those groups most often occur in mental health agencies and institutions.

Waldo and Bauman (1998) find those categories of group insufficient and propose the dimensions of process and goal as a more useful way to understand variations in groups. They have designed a matrix that maps the goals, pur-poses that guide group direction, and process, type of interaction characteristic of the group. Goals may be development—promoting growth, or remediation—correcting problems, or coping—effectively facing the unalterable. Process may be guidance—giving information and building skills through planned exercises; counseling—interpersonal support, interactive feedback, and here-and-now focus; and therapy—evoking emotional responses and exploring concerns in depth. Their classifications may be helpful as counselors plan for groups.

Two other types of groups merit attention. Support and self-help groups are most often formed by and for people who share concerns. They may be psycho-educational, psychotherapeutic, and perhaps task oriented. Alcoholics Anonymous may be the most recognized self-help group, but readers should know that over 800 self-help organizations exist in the United States so that an organization has been built for major chronic conditions and for shared experiences such as natural disasters. A clearinghouse for those groups can be found at http://www.mentalhelp.net/selfhelp/. With similar characteristics but with a differing media, online sup-port groups offer "encouragement, acceptance and virtual companionship to offset social and special isolation" (Rier, 2007, p. 1043). A Google search for online groups in 2013 revealed 1.4 million online support groups. Those different types are general sites sponsoring multiple groups, sites that recruit the Internet user to form a group, social networking sites, geographic communities, health- or medically related groups, mental health-related groups, parenting groups, politi-cal groups, ecology groups, business/enterprise groups, teaching- or academically focused groups, and interest-focused groups.

Some useful reviews of these online groups include summaries of interactive e-journaling (Haberstroh, Parr, Gee, & Trepal, 2006); internet support groups (Lieberman, Wizlenberg, Golant, & Minno, 2005); synchronous and asynchro-nous online discussions (Romano & Cikanek, 2003); and videos and computer simulations (Smokowski, 2003). Page (2011) summarized results of many online group formats.

THEORETICALLY ORIENTED GROUP COUNSELING

The number of group counseling methods almost equals the number of counseling theories, most of which can be adapted to a group counseling setting. The following summaries of theoretical approaches to groups can guide practitioners who form groups with children.

Gestalt therapy (see Chapter 7) focuses on the here and now and on maintaining personal awareness. The emphasis is on healing through the recognition of blocks that are interfering with the full experience of the here and now and the integration of those unacknowledged parts (Jacobs et al., 2012). Some Gestalt counselors ask for volunteers and focus on one client at a time within the group; for example, the hot seat technique requires the counselor to work with one person in the presence of the other group members. Structured interaction between other group members may be encouraged at certain times. Gestalt group leaders must be skillful enough to find the appropriate technique to help children gain awareness.

The principles of *behavioral counseling* (see Chapter 8) are also used in groups when the clients' goals are similar or members can help one another by providing feedback, support, or reinforcement to alter maladaptive behaviors, learn new behaviors, or prevent problems. Relaxation training, assertion training, modeling techniques, and self-management programs to control overeating or other negative behaviors are examples of behavioral techniques that can be used effectively in group settings. Behavioral group counseling is a type of education, so leaders must assume an active, directive role in the group, applying their knowledge and skills to the resolution of problems. Leaders emphasize current experiences, learning, and defining goals specifically. Leaders choose group procedures that are adapted to members' needs and that are scientifically verified. Gladding (2012) notes the prevalence of the use of positive reinforcement, extinction, desensitization, and modeling in behavioral group counseling.

Reality therapy (see Chapter 9) originally was used more extensively in groups than with individuals. The principles adapt effectively to group work because the group is a microcosm of the real world. The psychological needs of belonging, power, freedom, and fun can all be met by group members in that setting. Also, the members provide feedback about the reality of their behavior and plans for change. They reinforce one another in their commitments and check on the completion of homework assignments. The group leader focuses on helping the group members take responsibility for what they do, find better ways to have their needs met, and change their inappropriate or destructive behaviors (Glasser & Breggin, 2001). Fuller (2007) explained that reality therapy group leaders become involved quickly, focus on reality, help make plans, and establish rules to keep the group working well.

Wubbolding (2007) used the acronym WDEP to guide the counseling process. Identifying wants (W) starts the clarification of the concern. Once that focus has been identified, group members talk about what is being done (D) and the evaluation (E) of the effects of that behavior. The final part of the process is planning (P) for short- and long-term changes. Group members help throughout the process. Leaders may find it helpful to have the acronym posted to guide the group through those steps. Reality therapy has been a popular method for helping groups of children and adolescents in schools, those confined to correctional institutions, substance abusers, and those with handicaps.

Solution-focused (see Chapter 10) therapy emphasizes a person's strengths, positive coping, and solutions. Sharry (2007) applies solution-focused principles to groups. He proposes leaders focus on discussions that do not highlight pathology and change the conversations about problems to one about possibilities, reminding group leaders to highlight exceptions to problems and participants' strengths and positive coping. Group members look for what is right and what is working, and leaders help members find simple solutions and coach them to ease into these solutions. The group should be one of cooperation, collaboration, and opportunities. The benefits include group support, learning, optimism, opportunity to help others, and empowerment. Leaders can use the miracle questions, exception questions, and scaling and coping questions to keep the focus on possibilities.

Adlerian counselors used group work in their child guidance center in the early 1900s for group discussions involving parents (see Chapter 11). Adlerians believe that people are essentially social and need to belong to a community or group. Consequently, Adlerians see group counseling as a natural environment for helping children see the reality of the situation and meet their needs through social interactions in the group. As in individual counseling, Adlerian group counselors rely on investigation and interpretation of the child's life by establishing the relationship, exploring the dynamics operating in the child's life, communicating back to the child an understanding of self, and reorienting the child's behavior in new directions (Corey, 2012).

Adlerian groups emphasize the interpretation of a person's early history so that group members recognize and understand the ways they have created their own lifestyles. The group leader may focus participants on their private logic, their mistaken goals and the scripts they have about themselves, the world, and other people (Jacobs et al., 2012). Adlerian group leaders assume that if people can understand the reasons for their behaviors, they have a better chance to alter the actions that are not helpful. Adlerian groups also include the practice of having individual, interpersonal, and group process goals throughout the duration of the group. Gladding (2012) explains that individual goals involve developing insight, interpersonal goals revolve around becoming socially oriented and involved, and group process goals entail promoting and experiencing a cooperative group environment. Adlerian group leaders focus on understanding the current patterns of behavior of group members and challenging them to modify those patterns. When working with children in groups, the leaders may use encouragement to imply their faith in the child's ability to change. They may also emphasize natural consequences of behavior.

Rational emotive behavior therapy (REBT) (see Chapter 12) attempts to teach people to think rationally about events and to assume responsibility for their feelings. The techniques of this theory can be applied effectively in groups because members can learn the ideas quickly and discover how to apply those concepts in the group. Members are encouraged to recognize and confront their irrational thoughts and feelings, take risks, try new behaviors, and use others' feedback to learn new social skills. Members are taught to apply REBT principles to one another. Jacobs et al. (2012) explained that REBT helps children and adolescents feel more in control.

REBT leaders provide information, discuss problem-solving strategies, and may use many cognitive and/or emotive techniques. Leaders teach the ABC model of understanding behavior. As a reminder, C represents the consequences or emotional reaction, B represents the beliefs used in assessing the activating event—A—and connects A and C. Thus, group members learn that it is not what has happened to them but their interpretation of the situation that causes feelings. Group members can then learn to change their feelings by changing their self-talk. The group leader should be a role model for responsible and reality-oriented behavior, show care and respect, and teach participants to evaluate their present behaviors, as well as those planned.

Cognitive-behavioral (see Chapter 13) groups have several advantages. They create places with real-world interactions. They allow people to practice new behaviors and receive immediate feedback. The potential for role-plays exists and participants can test their beliefs with other group members (Gilman & Chard, 2007). The goals of cognitive therapy are to correct faulty information processing and to modify assumptions that maintain dysfunctional emotions and behaviors (Beck & Weishaar, 2008).

In a cognitive therapy approach the group leader creates an agenda with group members, discusses prior sessions, introduces topics, and teaches new information relative to the subject (Christner, Stewart, & Freeman, 2007; Scott, 2012). Group models have been outlined for working with children with depression, anxiety, PTSD, bereavement, eating disorders, and attention-deficit disorders. Group counseling is also effective for parent training and teaching children social skills (Gilman & Chard, 2007).

Ruffolo and Fischer (2009) provide an overview of translating a CBT evidence-based protocol for adolescents with depression to a school setting. Sommers-Flanagan, Barrett-Hakanson, Clarke, and Sommers-Flanagan (2000) have discussed a school group designed to improve social and coping skills of middle school students. Based on cognitive-behavioral theory, the groups included interventions to help students understand moods, identify pleasant events, reduce tension, increase strength, and solve problems.

Transactional analysis (TA) (see Chapter 14) is an ideal counseling method for groups; in fact, most counselors adhering to the principles of TA prefer treatment in groups. This method focuses on analysis of life scripts, strokes, games, and interactions among people, and the ideal setting for this teaching and learning is within a group that simulates life's interactions. Group members facilitate the counseling process by representing other individuals with whom past and present transactions can be analyzed. Group members can be taught the three ego states of Parent, Adult, and Child and the messages that accompany those states. Jacobs et al. (2012) suggest teaching TA by using a group member's situation as an illustration.

Table 18-1 contains the goals of these theories as related to group counseling. Other counseling methods have their place in group work but do not adapt to it as readily as those already mentioned. The relationship skills set forth by

TABLE 18-1 OVERVIEW OF THEORY GOALS IN GROUP COUNSELING

Theory	Goals
Gestalt	To help participants focus on the present so they can recognize and integrate the unknown parts of themselves.
Behavioral	To help group members eliminate unwanted behaviors and learn new ways of acting.
Reality therapy	To guide participants to realistic and responsible behavior. To help group members evaluate their behavior and determine a plan of action for change.
Solution-focused	To discover strengths, exceptions, and positive coping in the group members and to use those in finding solutions to the problem.
Adlerian	To create an environment that encourages group members to investigate their assumptions about life and to reach a fuller understanding of lifestyles.
Rational emotive behavior therapy	To teach group members they are responsible for their disturbances and to help them eliminate the irrational thoughts and self-defeating outlook and replace them with more rational ideas.
Cognitive behavioral	To help group members uncover their cognitive distortions and move to a more functional way of thinking.
Transactional analysis	To help participants give up scripts and games in their interactions.

person-centered counselors are appropriate in an individual or group setting. The therapeutic relationship is an essential ingredient for all clients to feel free enough to explore their world and make changes.

GROUP LEADERSHIP SKILLS

In groups for children and adolescents, counselors primarily work as leaders of the group process taking responsibility for structuring and conducting the groups as well as demonstrating caring, empathy, respect, and the importance of working together. Counselors will complete the following tasks: assess the needs for a group, define the purposes of the group, select participants, arrange permission for participants, organize the schedule, plan the activities, and arrange for materials and space to meet. DeLucia-Waack (2006) has provided many strategies and forms to help complete those tasks.

Conyne (2012) gives an integrative definition of group leadership that includes three central tasks: to create and maintain the group, to build a group culture, and to activate and illuminate the here and now. Leadership involves the ability to draw from best practices and professional judgment to create a group and, in collaboration with members, build and maintain a positive group climate that serves to nurture here-and-now interaction and its process by leader and members, all aimed at producing lasting growth and change (Yalom & Leszcz, 2005). Leaders contribute to building and maintaining either a healthy or unhealthy group climate. Trotzer (2011) says leaders who behave consistently with members in a caring and empathic manner, who constructively confront, and who maintain a supportive therapeutic relationship with members add greatly to positive group climate. Burlingame (2010) emphasized that encouragement is a critical leadership practice in groups with children.

According to the Association for Specialists in Group Work (2000), to lead effective groups, leaders must be able to do the following:

- Collaborative consultation with targeted populations to enhance ecological validity of planned group interventions
- Planning for a group work activity including such aspects as developing overarching purpose, establishing goals and objectives, detailing methods to be used in achieving goals and objectives, determining methods for outcome assessment, and verifying ecological validity of plan
- Encouraging participation of group members
- Attending to, describing, acknowledging, confronting, understanding, and responding empathically to group member behavior
- Attending to, acknowledging, clarifying, summarizing, confronting, and responding empathically to group member statements
- Attending to, acknowledging, clarifying, summarizing, confronting, and responding empathically to group themes
- Eliciting information from and imparting information to group members
- Providing appropriate self-disclosure
- Maintaining group focus; keeping a group on task
- Giving and receiving feedback in a group setting

- Contributing to evaluation activities during group participation
- Engaging in self-evaluation of personally selected performance goals
- Evidencing ethical practice in planning, observing, and participating in group activities
- Evidencing best practice in planning, observing, and participating in group activities
- Demonstrating diversity-competent practice in planning, observing, and participating in group activities (pp. 6–8)

Corey (2012) contends that the group leadership's personal characteristics and skills cannot be separated from the techniques used. Those authors believe that "leaders bring to every group their personal qualities, values, and life experiences . . . the most effective group direction is found in the kind of life the group members see the leader demonstrating and not in the words they hear the leader saying" (p. 53). Corey et al. (2014) suggest the following personal characteristics as essential to a group leader:

- *Presence*—genuine caring in "being there" for clients
- *Openness*—revealing enough of yourself to let the group members have an idea of who you are as a person
- *Willingness to model*—showing the desired behaviors in the group setting
- *Courage*—ability to take risks and be vulnerable
- *Goodwill, genuineness, and caring*—sincere interest in well-being of others; behaving without pretense
- *Nondefensiveness in coping with criticism*—knowing one's values, strengths, and limitations and dealing frankly with challenges
- Belief and enthusiasm for the group process
- *Being aware of subtle culture issues*—increasing awareness of our own prejudices and biases and confronting prejudicial attitudes or remarks in the group
- Being able to identify with a person's pain
- *Personal power*—knowing who you are and what you want, a sense of confidence in self
- *Stamina*—physical and psychological vitality
- Sense of humor
- *Inventiveness and creativity*—open to new ideas and experiences (pp. 31–38)

Jacobs et al. (2012) explained that leaders of groups for children and adolescents need some special skills. Leaders will need to vary the group format and use many different approaches such as puppets, drawings, and skits. Leaders must learn to hold the focus on the topic long enough for some impact, which may mean cutting off one child's talking to let someone else share. Leaders should use enthusiastic voices, be clear about the purpose of the group, and have specific knowledge about the topic of the group. With groups of adolescents, leaders need to take charge and be interesting to keep the participants' attention. Also, group leaders need to use structure to reach the group goals.

The professional skills needed by group leaders, as identified by Corey (2012), include active listening, reflecting, clarifying, summarizing, questioning, interpreting, confronting, supporting, empathizing, facilitating communication, initiating direction, setting goals, evaluating, giving feedback, suggesting, protecting, self-disclosing, modeling, linking (looking for themes), blocking (stopping counter-productive behaviors by confronting them), and terminating.

Gladding (2012) explains that three specific skills are significantly different in group counseling. He states that leaders in groups facilitate by helping group members communicate among themselves. Group leaders protect members by barring unnecessary attacks from others in the group, a skill unnecessary in individual counseling. A related skill, blocking, entails a group leader intervening in a group activity to stop counterproductive behavior. Group leaders also encourage participation, keep the group on task, and move the group in the direction of the stated objectives (Greenberg, 2003).

Johnson and Johnson (2013) and Yalom and Leszcz (2005) identified the functions of a group leader. The leader provides emotional stimulation, caring, praise, protection, acceptance, interpretations, and explanations. The leader serves as an example as well as the person who establishes limits, enforces rules, and manages time (Jacobs et al., 2012).

Corey et al. (2014) highlight the importance of developing diversity competence and the Association for Specialists in Group Work (2000) "Principles for Diversity-Competent Group Workers" as guidelines. Leaders do not allow their personal beliefs to interfere with work. They are aware of their own cultural background and their view of health. They are moving to an increasing awareness of all aspects of culture and they value and respect differences. They try to investigate and understand the world-view of their clients including religious and spiritual beliefs. Diversity-competent group leaders recognize their sources of discomfort with differences. They accept and value diversity, identify and understand cultural constructs, and avoid imposing their own constructs. Finally, culturally effective group leaders monitor themselves through consultation, supervision, and continuing training and education. Some excellent examples of the effectiveness of a culturally competent group leader can be found by examining work with African American males and other ethnic groups (Bailey & Bradbury-Bailey, 2007; Dowden, 2009; Shen, 2007; Steen, 2009; White & Rayle, 2007).

In summary, Jacobs and Schimmel (2005) have identified the knowledge and skills needed by group counselors. Group leaders need to be clear about the purpose of the group and must know the theory from which they are working. Group leaders should be familiar with the topics being covered and should be creative. Finally, the authors recommend that group leaders understand and accommodate students from diverse cultures.

GETTING STARTED

Choice Model

Conyne, Crowell, and Newmeyer (2008) talked about three Ps for running effective groups—planning, performing, and processing. The planning component includes identifying the group type (psychoeducational, counseling, or therapy), the stage of the group, and a best practice that is applicable. Group leaders are encouraged to analyze situations looking at context, connections, system maintenance, collaboration, sustainability, and making meaning. Then leaders review possible techniques. Leaders consider whether the focus will be cognitive, affective, behavioral, or structural. Group leaders also look at the level of impact being either individual, interpersonal, or group. Leaders then make selections with attention to the criteria of adequacy, appropriateness, effectiveness, efficiency, and side effects. Finally, leaders implement the strategy and evaluate its effectiveness. Those authors have an appendix, a "toolbox," that charts all those details: group types, best practice area, group stage, concepts, focus, and level. Using that toolbox would greatly enhance planning any type of group.

Group Focus

Counselors may use multiple sources of information to decide about group topics. A primary consideration should be the need of students as determined by reports from students, caretakers, and teachers. Counselors may also analyze available data such as school records for trends and recurring problems. Circumstances in the community may also drive the decision about the types of groups to offer. For example, a crisis in the neighborhood, military deployment, or a significant loss would be situations needing a counseling response that might include small groups. Whether using a formal or informal needs assessment, counselors use care in deciding the focus of groups they deliver.

Counselors determine the logistics of a group based on the type of group being held. Some groups may include materials that relate to a wide range of individuals. Others may focus on specific areas such as divorce or grief. In addition, resources chosen for a group may be chosen principally with the age of the participants in mind. The counselor could identify a topic by his or her perception of what is needed, from the results of a needs assessment, or by the special needs of the school and/or community (Greenberg, 2003). The topics will vary according to the children's ages and the settings in which the groups are to be held. Webb has identified the most common types of groups offered by school counselors. Those groups focus on social skills, learning skills, self-control or anger management, divorce, loss, and school adjustment/transitions. See Table 18-2 for a more comprehensive list of possible topics that would be suitable for children and adolescents.

Gazda, Ginter, and Horne (2001) recommend that children younger than 12 should take part in groups that include play and action with counselors using techniques such as sociodrama, child drama, and psychodrama. Ginott (1968; as cited in Gladding, 2003) recommends the use of watercolors, finger paints, clay, and sand for children younger than 9. Therefore, groups for children and young adolescents may be more action oriented than those for teenagers. Bergin and Klein (2009) suggest that structured exercises may help individuals in adolescent groups form trust and cohesion and become more open in their communication. Theme-oriented groups may also help adolescent groups. Gladding (2012) suggests having young people check off a list of interests and/or problems to determine a theme for a group.

Bergin and Klein (2009) note some elements basic to all groups. Groups must have purposes that are defined and reflected in the goals and objectives prepared before group participants are selected. The goals direct the group process and the objectives clarify that focus by outlining anticipated outcomes for group members. The objectives also help the counselor determine the activities and discussion procedure to use, as well as how to determine whether the purpose(s) has (have) been attained. Continuing with a note that all groups must have requirements for membership, they advocate for counselors incorporating structured activities to stimulate group interaction and self-reflection. The elements discussed by Bergin and Klein will be influenced by the type of group discussed next.

Greenberg (2003) classifies groups as remedial, support, or preventive groups. Remedial groups concentrate on the problems faced by most students such as study skills, listening skills, and overcoming test anxiety. Support groups deal with more personal problems and allow children to realize that others face similar challenges. Examples include groups about parental divorce, stopping a habit, or being new to the school. Preventive groups focus on avoiding difficulties. Problem solving, anger management, and handling stress could be topics of preventive groups. Wilson and Owens (2001) explain that prevention groups have focused on preventing

TABLE 18-2   POSSIBLE SMALL-GROUP TOPICS FOR SCHOOL-AGED CHILDREN

Group Topics

Academics	Personal/Social Development	Personal/Social Development	Future Planning
Academic achievement	Anger management/ aggression	Health concerns	Decision making
Attention-deficit disorder	Anxiety	Peer pressure	Goal setting
Attitudes about school	Body image	Pregnancy, in-school mothers	Work habits
Career awareness	Breaking a bad habit	Problem solving	Working as part of a team
Learning styles	Bullying preventions	Recognizing and dealing with emotions	
Motivation	Communication skills	Self-concept, identity, efficacy	
New to school	Conflict management	Social skills	
Overcoming test anxiety	Death, grief, loss	Stress management	
Responsible school behavior	Depression	Substance abuse	
Study skills	Family issues such as divorce	Valuing diversity	
Time management	Friendships		

Adapted from Cobia, D. C., & Henderson, D. A. (2007); Corey, Corey, & Corey (2014).

psychological disorders, difficulties in relationships, failure in roles, failure in work groups, and physical distress. Kulic et al. (2004) outline concepts and methods for counselors who use prevention groups with children and adolescents.

Activities in these groups may incorporate videos, books, games, worksheets, simulations, and role-plays. The Life Skills Training program incorporates activities related to self-identity, problem solving, decision making, social skills, and physical health (Shechtman, 2004).

According to Bergin and Klein (2009), problem-centered groups are more open ended, with topics determined by the concern of the group participants at the time of the meeting. These groups focus on the here-and-now experience. Members have the opportunity to engage every other member in exploring their problems, examining potential alternatives and the consequences of those possibilities, and deciding on a course of action. These groups may be more appropriate for older children who have the ability to state their concerns and to attend to others. Some topics that may concern elementary students include relationships with family and friends, conflicts with authority figures, relationships with peer groups, and moving into middle school. Adolescents may be troubled by relationships, dating, sexual matters, teachers, homework, and school; balancing commitments; and planning for the future. Two successful group formats that may be used in problem-solving groups are Shure (1992) *I Can Problem Solve* and Goldstein and McGinnis (1997) *Skillstreaming Curriculum*. Both focus on improving the social competence of children and adolescents.

Topic-specific groups focus on the needs of young people who have a situational difficulty that is causing negative feelings and stress (Bergin & Klein, 2009). The group members share some serious, immediate concerns. The group setting allows members to understand the issue in depth, to explore feelings, and to find coping strategies. This type of group may arise from a crisis event such as a death. In that case, the group purpose is to provide support in dealing with the crisis. The following concerns may be addressed by topic-specific groups: physical abuse, grief and loss, sexual abuse, aggressive behavior, divorce and separation, fear and stress, children of alcoholics, suicide, and teen parenting. The Children of Divorce Intervention Program (Pedro-Carroll & Cowen, 1985) is an example of a multimodal group developed to support children in sharing their divorce-related feelings and in building their competence.

Developing a Proposal

Corey et al. (2014) explained the procedure for developing a group proposal. Planning a group requires deciding on five general areas that are well documented. Leaders need to have a clear rationale for the group that includes the benefits of the group approach. The objectives of the group should be articulated with the strategies for achieving them identified. Objectives should be specific, measurable, and reachable within the specified time period. Practicalities such as membership criteria, meeting times, place, frequency, and duration need definition. The procedures chosen should be tied to the objectives and be appropriate and realistic (see Conyne et al., 2008, for a valuable resource). Finally, the proposal for a group should include the evaluation methods, which are chosen with objectivity, practicality, and relevance in mind.

The topic of groups will determine the criteria for selecting members to participate. Some general guidelines for that process are included in this section.

Selecting Group Members

Shechtman (2004) states the most relevant variables in forming groups are age, sex, problem topic, and size of group. Some counselors, such as Adlerians, hold that anyone who wishes to participate in a group should be allowed to do so, given similar, age-related levels of interest and intellectual abilities. Other counselors attempt to select members for either heterogeneity or homogeneity. Some counselors prefer a balance of boys and girls in the same group unless the presence of the opposite sex would hinder discussion (e.g., on some sex education topics). Other counselors prefer to eliminate tension by holding same-sex groups.

Homogeneity may be desirable for common-problem groups, such as children whose parents are divorced. However, a homogeneous group of underachievers or anger management concerns probably would be counterproductive because no peer model and peer reinforcement for improved behaviors would be present. Riva and Haub (2004) also caution that a group format may increase the likelihood of early adolescents learning deviant behaviors unless more socially adept young people are also included in the groups. Parents and adult caregivers should also be part of that type of treatment. For children who act out or withdraw, a heterogeneous group provides active discussion and role models.

The counselor should seriously consider the possible consequences of including children with highly dissimilar interests or maturity levels and extremely dominating, manipulative, gifted, or mentally retarded children. Children with extreme behaviors may be better candidates for individual counseling, especially during the initial stages of therapy. Riva and Haub (2004) suggest that extremely shy or anxious young people may find the group format too stressful.

Forming a Group

Counselors may begin by recruiting members for groups. Ritchie and Huss (2000) suggest that counselors avoid labeling groups with names that imply a diagnosis or dysfunction. Children may be identified by giving to adults some type of behavioral checklists to assess target behaviors. Counselors may also have children volunteer for group interactions by forming groups as responses to needs of assessments they have conducted. Corey et al. (2014) remind counselors that some children are not ready to be members of groups. The severity of the children's problems should also be considered in the selection process. Counselors need to establish clear criteria for all group participants.

Some reports of people being verbally attacked and hurt in groups that use extreme methods may leave parents or children with reservations about participating in a group. Counselors should explain fully the purpose of the group and the experiences planned to allay fears and clarify possible misconceptions. By providing this information to children before starting the group, the counselor can inform the children of their roles and what is expected of them and explain the role and expectations of the counselor as well. Explaining the process provides the structure needed to facilitate interaction once the group has begun. Following is an example of an informative statement:

> We are forming a group made up of young people about your age to talk about things that bother or upset us. Many of us have similar concerns, and it is often helpful to share these worries and help each other try to find ways of solving them. Each member will be expected to talk about what bothers him or her and try to figure out what can be done about these situations. In addition, members will be expected to listen carefully to each other and to try to understand the other members' worries and help them solve their problems. The counselor, too, tries to understand what all the members are saying or feeling, to help them explain and clarify their thoughts and feelings and to find solutions to their concerns.
>
> Most group members learn they can trust the others in the group and feel free to discuss things that worry them. Members are free to talk about anything or anyone that bothers or upsets them. However, the group will not be a gripe session, a gossip session, or a chatting session. We will be working together to find solutions to what is upsetting you. There may be very personal information or feelings that you would prefer not to discuss in the group. You should not feel pressured to disclose these feelings or thoughts to the group. Whatever is said in the group cannot be discussed with anyone except the counselor. If there is anyone you would rather not have in a group with you, discuss this with the counselor.

Screening Interview

Many group leaders prefer to hold an individual conference or intake interview with prospective members before forming the group. Other group leaders think that anyone should be eligible to join a group and that the intake interview is unnecessary. An intake interview allows the leader an opportunity to talk privately with prospective members, to learn a little about them and their concerns, and to define some possible goals. The leader also has an opportunity to determine whether the child will benefit from a group experience or whether individual counseling would be more helpful. The group leader would begin by identifying the characteristics of the group members that would be beneficial to the process, as well as criteria that would signify the person should be excluded (Ritchie & Huss, 2000). Children who are overly aggressive and children who are overly sensitive to criticism would probably not benefit from group counseling. Overly angry, hyperactive, self-centered, unstable children should also be helped with other types of interventions (Ritchie & Huss, 2000; Shechtman, 2004).

During the screening interview, the counselor can check the young person's willingness to engage in self-improvement, the desire to help others, the commitment to group progress, and compatibility with other group members (Bergin & Klein, 2009). Greenberg (2003) states other criteria for group members. The child should have the language skills to communicate with other group members and should be willing to participate in group interactions. The young people should be prepared to share their individual feelings and experiences. They should accept and abide by group rules and be committed to the group members. Greenberg suggests that counselors ask potential group participants about each of these areas.

Holcomb-McCoy (2003) emphasizes the importance of counselors being attuned to cultural beliefs and how culture affects the child's concerns. She suggests asking potential group members to discuss their perceptions of counseling and their expectations of the group. Group activities and structure could be modified accordingly. DeLucia-Waack and Donigian (2004) outlined the practice of multicultural group work in their book that contains perspectives from group leaders.

Ritchie and Huss (2000) list the following as possible screening questions:

How does this concern affect you at school, at home, at play?

Do you spend time worrying about this concern?

Would you like to talk with someone about this issue?

Do you feel comfortable talking about your feelings in a group? (p. 150)

Size of Group

The number of children in the group depends on age, maturity, and attention span. Children ages 5 and 6 years have very short attention spans and are unable to give much attention to others' concerns. Counselors may want to limit group size at this age to three or four and to work with the children for only short time periods at frequent intervals—for example, 20 minutes twice a week. Counselors can work with a larger number of older, more mature children for longer periods—for example, six children, ages 10 and 11, for 30 minutes twice a week. Corey et al. (2014) suggest keeping within two grade levels when forming a group such as first and second graders, ninth and tenth graders. The maximum number of children in a group that functions effectively seems to be eight.

Group Setting

A room away from noise and traffic is the best setting. In addition, children should not fear being overheard if they are expected to talk openly about their concerns. Groups should be conducted with all members sitting in a circle so that everyone can see everyone else's face. Some counselors prefer to have the children sit around a circular table; others think tables are a barrier to interaction. Many counselors prefer to have groups of children sit in a circle on a carpeted floor, which provides easy access for counselors to move the group into play therapy.

GROUP STAGES

The interactions in groups change as participants continue to meet. Several authors have explained these different group stages and most include a movement through stages of beginning, transition, working, and leaving. Gladding (2012) and Corey (2012) have identified four stages of group counseling.

Beginning

The initial stage—orientation and exploration—is one of getting acquainted, determining the structure of the group, and exploring the members' expectations. Bingman and Goodman (2008) stated that the tasks are determining who is here and what is going to happen and then questioning fit and trust. Group leaders focus on creating a safe environment for the participants. Members are somewhat tentative and reserved at this point; therefore, the leader should focus on making sure they feel included and on developing trust. The leader and the group establish ground rules and group procedures. In almost all groups, the leader should clarify the purpose of the group and the responsibilities of the group members. The leader should emphasize the need for confidentiality and other crucial guidelines. Some common procedures for groups with children include having only one person speak at a time, listening to the speaker, taking turns, and not making fun of each other. During the beginning of the group, the goal is for members to build rapport and to learn to participate in the group.

Corey et al. (2014) discussed this early stage as a time to become familiar with other people and with the group format. Risk taking will be low and exploration tentative. Members will be concerned with whether they belong or not, and they will try to define their place. The critical issue is trust or mistrust. Leaders in the initial stage teach guidelines and group process, model interpersonal skills, and assess the needs of the group. Jacobs and Schimmel (2005) recommend that group leaders pay attention to the ways group members relate to each other, as well as their connection with the purpose and content of the group in this and all other stages of the group.

Transition

The transition phase of the group involves members testing each other and perhaps the leader. They experiment with the new relationships and with the process of the group to determine who and how much to trust. Bingman and Goodman (2008) characterized the tasks of the transitions stage as developing norms about the rules of behavior, participation, and disagreement. Members are wondering if they have any influence, choice, and power. Corey (2012) characterizes this phase as one of dealing with resistance, in which feelings of anxiety may increase and the group leader may be challenged. The members will test the leader to determine whether the counselor can be trusted and decide whether to get involved. The leader structures the group, clarifies the purpose, and models trust.

Corey et al. (2014) talked about this group period as one of anxiety and defenses. Members worry about themselves and test the leader and other members for safety. The dilemma for members is whether to risk or to play it safe. The major issues are power and control. The leader teaches the value of recognizing and dealing with conflict situations and constructive self-preservation, helping members become both interdependent and independent.

Working

As the members begin to accept each other, they move to the working stage. This is the stage of cohesion and productivity. Bingman and Goodman (2008) identified the tasks of this phase as getting things done and solving problems as well as having a connection to other group members. During this stage, the members focus on identifying their goals and concerns, and they are willing to work both in the group and outside to address these concerns. As they focus on the issues on which they are working, they explore and clarify the concerns, set goals, and practice new behaviors. In a group that meets for eight sessions, the working phase often occurs between session 4 and 6.

Corey et al. (2014) characterized this stage as one of open communication with members interacting freely and directly. Conflict, if it occurs, is named and dealt with effectively. Feedback is given, accepted, and acted upon. Group members feel supported and hopeful. The leader continues to model and provides a balance between support and confrontation. When common themes emerge, the leader links them to engender the sense of universality among members. The focus at this group stage is moving from insight to action. Questions that may help this productive group period are the following: How did you feel during this activity? What did you learn? How can you apply what you learned? What will you do to practice? (Bingman & Goodman, 2008). Conyne et al. (2008) have resources for leaders to determine the most effective techniques to use at this and other group stages.

Ending

The last stage of group work includes the members evaluating what has been accomplished and then exiting the group experience. The final stage—consolidation and termination—is extremely important, according to Corey (2012), because integration of learning takes place and members must be able to transfer what they have learned to other situations outside the group. Bingman and Goodman (2008) explained the tasks at this stage are to end the group, apply what has been learned, and let go of the group experience. Group members may have some anxiety and reluctance to terminate; therefore, the leader must deal with these feelings and any other unfinished business, and then prepare members to use their new skills in their daily lives. The leader should make arrangements for some follow-up and evaluation of the group process to determine the effectiveness of the group and its effects on the member. A final group session, an individual session, or a questionnaire may be used for this purpose.

Corey et al. (2014) highlighted that some sadness may occur with the impending separation and that group members may retreat as they decide what actions to take. Members may talk about their fears, hopes, and concerns for one another. Group members also evaluate the group activity during this phase. The group leader helps consolidate by providing a structure to help participants clarify the meaning of their experiences and to connect their learning to everyday life.

Bingman and Goodman (2008) offered some questions for the closing stage of group counseling.

- What important things have you learned about yourself during our time together?
- How can you continue to practice what you have learned?
- What has been the most helpful part of the group for you?

Jones and Robinson (2000) have created a model for choosing topics and exercises appropriate for the different group stages. Their framework involves generating activities appropriate for the group theme, and then matching the activities to the goals and stages of the group. They discuss intensity, creating a climate of work, and building relationships through all the phases of group work.

GROUP COUNSELING PROCESS

The First Session

Early sessions should include introductions, discussion of the group purpose, and explanations about confidentiality. The members learn how the group functions, define their goals and expectations, and find their place in the group. Part of the first group counseling session will be devoted to establishing ground rules and agreeing on some guidelines for the group. The group or the leader determines the frequency of the meetings, the length of each meeting, the setting, and the duration of the group. Members also need to discuss confidentiality and what might be done if confidentiality is broken by a member, what to do about members who do not attend regularly, and whether to allow new members should a member drop out.

Confidentiality is an important concept to discuss with children. They often do not understand the necessity for "keeping what is discussed in our group among us" and not talking to others about what happens. The leader can provide specific instances of other children asking about their group and have participants role-play their responses.

The group leader also has to remind members to listen carefully to each other, to try to understand each other's feelings and thoughts, and to help one another explore possible solutions to problems. The children can be encouraged to wait until members appear to have explored and discussed their concerns thoroughly before changing the subject. The group leader can provide the role model for listening and reflecting feelings and content, and then reinforce these behaviors in group members.

By establishing ground rules and structuring the group during the initial session, the group leader defines expected behaviors. When inappropriate behaviors occur, the leader can ask the group, "What was the ground rule?" or present the problem to the group for discussion and resolution.

Group members may be reluctant to begin by bringing up concerns or worries for discussion, especially if the participants are not acquainted. The leader can reflect their feeling of reluctance and, if appropriate, try an icebreaker counseling technique; for example, the leader might ask members to introduce themselves and describe themselves with three adjectives, or members might be asked to introduce themselves and complete a statement such as "If I had three wishes, I would wish for _____." Another icebreaker is to complete the statement "I am a (n) _____, but I would like to be a (n) _____," using animals, vegetables, automobiles, flowers, or other nonhuman categories; for instance, "I am a dandelion, but I'd like to be a long-stemmed rose." These activities can be done in the entire group or in dyads; either method eases the tension of the first session and promotes interaction.

Building cohesiveness and trust is important for counselors. Children have had little experience listening to one another and trying to help one another solve problems. Unless these behaviors are taught, the group experience can become little more than unstructured play and chatter.

Guidelines for the Remaining Sessions

Before the second group session, the counselor reviews thoroughly the content of the first meeting (names, behaviors, concerns, other personal information) and develops a plan for guiding the second meeting. At this point, the counselor should have tentative goals in mind for each member, based on the initial interview, and should be aware of who in the group will facilitate the group process—a good listener, encourager, or problem solver—and who will distract—dominating, too talkative, silly, or confrontational. The counselor may want to develop plans for dealing with distracting behaviors, should they occur.

Corey et al. (2014) advise counselors that providing structure is particularly important in groups with children. One way to accomplish that is to use a standard format. Gilbert (2003) recommends that group leaders begin each meeting with a routine that may include welcomes, reviews of rules and previous sessions, focus on current topic, an exercise related to the topic, discussion about the exercise, and a closing activity in which participants talk about what they have learned or experienced.

The second session opens with a brief summary of the initial meeting. If homework was assigned, the results should be shared. The group is then ready to address a member's concerns, either one that was identified earlier or a situation that occurred between meetings that may be concerning a member. If no one volunteers to discuss a problem or concern, those identified in the pregroup interviews can be suggested by the counselor: "When we talked in our interview before the first meeting of the group, some of you shared with me that you were worried because you are going to high school next year. Who would like to start by telling the group about what frightens you about that change?"

Just as in individual counseling, a group leader establishes a therapeutic counseling atmosphere by demonstrating the facilitative skills of empathetic understanding, genuineness, and respect for group members. Counselors can demonstrate their caring by being nonjudgmental and accepting and by providing encouragement, support, and guidance. Counselors need to be adept at identifying, labeling, clarifying, and reflecting group members' feelings and thoughts. This process becomes difficult as the group size increases. The counselor-facilitator must be concerned about and aware of the reactions of each child in the group. As the leader models facilitative behaviors, group members begin to participate in the helping process and become more effective helpers for one another.

The group counseling process closely follows the format for individual counseling:

1. Establishing a therapeutic relationship
2. Defining the problems of the member or members
3. Exploring what has been tried and whether it has hurt or helped

4. Deciding what could be done and looking at the alternatives
5. Making a plan—goal setting
6. Trying new behaviors by implementing the plan
7. Assigning homework
8. Reporting and evaluating the results

Also, as in individual counseling, the counselor-facilitator is responsible for helping children identify and define their problems and the accompanying feelings and thoughts. The process of defining what is happening in the child's life and looking at alternatives for solving the conflict is enhanced in the group setting because of the other group members. Ideally, the group participants serve as several counselors to listen, understand, and help the child search for solutions. All group members can enjoy the acceptance, encouragement, support, and feedback from each other. The counselor must be skilled in facilitating these interactions and suggesting appropriate interventions. The counselor must also know about group dynamics and counseling skills to intervene and facilitate progress through the various steps of the counseling process.

Implications for Different Ages

The role of group counselors varies with different aged children. For instance, elementary school counselors work with children who are in their formative years. Group counseling can help these children acquire social skills and shape a positive attitude toward school. Gilbert (2003) suggests topics that should be routinely offered to this age group. These topics include children dealing with divorcing parents, children with attention-deficit/hyperactivity disorder, friendship, loss, academic achievement, and single-parent homes. She provides outlines for these groups. Ingley-Cook and Dobel-Ober (2013) have outlined a group counseling process for adopted children to help them with their questions and concerns. Children involved reported knowing others who had similar experiences was the most helpful part of the groups. Groups for elementary students have been used to help children build skills in empathy (Akos, 2000) and wellness (Villalba, 2007), reduce aggression (Choi, Lee, & Lee, 2010; Shechtman, 2001), deal with divorcing parents (DeLucia-Waack & Gellman, 2007), loneliness and anxiety (Bostick & Anderson, 2009), and live with a cancer patient (Stanko & Taub, 2002). Children at risk (Sherrod, Getch, & Ziomek-Daigle, 2009) and children with deployed parents (Rush & Akos, 2007) have also been supported in counseling groups. Ziff, Pierce, Johanson, and King (2012) explain a creative group counseling program that revolves around art media.

McEachern and Kenny (2007) conducted a group for high school students with disabilities who reported benefits in learning to move from high school into postsecondary opportunities. White and Rayle (2007) used a small-group counseling format to promote social interaction and wellness among African American male high school students. Paone, Packman, Maddux, and Rothman (2008) compared group activity therapy with group talk therapy on the moral reasoning of at-risk ninth graders.

Cooper and Whitebread (2007) explain nurture groups that focus on collaborative efforts and academic success of children who are categorized as "at risk."

The children's needs for attachment and relationships are met in the groups. The promising results have been replicated in countries other than the United Kingdom, where Cooper and Whitebread have developed this program.

Evaluation of Groups

The effectiveness of group work can be measured in many ways. Questions that can guide these decisions and their purpose are discussed in the following paragraphs.

What did we set out to accomplish? As stated earlier, the purpose of the group determines the type of group being led. During the planning process, the goal of the group is identified as well as the means for determining whether the goal was met. For example, in a friendship group, the goal may be for each member to initiate a conversation with a stranger. For an educational group, an assessment of the change in the participants' knowledge about the subject would be an evaluation possibility.

How did the participants respond? Feedback from the group members helps the leader monitor the progress and adapt the procedures as needed. Participants can respond to open-ended questions, rating scales, and summary statements to sum up their reflections and reactions.

What behaviors changed outside the group setting? The group leader may involve other adults in assessing changes in children who participated in groups. Teachers and parents may be asked to complete behavioral observations before, during, and after the group. They may be given a rating sheet about the behaviors that have been targeted. The group leader can interview the adults and ask for observations about the child's behavior.

How effective was the leader? One way to assess the group leader's effectiveness is to consider the answers to the previous three questions. Observations by colleagues, self-reflections, and input from the group members on rating scales or other instruments can also provide useful data. Bruckner and Thompson (1987) provide a model for evaluating weekly group counseling sessions with children in elementary school that could be adapted for use with group counseling programs in any setting. They developed an instrument containing the following six incomplete statements and two forced-choice items:

1. I think coming to the group room is _____.
2. Some things I have enjoyed talking about in the group room are _____.
3. Some things I would like to talk about that we have not talked about are _____.
4. I think the counselor is _____.
5. The counselor could be better if _____.
6. Some things I have learned from coming to the group room are _____.
7. If I had a choice, I (would) (would not) come to the group room with my class.
8. Have you ever talked with your parents about things that were discussed in the group? (yes) (no)

Some of these items may be used as a needs survey for future group sessions. Someone other than the group leader checks the results of the survey. Two independent people rate student responses on a five-point scale, ranging from 5 for statements showing an outright positive, accepting attitude toward the item to a rating of 1 for statements showing an outright rejecting, negative attitude toward the item. A rating of 3 is awarded to neutral, ambivalent, or evasive responses. Limited positive and negative responses receive ratings of 4 and 2, respectively. Raters should reach 85 percent levels of agreement and generally experience little difficulty in obtaining agreement on the remaining 15 percent.

Group Counseling Example

The process and techniques used in individual counseling (such as role-playing, role rehearsal, play therapy, homework assignments, and contracting) are just as appropriate for group counseling. In fact, individual counseling often is conducted in groups, as the following example shows. Karen, Susan, Peggy, Mark, Ken, and Mike are 11-year-old children in their fourth session in a counseling group. Following is an excerpt from this session:

COUNSELOR: Last time we met, Susan told us about the misunderstanding she was having with her neighbor, Mrs. Jackson. As I remember, Susan, you were going to offer to use your allowance to replace the storm window you broke playing baseball or offer to babysit free of charge for her until the bill was paid. Can you bring us up to date on what's happened?

SUSAN: Well, she decided she would rather have me babysit for her to pay for the window. I babysat 1 hour last week. We are keeping a list of the times I sit and how much will go toward the cost of the window.

COUNSELOR: It sounds as though you and Mrs. Jackson have worked things out to the satisfaction of both of you.

SUSAN: Yeah, she really liked the idea of my babysitting to pay for the window.

COUNSELOR: Good. Is there anyone else who has something they would like to discuss today?

ALL SIX CHILDREN: Mr. Havens!

COUNSELOR: You all sound pretty angry at Mr. Havens. Could one of you tell me what's happened?

KEN: We were all going on a trip to the ice-skating rink next week. Yesterday, somebody broke some equipment that belonged to Mr. Havens. No one would tell who did it, so he is punishing us all by not letting us go ice-skating.

COUNSELOR: You think Mr. Havens is being unfair to punish everyone because of something one person did. You'd like to find out who broke the equipment.

KAREN: That's right. We didn't break his equipment, so why should we have to miss the trip?

COUNSELOR: Have you thought of anything you could do to work this out?

MIKE: Yeah, break the rest of his old equipment!

COUNSELOR: How would that help you get to go skating?

MARK: It wouldn't. It would just make him madder.

PEGGY: [timidly] We could tell him who did it.

OTHER FIVE CHILDREN: You know who did it? Who?

PEGGY:	[very upset] If I tell, I'll be called a tattler, and no one will like me. Besides, I don't want to get anyone in trouble.
COUNSELOR:	Peggy, it sounds as though you are really feeling torn apart by this. You just don't know what to do. If you don't tell, the whole group will miss the skating outing. If you do tell, you'll get someone in trouble, and your friends might think you're a tattler and not want you around.
PEGGY:	Yeah, I don't know what to do!
COUNSELOR:	What do you think you could do?
PEGGY:	Well, I could tell who did it.
COUNSELOR:	What would happen if you told? [Silence.] Let's help Peggy think of all the things that could happen if she told who broke Mr. Havens' equipment. [The group thinks of all the possible positive and negative results of Peggy telling who broke the equipment: the group might still get to go skating, the person might beat up Peggy or try to get back at her in some other way, she might not be believed, the person could deny it and say Peggy broke the equipment, and so on.]
COUNSELOR:	We've listed all the things that could happen if Peggy told. What will happen if Peggy does not reveal who broke the equipment?
KAREN:	We won't get to go skating, and the person will get away with it! [Other possibilities— such as Mr. Havens's distrust of the whole group or the person thinking he or she "can get away with anything"—are discussed.]
COUNSELOR:	Can anyone think of any alternatives to solve this other than Peggy telling or not telling Mr. Havens?
KEN:	She could write him an anonymous letter telling him who did it.
COUNSELOR:	What would happen if she did?
MIKE:	He probably wouldn't believe an anonymous letter.
COUNSELOR:	What do the rest of you think about that? [They all agree by nodding their heads that Mike is probably right.]
COUNSELOR:	Is there anything else you could do to straighten this out?
SUSAN:	Peggy could tell you [the counselor], and you could tell Mr. Havens.
COUNSELOR:	How would my telling Mr. Havens help you all solve your problem?
MARK:	Mr. Havens would believe you, and we'd get to go skating!
COUNSELOR:	I would have to tell Mr. Havens how I knew and give him some details to assure him that I was right. I really think this is the group's problem. What can you do to work it out?
KAREN:	Seems like it's up to Peggy, then.
COUNSELOR:	You all think it's up to Peggy to decide whether to tell. [The group agrees it is Peggy's decision.]
COUNSELOR:	Peggy, we have looked at the consequences of your telling on the other person and not telling, and we've tried to think of other alternatives. Have you made any decision about what to do?
PEGGY:	No, I still don't know.

COUNSELOR: So far, it seems that we have come up with two possible alternatives—to tell on the person or not to tell. I wonder if you can think of any other alternatives that might help Peggy. [Silence.] Well, our time is about up for today, but this topic is really important. Let's meet together tomorrow and try to help Peggy come to some decision at that time. Peggy, I wonder if you would go over the list of alternatives and think about them before tomorrow. [Peggy agrees.] How would the rest of you feel about trying to put yourselves in Peggy's place and think of what you would do if you knew who broke Mr. Havens's equipment? Also, you might think about how you would feel if you were the person who broke the equipment. What would you want Peggy to do? [The group agrees and adjourns.]

The counselor checked on the results of the last homework assignment for the group, listened, and reflected the group members' angry feelings that Mr. Havens was being unfair. The counselor then helped them clarify and define the problem, look at possible alternatives, and consider the consequences of these alternatives. No decision has been reached, but the group has agreed to a homework assignment of thinking further about the problem. Possibly, the next session will bring new ideas and a resolution.

Classroom Meetings

School counselors may want to show teachers ways to use group meetings in their class. Glasser (1969) discusses three types of meetings. Educational-diagnostic classroom meetings are used to determine how much students know about a topic before a new unit is begun or at the conclusion of a unit of study. Social-problem-solving meetings are designed to help the classroom group solve their concerns. Teachers help students consider how their behaviors are helpful, not helpful, or perhaps harmful to themselves and/or to others. Classroom members in the problem-solving meetings follow the reality therapy questions to determine action to resolve the difficulty. Open-ended classroom meetings allow students opportunities to introduce and discuss thought-provoking questions related to their lives. Teachers can use the following guidelines to lead those meetings.

GUIDELINES FOR LEADING CLASSROOM MEETINGS

1. Identify the topic clearly:
    a. The topic for today is _____.
    b. Would someone restate what we will discuss today?
    c. Today we can discuss _____ or _____. Which will it be?

2. Ask for definitions:
    a. What do you mean by _____?
    b. What is _____?

3. Ask for specifics:
    a. What else do you need to know about _____?
    b. Tell me more about _____?

4. Ask for personal examples:
   a. Who do you know who has _____?
   b. Have you ever _____?
   c. How does _____ relate to your life?

5. Ask for agreements and disagreements:
   a. Who agrees with you?
   b. Who disagrees with you?
   c. Why?

6. Challenge the group:
   a. How can you find out more about that?
   b. What would you like to learn more about that idea?

7. Present hypothetical situations involving the topic:
   a. What would happen if we did not have _____?

8. Withhold personal judgment of right and wrong in students' answers and opinions. Help them arrive at their own evaluation of their thinking and behaving.
9. Refrain from asking any embarrassing questions or questions the person asking would be unwilling to answer. Each person always has the right to pass on responding to any question.
10. Uphold the right to state an opinion without being ridiculed.
11. Use the reality-therapy problem-solving model to reach a resolution to a specific concern.

GROUP CRISIS INTERVENTION

Two classmates are killed in a fiery car wreck.

A 12-year-old puts a gun to his head and commits suicide.

The mother of a 9-year-old dies of cancer.

The father of a 7-year-old is murdered.

War breaks out, and the television shows bombings on 24-hour newscasts.

Economic recession hits, and many parents lose their jobs.

Reports of an earthquake forecast send feelings of fear and panic throughout the population.

A hurricane devastates an entire section of the state.

In recent years, professionals have been asked to provide crisis counseling to children in schools, churches, and clubs. Incidents such as these stimulate fear, helplessness, loss, sadness, and shock. Children worry about the loss of their parents (their safe haven), their friends ("Could it happen to me? Why did it happen?"), and their security ("Where will I go if I lose my home?"). In some cases, their parents may be coping with their own loss or grief and be unable to help the children. In other cases, the situation may be related to the school, church, or an organizational group, and children may feel that their parents do not really understand the situation. Some parents may not realize their children are worried; some children are not able to verbalize their pain.

Those who work with children recognize that young people cannot learn or perform their daily activities with these fears and concerns. They become irritable, restless, or agitated. They have difficulty concentrating and sleeping. They may experience physical symptoms such as nausea or diarrhea. Someone has to help them cope, which is usually effected through group discussion and group counseling.

James and Gilliland (2012) propose six steps for crisis counseling that are similar to the reality therapy model described in previous chapters of this book. These steps include: (1) defining the problem, (2) ensuring the client's physical and psychological safety, (3) providing support through verbal and nonverbal means, (4) examining alternatives, (5) making plans—definite action steps, and (6) obtaining the client's commitment to take positive action. They urge counselors to evaluate the severity of the crisis in the clients' eyes; appraise clients' thinking, feelings, and behaviors; determine the danger and the length of time in a crisis mode; look for contributing factors; and evaluate resources, coping mechanisms, and support systems. James and Gilliland suggest that counselors may want to begin sessions with a nondirective approach but shift to more directive counseling as the need arises. Crisis counseling is short term, and counselors should carefully consider some children's need for referrals or other arrangements to ensure that each client successfully copes with the crisis in the days and weeks to follow.

Crisis counseling is focused on decreasing the stress of the event, giving support to the person involved, and increasing the person's coping abilities. Myer, Lewis, and James (2013) propose a task model of crisis response with the continuous task of assessment, safety, and support as the ongoing work of people who intervene. Counselors work to discover what the person needs and to ensure physical and psychological safety while encouraging and accepting. People need information about the current situation and the steps they can take. Counselor listens carefully, try to help people identify their pressing needs, and whether or not a solution is possible (Hendricks, McKean, & Hendricks, 2010). Crisis helps facilitate people developing coping skills to deal with their circumstances, hopefully reducing their distress and working toward a positive future.

Graham (1990) presents a plan for helping children after a trauma such as a hurricane or plane crash. Incorporating ideas presented by Graham with those of James and Gilliland (2012) and Greenstone and Leviton (2010), we suggest the following outline for group crisis counseling:

I. Introductory phase
   A. Ask members to introduce themselves and tell why they are in the group.
   B. Help members clarify their goals regarding what they would like to accomplish in the meeting.
   C. Discuss confidentiality—what group members talk about stays in the group. Get a commitment from all members to maintain confidentiality.
   D. Discuss basic rules:
      1. Take a bathroom break first because no one can leave the room after the group begins.
      2. Encourage group members to stay the entire time. The group generally runs for 2 hours; the time depends on the ages of the children.

      3. Elect or appoint a co-leader or a peer leader to keep the gate (i.e., not let people in or out).

      4. Remind the group that no group member holds rank over any other group member and that everyone's participation is valued equally.

II. Fact phase
   A. Focus on discussing what happened.
   B. Encourage everyone to participate.

III. Feeling phase
   A. Ask "What happened then?"
   B. Ask "What are you experiencing now?"

IV. Clients' symptoms
   A. Ask "How is this affecting you?" (Is the member having trouble sleeping or studying, or is the member worrying too much?)
   B. Ask "How is this affecting your grades, your studies, your health?"

V. Teaching phase
   A. Explore the common responses to this incident.
   B. Brainstorm about how people have been responding to the incident.
   C. Discuss how each response is helpful or not helpful to people.

VI. Summary phase
   A. Raise questions and provide answers.
   B. Summarize what has been learned and shared.
   C. Develop action plans for individuals and/or the group, if needed.
   D. Provide support for group members to ensure their physical, emotional, and psychological safety. An action plan should be made to protect any group member needing protection.
   E. Conduct a follow-up meeting in 3 to 5 days to see how well the group members are coping.
   F. Arrange individual counseling sessions for group members who need further assistance.

SUMMARY

In conclusion, group counseling can be a highly effective method for changing children's lives or, better still, preventing excess stress and conflict in their lives. Group counseling helps practitioners serve more students. Group members grow when they make commitments to each other to improve their behavior, when they accomplish specific personal goals, when they take appropriate risks in the group, and when they accept responsibility for themselves and for the growth of others. Finding their place in a group and helping one another are rewarding accomplishments for children, skills that will improve their lives at school and at home. Watching groups may be

built around remedial topics so that areas in which members have problems are addressed. Groups may be supportive in which meetings revolve around emotional or psychological support and understanding. Groups may also be focused on education around common issues. In all these categories groups provide a forum for children discussing concerns, developing goals and plan to reach those goals, and also practicing new behaviors. Watching children grow and develop into caring, functioning group members is rewarding for the group counselor. Without doubt, well-planned and delivered group counseling is an effective, efficient intervention to improve children's worlds.

WEB SITES FOR GROUP COUNSELING WITH CHILDREN

Internet addresses frequently change. To find the sites listed here, visit www.cengage .com/counseling/henderson for an updated list of Internet addresses and direct links to relevant sites.

Association for Specialists in Group Work

National Center for PTSD

REFERENCES

Akos, P. (2000). Building empathic skills in elementary school children through group work. *Journal for Specialists in Group Work, 25,* 214–223.

Akos, P., Goodnough, G. E., & Milsom, A. S. (2004). Preparing school counselors for group work. *Journal for Specialists in Group Work, 29,* 127–136.

Arman, J. F. (2000). In the wake of tragedy at Columbine High School. *Professional School Counseling, 3,* 218–220.

Association for Specialists in Group Work. (2000). *Professional standards for the training of group workers.* Alexandria, VA: Author. Retrieved from http://www.asgw.org/

Bailey, D. F., & Bradbury-Bailey, M. E. (2007). Promoting achievement for African American males through group work. *Journal for Specialists in Group Work, 32,* 83–96.

Beck, A. T., & Weishaar, M. E. (2008). Cognitive therapy. In D. Wedding & R. J. Corsini (Eds.), *Current psychotherapies* (10th ed., pp. 231–298). Belmont, CA: Thomson.

Bergin, J. J. & Klein, J. F. (2009). Small-group counseling. In A. Vernon (Ed.), *Counseling children and adolescents* (4th ed., pp. 359–386). Denver, CO: Love Publishing.

Bingman, G., & Goodman, B. (2008). *Group counseling for school counselors: A practical guide* (3rd ed.). Portland, ME: Walch.

Bostick, D., & Anderson, R. (2009). Evaluating a small-group counseling program—A model for program planning and improvement in the elementary setting. *Professional School Counseling, 12*(6), 428–433. doi:10.5330/PSC.n.2010-12.428

Boutwell, D. A., & Myrick, R. D. (1992). The go for it club. *Elementary School Guidance and Counseling, 27,* 65–72.

Bruckner, S., & Thompson, C. (1987). Guidance program evaluation: An example. *Elementary School Guidance and Counseling, 21,* 193–196.

Burlingame, G. M. (2010). Small group treatments: Introduction to special section. *Psychotherapy Research, 20,* 1–7.

Choi, A., Lee, M. S., & Lee, J. (2010). Group music intervention reduces aggression and improves self-esteem in children with highly aggressive behavior: A pilot controlled trial. *Evidence-Based Complementary and Alternative Medicine, 7*(2), 213–217. doi:10.1093/ecam/nem182

Christner, R. W., Stewart, J. L., & Freeman, A. (2007). *Handbook of cognitive-behavior group therapy with children and adolescents: Specific settings and presenting problems.* New York: Routledge.

Conyne, R. K. (2012). Group counseling. In E. M. Altmaier & J. C. Hansen (Eds.), *The Oxford handbook of counseling psychology* (pp. 611–646). New York: Oxford University Press.

Conyne, R. K., Crowell, J. L., & Newmeyer, M. C. (2008). *Group techniques: How to use them more purposefully.* Upper Saddle River, NJ: Merrill.

Cooper, P., & Whitebread, D. (2007). The effectiveness of nurture groups on student progress: Evidence from a national research study. *Emotional & Behavioural Difficulties, 12*(3), 171–190. doi:10.1080/13632750701489915

Corey, G. (2012). *Theory and practice of group counseling* (8th ed.). Pacific Grove, CA: Brooks/Cole.

Corey, M. S., Corey, G., & Corey, C. (2014). *Groups: Process and practice* (9th ed.). Pacific Grove, CA: Brooks/Cole.

DeLucia-Waack, J. L. (2006). *Leading psychoeducational groups for children and adolescents.* Thousand Oaks, CA: Sage.

DeLucia-Waack, J. L., & Donigian, J. (2004). *The practice of multicultural group work: Visions and perspectives from the field.* Belmont, CA: Thomson.

DeLucia-Waack, J. L., & Gellman, R. A. (2007). The efficacy of using music in children of divorce groups: Impact on anxiety, depression, and irrational beliefs about divorce. *Group Dynamics: Theory, Research, and Practice, 11*(4), 272–282. doi:10.1037/1089-2699.11.4.272

Dowden, A. R. (2009). Implementing self-advocacy training within a brief psychoeducational group to improve academic motivation in Black adolescents. *Journal for Specialists in Group Work, 34,* 118–136.

Durlak, J. A., & Wells, A. M. (1997). Primary prevention mental health programs for children and adolescents: A meta-analytic review. *American Journal of Community Psychology, 25*(2), 115–152. doi:10.1023/A: 1024654026646

Dye, A. (2002). Designing a counseling group. *Group Work Practice Ideas, 7,* 9–12.

Fall, K. A., Landreth, G. L., & Berg, R. C. (2013). *Group counseling.* Abingdon, Oxon, UK: Taylor and Francis. doi:10.4324/9780203114629

Forsyth, D. R. (2010). The nature and significance of groups. In R. K. Conyne (Ed.), *Oxford handbook of group counseling* (pp. 19–35). New York: Oxford University Press.

Fuller, G. B. (2007). Reality therapy approaches. In H. T. Prout & D. T. Brown (Eds.), *Counseling and psychotherapy with children and adolescents: Theory and practice for school and clinical settings* (pp. 332–387). Hoboken, NJ: Wiley.

Furr, S. R. (2000). Structuring the group experience: A format for designing psychoeducational groups. *Journal for Specialists in Group Work, 25,* 29–49.

Gazda, G. M., Ginter, E. J., & Horne, A. M. (2001). *Group counseling and group psychotherapy: Theory and applications.* Boston, MA: Allyn & Bacon.

Gerrity, D. A., & DeLucia-Waack, J. L. (2007). Effectiveness of groups in the schools. *Journal for Specialists in Group Work, 32*(1), 97–106.

Gilbert, A. (2003). Group counseling in an elementary school. In K. R. Greenberg (Ed.), *Group counseling in K-12 schools: A handbook for school counselors* (pp. 56–80). Boston, MA: Allyn & Bacon.

Gilman, R., & Chard, K. M. (2007). Cognitive-behavioral and cognitive approaches. In H. T. Prout & D. T. Brown (Eds.), *Counseling and psychotherapy with children and adolescents: Theory and practice for school and clinical settings* (pp. 241–278). Hoboken, NJ: Wiley.

Ginott, H. (1968). Group therapy with children. In S. T. Gladding (Ed.), (2003). *Group work: A counseling specialty* (4th ed.). Upper Saddle River, NJ: Merrill.

Gladding, S. T. (2012). *Group work: A counseling specialty* (6th ed.). Upper Saddle River, NJ: Merrill.

Glasser, W. (1969). *Schools without failure*. New York: Harper & Row.

Glasser, W., & Breggin, P. R. (2001). *Counseling with choice theory*. New York: HarperCollins.

Goldstein, A. P., & McGinnis, E. (1997). *Skillstreaming the adolescent: New Strategies and perspectives for teaching prosocial skills*. Champaign, IL: Research Press.

Goodnough, G. E., & Lee, V. V. (2010). Group counseling in schools. In B. T. Erford (Ed.), *Professional school counseling: A handbook of theories, programs and practices* (2nd ed., pp. 435–443). Austin, TX: ProEd.

Greenberg, K. R. (2003). *Group counseling in K-12 schools*. Boston, MA: Allyn & Bacon.

Greenstone, J. L., & Leviton, S. C. (2010). *Elements of crisis intervention* (3rd ed.). Belmont, CA: Cengage.

Haberstroh, S., Parr, G., Gee, R., & Trepal, H. (2006). Interactive E-journaling in group work: Perspectives from counselor trainees. *The Journal for Specialists in Group Work, 31*(4), 327–337. doi:10.1080/01933920600918840

Hendricks, J. E., McKean, J. B., & Hendricks, C. G. (2010). *Crisis intervention: Contemporary issues for on-site interveners*. Springfield, IL: Charles C Thomas Publisher.

Hoag, M. J., & Burlingame, G. M. (1997). Evaluating the effectiveness of child and adolescent group treatment: A meta-analysis review. *Journal of Clinical Child Psychology, 26*, 234–246.

Holcomb-McCoy, C. C. (2003). Multicultural group counseling in the school setting. In K. R. Greenberg (Ed.), *Group counseling in K-12 schools: A handbook for school counselors* (pp. 150–164). Boston, MA: Allyn & Bacon.

Ingley-Cook, G., & Dobel-Ober, D. (2013). Innovations in practice: Group work with children who are in care or who are adopted: Lessons learnt. *Child and Adolescent Mental Health, 18*(4), 251–254. doi:10.1111/j.1475-3588.2012.00683.x

Jacobs, E. E., Masson, R. L., Harvill, R. L., & Schimmel, C. J. (2012). *Group counseling: Strategies and skills* (7th ed.). Belmont, CA: Thomson.

Jacobs, E., & Schimmel, C. (2005). Small group counseling. In C. Sink (Ed.), *Contemporary school counseling: Theory, research, and practice* (pp. 82–115). Boston, MA: Lahaska Press.

James, R. K., & Gillaland, B. E. (2012). *Crisis intervention strategies* (7th ed.). Pacific Grove, CA: Brooks/Cole.

Johnson, D. W., & Johnson, F. P. (2013). *Joining together: Group theory and group skills* (11th ed.). Boston, MA: Allyn & Bacon.

Jones, K. D., & Robinson, E. H., III. (2000). Psychoeducational groups: A model for choosing topics and exercises appropriate to group stage. *Journal for Specialists in Group Work, 25*, 356–365.

Kulic, K. R., Horne, A. M., & Dagley, J. C. (2004). A comprehensive review of prevention groups for children and adolescents. *Group Dynamics: Theory, Research, and Practice, 8*(2), 139–151. doi:10.1037/1089-2699.8.2.139

Lieberman, M., Wizlenberg, A., Golant, M., & Minno, M. (2005). The impact of group composition on Internet support groups: Homogeneous versus heterogeneous Parkinson's groups. *Group Dynamics: Theory, Research, and Practice, 9*, 239–250.

McEachern, A. G., & Kenny, M. C. (2007). Transition groups for high school students with disabilities. *Journal for Specialists in Group Work, 32*, 165–177.

Myer, R. A., Lewis, J. S., & James, R. K. (2013). The introduction of a task model for crisis intervention. *Journal of Mental Health Counseling, 35*(2), 95–107. Retrieved from http://search.proquest.com/docview/1346367814?accountid=14868

Orton, G. L. (1997). *Strategies for counseling with children and their parents.* Pacific Grove, CA: Brooks/Cole.

Page, B. (2011). Online groups. In R. K.Conyne (Ed.), *The Oxford handbook of group counseling* (pp. 520–533). New York: Oxford University Press.

Paone, T. R., Packman, J., Maddux, C., & Rothman, T. (2008). A school-based group activity therapy intervention with at-risk high school students as it relates to their moral reasoning. *International Journal of Play Therapy, 77,* 122–137.

Pedro-Carroll, J. L., & Cowen, E. L. (1985). The children of divorce intervention program: An investigation of the efficacy of a school-based prevention program. *Journal of Consulting and Clinical Psychology, 53,* 603–611.

Rier, D. A. (2007). Internet support groups as moral agents: The ethical dynamics of HIV+ status disclosure. *Sociology of Health & Illness, 29*(7), 1043–1058.

Ritchie, M. H., & Huss, S. N. (2000). Recruitment and screening of minors for group counseling. *Journal for Specialists in Group Work, 25,* 146–156.

Riva, M. T., & Haub, A. L. (2004). Group counseling in schools. In J. L. DeLucia-Waack, D. Gerrity, C. R. Kalodner, & M. T. Riva (Eds.), *Handbook of group counseling and psychotherapy* (pp. 309–321). Thousand Oaks, CA: Sage.

Romano, J. L., & Cikanek, K. L. (2003). Group work and computer applications: Instructional components for graduate students. *Journal for Specialists in Group Work, 28*(1), 23–34. doi:10.1080/714860147

Ruffolo, M. C., & Fischer, D. (2009). Using an evidence-based CBT group intervention model for adolescents with depressive symptoms: Lessons learned from a school-based adaptation. *Child & Family Social Work, 14*(2), 189–197. doi:10.1111/j.1365-2206.2009.00623.x

Rush, C. M., & Akos, P. (2007). Supporting children and adolescents with deployed caregivers: A structured group approach for school counselors. *The Journal for Specialists in Group Work, 32*(2), 113–125. doi:10.1080/01933920701227034

Scott, M. J. (2012). *Simply effective group cognitive behaviour therapy.* Abingdon, Oxon, UK: Taylor and Francis.

Sharry, J. (2007). *Solution-focused group work.* Los Angeles, CA: Sage.

Shechtman, Z. (2001). Prevention groups for angry and aggressive children. *Journal for Specialists in Group Work, 26,* 228–236.

Shechtman, Z. (2002). Child group psychotherapy in the school at the threshold of a new millennium. *Journal of Counseling and Development, 80,* 293–299.

Shechtman, Z. (2004). Group counseling and psychotherapy with children and adolescents: Current practice and research. In J. L. DeLucia-Waack, D. Gerrity, C. R. Kalodner, & M. T. Riva (Eds.), *Handbook of group counseling and psychotherapy* (pp. 429–444). Thousand Oaks, CA: Sage.

Shen, Y. (2007). Developmental model using Gestalt-play versus cognitive-verbal group with Chinese adolescents: Effects on strengths and adjustment enhancement. *Journal for Specialists in Group Work, 32,* 285–305.

Sherrod, M. D., Getch, Y. Q., & Ziomek-Daigle, J. (2009). The impact of positive behavior support to decrease discipline referrals with elementary students. *Professional School Counseling, 12*(6), 421–427. doi:10.5330/PSC.n.2010-12.421

Shure, M. (1992). *I can problem solve (ICPS): An interpersonal cognitive problem solving program for children.* Champaign, IL: Research Press.

Smokowski, P. R. (2003). Beyond role-playing: Using technology to enhance modeling and behavioral rehearsal in group work practice. *Journal for Specialists in Group Work, 28*(1), 9–22. doi:10.1080/714860206

Sommers-Flanagan, R., Barrett-Hakanson, T., Clarke, C., & Sommers-Flanagan, J. (2000). A psychoeducational school-based coping and social skills group for depressed students. *Journal for Specialists in Group Work, 25,* 170–190.

Stanko, C. A., & Taub, D. J. (2002). A counseling group for children of cancer patients. *Journal for Specialists in Group Work, 27,* 43–58.

Steen, S. (2009). Group counseling for African American elementary students: An exploratory study. *Journal for Specialists in Group Work, 34,* 101–117.

Trotzer, J. (2011). Personhood of the leader. In R. K. Conyne (Ed.), *The Oxford handbook of group counseling* (pp. 287–306). New York: Oxford University Press.

Villalba, J. A. (2007). Incorporating wellness into group work in elementary schools. *Journal for Specialists in Group Work, 32,* 31–40.

Waldo, M., & Bauman, S. (1998). Regrouping the categorization of group work: A goals and process (GAP) matrix for groups. *Journal for Specialists in Group Work, 23*(2), 164–176. doi:10.1080/01933929808411388

Whiston, S. C., & Sexton, T. L. (1998). A review of school counseling outcome research: Implications for practice. *Journal of Counseling & Development, 76*(4), 412–426. doi:10.1002/j.1556-6676.1998.tb02700.x

Whiston, S. C., WendiLee, T., Rahardja, D., & Eder, K. (2011). School counseling outcome: A meta-analytic examination of interventions. *Journal of Counseling & Development, 89,* 37–55.

White, N. J., & Rayle, A. D. (2007). Strong teens: A school-based small group experience for African American males. *Journal for Specialists in Group Work, 32,* 178–189.

Wilson, F. R., & Owens, P. C. (2001). Group-based prevention programs for at-risk adolescents and adults. *Journal for Specialists in Group Work, 26,* 246–255.

Wubbolding, R. (2007). Reality therapy theory. In D. Capuzzi & D. R. Gross (Eds.), *Counseling and psychotherapy: Theories and interventions* (4th ed., pp. 289–312). Upper Saddle River, NJ: Pearson.

Yalom, I., & Leszca, M. (2005). *The theory and practice of group psychotherapy* (5th ed.). New York: Basic Books.

Ziff, K., Pierce, L., Johanson, S., & King, M. (2012). ArtBreak: A creative group counseling program for children. *Journal of Creativity in Mental Health, 7*(1), 108–121. doi:10.1080/15401383.2012.657597

CHAPTER 19

Counseling Children with Special Concerns

I have found the paradox that if I love until it hurts, then there is no hurt, but only more love.
—MOTHER TERESA

In previous chapters, we described some of the challenges inherent in our complex society—difficulties with which children must cope during their major years of growth and development. Counselors obviously cannot supply all the answers to these problems; however, several concerns of children are pressing, and children facing those challenges are seen frequently by counselors. This chapter suggests ways of working with children with some of these special needs and problems. The suggestions should be incorporated into a caring, accepting counseling atmosphere and modified to meet the unique needs of the child and the presenting concern. This chapter examines the following problems: child maltreatment; substance abuse in the family; children who encounter death, depression, and suicidal behaviors; family complications such as divorce and separation, single-parent homes, stepfamilies; and, finally, children and violence.

After reading this chapter, you should be able to:

▸ Define child maltreatment, its causes, and factors that protect against abuse and neglect
▸ Explain interventions for child maltreatment
▸ Discuss the difficulties of children of substance-abusing parents
▸ Outline treatment for children and parents in alcoholic families
▸ Explain children's reactions to death and interventions to help them as they grieve
▸ Talk about depression and suicide and responses to those problems
▸ Describe concerns of children in divorce, in stepfamilies, and with single parents
▸ Define treatment options for children in those family constellations
▸ Discuss children with violent tendencies and ways to work with them

CHILD MALTREATMENT

Practitioners who work with children are likely to encounter a child who has been subjected to maltreatment. Child maltreatment is a general term that includes four primary acts: physical abuse, neglect, sexual abuse, and emotional abuse. Unfortunately, those acts occur too frequently.

Over 3 million reports of maltreatment are made each year in the United States, yet some experts estimate the actual incidents are more than three times greater than reported (Childhelp, 2014). Between four and seven children die every day as a result of child abuse and neglect. In 2012, there were 686,000 victims of child maltreatment or about 9.2 children per 1000. Child neglect was the most prevalent pattern of maltreatment (78 percent), followed by physical abuse (19 percent), sexual abuse (8 percent), psychological abuse and neglect (8.5 percent), and other forms (10 percent) of abuse. Four-fifths (81.5 percent) of the victims were maltreated by one or more parents (U.S. Department of Health and Human Services, 2013).

Definitions

All states have laws requiring people in contact with children as part of their job or volunteer work to report known or suspected abuse to the police or child welfare agencies. State governments are charged with protecting children from maltreatment. Federal legislation presents a foundation for states by identifying a minimum set of acts or behaviors that define child abuse and neglect in the Federal Child Abuse Prevention and Treatment Act (CAPTA) (42 U.S.C.A. § 5106g), as amended by the CAPTA Reauthorization Act of 2010. That federal legislation provides guidance to states by identifying a minimum set of acts or behaviors that define child abuse and neglect at a minimum as:

- "Any recent act or failure to act on the part of a parent or caretaker which results in death, serious physical or emotional harm, sexual abuse or exploitation"; or
- "An act or failure to act which presents an imminent risk of serious harm" (https://www.childwelfare.gov/can/defining/federal.cfm).

This definition of child abuse and neglect refers specifically to parents and other caregivers. A "child" under this definition generally means a person who is younger than age 18 or who is not an emancipated minor.

While CAPTA provides definitions for sexual abuse and the special cases of neglect related to withholding or failing to provide medically indicated treatment, it does not provide specific definitions for other types of maltreatment such as physical abuse, neglect, or emotional abuse. Each state provides its own definitions of maltreatment within civil and criminal statutes.

State laws differ in the specificity of who is to report and under what conditions reports should be filed. For example, the standards for what constitutes an abusive act vary among the states. Some states define abuse in terms of harm or threatened harm to a child's health or welfare. Other standards may be written to include "acts or omissions," "recklessly fails or refuses to act," "willfully causes or permits," and "failure to provide." Some laws include abandonment and parental substance abuse as forms of child abuse and neglect. These standards guide mandatory reporters in deciding whether to make a report to child protective services. In addition, the state laws are reviewed and revised periodically. Relevant information for the state reporting law can be accessed through the Child Welfare Information Gateway (www.childwelfare.gov). The Child Welfare Information Gateway (2014) and other authors provide definitions of child maltreatment (Mash & Wolfe, 2013). For example:

Physical abuse causes nonaccidental physical injury to the child; the multiple acts of aggression may include punching, beating, shaking, striking, kicking, burning, or biting the child or some other action that results in substantial risk for physical or emotional harm to the child. The severity and nature of the injuries range from minor indications such as bruises to moderate signs such as scars to severe injuries like burns, sprains, or broken bones to death. Most of the injuries are not intentional but the result of severe physical punishment. According to the Child Welfare Information Gateway (2014) in approximately 38 states the definition of abuse also includes acts or circumstances that threaten the child with harm or create a substantial risk of harm to the child's health or welfare.

Emotional abuse refers to actions, such as intentional and frequent rejection, criticism, punishment for minor infractions, belittling, and threatening that damage the child cognitively, emotionally, or in their social interactions. According to the Child Welfare Information Gateway (2014) all states except Georgia and Washington include emotional maltreatment as part of their definitions of abuse or neglect. Approximately 32 states and the District of Columbia provide specific definitions of emotional abuse or mental injury to a child. Typical language used in these definitions is "injury to the psychological capacity or emotional stability of the child as evidenced by an observable or substantial change in behavior, emotional response, or cognition," or as evidenced by "anxiety, depression, withdrawal, or aggressive behavior." Brassard and Donovan (2006) classify psychological maltreatment as spurning, terrorizing, isolating and/or exploiting/corrupting the child. We would add criticizing the child's qualities and abilities, witnessing violence and age-inappropriate demands.

Physical neglect refers to failing to provide a child's basic needs such as food, clothing, shelter, medical attention, supervision, and hygiene. Delaying medical care, refusing to keep the child in the home, not allowing a runaway to return home, and abandoning a child are all examples of physical neglect. According to the Child Welfare Information Gateway (2014), seven states further define medical neglect as failing to provide any special medical treatment or mental health care needed by the child. In addition, four states define as medical neglect the withholding of medical treatment or nutrition from disabled infants with life-threatening conditions.

Abandonment Many states now have definitions for child abandonment in their reporting laws. Approximately 17 states and the District of Columbia include abandonment in their definition of abuse or neglect with 13 states providing separate definitions for establishing abandonment. In general, the following conditions are considered abandonment of the child: the parent's identity or whereabouts are unknown, the child has been left by the parent in circumstances in which the child suffers serious harm, or the parent has failed to maintain contact with the child or to provide reasonable support for a specified period of time (Child Welfare Information Gateway, 2014).

Educational neglect means allowing chronic truancy, not enrolling a school-aged child, and failing to pay attention to a child's special educational needs. According to the Child Welfare Information Gateway (2014), 21 states and American Samoa, Puerto Rico, and the Virgin Islands include failure to educate the child as required by law in their definition of neglect.

Emotional neglect is the category most difficult to define. It refers to the failure to provide children's needs for affection and emotional support. Examples are spousal abuse in the child's presence, not providing needed psychological care, and permitting drug or alcohol use by the minor.

Neglected children may have health problems such as growth deficiencies and complications to diabetes, allergies, and other diseases (Lyons-Ruth, Zeanah, & Benoit, 2003). They may exhibit a range of behaviors from undisciplined activity to extreme passivity based on the ways they have adapted to the neglectful caretaker (Hildyard & Wolfe, 2002). Young children may be fearful with sleep problems, headaches, and other physical signs of distress. Older boys may be more aggressive and girls more passive (Crooks & Wolfe, 2007).

Sexual abuse is defined as the use of a child for sexual gratification. All states include sexual abuse in their definitions of child abuse. Some states refer in general terms to sexual abuse, while others specify various acts as sexual abuse. Sexual exploitation, allowing the child to engage in prostitution or in the production of child pornography, is an element of the definition of sexual abuse in most jurisdictions. Sexual abuse may vary in intrusiveness (from viewing to oral/anal/genital penetration) and frequency (from a single incident to frequent abuse). Berliner (2010) explained that sexually abused children may have significant behavior and developmental consequences. The duration, frequency of abuse, the use of force, penetration, and relationship to the abuser all impact the child's reactions. Physical complications may be urinary tract problems, gynecological problems, sexually transmitted diseases, and pregnancy (Mash & Wolfe, 2013). The child's reactions are impacted by the nature of the assault and the response of other people, especially the mother (London, Bruck, Wright, & Ceci, 2008). Fears, anger, anxiety, fatigue, depression, passiveness, trouble focusing, and withdrawing may occur with victims of child sexual abuse. Mash and Wolfe (2010) stated that physical abuse and neglect are connected to parenting, discipline, or lack of attention to needs. Sexual abuse, however, is a breach of trust and involves deception, intrusion, and exploitation of the child's innocence.

All statistics underestimate the prevalence of child maltreatment. Those miscalculations are caused by variations in definitions of child abuse across the nation, as well as the fact that many incidents of child abuse are unreported or misreported. The more complete measure of the scope of maltreatment is the National Incidence Study of Child Abuse and Neglect (NIS) (McPherson, Greene, & Li, 2010).

Leeb, Paulozzi, Melanson, Simon, and Arias (2014) prepared a brief for the Centers for Disease Control that proposed uniform definitions for child abuse and neglect in order to provide better surveillance of the problem. These descriptions may become part of child maltreatment laws in multiple states.

Their proposed definitions are as follows.

Child Maltreatment: Any act or series of acts of commission or omission by a parent or other caregiver that result in harm, potential for harm, or threat of harm to a child.

Acts of Commission (Child Abuse) are words or overt actions that cause harm, potential harm, or threat of harm to a child. Acts of commission are deliberate and intentional, but the harm to a child may or may not be the intended consequence.

Intentionality only applies to the caregivers' acts—not the consequences of those acts. For example, a caregiver may intend to hit a child as punishment (i.e., hitting the child is not accidental or unintentional) but not intend to cause the child to have a concussion.

The following types of maltreatment involve acts of commission: physical abuse, sexual abuse, psychological abuse.

Acts of Omission (Child Neglect) are the failure to provide for a child's basic physical, emotional, or educational needs or to protect a child from harm or potential harm. Similar to acts of commission, harm to a child may or may not be the intended consequence. The following types of maltreatment involve acts of omission: failure to provide, physical neglect, emotional neglect, medical/dental neglect, educational neglect, failure to supervise, inadequate supervision, exposure to violent environments (http://www.cdc.gov/violenceprevention/childmaltreatment/definitions.html).

A growing menace in the maltreatment of children occurs with online relationships in which minors are enticed, invited, or persuaded to meet for sexual acts (National Center for Missing and Exploited Children, 2014). Predators may use e-mail, instant messages, bulletin boards, and chat rooms to gain the young person's confidence, and then to arrange a meeting. The federal government and all states have laws related to child pornography and other types of child sexual exploitation. Those statutes are summarized on the Web site of the National Center for Missing and Exploited Children (www.ncmec.org). Parents and other adults in protective roles should know the signs for children who may be at risk for online victimization and will find helpful hints for protecting their child at http://www.netsmartz411 .org/ and at http://www.missingkids.com/Safety.

Causes

Child abuse occurs at all levels of social, economic, and educational status and, unfortunately, in all countries of the world (UNICEF, 2013). In the United States, most cases involve one or both parents. The offender may use bribes, threats, guilt, or coercion to ensure secrecy. To protect the family and this relative or friend, the abuse may be ignored or hushed up in a variety of ways, the incidents are never reported or recorded, and the child and family never confront the issue or receive treatment.

Several hypotheses have been advanced to explain the causes of child abuse. Currently, the origins of child abuse are understood as the interacting variables of the child, the family, and community (Child Welfare Information Gateway, 2014). Goldman, Salus, Wolcott, and Kennedy (2003) summarized risk factors for child abuse. *Most important, children are never responsible for the maltreatment inflicted on them; it is never their fault.* Yet, Goldman et al. (2003) identified some individual factors related to maltreatment. Some child characteristics such as having disabilities significantly correlate with an increased risk for abuse or neglect. Younger children are more likely to be neglected, and the risk for sexual abuse increases with age. Female children and adolescents are more likely than male children and adolescents to be subjected to sexual abuse.

People who abuse have a few common characteristics. They may have low self-esteem; believe that events are determined by chance or outside forces beyond one's personal control; have poor impulse control, and be suffering from depression, anxiety, or antisocial behavior.

Some family characteristics are linked to child maltreatment. Substance abuse may be a contributing factor for between one-third and two-thirds of maltreated children in the child welfare system. Caregivers may have negative attitudes about a child's behavior and inaccurate understanding about child development. Caretakers may have unrealistic expectations of the child that result in harsh, inappropriate punishment when the child does not live up to the caretakers' standards. In 30 to 60 percent of families where spousal abuse takes place, child maltreatment also occurs. Children in violent homes may witness parental violence, be victims of physical abuse themselves, and be neglected by parents who are focused on their partners or unresponsive to their children due to their own fears (USDHHS, 2013). Even if children are not physically abused, they may experience harmful emotional consequences from the violence they witness. Finally, stress plays a role in family functioning, although its exact relationship with maltreatment is not fully understood. In various studies, physical abuse has been associated with stressful life events, parenting stress, and emotional distress. Similarly, some studies have found that neglectful families report more day-to-day stress than non-neglectful families. What is not clear is whether maltreating parents actually *experience* more life stress or, rather, *perceive* more events and life experiences as being stressful. In addition, specific stressful situations (e.g., losing a job, physical illness, marital problems, or the death of a family member) may exacerbate certain characteristics of the family members affected such as hostility, anxiety, or depression and may aggravate the level of family conflict and maltreatment.

Research on maltreating parents found that they were more likely to use harsh discipline strategies and less likely to use positive parenting strategies such as time-outs, reasoning, and recognizing and encouraging the child's successes. Some studies of physical abuse, in particular, have found that teenage mothers tend to perpetrate higher rates of child abuse than did older mothers. Other factors, such as lower economic status, lack of social support, and high stress levels may contribute to the link between adolescent mothers or young parents and child abuse (Goldman et al., 2003).

The family structure most associated with physical and sexual abuse is the child living with one parent who has an unmarried partner (not the child's parent) living in the household (McPherson et al., 2010). Families with conflict and marital violence and with substance abuse problems have a higher risk for abuse (Mash & Wolfe, 2013). The families are often rigid, authoritarian, and isolated from one another and the outside world. They may be experiencing marital, financial, or parent–child relationship problems but lack the resources and skills to cope with them. Poverty, unemployment, parents who were victims of abuse themselves, and stressful changes such as moving or marital separations are often associated with abuse. The community may also be one of social isolation with few gathering places such as parks, child care or recreational centers, and churches to serve as family supports. Societal factors such as the acceptance of domestic violence and corporal punishment may also contribute to the incidence of child abuse. The abused child is usually thought of in negative terms and may be isolated, rejected, ignored, or even terrorized.

Protective Factors

Buffers or conditions in families and communities can increase health and well-being of children and families. These protective factors allow parents to find resources, supports, or coping strategies that help them parent well even when they are stressed. Research (USDHHS, 2013) has shown these protective factors are linked to a lower incidence of child abuse and neglect. All positive aspects of development are enhanced when children are nurtured and have a chance to develop a close bond with a loving adult. The bond of strong, warm feelings for one another helps children trust that their caretakers will give them what they need—love, acceptance, positive guidance, and protection. This positive, consistent relationship with a caring adult in the early years correlates with school success, healthy behaviors, more friends, and better coping skills in adolescence. Children thrive when affectionate parents provide respectful communication and listening, consistent rules and expectations, and safe opportunities to promote independence. Effective parenting boosts children's psychological adjustment, helps children succeed in academics, encourages curiosity about the world, and motivates children to achieve (USDHHS).

Adults who can deal with the stresses of everyday life, as well an occasional crisis, have resilience. They demonstrate the flexibility and inner strength needed to cope when things are not going well. Stress-producing events, such as a family history of abuse or neglect, health problems, marital conflict, or domestic or community violence—and financial stressors such as unemployment, poverty, and homelessness—may reduce a parent's abilities to handle the typical day-to-day stresses of raising children.

Parents with a social network of emotionally supportive friends, family, and neighbors may find it easier to care for their children and themselves. Most parents need people they can call on once in a while when they need a sympathetic listener, advice, or concrete support. Caretakers who are isolated, with few social connections, are at higher risk for child abuse and neglect.

Many factors affect a family's ability to care for their children. Families who can meet their own basic needs for food, clothing, housing, and transportation—and who know how to access essential services such as child care, health care, and mental health services to address family-specific needs—are better able to ensure the safety and well-being of their children.

Counselors and others who partner with parents to identify and access resources in the community may help prevent the stress that sometimes leads to child maltreatment. Providing concrete supports such as referrals to food banks, transportation, other resources, or low-cost child-care facilities may also help prevent the unintended neglect that sometimes occurs when parents are unable to provide for their children. Counselors and others should work to create and augment protective factors as a response to the prevalence of child maltreatment.

Signs and Symptoms

Counselors will need to understand the signs and symptoms of abuse and the ways to support the young person who has been victimized. Victims of child maltreatment demonstrate a variety of responses to the abuse as the notes above indicate. The counselor may see constellations of symptoms that cross several areas of a child's functioning. Leeb, Lewis, and Zolotor (2011) discuss implications of those symptoms, and Siegel (1999) weaves ideas and research from attachment theory, child development, communication, systems, emotion, evolution, information process, and neurobiology to explain the interacting variables that affect all children and the impact of child abuse on a child's mind, body, and spirit.

Webb (2007) discusses two types of trauma: Type I, a traumatic, single event in an otherwise normal life, and Type II, or complex trauma, prolonged and repeated trauma in which anticipated and actual pain, violence, and chaos occur. The coping mechanisms of denial, numbing, self-hypnosis, dissociation, and shifts between rage and passivity are developed. Gil (2006) explains that children will demonstrate the impact of abuse either with internal or external behaviors. Children who internalize the trauma cope with the pain alone. They avoid interaction and may seem depressed, joyless, fearful, hypervigilant, and regressed. They may also have physical symptoms such as sleeping problems, headaches, and stomachaches. Severe cases may self-mutilate or become suicidal. Children who express their pain externally may be hostile, provocative, or violent. They may hurt animals, destroy property, and show sexualized behaviors.

The Child Welfare Information Gateway (2014) summarizes the most common physical, psychological, and behavioral consequences of child maltreatment and acknowledges that the categories often overlap. Table 19-1 contains an overview of those signs and symptoms.

One critical consideration is the effect of stress on the developing brain. Stien and Kendal (2004) explained that childhood experiences lead to the process of gene transcription, the ways genes are activated. Chronic stress may cause diminished left hemisphere development, decreased cortical integration, increased electroencephalographic (EEG) abnormalities, and a smaller corpus callosum. Therefore, abuse in early years may interrupt, alter, or overtax internal resources (Gil, 2006). The plasticity of the brain and the possibility of some recovery from trauma-related brain damage indicate there may be potential for stimulating growth in underdeveloped areas (Stien & Kendall, 2004), particularly with positive experiences such as nurturing from a caring adult.

Long-Term Consequences

Two ongoing research efforts follow the impact of child maltreatment. The Longitudinal Studies of Child Abuse and Neglect (LONGSCAN) studies the impact of maltreatment and the effectiveness of child protection services (www.iprc.unc.edu /longscan). In addition, the National Survey of Child and Adolescent Well-Being (NSCAW) focuses on the child welfare system and child and family experiences with that system as well as the life course of these children (www.acf.hhs.gov/programs /opre/abuse_neglect/nscaw/index.html). English et al. (2005) remind us that not all children who suffer abuse or neglect will have long-term negative consequences. Individual outcomes vary and are affected by the combination of variables like the child's age and development status when the abuse happened; the type of abuse; the frequency, duration, and severity of the abuse; and the relationship between the victim and the abuser.

In spite of the encouraging concept of resilience in children, many do suffer long-term consequences of maltreatment. For example, more than 25 percent of children who had been in foster care for more than a year had some lasting or recurring health problem (Office of Planning, Research and Evaluation, n.d.). Other physical consequences of abuse are shaken baby syndrome, impaired brain development, and poor health. Adults who were abused or neglected in childhood are more

TABLE 19-1 SIGNS OF MALTREATMENT

	Maltreatment	Physical Abuse	Neglect	Sexual Abuse	Emotional Maltreatment
Child	Shows sudden changes in behavior or school performance	Unexplained burns, bites, or bruises	Frequently absent from school	Has trouble walking or sitting	Extremes in behavior, overly passive or aggressive
	Has not received help for physical problems brought to the parents' attention	Fading bruises or other marks after absence	Begs or steals food or money	Suddenly refuses to change for gym or to take part in physical activities	Either inappropriately adult or infantile
	Has learning difficulties not from specific physical or psychological causes	Seems frightened of parents, protests when time to go home	Lacks needed medical or dental care, immunizations, or glasses	Reports nightmares or bedwetting	Delayed in physical or emotional development
	Is always watchful, as though preparing for something bad to happen	Cringes as adults approach	Is consistently dirty and has severe body odor	Has sudden changes in appetite	Has attempted suicide
	Lacks adult supervision		Does not have sufficient clothing for the weather	Shows bizarre, sophisticated, or unusual sexual knowledge	Reports lack of attachment to parent
	Is overly compliant, passive, or withdrawn		Abuses alcohol or other drugs	Becomes pregnant or has a venereal disease, especially if younger than 14	
	Comes to school early, stays late, and does not want to go home		Says there is no one at home to give care	Runs away	

Parent			
Shows little concern for the child	Offers conflicting or unconvincing explanations about child's injuries	Appears to be indifferent to the child	Unduly protective of the child or severely limits the child's interactions with other children
Denies problems or blames others for the child's troubles at school or home	Describes child as "evil" or other negative way	Seems apathetic or depressed	Is secretive and isolated
Recommends harsh physical discipline if the child misbehaves	Uses harsh physical discipline	Behaves irrationally or in bizarre ways	Is jealous or controlling with family members
Talks about the child as entirely worthless or bad or a burden		Is abusing substances	
Demands a physical or academic performance level beyond the child's abilities			
Leans on the child for care, attention, and satisfaction of the parent's emotional needs			

Adapted from Goldman, J, Salus, M. K., Wolcott, D., & Kennedy, K. Y. (2003). *A coordinated response to child abuse and neglect: The foundation for practice.* Washington, DC: U.S. Department of Health and Human Services. Retrieved September 2009 from http://www.childwelfare.gov/pubs/usermanuals/foundation/foundatione.cfm

likely to suffer from allergies, arthritis, asthma, bronchitis, high blood pressure, and ulcers (Springer, Sheridan, Kuo, & Carnes, 2007). The emotional effects that are quickly apparent—isolation, fear, and lack of trust—can become long-term habits of low self-esteem, depression, and problems with relationships. In one study, as many as 80 percent of young people who had been maltreated displayed the criteria for a psychiatric disorder by the time they were 21. The poor emotional health included problems such as depression, anxiety, eating disorders, suicide attempts, panic disorder, dissociative disorders, anger, post-traumatic stress disorder, and others (Springer et al., 2007). Cognitive difficulties included lower scores than the general population on capacity, language development, and academic achievement as well as poor academic performance and school functioning (Child Welfare Information Gateway, 2014). Children who have been abused may also demonstrate behavioral consequences such as delinquency, teen pregnancy, lower grades, drug use, and mental health problems (Johnson, Rew, & Sternglanz, 2006). Without doubt abused and neglected children have greater probabilities of difficulties throughout life.

ASSESSMENT

Practitioners begin with all children by assessing their abilities and needs. With children who are maltreated, a primary concern is the feasibility of the child and family staying together. Gil (2006) explains that counselors who specialize in childhood trauma must balance providing mental health services while monitoring safety issues and the best interests of the child. Counselors may be asked to give opinions about placements, the impact of the child testifying in court, the physical and emotional safety of the child's environment, and the families' capacity and readiness for decreasing high-risk factors like substance abuse and domestic violence. Azar and Wolfe (2006) outlined risk-assessment strategies to aid in that determination that is contained in Table 19-2.

The goals of an assessment process are to determine the child's overall functioning, identify current symptoms or problems; assess any traumatic impact; find the child's internal resources such as coping strategies; discover the child's ideas about parent support; and encourage parental support, nurturance, and guidance for the child (Gil, 2006).

Powell and Wilson (2012) have compiled a valuable guide to interviewing children about traumatic event, and James and Burch (1999) offer suggestions for interviewing a child who may be abused:

1. Use statements and questions such as "Tell me about a time something happened to you that made you feel uncomfortable." "Tell me what happened to you." "Has anyone tried to touch your private parts?" (Counselors can define "private" as parts of the body covered by a bathing suit.)
2. Pay attention to the child's body language as the interview progresses. The child may tell more nonverbally than with words.
3. Let the child tell his or her own story.
4. Be empathic but neutral.
5. Use clarification and summary skills.
6. Use the child's terms when paraphrasing (p. 215).

TABLE 19-2   CHILD ABUSE AND NEGLECT ASSESSMENT STRATEGY: AN OVERVIEW

1. Determining dangerousness and risk to the child in cases of detected or undetected maltreatment decisions
   - Apprehension of child risk
   - Alternative placement of child

   Precautions
   - Removing and returning child to the family is highly stressful
   - Initial impression of family may be distorted

2. Identifying general strengths and problem areas of the family system decisions
   - Family background
   - Marital/couple relationship
   - Perceived areas of stress and supports
   - Symptom pattern
   - Major factors (antecedents, consequences, and individual characteristics) suspected to be operative within the family
   - Directions for protective services, supports, additional community services

   Precautions
   - Involvement of too many professionals may overwhelm family
   - "Crises" that family members report may change dramatically
   - Parent–child problems may be embedded in chronic family problems (e.g., financial, marital/couple) that resist change

3. Identification of parental needs vis-á-vis child-rearing demands decisions
   - Child-rearing methods and skills
   - Anger and arousal toward child
   - Perceptions and expectations of children
   - Behavioral intervention planning and establishing priority of needs

   Precautions
   - Parental behavior toward child may be a function of both proximal (e.g., child behavior) and distal (e.g., job stress) events
   - Numerous factors that may interfere with treatment must be identified (e.g., resistance, socioeconomic status, marital/couple problems)

4. Identification of the child's needs decisions
   - Child behavior problems with family members
   - Child adaptive abilities and cognitive and emotional development
   - Referral to school-based intervention
   - Behavioral interventions (e.g., parent training)
   - Returning child to family
   - Unclear or delayed expression of symptoms/impairments

   Precautions
   - Child's behavior may be partially a function of recent family separation and change

From Azar, S. T., & Wolfe, D. A. (2006). Child physical abuse and neglect. In E. J. Marsh & R. A. Barkley (Eds.), *Treatment of childhood disorders* (3rd ed., p. 605). New York: Guilford.

Treatment Goals

The following points indicate child and family characteristics that must be considered when establishing treatment goals for children who have been maltreated.

Child needs

1. Social sensitivity and relationship development such as problems connecting with others, empathy, trust, and affective expression
2. Cognitive, language, and moral development, particularly poor social judgment, communication skills, and school performance
3. Self-control and aggression
4. Attention to concerns about health, safety, and protection from harm

Parent needs

1. Symptoms of emotional distress, learning problems, parent psychopathology, and personality deficits that limit adjustment and coping
2. Emotional arousal and reactivity to the child, poor control of anger, and hostility
3. Inadequate and inappropriate methods of teaching, discipline, and child stimulation
4. Inappropriate perceptions and expectations of children that emerge in rigid and limited beliefs about child rearing and in negative bias
5. Negative lifestyle and habits such as use of alcohol and drugs, prostitution, subcultural peer groups that interfere with the parent–child relationship and with problem-solving abilities

Family/situational needs

1. Couple distress
2. Chronic economic troubles and stressors
3. Social isolation and inability to establish social support (Azar & Wolfe, 2006, p. 610)

Gil (2006) reviewed treatment goals and approaches, concluding that counselors serve children who have been maltreated by building a trusting relationship, offering psychoeducational information, addressing their problems in relationships with others, and helping them discuss their traumatic memories. Gil recommends an integrated approach of CBT, expressive therapies, and education to accomplish those goals with children. Allen and Kronenberg (2014) provide extensive case study presentations of these effective therapies for traumatized children and their caregivers: trauma-focused cognitive-behavioral therapy (TF-CBT), child–parent psychotherapy (CPP), and parent–child interaction therapy (PCIT).

Carr (2009) cites practice interventions for survivors of child abuse involving the child and the nonabusing parent concurrently in group or individual sessions. The child-focused counseling involves identifying the complex emotions associated with the abuse, relaxation, and coping skills training, assertiveness, and safety skills. PCIT (Timmer, Urquiza, Zebell, & McGrath, 2005) and other types of parent-involved treatment (Corcoran & Pillai, 2008) for victims of physical abuse have been noted as effective treatment (Carr, 2009). Behavioral parent training builds child management skills and handling negative emotions such as anger, anxiety, and depression (Valle & Lutzker, 2006). Timmer and Urquiza (2014), in an indispensable volume for practitioners, outline effective treatments for traumatized children and their caretakers across age spans.

Lev-Wiesel (2008) explained that most treatment approaches for traumatized children have one or more goals. One goal is *symptom relief*, accomplished by encouraging the child to think differently or by teaching the child to manage behaviors, facilitating the expression of negative emotions, affirming the child's experience, and providing emotional support. Another goal is *de-stigmatization*, which may be achieved by affirmation from other child victims and by the counselor's emotional support. A third goal involves *increasing self-esteem* by using cognitive and interpersonal exercises, role-plays, and games. The fourth goal is *preventing future abuse* by changing the child's environment, behaviors, and awareness of danger. Each or all of these goals may help guide treatments for traumatized children.

General Counseling Strategies for Working with Children Who Have Been Abused

Counselors who work with abused children may find it helpful to consider this question: What does this child need to understand about the traumatic situation that he or she does not know right now? (Shapiro, Friedberg, & Bardenstein, 2006). The answers to that query can guide an educational component of the treatment directed toward helping the abused child revise some of his or her misunderstandings about the victimization. As Shapiro and his colleagues explain, molestation violates our ideas about privacy, pleasure, adult–child relationships, and trust. To counter the self-blame children may be experiencing, the victims need to know that abuse has also happened to some other young people and that they are not alone in suffering with being maltreated. Those authors suggest some resources: *My Very Own Book about Me: A Personal Safety Book* (Dietzel, 2000); *Something Happened and I'm Scared to Tell: A Book for Young Victims of Abuse* (Kehoe & Deach, 1987); *It Happened to Me: A Teen's Guide to Overcoming Sexual Abuse* (Carter, 2002); *The Rainbow Game* (Rainbow House, 1989); and therapeutic stories by Davis and Sparks (1988). More possibilities for this and other topics can be found at the Carnegie Library of Pittsburgh Web site (http://www.carnegielibrary.org/research/parentseducators/parents/bibliotherapy/).

Miller-Perrin (2001) noted self-protection training for physically abused children includes having them identify potentially harmful situations and move to safer locations. She has outlined some other ways of intervening with children who have been victims of abuse. One goal suggested was to help the child learn to manage the negative cognitions and emotions associated with the incident(s). Emotions such as guilt, shame, anger, stress, stigma, and fear occur as a result of abuse. Relaxation training, anger management, problem-solving skills, positive coping statements, and the use of imagery are possible techniques for addressing those emotions. Cognitive-behavioral approaches are useful to help victims change their ideas about being different from other children, as well as feeling they are somehow responsible for the abuse. Group therapy to counter such beliefs and to confront secrecy is helpful to children who are able to discuss their abuse with peers who have also been abused. Children also need to know they have a right to say no to inappropriate touching and to talk about incidents that make them uncomfortable.

James and Burch (1999) suggest some activities that can be conducted in schools:

1. Prepare school personnel by teaching about normal sexual development, symptoms of abuse, state law, school policy, and reporting procedures.
2. Deliver an abuse prevention program at school that educates children to danger signs, preventions skills, and the importance of telling adults about abuse.
3. Develop a network of professionals to build skills in assessment and knowledge base of ways to work with abused children. The network should include child protection workers, other counselors, therapists, and agencies that diagnose and treat victims.
4. Have toys, books, and games in the counseling office to ease discussions of family, feelings, or trauma.
5. Have resources about testifying in court.
6. Keep accurate professional records that are clear and objective (p. 216).

Some specific ideas for working with abused children are as follows:

- In counseling all abuse victims, counselors must be prepared to become totally involved with the child client, including the child's repeated testing of the counselors' caring.
- Relaxation and visualization may help the child develop a more positive attitude toward self and life.
- Play therapy may help abused children to communicate their thoughts and feelings. Gil (2006) has specific ideas about using art, play, and the sand tray with abused and traumatized children.
- Sexually abused children require extra consideration, understanding, and support from the counselor. Often, the children initially are unable to discuss the problem with the counselor because of intense feelings of guilt. They believe that somehow they provoked the attack or that they could have done something to prevent it. They may feel worthless and ashamed of having been abused in such a manner. They may be more affected by the questions and reactions that follow than by the act itself. Furthermore, they often feel intense guilt at having gotten a parent or other adult in trouble, in jail, or barred from the home because the child "told." Empathetic listening and clarification of words and nonverbal expressions are essential.
- Specific techniques such as bibliocounseling, role-playing, or group counseling may be considered, depending on the child's maturity. Placing sexually abused children in groups requires caution, especially if the trauma is recent. The child may not be ready to share intense feelings.
- Children may need information about what is appropriate and inappropriate touching or treatment and to be assured that certain parts of their bodies are private. They may need to be told that the adult's sexual or punishing behavior was inappropriate. Because of children's limited cognitive development and understanding, and to allay the anxiety surrounding the topic, most programs designed to teach children about child abuse

use role-play, puppets, coloring books, filmstrips, movies, and so on. The vocabulary used is not explicit, but instead refers to *touching* and *private areas*. The programs are designed not for sex education, but to give children information and strategies for coping with abusive situations.

- Children may need to learn how to say no or how to handle potentially abusive situations. The child needs help to determine the warning signs of abuse and to plan ways for coping with the situations (e.g., calling a special person when the father or mother begins to drink). Role-playing these strategies prepares children to handle such situations more effectively. Counselors need to do a careful assessment of the child's situation so that the new skills would not place the child at an increased risk.
- Encourage children to tell someone right away when an abusive situation occurs. Adults who abuse children sexually often warn the children to keep "their secret." Children need help discerning when they should tell a secret and when information should be kept confidential and also in deciding whom they should tell and what to do if the adult does not believe their story.
- Counselors must deal with issues of trust at some point in work with abused children. Developmental theorists have emphasized that children must develop trust in people and their interactions to live effectively, yet children receive a multitude of daily messages, designed to protect them, that imply that the world and the people in it are dangerous.

Caretakers

Childhood abuse is a part of an overall pattern of abusive behavior. The family network, as well as the personality of the abuser, must be considered. In addition, family reactions to the child who has been abused will enhance or interfere with counseling treatment and progress. Counselors should consider family therapy at an appropriate time in their treatment plans. Some treatments for the family and for the nonabusing parent have been noted previously.

Counselors working with abused children must be prepared to provide understanding and support for all persons involved. The natural reaction is anger at anyone who hurts a child; however, these feelings must be recognized and resolved for the counselor to work effectively with the child and the family, particularly the abuser. Counselors who are overly sympathetic with abused children lose objectivity and their ability to help the child; counselors who are extremely angry and judgmental toward the family of an abused child (for allowing this to happen) or toward the abuser can never establish the relationship necessary to help these individuals. Before beginning counseling with victims of abuse, counselors may need to examine their own feelings and views about the case.

Parent-focused interventions that focus on physical abusive and neglectful parents involve:

- Teaching parents about normal child development to correct unrealistic expectations
- Educating parents about appropriate discipline procedures and other child management strategies

- Practicing anger-control techniques and coping skills
- Discussing stress management techniques (Schellenbach, 1998)

Other Steps

Media accounts of child abuse tragedies are sometimes followed by neighbors or others saying they knew something was wrong but did not report it. A surprising discrepancy was discovered in a survey (Childhelp, 2014) with results showing that the majority of Americans who responded believe that everyone should play a role in stopping child abuse, yet many people also admitted witnessing child abuse and doing nothing about it. People said they did not know where to call or what would happen if they did report their suspicion. Their misperceptions included believing that children would be removed from their homes, that reports cannot be anonymous, and that the person who is accused would know who made the report. Those misperceptions may help perpetuate the epidemic of child maltreatment. Counselors may impact these faulty beliefs by predominately displaying child abuse reporting local numbers or the Childhelp® National Child Abuse Hotline at 1-800-4-A-CHILD® (1-800-422-4453). The hotline is staffed by degreed professionals 24 hours a day who accept calls from the United States, Canada, Guam, Puerto Rico, and the U.S. Virgin Islands. Calls are anonymous and toll-free. Their state-of-the-art technology provides translators in 140 languages.

In addition, counselors can take the lead at educating other adults about child maltreatment signs, symptoms, and reporting procedures. Kenny (2007) studied the effectiveness of brief online tutorials to provide information and found significant gains from pretest to post-test scores.

Child maltreatment is a tremendous problem in our world. Victims need extra care and attention to overcome the effects of their trauma. Counselors can be instrumental in protecting the child's safety and providing helpful interventions for enhancing the child's life.

CHILDREN IN CHEMICALLY DEPENDENT FAMILIES

Children living in families affected by chemical dependency may have special needs. According to the Substance Abuse and Mental Health Services Administration (2009), alcoholism and drug addiction affects approximately 8.3 million children; about 13 percent of young people under the age of 18 live with someone who needs treatment for chemical dependency. Adverse childhood experiences (ACEs) are probable traumatic events that have the potential for negative effects on a child's well-being. A key finding of the recent survey (http://www.acestudy.org/) about prevalence of these experiences indicate that exposure to the abuse of alcohol or drugs in the family was one of the most commonly reported ACE in every state (Sacks, Murphey, & Moore, 2014).

Yet children are often left out of an alcoholic parent's treatment even though the entire family is affected. Those children have significant risks for mental illness or emotional problems, physical health difficulties, and learning problems. Compared with other children, they are three times more likely to be abused and four times more likely to be neglected (Substance Abuse and Mental Health Services Administration). Baruth, Gibbons, and Guo (2006) studied the correlation of parents receiving substance abuse treatment with the recurrence of maltreatment among caregivers and found re-reports greater among those who had received treatment, emphasizing the need for a better system to serve children who have substance abusing parents. Those conclusions were echoed by Straussner and Fewell (2011).

Children of chemically dependent parents frequently do not have their physical or psychological needs met in the family. Money needed for food and shelter may be spent on alcohol or drugs; even if there is money, the parents may be too preoccupied with their chemical dependency to attend to the child's physical needs. Parents who have lost control of their lives frequently dislike themselves. They cannot meet the child's need for love, belonging, and security. Children who live in homes where rules are consistently broken and with family members who cannot be relied on to provide love and nurturance cannot be expected to grow and develop into fully functioning, well-adjusted individuals.

These children frequently are the victims of abuse and neglect, have little structure in their lives, receive inconsistent discipline, and cope with constant conflict in the home. Households with alcoholic residents often are described as turbulent and lacking in parental warmth and affection. Children adapt the roles they need to survive in this environment and often fail to learn the variety of roles children from homes with open communication and consistent lifestyles master (James & Gilliland, 2013). The adverse effects of conflicted home environments are seen in behavior such as school absenteeism, poor academic performance, isolation from peers, physical symptoms such as headaches and stomachaches, psychological symptoms (fears, moods, regressive behaviors), and "people-pleasing behaviors" (American Academy of Child & Adolescent Psychiatry, 2011). Sciarra (2004) summarizes seven problems that may occur for children in families with chemically dependent members: family conflict, abuse and neglect, inconsistent discipline and inadequate structure, disruption of family rituals, role reversal and parentification, distortion, and the denial of reality and isolation.

The American Academy of Child and Adolescent Psychiatry (2011) summarized the variety of problems children of alcoholics may have:

- Guilt: Children may feel they are responsible for the drinking.
- Anxiety: Children may worry constantly about the home situation.
- Embarrassment: Children may be ashamed of their home lives and avoid having friends visit.
- Unable to have close friendships: Children who have been disappointed frequently by parents who drink may not trust other people either.
- Confusion: An alcoholic parent will switch from a loving to an angry stance quickly, confusing the child. The home schedule is also chaotic with no consistent bedtimes or mealtimes.
- Anger: Children may be angry at the parent who is drinking and angry at the nonalcoholic parent for not supporting or protecting them.
- Depression: Children of substance-abusing parents are lonely and feel helpless to change the situation.

Sciarra (2004) outlined roles children of chemically dependent families may assume to cope with their parents' dependence: chief enabler (the addict's confidant and support); family hero (overly responsible, mature); scapegoat (one who is blamed for all problems); lost child (scared and isolated); placater ("people pleaser"); or mascot (the clown). In addition to these roles children assume, they also learn the family's unspoken rules. Those guidelines for surviving in an alcoholic family have been summarized by Doweiko (2011) and James and Gilliland (2013):

- *Don't talk/Don't have problems.* This stems from the denial of the problem of alcoholism, as well as the lack of recognition of the child's problem. Doweiko (2011) explains that the family will make clear no problem exists and you better not discuss it. Some may believe that if one does talk, bad things will happen.
- *Don't trust.* Children cannot depend on the drinking parent and often cannot depend on the nondrinking partner who is so busy meeting the needs of the alcoholic.
- *Don't feel.* Children learn that expressing fear, guilt, anger, sadness, or other feelings will bring more pain to the family.
- *Don't behave differently.* Shifting roles is not allowed.
- *Don't blame chemical dependency.* Blame typically is assigned to people, situations, or things outside the family. Denial of personal responsibility for actions is the norm.
- *Do behave as I want.* If a child does not comply with the wishes of the alcoholic, the threats of losing love or support, abuse, and increased drinking may occur.
- *Do be better and more responsible.* No matter what a family member does, it will never be enough to satisfy the alcoholic.
- *Don't have fun.* Broken promises, angry recriminations, embarrassment of the family situation, unpredictable outbursts, and exhaustion keep children from enjoying life.

Moe, Johnson, and Wade (2007) used qualitative methods to study children of alcoholics. The researchers asked "What helps kids (in alcoholic homes) have lives that are good?" The children's thematic responses indicated the ability to express feelings, knowing the truth about addictions, and making different life choices contribute to a good life. The authors concluded that individuals who coped effectively with the trauma of growing up in a family with addiction relied on support systems more than those who did not cope well and reported problems.

Interventions for Children from Chemically Dependent Families

One method to screen children of alcoholics is the Children of Alcoholics Screening Test (CAST) (Jones, 1985). This 30-item inventory measures negative life events associations with alcoholic families such as emotional distress, marital discord, attempts to control parental drinking, efforts to escape from alcoholism, exposure to drinking-related violence, and desire for help. CASTD (Pidcock, Fischer, Forthun, & West, 2000) is the shortened version of the instrument that has 14 items and has been adapted to include other types of substance use. Family CAGE (Price & Emshoff, 1997) is also a useful diagnostic tool.

Adger et al. (n.d.) have identified core competencies for all health care providers who care for children and adolescents. Those authors list these requirements for Level I competencies:

- A basic understanding of the physical, psychiatric, and behavioral symptoms of children and adolescents in families affected by substance use disorders
- Knowledge of local resources

- Routine screening of family history/current use of alcohol and other drugs
- Examination of whether family resource needs and services are adequate
- Ability to express an appropriate level of concern and offer support and follow-up

Fundamental to all work with children who live in homes with substance abuses are messages to counteract the negative effects (Adger et al., n.d.). Children need to know they are not alone. They need to understand it is not their fault. Children need to be reassured that their concern is valid—there is a problem. Finally, these young people need to know where to go for help where they can begin to understand they can love someone without liking the behaviors being exhibited.

Small groups for children provide a forum for those messages to emerge. O'Rourke (1990) provides an outline for a children's support group that includes attention to the preceding needs and provides information about alcoholism for young participants. These children also need activities to improve their self-esteem, assertiveness training to teach them to say no to drugs and alcohol, and help with developing problem-solving and decision-making skills. Arman and McNair (2000) outline a nine-session group that also incorporates the identified needs of children from chemically dependent families. O'Rourke and Worzbyt (1996) caution that prevention programs should respect the conditions under which the children of alcoholics live and understand that they live in a world with limited choices. They encourage counselors to focus on strengthening self-esteem and building strengths, resources, and resiliencies. Jacobus-Kantor and Emshoff (2010) provide another useful summary of working with children of alcoholics using play therapy both in groups and individually.

Treatment Goals

James and Gilliland (2013) summarizes treatment goals for children from substance-abusing families. In working with these children, counselors will want to accomplish the following goals:

- Give emotional support to the children
- Provide accurate, nonjudgmental information about chemical dependency
- Correct children's perceptions of being the cause of the parental problems and the attached guilt and shame
- Help children focus on their own behavior to gain a sense of control, to make responsible choices, and perhaps to teach them to have fun
- Help children learn to cope with possible situations that may occur because of the abuse
- Reduce children's isolation
- Reduce the children's risk for abusing

Children who are living in families with addictions need support, access to helpful resources, and adults who refuse to keep the secret of alcoholism and work to eliminate its negative effects on children.

DEATH AND BEREAVEMENT

When asked about death or dying, most adults try to avoid the subject or excuse themselves by expressing their inadequacy to discuss such a subject with young people. Discussions about death may be accompanied by a great deal of adult discomfort, anxiety, vagueness, and avoidance behavior. Yet talking about death may help people accept it as a part of life and cope with the feelings that accompany it. Children often are affected by the death of pets or grandparents, if not by loss of parents, friends, or siblings. Counselors need to be prepared to help children accept the reality of death as a part of life. To work effectively with children on the issue of death, counselors must first examine their own attitudes toward death so that they can be open to a child's grieving process.

Children's adjustment to the loss of an important person in their lives depends on their ability to make sense of the concept of death and their previous experiences with bereavement. Wagner (2008) recognizes that counselors who treat young clients who have a loss must consider the child's ability to master the concepts of irreversibility, finality, causality, and inevitability. Irreversibility refers to the recognition that death is something that cannot be fixed or reversed; the person cannot be mended or glued back together as other things in life have been. Finality means that children understand death is a permanent condition. Children must have a realistic concept about time for permanence to have meaning for them. Causality refers to understanding the actual reason for the death, the understanding that some things happen over which they have no control. Inevitability is that recognition of the cycle of life with death being a natural, unavoidable process for all living things. Some (Huss & Conklin, 2010; Salek & Ginsburg, 2014) outline generalizations about the notions that children may hold about death at certain ages. The following paragraphs contain a summary of those ideas about the varying ways children experience grief.

Early Childhood

Preschool children do not understand the finality of death. They regard it as temporary and reversible. They may explain that the deceased person is on a trip or asleep. They do not understand the difference between dying and going away. Their magical thinking may cause them to believe that their thoughts can make things happen. Therefore, they may either blame themselves or believe if they are "good" enough, the dead person will return. These young children may show few reactions to the loss, they may revert to behavior from an earlier stage of development, or they may have nightmares, physical ailments, or a great deal of confusion. Their caretakers need to provide a secure, supportive environment for these youngsters (Wagner, 2008). Sciarra (2004) says these children need to know who will take care of them and that the death is not their fault. They also need to know that they have their own feelings that may be different than the feelings of people around them, and that they can have as much time as they need to figure things out; they do not need to rush or pretend to feel differently.

Around age 5 or 6, children may believe that death is a creature, a monster. They may think that death can be avoided if they can outsmart it. They also may think it happens only to those who are very old or who are in an accident, things that do not affect them. They begin to comprehend the irreversibility of death.

They may be unusually interested in the details of the death and may ask very concrete questions. They may ask many questions as they try to understand. As they develop socially, they may watch to see how others respond to the death, mirror those adult reactions, and may ask how they "should" act. James and Gilliland (2013) explain that for children this age, death is more specific and factual.

Middle Childhood

By ages 9 and up, children know that death is final and irreversible. They begin to grasp the idea that everyone eventually dies and may be frightened when they realize they will die too. These children may be overwhelmed by their realizations. They may think they caused the death. They probably will want facts about the loss. Children after the age of 11 or 12 may have trouble concentrating on their school work, may withdraw from friends and family, and may seem angry and sad, as well as being tired and drowsy (Sciarra, 2004). As with younger children, they may exhibit psychosomatic symptoms of sleeplessness, loss of appetite, and agitation. Adults should remember that children are concerned about whether they somehow caused the death, whether they will be cared for, and whether they will die soon. Pictures, scrapbooks, videos, and other aids help children anchor their memories of the deceased. Many resources and activities can be found at the Doughy Center (http://www.dougy.org /grief-resources/activities/) Web site. With these elementary age students, counselors can focus on their feelings about the permanence of their loss (Wagner, 2008).

Adolescence

Adolescents are more capable of understanding cognitively and may experience deep fear, guilt, helplessness, and grief. Like younger children, they also may not know how to express those emotions. They may show more variations in their responses to death. Teens may rely more on their friends for support than on adults even though they may also feel pressured to assume more adult roles. They may distract themselves by becoming intensely involved in sports or social activities or music (Sheller & Watts, 1999). Sciarra (2004) recommends these books to help adolescents deal with loss: *Say Goodnight, Gracie* (Deaver, 1988), *Shira: A Legacy of Courage* (Grollman, 1988), *The Sunday Doll* (Shura, 1988), and *Tiger Eyes* (Blume, 1981). Sciarra cautions adults to be alert to teens who appear to be "perfectly fine" after the death of a family member or friend. Those adolescents may be hiding their grief as they attempt to appear mature and independent.

Children of all ages who are grieving may have trouble concentrating, completing school assignments, and learning new material. All children need patience and understanding to get through these temporary setbacks. They also need adults to help them understand their hurt and validate their experiences. Children may grieve longer than adults and may have periods of normal activities intermittent with their sadness (American Academy of Child & Adolescent Psychiatry, 2013).

Stages and Phases

From her work with terminally ill patients, Kübler-Ross (1969) defines the stages that most patients and their families go through in facing death. The first reaction is denial: "This is not happening to me." Second, the patient and family experience anger over the situation: "Why did this have to happen to me and not to somebody else?" The next stage includes bargaining. People may try to bargain to be a better person if they or their loved one can live. When the inevitability of death must be faced and the pressures become a harsh reality, depression is common. Eventually, the patient comes to the realization of the inevitability of death and often a peaceful acceptance.

Freeman (2001) discusses the grief experience as a progression through 10 stages. The person moves from shock, to an emotional release, to depression, and often to physical symptoms of distress. The bereaved shows anxiety, hostility, and then guilt and fear. The last two stages include healing through memories and acceptance of the death. He states that the tasks of mourning involve expressing the reality of the death, tolerating the suffering, and converting the relationship from the present to one of memory. The final tasks are developing a new identity of self without the deceased and finding some meaning in grief. Moore and Carr (2000) provide examples (Table 19-3) of the child's statements that might indicate these stages.

Interventions for Children Who Are Grieving

Wolfelt (2004) lists tasks for grieving children to accomplish: (1) understanding and accepting the reality of the loss; (2) grieving or facing the pain of death; (3) experiencing the pain or emotional aspects of the loss; (4) building memories or commemorating the deceased; (5) adjusting to an environment in which the significant one is missed; and (6) making sense of the loss or meaning; and then (7) moving on with life. These tasks do not necessarily occur in that sequence.

Shapiro et al. (2006) outline three immediate needs of children after a loss: having their emotions validated, being given accurate information, and reassurance about the future. First, children should be given permission to experience the emotions they have, not what they "should" have. That reaction helps the children know their emotions are valid responses to the loss. Second, children should be given an age-appropriate explanation of death that is respectful of the family's religious beliefs. Finally, children's concerns about what the death will mean for their lives should be addressed. Adults should help children express their fears and reassure them about their future.

Some situations may point to a need for professional help for children who have suffered a loss such as consistent problems of pain or withdrawing, intensification of symptoms over time, a dramatic or sudden behavioral change, an adult who cannot cope, and extremes in the child's behavior. Other concerning situations are extended periods of depression in which the child loses interests in everyday pleasures, exhibits prolonged fear of being alone, and refuses to attend school (American Academy of Child & Adolescent Psychiatry, 2013).

Bereavement is often a family transition, and each member's grieving affects others (Shapiro et al., 2006). Moore and Carr (2000) suggest a six-session family therapy that focuses on grief work for all family members to improve the child and parent adjustment. Webb (2002) lists the advantages of family counseling, including that it gives the counselor the opportunity to observe the child's role in the family, to assess the availability of other family members to the child, and to observe how

TABLE 19-3 THEMES UNDERLYING CHILDREN'S GRIEF

Grief Process	Underlying Theme	Behavioral Expressions of Grief Processes
Shock	• I am stunned by the loss of this person.	• Complete lack of affect and difficulty engaging emotionally with others • Poor concentration and poor school work
Denial	• The person is not dead.	• Reporting seeing or hearing the deceased • Carrying on conversations with the deceased
Yearning and searching	• I must find the deceased.	• Wandering or running away • Phoning relatives
Sadness	• I am sad, hopeless, and lonely because I have lost someone on whom I depended.	• Persistent low mood, tearfulness, low energy, and lack of activity • Appetite and sleep disruption • Poor concentration and poor school work
Anger	• I am angry because the person I needed has abandoned me.	• Aggression, tantrums, defiance, delinquency • Conflict with parents, siblings, teachers, and peers • Drug or alcohol abuse • Poor concentration and poor school work
Anxiety	• I am frightened that the deceased will punish me for causing their death or being angry at them. I am afraid that I too may die of an illness or fatal accident.	• Separation anxiety, school refusal, regressed behavior, bedwetting • Somatic complaints, hypochondriasis, and agoraphobia associated with a fear of accidents • Poor concentration and poor school work
Guilt and bargaining	• It is my fault that the person died so I should die.	• Suicidal behavior
Acceptance	• I loved and lost the person who died and now I must carry on without them while cherishing their memory.	• Return to normal behavioral routines

Note: Reprinted from Moore, M., and Carr, A. (2001). Depression and grief. In A. Carr (Ed.), *What works with children and adolescents? A critical review of psychological interventions with children, adolescents, and their families* (p. 209). Andover, UK: Routledge. Reprinted with permission of Taylor & Francis.

the reality of death is shared with other family members. Family counseling gives the family the opportunity to understand the pace and form of the child's grieving process. The disadvantages include the possibility of the child not being focused on because of grieving adults in the family, and that the family may be so grief stricken they cannot empathize with the child. Webb (2011) includes cognitive-behavioral therapy, play therapy, conjoint therapy with caregiver and child, groups and storytelling as effective interventions with children who are grieving. In addition, in a meta-analytic review of bereavement interventions, Currier, Holland, and Neimeyer (2007) concluded that child grief interventions do not lead to the positive outcomes of some other interventions. They noted that the time sensitivity of the interventions and the implementation of specific selection criteria generated better outcomes than the studies that did not include those factors.

Counselors can help children who grieve by providing information as they answer the children's questions, validating all their feelings about the death and giving them the time and opportunities they need to incorporate their memories of the significant person into their lives.

Counselors may not only be working with children individually or in small groups but may also be acting as a resource for the caretaking adults in the child's life. Those adults will need to understand that children may have grief reactions for an extended period of time, particularly at triggers such as birthdays, anniversaries, and holidays.

Information

Children need to know that caring adults can help them understand the intense feelings they are experiencing. The young people may need permission to express themselves. They need to know that it may take some time for them to feel better. They should be reassured that they did not cause the death. Counselors should use clear language rather than euphemisms—referring to the loss as *death* rather than *sleeping* or *passed away*. Counselors should be particularly careful with language that is appropriate to the culture of the child.

Children may not share their concerns with other adults because they are afraid they are adding to the problems surrounding those adults. Talking about death may be helpful because children may not have had the opportunity to ask questions in the chaos that has surrounded them. They may have many questions and may need to ask them repeatedly. Their first concern will probably be who will take care of them and how the death impacts them.

One helpful conversation with children would be clarifying what they have heard from the adults that surround them. Another valuable dialogue would be reviewing the children's routines and allowing them to ask questions as they plan for the next days and determine how and from whom they could get their answers.

Counselors should listen carefully to the child's thoughts, feelings, and concerns. They should remember the child's level of understanding and then answer clearly and objectively. Some questions could have a double meaning or could suggest a hidden concern. Counselors should clarify and respond to both the explicit and implicit meaning.

Some of the questions children ask may be difficult. For example, children may not understand abstract concepts such as heaven and eternity. Counselors will want to be respectful of the child's family's beliefs and may need to consult with family members or clergy for assistance in dealing with such sensitive topics. Counselors may find a response such as "What have you heard your __ say about that?" or "Who has explained that best to you and what did that person say?" will elicit information about the family's traditions and faith base.

Counselors should welcome the child's questions but also recognize they may not have answers. Children may ask counselors for details about what caused the death, whether it could have been avoided, who is responsible for the accident, why this happened to their loved one. They may want to know what happens during an autopsy, what happens after the casket is in the ground, or what the cremation process involves. Counselors should answer these queries honestly but carefully, always respecting the family's beliefs. Counselors can also respond by acknowledging they do not know the answers.

Adults may ask the counselor's recommendation about whether or not the child should attend the funeral. The answer depends on the age of the child, relation to the deceased person, and the child's reaction(s) to the death. The child may need the opportunity a funeral offers to say good-bye to the loved one. If the young person is going to attend and the loss was a family member, an adult who will not be intensely mourning should accompany the child and help him or her leave if overwhelmed by the ceremony. The child should be prepared in advance for what will be seen and heard at the funeral.

Validation

Counselors should provide ways to express grief both verbally and nonverbally. Drawing pictures, writing poems, reading books, playing in a sand tray, manipulating clay, or other expressive activities may create outlets for children to communicate their distress.

These incomplete sentences may help begin the conversations:

What makes me saddest is …

If I could say one more thing to the person who died, I'd say …

When the person died, I …

Since the death …

When I'm alone …

Counselors can help children realize that grieving may take longer than they expect. Children can be encouraged to be patient with themselves and with others who are sad, not expecting too much in a short period of time. They can also be encouraged to take breaks, spending time with friends and playing (Parsons, 2007).

Memories

Reconciliation describes the process of adjusting to the loss and accepting the reality of life without the loved one. Cohen and Mannarino (2004) explain that in order to accomplish reconciliation, children must accept the loss, experience the pain of the death, adjust to the world and their self-identity without the deceased, convert the relationship to one of memory, find meaning in the loss, and enjoy the comfort of other people in their lives. Shapiro et al. (2006) point out that memory is the central issue in bereavement. Counselors can offer memory-enhancing opportunities such as those described shortly.

Cohen and Mannarino (2004) describe an activity to help children talk about the deceased person. The counselor writes the dead person's name on a blank sheet of paper with one letter for each horizontal line. Then the counselor asks the child to fill in a word or phrase for each letter of the person's name. The following example was completed by Tessa, a first-grader whose classmate had been killed in an automobile accident:

Really fun

I liked him a lot

Could read me stories

Kept me laughing

Counselors could provide fill-in-the-blank sheets that can be custom designed for the deceased. Examples of things to be included would be "What was the happiest time you had with him/her?" "What did s/he do best?" "What did s/he do to make you laugh?" (Cohen & Mannarino, 2004).

Wagner (2008) recommends counselors use concrete activities that encourage children to remember and to express their feelings about the deceased. Children can use puppets or felt figures on a board to act out the funeral, their memories, or some other story about the deceased. Music is an effective way to help children deal with death (Willis, 2002). Children can also write a good-bye letter or make a farewell drawing. The National Association of School Psychologists (n.d.) lists books helpful for grieving children at all ages.

Children could collect objects that are reminders of the loved one. Creating collages and pictures and writing poems or other creative writing projects may also help children organize their reminiscences. A memory book, box, or scrapbook or other collection could contain chapters or sections about significant events the children experienced with the deceased. They may illustrate or write about places they went together, shared rituals, and other special times. The children may also want to include future plans they had with the deceased (Cohen & Mannarino, 2004).

Bereavement Groups

Children can find a natural support system when counselors form small groups of children who have suffered a loss. Huss and Conklin (2010) and Sciarra (2004) suggest that small-group counseling is the recommended intervention for bereaved children. A summary of their suggestions follows.

The first group session can be titled "telling our stories." The group focuses on each member's experience—who died, how it happened, and other details about the situation. Huss and Conklin (2010) recommend using folders on which the children place a picture or word that relates to the deceased. The rest of the folder holds pictures and words that describe the group member.

The next group focuses on the emotional aspect of the loss. The goal is to have members identify their varied emotions. After generating a list of emotions, group members discuss and compare the feelings they have had. The counselor will acknowledge the differences and similarities and the legitimacy of all their experiences.

"What life is like now" would be a subsequent session. Group members would explain how their lives are different since the death. They can draw a before-and-after picture of their family, friendship circle, classroom, or whatever is appropriate to illustrate the changes. Group members are encouraged to identify both positive and negative changes. They may also be asked to talk about someone they would like to be able to tell about the person who died and their feelings.

At some point during the session, a memorial service can be conducted. Group members bring something that either belonged to the deceased or reflects that person. Photographs, jewelry, and other mementos are possibilities. Each member has the chance to talk about what has been brought, the circumstances around it, and their feelings. Some members may prefer to create their own memento by drawing a picture, writing a story or poem, or just talking about the individual who has died. This session design communicates that remembering honors the deceased.

Moving on represents the group sessions in which the members plan for their future. They may want to share how they are going to recognize holidays, birthdays, and other special occasions without the person who died. They can discuss how at those times the painful emotions may resurface and identify who they can turn to for support during those difficult occasions. The group members can also be asked to make three goals for the next few weeks. Older children may also make some long-term goals.

The last group should involve recognition of the accomplishments of sharing and planning. A review of the coping strategies that have been heard and used should occur and follow-up meetings should be scheduled to determine if more services are needed for any member who still seems to be suffering.

Eppler (2008) identified themes of resilience in children who had lost a parent. Her research led her to the recommendations of infused strengths into small grief groups and into collaboration to support bereaved children. Holland (2008) talked about other ways schools can support grieving children.

Carr (2009) concluded that with young people who have suffered bereavement, the preferred treatment is a combination of child- and family-focused interventions to facilitate the grief process and help the adjustment of the new family structure. He recommended these evidence-based treatment manuals to guide counseling: *Family Focused Grief Therapy* (Kissane & Bloch, 2002) and *Treating Trauma and Traumatic Grief in Children and Adolescents* (Cohen, Mannarino, & Deblinger, 2006).

In summary, counseling strategies for helping children who have experienced loss through death include listening and being patient and sensitive to their unique way of dealing with grief. Grieving children need a chance to be heard and understood. They need reassurances that they are loved and will be cared for. They need honesty when they ask questions. They should have opportunities to say what they are feeling and to experience the emotions provoked by their loss. Children need ways to remember and honor the loved one who has died. Counselors can support children by listening, validating, and encouraging these chances to heal.

DEPRESSION AND SUICIDE

About 5 percent of children and adolescents suffer from depression, and in 2012, an estimated 2.2 million adolescents aged 12 to 17 in the United States had at least one major depressive episode in the past year. This represented 9.1 percent of the U.S. population aged 12 to 17 (National Institute of Mental Health, 2014). Persisting sadness and hopelessness are troubling predictors of clinical depression, which is significantly linked to suicidal behavior.

Signs of depression include persistent sadness, hopelessness, loss of interest in normal activities, changes in eating or sleeping habits, school absenteeism or poor performance, aches and pains that do not get better with treatment, and thoughts about death or suicide. The American Academy of Child and Adolescent Psychiatry (2013) outlines symptoms for children:

- Sadness, tearfulness, crying
- Hopelessness
- Decreased interest in activities
- Persistent boredom and low energy
- Social isolation, poor communication
- Low self-esteem and guilt
- Extreme sensitivity to rejection or failure
- Increased irritability, anger, or hostility
- Relationship problems
- Drastic changes in eating and/or sleeping patterns
- Thoughts or talk of suicide or self-harm

Adolescents may appear to be angry rather than sad. McWhirter, McWhirter, McWhirter, and McWhirter (2012) report that children and adolescents may have frequent physical complaints such as headaches, stomachaches, muscle aches, or fatigue. They may often be absent from school, may be unsuccessful in academics, and may have outbursts of anger, irritability, or crying. These troubled young people may have no interest in previously engaging activities, abuse substances, and have problems with their relationships.

Symptoms can vary in degree, intensity, and duration. Sciarra (2004) explains that the variations help in the identification of four different types of depression. Normal depression, the least severe type, occurs in everyone from time to time as a response to setbacks. Chronic depression is a more persistent feeling of sadness that may occur after an event or for no apparent reason. Crisis depression is a response to an external event and interferes with a person's life in a debilitating way. Finally, clinical depression is the most severe form, with extreme psychosocial impairment and thoughts of suicide occurring often. A three-part typology for depression outlines an affective type dominated by sadness and helplessness, a self-esteem type dominated by discouragement and negative self-esteem, and a guilt type dominated by guilt and self-destructive thoughts.

Some assessment instruments help screen for symptoms of depression. The Reynolds Adolescent Depression Scale (Reynolds, 1987) and the Reynolds Child Depression Scale (Reynolds, 1989) are self-report measures that are both easy to administer and to take. The Beck Depression Inventory (Beck & Steer, 1993) and the Children's Depression Inventory (Kovacs, 1985) are two other possibilities.

Interventions for Depression

Mash and Wolfe (2013) discuss antidepressant medication for young people with depression. Selective serotonin reuptake inhibitors (SSRIs) such as fluoxetine (Prozac), sertraline (Zoloft), and citalopram (Celexa) are prescribed frequently for depressed young people. David-Ferdon and Kaslow (2008) reported that SSRIs are effective in reducing symptoms of depression in children and adolescents; however, concerns about the side effects of suicidal thoughts and self-harm as well as the lack of information about long-term effects of the drugs have led to warnings. Antidepressant medications include a black-box warning and Patient Education Guide to tell users about the increased risks associated with the depressant. Counselors who work with depressed youth should ask them whether they are taking any medicine, how long they have been taking it, and who prescribed it. Sommers-Flanagan and Campbell (2009) conclude from their review of research pertaining to antidepressants that medication should be used in conjunction with psychosocial treatment interventions.

McWhirter and Burrow-Sanchez (2006) and Jacobson and Mufsor (2010) provide treatment protocols using interpersonal theory (IPT) for working with adolescents with depression. Interpersonal therapy assumes depression as a conflict in relationships. Five problem areas and treatment foci in interpersonal therapy are grief, interpersonal role disputes, role transitions, interpersonal deficits, and single-parent families. The goals of therapy are reduction in depression and resolving the underlying conflicts. According to David-Ferdon and Kaslow (2008), IPT has been identified as a well-established intervention for adolescents. Similarly, Weitz, Hollon, Kerkhof, and Cuiipers (2014) conclude that IPT and medication reduce suicidal ideation in people who are depressed.

Others (Seligman, 1998) have linked depression to a model of learned helplessness, a response to failures to solve a problem or to improve a situation. Pryce, Azzinnari, Spinelli, Seifritz, Tegethoff, and Meinlschmidt (2011) in their review of the concept found learned helplessness a concept that had potential for improving the treatment of depression. According to that model, a person becomes convinced nothing attempted will make a difference; therefore, the individual gives up and depression occurs. One recommendation for working with students who exhibit learned helplessness is to work in small steps so the child can develop a sense of mastery. Another strategy includes providing opportunities for selecting assignments or other choices. Giving feedback and explanations that help a child see cause-and-effect relationships may also help. Finally, encouraging depressed children to increase their sense of confidence by allowing them to identify their helpful behaviors and outcomes will support their overcoming learned helplessness (Sciarra, 2004). The Penn Prevention Program, also known as the Penn Optimism Program, has also been found to be efficacious for depressive symptoms (David-Ferdon & Kaslow, 2008).

Cognitive models to treat depression (Capuzzi & Gross, 2014; Clarke & DeBar, 2010; McWhirter & Burrow-Sanchez, 2006; Weersing & Brent, 2010) focus on replacing negative self-statements with positive self-talk and on developing other coping skills. Counseling with a behavioral approach might begin with behavior approaches such as scheduling pleasant activities, relaxation training, social skills training, role-plays, and behavioral rehearsals to increase the young person's activity. Then emphasis would move to identifying, testing, and modifying cognitive distortions. McWhirter and Burrow-Sanchez suggest two techniques they have found helpful. One is to ask the young person to repeat a standard, positive phrase such as "I am a good person" every time the child takes out a writing instrument. The other idea is to have the child or adolescent write an affirming self-statement on three or four note cards. The cards are placed in the child's notebook and every time it is used, the child silently reads one of the cards. Cognitive behavior treatment with the child, a small group, and the child plus a parent component were identified as well-established, resulting in significant benefits in a summary of evidence-based treatment of childhood depression (David-Ferdon & Kaslow, 2008).

The ACTION program (Stark, Streusand, Krumholz, & Patel, 2010) has also been created for working with young girls who are depressed. Children are taught the acronym that stands for:

A—Always find something to do to feel better.

C—Catch the positive.

T—Think about it as a problem to be solved.

I—Inspect the situation.

O—Open yourself to the positive.

N—Never get stuck in the negative muck.

Interventions can be with the individual or groups. The ACTION workbook contains situations in which children identify negative thinking and change it to a coping response.

Counselors will want to teach life skills to any young person who is struggling. A life skills training program would include interpersonal communication skills, cognitive change strategies, and anxiety-coping approaches. Interpersonal communication skills would include listening, reading social cues, and learning to say no. Cognitive change strategies involve problem solving, decision making, self-control, and reframing thoughts. Relaxation, exercise, and imagery would be included in anxiety-coping approaches. Counselors could help children improve in those areas by teaching, modeling, allowing the children to practice, giving feedback and reinforcement, and providing ways to practice the skills (Capuzzi & Gross, 2014; McWhirter & Burrow-Sanchez, 2006).

After his review of research studies, Carr (2009) concluded that the family-based component of effective counseling for depression includes education, help in family understanding and supporting the depressed youngster, and organizing liaisons between home and school to re-establish routines. The individual component involves identifying the contributing factors; mood monitoring; increasing physical exercise, social activity, and pleasant events; altering depressive thinking and patterns of social interaction; learning and using social problem-solving skills; developing relapse prevention skills. Stice, Shaw, Bohon, Marti, and Rohde (2009) reviewed depression prevention programs and identified larger effect sizes for programs targeting high-risk individuals, samples with more females, older adolescents, programs with shorter duration and homework assignments, and programs delivered by professionals. Sommers-Flanagan and Campbell (2009) recommend the following for working with depressed young people:

1. Children with significant depression should be offered counseling. CBT and IPT approaches, family therapy, parent consultation, activities that build positive affect, and group counseling are appropriate interventions. Homework assignments should emphasize pleasant activities and thought monitoring.
2. Young people who have severe depression should be monitored closely for suicidal thoughts and impulses, especially if they are taking medications such as SSRIs.
3. If symptoms have not reduced by 8 to 12 weeks of counseling, SSRIs may be considered to augment counseling. Referral to another counselor may also be considered.
4. Weekly sessions should continue with SSRI medication because therapy along with medication may reduce suicide risk.
5. The counselor and health care provider should communicate regularly.

Certainly depression itself is devastating to the struggling person and to others who are close. When depression leads to suicide, no one remains unscathed.

Suicide

Suicide is the third leading cause of death for 10- to 24-year-olds and results in the loss of approximately 4600 lives each year. Young people complete suicide by the use of firearms (45 percent), suffocation (40 percent), and poisoning (8 percent). The prevalence of suicidal behavior may be even greater because some may be reported as accidental deaths. These figures do not reflect suicide attempts, which may outnumber deaths by at least eight to one (Center for Disease Control and Prevention, 2014).

The reason a child attempts suicide is a complex question. James and Gilliland (2013) offers two theories: Freud's theory of inward aggression and Durkheim's social integration approach. Theories such as biochemical malfunction, mental deficiencies, escape, and interactional explanations also offer answers. Capuzzi and Gross (2014) add psychiatric disorders, poor self-efficacy, sexual or physical abuse, concerns over sexual identity, and other issues. Granello and Granello (2007) explain that people who attempt or commit suicide are making a desperate effort to say something (communicate), to ease some suffering either present or future (avoidance), or to take charge of a situation in which they feel helpless (control). Those three major categories may guide and organize thinking about the problem of child and adolescent suicide.

Granello and Granello (2007) summarized risk factors in children and adolescents as biological, emotional, cognitive, and environmental. Biological risk factors include impulsivity, aggression, hyperactivity, and brain damage. Emotional risk factors are depression and all other mental disorders, anger, identity problems, and the belief they are expendable. Cognitive factors include rigid cognitive structures, immature views of death and suicide, poor coping skills, limited problem-solving skills, inability to envision a future, and attraction to death and repulsion of life. The environmental factors contain early loss, family problems, child maltreatment, bullying and victimization, social isolation, and few friends.

Sciarra (2004) included personality traits that may help identify children and adolescents at risk for suicide. He also incorporates suggestions for working with those students. Suicide may be seen as the only option for those who feel hopeless and helpless about improving their situation. Groups that focus on problem solving and building self-esteem may help these children. Students with a history of impulsive and aggressive behaviors may also be at great risk. Truancy, running away, and a lack of cooperation are warning signs of these problems, and groups that incorporate methods to control anger can help. Children who are isolated from peers and have no other support system are also a great risk. Small groups that include building relationship skills may be an important intervention for the alienated students. Low self-esteem is another trait that may indicate risk for suicide, with an obvious intervention being a self-esteem group. High stress and poor life skills are risk factors. A stress management group should be considered. The related trait of perfectionism also may indicate suicidal behavior with cognitive behavioral interventions aimed at changing the thoughts about having to be perfect. Students with cognitive deficits may have an increased risk for suicide. Finally, excessive, persuasive guilt is another risk factor, one that requires long-term counseling treatment.

Assessment

In considering risk factors, Capuzzi and Gross (2014) and Granello and Granello (2007) conclude that the single best predictor of suicide is persistent suicidal ideation even though many children think about suicide without making an attempt. Suicide attempts are another high-risk indicator. Capuzzi and Gross report that as many as 40 percent of people who have attempted suicide will make future attempts. Attempts that may be misclassified as accidents must also be considered. Parental suicide, depression, marital discord, family violence, child abuse and neglect, and poor academic performance were all identified as high-risk factors. Evaluations for suicide should include interviews with the child and family; observations of play that look for developmentally inappropriate activities, dangerous or reckless behaviors, or activities indicating death or violence fantasies; discussions about what the child is thinking and feeling; and perhaps psychological testing on instruments such as the Child Suicide Potential Scale.

Granello and Granello (2007) identify the essential features of suicide risk assessment. They remind us that each person is unique and that assessment is an ongoing, complicated, and challenging process. The best assessment uses many perspectives and tries to uncover any foreseeable risk. Clinical judgment is always involved, and assessment is a part of treatment. Those authors caution counselors to err on the side of caution—that is particularly true with children and adolescents. All threats, warning signs, and risk factors should be taken seriously. Assessment attempts should try to uncover the underlying message about communication, avoidance, or control. Another important feature of suicide risk assessment is that it is always documented.

The most common method to determine suicide risk is to simply ask the person if he is considering suicide. Barrio (2007) suggested this simple question: "Do things ever get so bad that you think about hurting yourself?" Counselors who want to assess the risk for suicide may use a suicide interview. McWhirter et al. (2012) state that interviews are the most effective way to assess suicide. With the young person counselors will probe for suicidal ideation (the frequency, duration, and intensity of thoughts of suicide), suicidal volition, a suicide plan and the accessibility of the means, the person's mood, family history and current mental state, and the history of attempted suicide (Granello & Granello, 2007; Sciarra, 2004). Worchel and Gearing (2010) and Barrio (2007) explain that the assessment interview may alternate between problem solving, structuring the environment, and assessing the need for services. Jacobsen, Rabinowitz, Popper, Solomon, Sokol, and Pfeffer (1994) suggest questions such as the following to interview children about suicidal ideation and behaviors:

- Did you ever feel so upset that you wished you were not alive or wanted to die?
- Did you ever do something that you knew was so dangerous that you could get hurt or killed?
- Did you tell anyone that you wanted to die or were thinking about killing yourself?
- What would happen if you died? What would that be like?
- How do you remember feeling when you were thinking about killing yourself or trying to kill yourself?
- Has anything happened recently that has been upsetting to you or your family?
- Have you had a problem with feeling sad, having trouble sleeping, not feeling hungry, losing your temper easily, or feeling tired all of the time recently? (p. 450)

Barrio (2007) talks about the "free narrative account" that consists of open-ended prompts and reflects to help the child get the story told without being overwhelmed by questions. Other interview protocols can be found in the guides of Goldston (2003) and Worchel and Gearing (2010). The Adapted SAD PERSONS Scale (Junhke, 1996), the Suicide Ideation Questionnaire (Reynolds, 1988), the Suicide Risk Screen (Thompson & Eggert, 1999), and the Scale of Suicide Ideation (Beck, Kovacs, & Weissman, 1979) are other inventories. Although it is difficult to determine the factors associated with a child's potential for suicide, guidelines such as these give counselors some basis for assessment of risks.

Interventions for Suicide

Strategies for counselors working with suicidal children include those offered by Capuzzi and Gross (2014), James and Gilliland (2013), McWhirter et al. (2012), and Sciarra (2004):

1. Trust your suspicions if you think the young person may be self-destructive.
2. Never ignore threats, hints, and continued comments about destroying oneself, "leaving this world," "you're going to miss me," or "life is not worth living." These comments may be attention-getting, but children who use these techniques to get attention need help. Follow up the threat immediately with active listening in an attempt to discover the feelings or events that brought on the self-destructive feelings.
3. Tell the young person you are worried and listen to him or her in a nonjudgmental and supportive way. Reinforce the youngster for seeking help.

4. Ask direct, specific questions about whether the child is considering suicide and whether there is a plan. Confront the child with your thoughts and feelings. You are not placing the thought in the child's mind, but you may provide an opening and opportunity for the child to discuss troublesome thoughts and feelings.

5. If suicidal children admit to self-destructive thoughts, ask about their plan. A well-thought-out plan is a significant danger signal.

6. Do not debate whether suicide is right or wrong.

7. Do not promise to keep the suicidal intentions a secret.

8. Do not leave the youngster alone if you think the threat of suicide is imminent. Ensure the safety of the child and that the appropriate adults who are responsible for the child have been notified.

9. You should remain actively involved with the youngster. Take an active, directive role to protect the youngster. In a crisis situation, do not attempt in-depth counseling until more stability is established. Monitor progress.

10. If you believe a child could be seriously contemplating suicide, suggest to the parents that they consult a doctor or psychiatrist. Hospitalization may be indicated for consistent care and monitoring. Inpatient treatment should be considered if the youngster is agitated, has not been eating, is overly tired or dehydrated, or has some other physical condition.

11. Use the resources that are available. Never hesitate to consult with someone thoroughly trained in suicide prevention—suicide-prevention centers, clinics, or psychiatrists—or refer suicidal children to them.

12. Assure the young person that something is being done, that the suicidal urges are serious, and that you are with them through this emergency. Tell them that survival is a step-by-step process, that help is available, and that asking for help directly is critical when the urges are strong.

13. Use techniques to enhance the self-concept of children who exhibit suicidal tendencies.

14. At a time of crisis, listen to the child carefully in a nonjudgmental manner. Have the child tell you everything that has happened during the previous few hours or days. You may gain some understanding or knowledge of factors contributing to the depression.

15. Suicidal children need permission to call, and the phone number of, a person (the counselor or another close and understanding friend) they feel they can talk with in times of distress.

16. The parents of a suicidal child should be made aware of the child's feelings and thoughts and helped to understand the situation without panic or guilt. Counsel them about how to listen to and talk with the child. Consult with them concerning danger signals and make a plan for handling crises, should they arise.

17. Talk with suicidal children about what has happened in their lives recently. Losses of loved ones, pets, and other significant objects in the children's lives; feelings of personal failure; feelings of extreme shame or grief; and other traumatic events contribute to suicidal thoughts. Allow children to express their feelings without being judgmental, glossing over, or denying their right to these feelings.

18. Ask suicidal children to tell you about their fantasies or dreams. Ask them to draw a picture or write out their thoughts. These techniques often give the adult some insight into the child's thoughts and feelings.

19. Often, children do not understand death as final and irreversible; therefore, any child who is seriously disturbed or depressed needs careful attention.
20. The months after the threat also are crucial, and careful attention should continue until the conflict is completely resolved. A sudden recovery after severe depression may be a warning signal that the client has made a decision to end his or her life.

Postsuicide Interventions

Although Szumilas and Kutcher (2011) found little evidence of effectiveness of postsuicide interventions, many institutions have protocols for dealing with the aftermath of a completed suicide. Kerr (2009) lists factors to consider when planning a postvention. Previous tragedies and how the school has dealt with those losses should be taken into account. How long the person was in the school and how well known and liked the person was are other considerations. The way the death has been reported and how many students witnessed the tragedy must be concerns as well as other students who may be at risk, the ages of the students, and whether the school is in session or not. The postvention program must be implemented quickly—as well as over a longer time. Surviving students may need support. Various opportunities should be available such as individual, small-group, and classroom sessions. All members of the postvention team should be careful to be factual and not to dramatize the suicide—surviving students need to know suicide is a bad choice and other options are available (Granello & Granello, 2007). Suicide contagion may lead to further suicidal behavior or deaths, especially with adolescents who are highly vulnerable (Kerr). McWhirter et al. (2012) explain issues that should be addressed after a nonfatal suicide attempt.

Many writers in this area suggest psychological education and peer-group counseling as preventive measures to suicide. The Suicide Prevention Resource Center provides information about evidence-based practices in suicide prevention, and Granello and Granello (2007) have an outline of classroom activities to help teens understand suicide risks and learn how to help their friends and themselves. The Multisystemic Treatment of Children and Adolescents with Serious Emotional Disturbance (Henggeler, Schoenwald, Rowland, & Cunningham, 2002) combines family therapy with skills training for the teen as well as interventions in the school and other networks. The program decreased rates of attempted suicide in a one-year follow-up with adolescents at risk for suicide.

Kerr (2009), Capuzzi and Gross (2014), and James and Gilliland (2013) suggest that all schools should have a disaster plan to use in the event of a suicide, just as schools have a plan for hurricanes, tornadoes, earthquakes, and other traumatic events. Some of their suggestions include:

1. Develop a team of resource people to handle the emotional crisis.
2. Present in-service training programs to the entire staff on the causes of suicide, warning signs, and sources of help for suicidal students.
3. Establish a network to inform all faculty members of the facts of the tragedy.
4. Designate special crisis centers for children needing additional help.

5. Develop a checklist of activities to be included in the classroom announcement.
6. Plan to communicate cautions about the dangers in the days following a suicide.
7. Carry out home visits.
8. Develop guidelines for media coverage.
9. Develop procedures to continue alertness for several months.

Helping professionals are aware that children may imitate other children who commit suicide and such a plan, together with psychological education and group counseling, may prevent further tragedies.

FAMILY STRUCTURES CHILDREN OF DIVORCE

The National Center for Health Statistics (2014) reports that almost 50 percent of all marriages in the United States end with divorce, a statistic that has remained stable for the last decade. That split may be devastating to the children involved who may feel confused, insecure, fearful, trapped, angry, unloved, and guilty (James and Gilliland, 2013). Counselors are often the support anchor the youngsters need in the midst of their changing world.

The lives and relationships of children in a divorcing family are profoundly affected—socially, economically, psychologically, and even legally. Papilia, Feldman, and Martorell (2014) outline the stresses of divorce as a chain of events. It begins with the conflict before the divorce and continues with the aftermath that may involve relocations, loss of friends, changes in socioeconomic status, redefining relationships with both parents, and perhaps adjusting to the remarriage of one or both parents. Children must adjust to separation from one parent and formation of a new and different relationship with the other. A change in the family's economic status, possibly a change in the home and school environment, different parenting styles, custody battles, and sometimes a totally different lifestyle create feelings that may be positive or negative. Often, mothers who were totally involved in the care of children and home may have to go to work; many are unskilled and accept low-paying jobs. The income loss may be compounded by increased work, job instability, and move to less desirable neighborhoods. Children may be torn by conflicting loyalties or learn to manipulate the parents to get their own way. Children of divorced parents may be asked to assume the role of the absent parent and to fulfill physical or emotional responsibilities beyond their maturity level.

Wallerstein (2008) identifies these concerns of young people. The children are afraid. They may not understand who will provide food, housing, clothes, and protection. They may be concerned that if the marriage can fail, the parent–child relationship could also be terminated. The children may be sad; may have changes in sleeping, eating, and paying attention; and may have emotional swings. They may want more contact with the absent parent and may continue to hope for reconciliation. The children may be lonely, overlooked by parents who are preoccupied with the divorce. The youngsters may feel rejected and may have conflicting loyalties. Finally, they may be angry about all the changes in their lives. Wallerstein notes that the primary peril of divorce is adverse effects on the child's development.

Several factors can be associated with a child's vulnerability to negative effects of parents separating. The child's adjustment before the divorce as well as the child's personality, temperament, gender, and the custody decision impact adjustment (Hetherington, 2006). Children in joint-custody situations adjusted better than those in sole-custody families; in fact, children in joint custody are often as well-adjusted as those in families who have not divorced (Bauserman, 2002). Numerous studies suggest that the child's developmental level is related to the reaction that follows the separation. Wallerstein (2008) suggests that infants respond mainly to the emotional reactions of their caretaker; for example, mothers or fathers under stress convey their feelings to the infant through their handling and verbal communication. Very young children appear to have many of their needs met regardless of the stress of the caretaker. Preschoolers (ages 3–5) have only a vague understanding of the family situation because of their limited cognitive development; thus, they often feel frightened and insecure, experience nightmares, and regress to more infantile behaviors. School-age children, who have more advanced cognitive and emotional development, see the situation more accurately. However, children ages 6 to 8 often believe the divorce was their fault ("If I had not been bad, Dad would not have left."), and children at this age often hold unrealistic hopes for a family reconciliation. They may feel loss, rejection, guilt, and loyalty conflicts. Ages 9 to 12 are a time when children are developing rapidly and rely on their parents for stability. They may become angry at the parent they blame for the divorce or may take a supportive role as they worry about their troubled parents. Because of their anxiety, they may develop somatic symptoms, engage in troublesome behaviors, or experience a decline in academic achievement. The parents' divorce during children's adolescent years brings a different set of developmental problems. Young people at this age are striving for independence and exploring their own sexuality. They need structure, limits, and guidance in dealing with their sexuality. They also may worry about their own relationships and the possibility of repeating their parents' mistakes. One intervention proposed by Thomas and Gibbons (2009) is to facilitate adolescents' decisions about their future with career counseling to help teens focus on their possibilities.

Most importantly, children who are socially mature and responsible and who have few behavior problems and easy temperaments cope better with their parents' divorce (Santrock, 2012), and within 2 to 3 years after a divorce, parents and children have adjusted to their new life.

Interventions with Children of Divorce

Wallerstein and Blakeslee (2003) describe "psychological tasks" that children of divorce must successfully resolve. These tasks are described in the following paragraphs.

ACKNOWLEDGING THE REALITY OF THE MARRIAGE BREAKUP   Supportive counseling techniques, including listening, reflection, clarification, and problem solving, and perhaps stress-reduction techniques such as relaxation or guided imagery are appropriate for children working through this task. The most critical factor in helping children through divorce is parental support. Both parents should talk with all the children together about the decision to divorce several days before one parent leaves the home. Children should be provided with a clear explanation about why their parents are divorcing, although they need not be told the details of an infidelity or other sexual problems. The parents should convey that, unfortunately, they have made a mistake in their marriage, but they remain committed to the family. According to the authors, understanding the divorce and its consequences is the first psychological task for children of divorcing families.

DISENGAGING FROM PARENTAL CONFLICT AND DISTRESS AND RESUMING CUSTOMARY PURSUITS   The resolution of this task calls for the children to distance themselves from the crisis in their household and resume their normal learning tasks, outside activities, and friendships. Parents must work to help children keep their lives in order and not let the divorce overshadow all their activities by keeping familiar routines and encouraging participation in extracurricular activities.

RESOLUTION OF LOSS   Divorce brings not only loss of a parent but also often loss of familiar surroundings and possibly a different lifestyle. A consistent pattern of visitation by the absent parent and an emphasis on building a new and positive relationship can help children through this stage. Individual and group sessions focusing on building self-esteem may be helpful—for example, strengths testing, peer teaching, finding the child a "buddy," and the techniques of cognitive restructuring.

RESOLVING ANGER AND SELF-BLAME   Divorce is a voluntary decision by one or both parents and often children tend to blame them for being selfish. Children may also blame themselves for the breakup of the family. The child's ability to forgive himself or herself for the divorce or lack of reconciliation is a significant step toward forgiving the parents and reconciling the relationship with parents. There are some excellent children's books that can help them understand the divorce process and the reality that they are not to blame for the divorce. Counselors can recommend specific books for the developmental level of their clients.

The child's intense anger often results in acting-out behavior. A consistent, structured environment at home and at school provides some of the security the child needs during this period of turmoil and change. Group counseling that focuses on role-playing, play therapy, drawing, and writing can help children express their anger and feelings of guilt. Group problem-solving discussions help children find constructive ways of handling their feelings.

ACCEPTING THE PERMANENCE OF DIVORCE   The fantasy of a reunited family persists tenaciously for children of divorce, even after the parents marry other partners. Reality therapy may help the child accept the permanence of divorce. Group counseling with other children who are going through divorce or who have experienced it may also help. Drawings of the family before the divorce and at the present time, family changes since the divorce, and filmstrips and books about divorce and other family lifestyles (the stepfamily or single-parent family) often stimulate excellent discussions.

ACHIEVING REALISTIC HOPE REGARDING RELATIONSHIPS   Children often feel rejected, unlovable, and unworthy because they feel guilty over the divorce or because they believe that one or both parents rejected them and cared little about their feelings and welfare. Wallerstein and Blakeslee (2003) note that some adolescents engage in acting-out behavior (promiscuity, alcohol or drug abuse, or other similar behaviors) that indicates low self-esteem. An important task for adolescents is realizing they can love and be loved. They must learn to be open in relationships while knowing that divorce or loss is possible. According to Wallerstein and Blakeslee, effective resolution of this last psychological task of "taking a chance on love" leads to freedom from the psychological trauma of divorce and provides second chances for children of these families.

Wallerstein and Blakeslee (2003) conclude that the effects of divorce are much more pervasive and longer lasting than originally thought. Twenty years after Wallerstein began her initial research, she found parents' continuing anger still a factor in their children's lives. Many of the sample of children, now adults, were underachievers or drank heavily; a few had been involved in serious crimes. One-third of the girls had relationship problems. Those findings indicate the need for interventions for children of divorce even though many children will overcome the difficulties within a few years.

Parents

Counselors working with the parents of children involved in a divorce can be of assistance by providing consulting advice. In their comprehensive article attempting to link intervention to basic research on children of divorce, Grych and Fincham (1992) also suggest helping parents understand how their behavior affects their children's adjustment and assist them in minimizing the effect of the divorce on children. Parents and counselors need to remember that adjustment after a divorce takes time for a child and requires continuing understanding and reassurance. Parent group meetings can help parents understand the problems their children are experiencing, learn new methods for communicating with their children, try new methods of discipline, and resolve some of their own frustration.

Grych (2005) stated the goals of parent education for divorcing adults was to decrease conflict and improve child adjustment. Some suggestions that counselors may want to offer parents follow:

1. Explain what has happened at the child's level of understanding and try to relate the experience to one that the child may have had. Emphasize that the child is not at fault. Keep the lines of communication open so the child's misconceptions or fears are recognized immediately. Avoid blaming or criticizing the other parent and relating all the unpleasant details.
2. Plan for ways to make the child's life as stable and consistent as possible, even though changes may be necessary. Household routines, school schedules, and consistent discipline help children understand that their world is not completely wrecked. Involve teachers, counselors, ministers, grandparents, and other support systems.
3. Avoid using the children as go-betweens to carry messages ("The child support check is late!") or to find out about the other parent's life ("What does the apartment look like?"). Children love both parents and are already torn by conflicting loyalties.

4. Arrange for regular visits from the absent parent to assure the children that they are loved by both parents. Children are sometimes disappointed by absent parents who fail to call or come for a visit. Custodial parents need to provide a lot of love and reassurance at these times.

5. Talk with the children about the future. Involve them in the planning without overwhelming them with problems. They need to know what to expect.

6. Children experiencing a divorce in their family are still children at a particular developmental level. Avoid asking them to assume responsibilities beyond their capabilities—being the man of the family, babysitting younger children, or taking on excessive household chores.

Outcomes

Carr (2009) noted that child-focused, parent-focused, and combined child-and-family-focused interventions all have beneficial effects on the adjustment of children after separation or divorce. Child-focused treatment helps children build coping skills within a supportive group. Parents learn parenting skills in the parent-focused programs and the combined treatment contains both elements. Programs positively impact mood, divorce-related beliefs, self-esteem, behavior problems at home and school, and family relationships.

Although many children of divorce do experience increased risks for social, emotional, and academic difficulties, others have successfully adjusted to the disruption and do not display significant signs of distress as a result of the experience. Gately and Schwebel (1992) have found some areas in which the children experienced favorable outcomes:

1. *Maturity*, because they tended to assume greater responsibility for chores;
2. *Improved self-esteem*, because they coped effectively with their changing life's circumstances;
3. *Empathy*, due to increased concern for family members;
4. *Androgyny*, as a result of seeing models not confined by stereotypical sex roles.

Positive factors in their lives that contributed to the development of these attributes were positive personality, supportive family environment, and supportive social environment (Gately & Schwebel, 1992).

Family courts have moved from who would have custody to decisions about ways time and access to children can be shared by the divorcing parents. Deutsch (2008) describes education, mediation, and evaluation services delivered by multidisciplinary teams that support the parents and courts in custody decisions as well as increasing the possibilities of children's adjustment.

Children in Stepfamilies

Many U.S. children live in a stepfamily. This combination of adults and a child or children from a previous relationship may also be referred to as a blended family. Joining two families into one presents children with another set of unique problems with which to cope at a time when the effects of the biological parents' divorce may still be troublesome. Because the stepfamily is not considered a "normal" family, expectations and relationships are more ambiguous and complex. Not only are cultural and social guidelines unclear but also children who are members of two households, moving in and out, have ambiguous and complex home guidelines and schedules. Adults and children experience changes in roles, alliances, parenting arrangements, household responsibilities, rules, expectations, and demands. For children who are attempting to regain stability after the first family breakup, this lack of structure may bring additional stresses and strains. Nevertheless, Wen (2008) used data from the 1999 National Survey of America's Families for an association between children's well-being among children aged 6 to 17; he found that both stepfamilies and intact families have more advantages than single-parent families.

MacFarland and Tollerud (2009) explain four categories of issues in blended families. In the early development of the new family, issues about loyalty, loss, attachment, and fantasies of reconciliation may occur as well as redefining roles and feelings of rejection. Developing family issues, a second category, includes discipline, family roles, sibling conflict, time with the noncustodial parent, and moving between families. A third category is feelings about self and others that may be influenced by negative images of stepfamilies. Children may act out their stresses in school and may hide their emotions. If the new parent has a child of his or her own, stepchildren may feel less valued and other difficulties may arise. Adult issues that relate to the new family involve financial support and alimony, competition among parents, continuing conflicts, and different parenting styles in the blended family.

Papernow (1995) outlines the following stages of stepfamily development:

I. Early stage
   a. *Fantasy stage*—there is the dream the new family will be ideal and everyone will love each other
   b. *Immersion stage*—reality indicates that something in the family is different and may not be right
   c. *Awareness stage*—identifying new position in the family structure and clarifying understanding of associated feelings

II. Middle stage
   a. *Mobilization*—more conflict may emerge as the new family begins to move toward a new structure
   b. *Action stage*—the new family reaches consensus on the family structure and operation

III. Later stages
   a. *Contact stage*—deeper stepfamily relationships are formed
   b. *Resolution stage*—step relationships become more intimate and solid; family norms and procedures are established

Families and individual members proceed through these stages at varying rates. Counselors need to help both parents and children in the stepfamily to find their appropriate roles and clearly define expectations of all members. Defining these new roles requires time and patience. Parents and children need to express and clarify their thoughts and feelings, establish routines and expectations, plan visitations with other parents, and agree on discipline guidelines. Play therapy is especially helpful for counseling with younger children. Drawings, journals, bibliocounseling, and group counseling with other children in stepfamilies may assist older children in working through their feelings and concerns. Family counseling is encouraged to help the newly organized family increase awareness and acceptance of each other and individual differences, facilitate problem solving, and build support for each other.

The stepparent has the power to impact or even shape the relationship of the biological parent and children. In Ahrons' (2007) interviews with adults who had been in stepfamilies, the majority discussed good relationships with stepparents. Her participants explained that positive connections may not have begun immediately but the relationships improved as the stepparent and child began to know each other better. Wallerstein and Lewis (2007) emphasize the urgent need for expanded parent education, conflict resolution, and opportunities inherent in changes as well as realistic advice for stepparents. Ahrons added providing information to parents about life course and family system perspectives. Early interventions with fathers have significant impact on improving parenting skills and increasing their involvement with their children.

Pasley and Garneau (2011) identified key components of successful stepfamilies as cooperation and appropriate boundary settings between the separate households. Counselors who can help clients increase cooperation and provide limits will also help increase satisfaction with the new family. Likewise, Greeff and Du Toit (2009) identified aspects of family resilience associated with adjustments in stepfamilies. The most important factors they found were supportive family relationships; affirming and supportive communication; a sense of control over outcomes in life; activities and routines that allow the family to spend time together; a strong marriage; support from others; redefining stressful events; and spirituality within the family.

Counselors need to give youngsters in blended families emotional support. The young people must come to terms with loss, their feelings of helplessness, role frustrations, and communication difficulties. Counselors may use creative arts to help children gain insight, consider relationships, and develop coping strategies. MacFarland and Tollerud (2009) recommend kinetic art, creative drama, role-play, bibliotherapy, and group counseling. Some books about step families include these:

Louie's Search (Keats, 2001)

My Family's Changing (Thomas, 1999)

All Families Are Different (Gordon & Cohen, 2000)

We have suggested that periodically counselors need to examine their own attitudes and beliefs about certain clients to maintain the highest levels of objectivity and efficiency. Because negative stereotypes of stepparents are common, people in the helping professions may sometimes unwittingly adopt stereotypical thinking and evaluate stepparents or stepchildren clients in light of these negative stereotypes.

In addition, schools need to evaluate their activities in light of their effects on stepfamilies—Do policies and activities allow stepparents' participation in the child's school life? Do special occasions such as Mother's Day and Father's Day include references to stepparents? Are living arrangements and name differences clearly indicated in records to avoid embarrassment? School may be the one place a child in a new stepparent home finds structure and familiarity. Counselors can help school personnel make the environment more comfortable and accepting for children in a changing world.

Children in Single-Parent Homes

Thirty-five percent of children in the United States live in single-parent families (KidsCount Databank, 2014) and 24 percent live in households headed by a single mother. Single mothers are vulnerable economically because their earnings are usually low and many do not receive child support. Single motherhood appears to be strongly related to poverty, and never-married mothers are particularly apt to end up receiving welfare. Poverty, of course, has a strong correlation with children's low academic achievement, conduct disorders, and even juvenile crime.

Counseling strategies to help children in single-parent homes are similar to many described for children of divorce and children in stepfamilies. The counselor must help the child deal with feelings of loss, whether the loss resulted from divorce, separation, or death. Emotions must be recognized and discussed. These children need stability, security, and consistency in their lives. Therefore, counselors may want to recommend to the child's parent and other family members that they join a support group to help the family reorganize effectively after the loss. Counselors in schools can provide group activities for children of single-parent homes to help them discuss their fears, concerns, and feelings about having only one parent in the home.

As stated earlier in this section, considerable research substantiates that children from single-parent homes have a higher rate of conduct disorders and other adjustment problems than children from intact homes. However, well-adjusted children live in single-parent homes. Counselors must be careful not to allow generalizations or personal bias to interfere with their objectivity in working with these children.

Children and Violence

Violent behavior in children can take many forms, from temper tantrums to intentional destruction of property. Parents and other adults may be concerned but uncertain about what to do. Violent behavior in children should not be ignored. Intense anger, frequent outbursts, extreme irritability and/or impulsiveness, and low frustration threshold are warning signs of children who need some help controlling themselves.

Antisocial behavior refers to behavior that conflicts with social norms. It may sometimes include criminal activity. McWhirter et al. (2012) list the most common antisocial behaviors of young people as: (1) aggression and coercive misbehaviors in the family; (2) problems in school that often lead to a diagnosis of conduct disorder; (3) community and school problems such as fighting and property destruction; (4) minor criminal activity such as vandalism, substance use, and running away; (5) major criminal activity such as robbery; and (6) violence and gang membership.

Antisocial behavior, aggression, delinquency, and violence have common antecedents and consequences. Kimonis, Frick, and McMahon (2014) explain that conduct problems and antisocial behaviors are terms that cover a range of actions and attitudes that violate the expectations of parents, society, and the personal or property rights of others. Children with conduct problems show a variety of rule-breaking behaviors from the annoying to more serious forms like vandalism, theft, and assault. The behaviors can be conceived on covert–overt dimensions and destructive–nondestructive dimensions.

The overt–covert ranges from visible acts like fighting (overt) to hidden acts like lying or stealing (covert). Mash and Wolfe (2013) describe children who exhibit overt antisocial behavior as irritable, negative, and resentful in reactions to hostile situations. They also have a higher level of family conflict. Those displaying covert antisocial behavior are less social, more anxious, and suspicious, and come from homes that give them little support. Many children show both overt and covert behaviors and are frequently in conflict with authority, have severe family discord, and have the poorest long-term outcomes. The destructive–nondestructive dimension ranges from acts like cruelty to animals and physical assault to nondestructive behaviors like arguing or irritability. Children who exhibit overt destructive behaviors, especially persistent physical fighting, have a high risk for later psychiatric disorders. Figure 19-1 illustrates these dimensions.

James and Gilliland (2013) outlined the reasons for violence in young people and the causes: poor parenting, disenfranchised students, lack of role models, hate crimes, bullying, and media violence. The U.S. Department of Health and Human Services (2001) disseminated a report of the Surgeon General's that included statistically relevant facts associated with youth violence such as a history of criminal offenses, substance abuse, weak social connections, antisocial delinquent peers, and gang membership. The report also identified subcategories. Late-onset characteristics of violent young people occur after puberty. Those variables include all of those above as well as risk-taking behaviors, criminal activities, and violence toward other people. Early-onset risk factors emerge before puberty. Factors such as poor parent–child relationships, little supervision or discipline, and neglectful parents, as well as poor school performance and attitude relate to the incidence of youth who are violent. McWhirter et al. (2012) summarize with a progressive model of aggression and violence that can be found in their book.

Mash and Wolfe (2013) also illustrate the pathway from disruptive to antisocial behavior from childhood to adolescence. The approximate order begins with a difficult temperament, a fussy child with irregular sleeping and eating patterns, and a low frustration for novel events. As the child ages, more hyperactivity may be evident and simple forms of oppositional and aggressive behavior may peak in the preschool years. Most children with conduct disorders add new forms of antisocial behavior as they grow. Poor social skills and social-cognitive problems lead to poor peer relationships and social isolation. Truancy, reading problems, and academic failure may characterize the school years. By ages 8 to 12, the child may be fighting, bullying, setting fires, stealing, being cruel to animals and humans, and vandalizing property. Across all cultures, conduct problems escalate in adolescence with an increasing association with deviant peers, more arrests and re-arrests, and convictions for criminal activity. This illustration does not fit every child; about 50 percent with early conduct problems improve as they grow. Those who improve have less extreme levels of early problems, higher intelligence and SES, fewer deviant friends, mothers who are not teenagers, and parents with more social skills and fewer problems (Lahey, Loeber, Burke, & Rathouz, 2002).

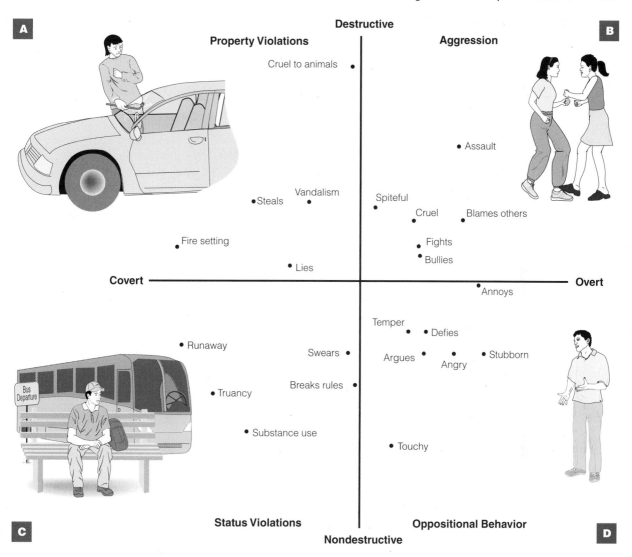

FIGURE 19-1   FOUR CATEGORIES OF CONDUCT PROBLEMS

From Mash, E. J., & Wolfe, D. A. (2013). *Abnormal child psychology* (5th ed., p. 157). Belmont, CA: Wadsworth. Reprinted with permission.

Some gender differences in conduct problems are apparent. Mash and Wolfe (2013) explain that when girls are angry they use indirect and relational forms of aggression like verbal insults, gossip, tattling, ostracism, threats, getting even, or third-party retaliation. As they become adolescents, girls' aggressive behavior revolves around group acceptance and affiliation while boys continue to be confrontational and physically violent. The relational aggression girls exhibit at school associates with adolescent's perceptions of a hostile school environment. Teens who witness high levels of relational aggression see school as less safe. In males, exposure to relational aggression was associated with carrying a weapon to school (Goldstein, Young, & Boyd, 2008).

Treatment and Prevention

The most promising treatments for children with violent tendencies use several approaches and include individual, family, school, and community settings (Kimonis, Frick, & McMahon, 2014). Family problems like depression, partner discord, abuse, and other stressors must also be addressed. Group treatments that bring together antisocial young people may exacerbate the problem since those like-minded people may encourage each other's misbehavior (Dishion & Dodge, 2005). Promising treatments also contain methods and goals appropriate to the child's developmental level and type and severity of the problems. The more advanced the child is on the antisocial pathway, the more intense treatment is indicated. Frick (2000) suggested a two-prong approach:

> *Early intervention/prevention* for young children just starting to exhibit problems.
> *Ongoing interventions* for older children and their families to cope with the many social, emotional, and academic problems.

Bay-Hinitz and Wilson (2005) suggest a group play therapy intervention for preschool children. The intervention involves cooperative games to reduce aggression and increase cooperation. PEACE (Salmon, 2003) is a school curriculum designed to increase empathy skills and to interpret social cues. Aggression Replacement Training focuses on the strengths and potential of children to help them change (Roth & Striepling-Goldstein, 2003). Finally, Promoting Alternative Thinking Strategies (PATHS) focuses on internal and interpersonal processes with the goal of reducing violence and risky behaviors, a curriculum that promotes emotional competence and empathy (Capuzzi & Gross, 2014).

Eyberg, Nelson, and Boggs (2008) have identified some successful treatment approaches—the parent management training (PMT), problem-solving skills training (PSST), and multisystemic treatment (MST).

Carr (2009) concludes that for children under age 12, parent training programs were significantly more effective than child-focused programs for deviant behavior. Parent management training (Brinkmeyer & Eyberg, 2003; McMahon & Forehand, 2003) teaches parents ways to manage their child's behavior at home and in other settings. The goal of PMT is for the parent to learn new skills. Parents learn to change their interactions with children, promote positive child behavior, and decrease antisocial behavior. They learn to recognize, define, and observe their child's behavior. Sessions include the use of commands, setting clear rules, using praise and tangible rewards, use of mild punishment, negotiation, and contingency contracting. Parents see the techniques, practice the behaviors, and review their progress at home in homework assignments. Their progress is carefully monitored and adjustments are made in the training if needed. This program has been evaluated more than any other treatment for conduct disorder (Eyberg et al., 2008) and has impressive success. Currently, some adaptations to the intervention are related to the importance of providing marital and social support, checking on the therapy style and engagement, and looking at ethnic and cultural factors in treatment (Yasui & Dishion, 2007).

The effectiveness of parent training programs may be enhanced when children increase their social and problem-solving skills (Carr, 2009). PSST concentrates on cognitive deficiencies and distortions that children with conduct problems show in interpersonal situations (Kazdin, 2003). This treatment can be used alone or with PMT. This approach is based on the assumption that the child's perceptions of events will trigger aggressive and antisocial responses and that adjusting faulty thinking will lead to change in behavior. Self-statements direct attention to parts of the problem that lead to better solutions. The treatment incorporates structured tasks like games, school activities, and stories. The problem-solving skills are applied to real-life situations. The counselor takes an active part, providing examples of the cognitive process as well as feedback and praise. The components of treatment are modeling, practice, role-playing, behavioral contracts, reinforcement, mild punishments, homework assignments, and parent involvement. The child learns five problem-solving steps to identify thoughts, feelings, and behaviors in difficult social situations. The steps (Kazdin, 1996, p. 383) with examples are the following:

Problem Situation

Mona, one of your classmates, took your dessert off your tray. What do you do?

Step 1: What am I supposed to do?

I want her to know that made me mad.

Step 2: I have to look at all my possibilities.

I can scream at her, take something from her, tell my teacher, or tell her she made me mad.

Step 3: I had better concentrate and focus.

If I scream I'll get in trouble. I might get caught if I take something from her and everyone will think I'm a tattle if I tell my teacher. If I tell her how mad I am, she might be sorry for taking my dessert.

Step 4: I need to make a choice.

I'm going to tell her I don't like her taking my things and that it makes me mad. If that doesn't work, I'll think about this some more.

Step 5: I did a good job or I made a mistake.

I made a good choice. I won't get in trouble but she just laughed at me. I may not want her for a friend any more if that's how she's going to act, but I can decide that later.

PPST is effective with children who have conduct problems, and parent and family relationships also improve (Kazdin, 2003).

MST combines intensive family- and community-based approaches for teens with conduct problems so severe the adolescent may be put in an out-of-home placement (Henggeler, Sheidow, & Lee, 2007). The assumption is that antisocial behavior happens because of the interconnected systems of family, school, neighborhood, court, and juvenile services. MST helps caregivers improve the functioning of the teen and the family. Assessment focuses on identifying the fit between the problem and the context. Interventions are action oriented and focus on specific, well-defined problems that are behavioral transactions within and between multiple systems. Treatment is modified for the developmental level and needs of the child. Interventions involve daily and weekly tasks by family members, continuous evaluation, and long-term maintenance. Treatment emphasizes the positive and makes use of system strengths as change levers. Finally, the interventions promote responsible behavior and decrease disruptive behavior (Henggeler & Lee, 2003). Mash and Wolfe (2013) commented that the outcome studies of MST are superior to usual services of individual counseling, community services, and hospitalization. The positive effects have lasted as long as 5 years after treatment.

The programs we have reviewed are treatment programs for children and teens exhibiting behavior problems. Prevention interventions try counteracting negative factors before the troubling behavior begins. An example of intensive and multifaceted early intervention programs is The Incredible Years program (Webster-Stratton & Reid, 2003), which is for parents and teachers and includes child management skills, self-control strategies, and building positive relationships. Several studies support the effectiveness of Incredible Years. Fast Track (Conduct Problems Prevention Research Group, 2007) began with kindergarten children who were identified from their disruptive behavior and poor relationships with peers. The interventions started in grade 1 and lasted until grade 10. Children learned social-cognitive and academic skills. Parents, teachers, and project staff are included. The efficacy of Fast Track was greatest for the children who had the highest risk factors for conduct problems.

BULLYING

One type of violent behavior is bullying. Finn (2014) recommends schools target bullying such as coercive verbal comments, physical intimidation, or a combination of these. The impact of bullying on the target children is that of chronic, systematic terrorism. The bully also suffers negative consequences, and schools in which bullying is tolerated are hostile environments (Olweus, Limber, & Mihalic, 1999).

Olweus (1993, 2001, 2002, 2004) explains that a person is bullied when exposed repeatedly to negative actions on the part of another person or persons and has trouble defending himself or herself. The significant aspects of this definition include the aggressive behavior, repeated over time as well as the imbalance of power or strength. Olweus argues that peer abuse should never be tolerated. Prominent examples of bullying include these:

- Verbal abuse including derogatory comments and inflammatory names
- Exclusion or isolation
- Hitting, kicking, shoving, and spitting
- Lies and false rumors
- Taking or damaging possessions of the student who is being targeted
- Threats or intimidation, being forced to do something
- Racial bullying

- Sexual bullying
- Cyber bullying

According to Olweus, young people bully because they have strong needs for power and dominance, they enjoy causing injury and suffering, and they are rewarded thorough material or psychological rewards.

The Olweus Bullying Prevention Program is designed to address bullying issues at the school, in the classroom, and with individuals, and it has had impressive outcomes (Finn, 2014). The U.S. Department of Health and Human Services has the Stop Bullying Now Web site (http://stopbullyingnow.hrsa.gov/adults/default.aspx) with resources for students and adults who are concerned about bullying behaviors and mental health information links at http://mentalhealth.samhsa.gov/15plus/aboutbullying.asp. Bullying behaviors should be addressed by knowledgeable adults, and young people should be taught effective responses to a bully.

Peer Mediation and Conflict Resolution

In addition to treatment, children need the tools to resolve their difficulties without resorting to violent behavior. Children who learn problem-solving skills or conflict resolution are less impulsive and aggressive than those who do not have those skills and tend to be more rational and patient. The basic principles of conflict resolution are similar to the problem-solving strategies described previously: Listen objectively to the other person, identify the problem, brainstorm for alternatives, agree on common grounds, and find a win–win solution. Most programs discuss the nature of the conflicts encountered by children, incorporate rules for attacking the problem (not the person) and treating others with respect, and emphasize accepting responsibility for one's behavior. Participants may also discuss issues related to diversity, power, and anger control. Role-plays, simulations, stories, and discussions provide practice for children learning the new skills required for conflict resolution.

Amatruda (2006) described her work with children in an elementary special education program. She used action techniques and psychodrama in biweekly sessions aimed to help students communicate more positively with each other and increase their conflict resolution and social skills.

Another way to work effectively with conflicts in schools includes children as collaborators. Peer mediators are trained to facilitate the conflict resolution process. Lane and McWhirter (1992, 1996) describe a peer mediation model for elementary and middle school children with 19 steps for the mediation. Peer mediators learn specific actions concerning introductions, listening, ascertaining "wants," and finding solutions. Peer mediators are trained in the steps of mediation and record their interactions. The Association for Conflict Resolution (2007) has published standards for school-based peer mediation programs that outline best practices in this area. Johnson and Johnson (2012) believe that all students should learn to negotiate and mediate and have the experience of serving as a mediator. They cite studies showing that conflict resolution and mediation training results in less student-to-student conflicts and increased student management of their conflicts without adult intervention. In fact, McWhirter et al. (2012) discuss the ripple effects of peer mediation program implementation. They cite improved school climate, less playground problems, less referrals to the principal's office or to the nurse, and less conflict in homes as benefits.

SUMMARY

Many children have special concerns, challenges that may create troubling situations in their lives. This chapter has highlighted a small portion of some of the more common difficulties some children may face. As with any young people, counselors begin by developing a knowledge base of relevant information and then listening to children to learn about their world and their needs. Counselors maintain a careful study of current practices and of valuable resources to be effective, efficient helping professionals. In the situations we have highlighted, many authors emphasize working with parents, teachers, and other people who touch the youngsters' lives. They also suggest building strong connections with the children as the counseling partnership develops. Children always need to receive respect and hope from their counselors, no matter how discouraging the world might be during difficult times.

WEB SITES FOR COUNSELING CHILDREN WITH SPECIAL CONCERNS

Internet addresses frequently change. To find the sites listed here, visit www.cengage .com/counseling/henderson for an updated list of Internet addresses and direct links to relevant sites.

Center for Missing and Exploited Children

Centers for Disease Control and Prevention (CDC)

National Institute of Mental Health (NIMH)

Substance Abuse and Mental Health Services Administration (SAMHSA)

U.S. Department of Health and Human Services

REFERENCES

Adger, H., Blondell, R., Cooney, J., Finch, J., Graham, A., Macdonald, D. I., Pfeifer, J., Wenger, S., & Werner, M. (n. d.). Helping children and adolescents in families affected by substance use. Retrieved from http://www.nacoa.org/pdfs/guide%20for%20health.pdf

Ahrons, C. (2007). Family ties after divorce: Long-term implications for children. *Family Process, 46*, 53–65.

Allen, B., & Kronenberg, M. (2014). Treating traumatized children: A casebook of evidence-based therapies. New York: The Guilford Press.

Amatruda, M. J. (2006). Conflict resolution and social skill development with children. *Journal of Group Psychotherapy, Psychodrama, & Sociometry, 58*, 168–181.

American Academy of Child and Adolescent Psychiatry. (2011). Children of alcoholics. Retrieved from http://www.aacap.org/AACAP/Families_and_Youth/Facts_for_Families /Facts_for_Families_Pages/Children_Of_Alcoholics_17.aspx

American Academy of Child and Adolescent Psychiatry. (2013). Children and grief. Retrieved from http://www.aacap.org/AACAP/Families_and_Youth/Facts_for_Families/Facts_for _Families_Pages/Children_And_Grief_08.aspx

Arman, J. F., & McNair, R. (2000). A small group model for working with elementary school children of alcoholics. *Professional School Counseling, 3,* 290–293.

Association for Conflict Resolution. (2007). *Standards for school-based peer mediation programs.* Retrieved from http://education4resilience.iiep.unesco.org/fr/node/560

Azar, S. T., & Wolfe, D. A. (2006). Child physical abuse and neglect. In E. J. Mash & R. A. Barkley (Eds.), *Treatment of childhood disorders* (3rd ed., pp. 595–646). New York: Guilford Press.

Barrio, C. (2007). Assessing suicide risk in children. *Journal of Mental Health Counseling, 29,* 50–66.

Baruth, R. P., Gibbons, C., & Guo, S. (2006). Substance abuse treatment and the recurrence of maltreatment among caregivers with children living at home: A propensity score analysis. *Journal of Substance Abuse Treatment, 30,* 93–104.

Bauserman, R. (2002). Child adjustment in joint-custody versus sole-custody arrangements: A meta-analytic review. *Journal of Family Psychology, 16,* 91–102.

Bay-Hinitz, A., & Wilson, G. (2005). A cooperative games intervention for aggressive preschool children. In L. A. Reddy, T. M. Files-Hall, & C. E. Schaefer (Eds.), *Empirically based play interventions for children* (pp. 191–211). Washington, DC: American Psychological Association.

Beck, A. T., Kovacs, M., & Weissman, A. (1979). Assessment of suicidal intention: The scale for suicidal ideation. *Journal of Clinical and Consulting Psychology, 47,* 343–352.

Beck, A. T., & Steer, R. A. (1993). *Beck depression inventory.* San Antonio, TX: Psychological Corporation.

Berliner, L. (2010). Child sexual abuse. In J. E. B. Myers (Ed.), *The APSAC handbook on child maltreatment* (3rd ed., pp. 215–232). Thousand Oaks, CA: Sage.

Blume, J. (1981). *Tiger eyes.* Scarsdale, NY: Bradbury.

Brassard, M. R., & Donovan, K. M. (2006). Defining psychological maltreatment. In M. Feerick, J. F. Knutson, P. K. Trickett, & Flanzer, S. (Eds.), *Child abuse and neglect.* Baltimore, MD: Brookes Publishing.

Brinkmeyer, M. Y., & Eyberg, S. M. (2003). Parent-child interaction therapy for oppositional children. In A. E. Kazdin & J. R. Weisz (Eds.), *Evidence-based psychotherapies for children and adolescents* (pp. 204–223). New York: Guilford Press.

Capuzzi, D., & Gross, D. R. (2014). "I don't want to live": The adolescent at risk for suicidal behavior. In D. Capuzzi & D. R. Gross (Eds.), *Youth at risk: A prevention resource for counselors, teachers, and parents* (6th ed., pp. 226–263). Alexandria, VA: American Counseling Association and Merrill Publishing.

Carr, A. (2009). *What works with children, adolescents, and adults? A review of research on the effectiveness of psychotherapy.* New York: Routledge.

Carter, W. L. (2002). *It happened to me: A teen's guide to overcoming sexual abuse.* Oakland, CA: New Harbinger.

Center for Disease Control and Prevention. (2014). *Suicide prevention.* Retrieved from http://www.cdc.gov/violenceprevention/pub/youth_suicide.html

Childhelp USA. (2014). *National child abuse statistics.* Retrieved from http://www.childhelp.org/pages/statistics

Child Welfare Information Gateway. (2014). *Child abuse and neglect.* Retrieved from http://www.childwelfare.gov

Clarke, G. N., & DeBar, L. L. (2010). Cognitive-behavioral group treatment for adolescent depression. In A. E. Kazdin & J. R. Weisz (Eds.), *Evidence-based psychotherapies for children and adolescents* (2nd ed., pp. 110–125). New York: The Guilford Press.

Cohen, J. A., & Mannarino, A. P. (2004). Treatment of childhood traumatic grief. *Journal of Clinical Child and Adolescent Psychology, 33,* 819–831.

Cohen, J. A., Mannarino, A., & Deblinger, E. (2006). *Treating trauma and traumatic grief in children and adolescents*. New York: Guilford Press.

Conduct Problems Prevention Research Group. (2007). Fast track randomized controlled trial to prevent externalizing psychiatric disorders: Findings from grades 3 to 9. *Journal of the American Academy of Child & Adolescent Psychiatry, 46*, 1250–1262.

Corcoran, J., & Pillai, V. (2008). A meta-analysis of parent-involved treatment for child sexual abuse. *Research on Social Work Practice. 18*(5), 453–464.

Crooks, C. V., & Wolfe, D. A. (2007). Child abuse and neglect. In E. J. Mash & R. A. Barkley (Eds.), *Assessment of childhood disorders* (4th ed., pp. 639–684). New York: Guilford Press.

Currier, J., Holland, J., & Neimeyer, R. (2007). The effectiveness of bereavement interventions with children: A meta-analytic review of controlled outcome research. *Journal of Clinical Child & Adolescent Psychology, 36*, 253–259.

David-Ferdon, C., & Kaslow, N. J. (2008). Evidence-based psychosocial treatments for child and adolescent depression. *Journal of Clinical Child & Adolescent Psychology, 37*, 62–104.

Davis, N., & Sparks, T. (1988). *Therapeutic stories to heal children* (Rev. ed.). Oxon Hill, MD: Psychological Associates.

Deaver, J. R. (1988). *Say goodnight, Gracie*. New York: Harper & Row.

Deutsch, R. (2008). Divorce in the 21st century: Multidisciplinary family interventions. *Journal of Psychiatry & Law, 36*(1), 41–66.

Dietzel, M. (2000). *My very own book about me: A personal safety book* (7th ed.). Spokane, WA: ACT for Kids.

Dishion, T. J., & Dodge, K. A. (2005). Peer contagion in interventions for children and adolescents: Moving toward an understanding of the ecology and dynamics of change. *Journal of Abnormal Child Psychology, 33*, 395–400.

Doweiko, H. E. (2011). *Concepts of chemical dependency* (8th ed.). Pacific Grove, CA: Brooks/Cole.

English, D. J., Upadhyaya, M. P., Litrownik, A.J., Marshall, J.M., Runyan, D.K., Graham, J. C., & Dubowitz, H. (2005). Maltreatment's wake: The relationship of maltreatment dimensions to child outcomes. *Child Abuse and Neglect, 29*, 597–619.

Eppler, C. (2008). Exploring themes of resiliency in children after the death of a parent. *Professional School Counseling, 11*(3), 189–196.

Eyberg, S. M., Nelson, M. M., & Boggs, S. R. (2008). Evidence-based psychosocial treatments for children and adolescents with disruptive behavior. *Journal of Clinical Child and Adolescent Psychology, 37*, 215–237.

Finn, A. (2014). Death in the classroom: Violence in schools. In D. Capuzzi & D. R. Gross (Eds.), *Youth at risk: A prevention resource for counselors, teachers, and parents* (6th ed., pp. 337–366). Alexandria, VA: American Counseling Association.

Freeman, S. J. (2001). Death and bereavement. In E. R. Welfel & R. E. Ingersoll (Eds.), *The mental health desk reference* (pp. 38–43). New York: Wiley.

Frick, P. J. (2000). A comprehensive and individualized treatment approach for children and adolescents with conduct disorders. *Cognitive and Behavioral Practice, 7*, 30–37.

Gately, D., & Schwebel, A. (1992). Favorable outcomes in children after parental divorce. In C. A. Everett (Ed.), *Divorce and the next generation* (pp. 25–48). Binghamton, NY: Haworth.

Gil, E. (2006). *Helping abused and traumatized children: Integrating directive and nondirective approaches*. New York: Guilford Press.

Goldman, J., Salus, M., Wolcott, D., & Kennedy, K. Y. (2003). *A coordinated response to child abuse and neglect: The foundation for practice*. Washington, DC: United States Dept. of Health and Human Services, Office on Child Abuse and Neglect.

Goldstein, S. E., Young, A., & Boyd, C. (2008). Relational aggression at school: Associations with school safety and social climate. *Journal of Youth and Adolescence*, 37, 641–654.

Goldston, D. B. (2003). *Measuring suicidal behavior and risk in children and adolescents*. Washington, DC: American Psychological Association.

Gordon, S., & Cohen, V. (2000). *All families are different*. Amherst, NY: Prometheus Books.

Granello, D. H., & Granello, P. F. (2007). *Suicide: An essential guide for helping professionals and educators*. Boston, MA: Allyn & Bacon.

Greeff, A., & Du Toit, C. (2009). Resilience in remarried families. *American Journal of Family Therapy*, 37(2), 114–126.

Grollman, E. A. (1988). *Shira: A legacy of courage*. New York: Doubleday.

Grych, J. H. (2005). Interparental conflict as a risk factor for child maladjustment: Implications for the development of prevention programs. *Family Court Review*, 43, 97–108.

Grych, J. H., & Fincham, F. (1992). Interventions for children of divorce: Toward greater integration of research and action. *Psychological Bulletin*, 111, 434–454.

Henggeler, S. W., & Lee, T. (2003). Multi-systemic treatment of serious clinical problems. In A. E. Kazdin & J. R. Weisz (Eds.), *Evidence-based psychotherapies for children and adolescents* (pp. 301–322). New York: Guilford Press.

Henggeler, S. W., Schoenwald, S. K., Rowland, M. D., & Cunningham, P. B. (2002). *Multi-systemic treatment of children and adolescents with serious emotional disturbance*. New York: Guilford Press.

Henggeler, S. W., Sheidow, A. J., & Lee, T. (2007). Multisystemic treatment of serious clinical problems in youth and their families. In D. W. Springer & R. A. Roberts (Eds.), *Handbook of forensic mental health with victims and offenders: Assessment, treatment, and research* (pp. 315–345). New York: Springer.

Hetherington, E. M. (2006). The influence of conflict, marital problem solving, and parenting on children's adjustment in nondivorced, divorced, and remarried families. In A. Clarke-Stewart & J. Dunn (Eds.), *Families count* (pp. 203–236). New York: Oxford University Press.

Hildyard, K., & Wolfe, D. A. (2002). Child neglect: Developmental issues and outcomes. *Child Abuse & Neglect*, 26, 679–695.

Holland, J. (2008). How schools can support children who experience loss and death. *British Journal of Guidance & Counselling*, 36, 411–424.

Huss, S. N., & Conklin, A. (2010). Bereavement in schools. In B. Erford (Ed.), *Professional school counseling: A handbook* (2nd ed., pp. 935–949). Austin, TX: ProEd.

Jacobsen, I., Rabinowitz, I., Popper, M., Solomon, R., Sokol, M., & Pfeffer, C. (1994). Interviewing prepubertal children about suicidal ideation and behavior. *Journal of the American Academy of Child and Adolescent Psychiatry*, 33, 439–452.

Jacobson, C. M., & Mufsor, L. (2010). Treating adolescent depression using interpersonal psychotherapy. In A. E. Kazdin & J. R. Weisz (Eds.), *Evidence-based psychotherapies for children and adolescents* (2nd ed., pp. 140–157). New York: The Guilford Press.

Jacobus-Kantor, L., & Emshoff, J. G. (2010). Play therapy for children of alcoholics. In A. A. Drewes & C. E. Schaefer (Eds), *School-based play therapy* (2nd ed., pp. 331–357). Hoboken, NJ: John Wiley & Sons. doi:10.1002/9781118269701.ch16

James, R. K., & Gilliland, B. E. (2013). *Crisis intervention strategies* (7th ed.). Pacific Grove, CA: Brooks/Cole.

James, S. H., & Burch, K. M. (1999). School counselors' roles in cases of child sexual behavior. *Professional School Counseling*, 2, 211–217.

Johnson, D. W., & Johnson, F. P. (2012). *Joining together* (11th ed.). Upper Saddle River, NJ: Pearson.

Johnson, R., Rew, L., & Sternglanz, R. W. (2006). The relationship between childhood sexual abuse and sexual health practices of homeless adolescents. *Adolescence*, 41, 221–234.

Jones, J. W. (1985). *Children of alcoholics screening test*. Chicago: Camelot.

Junhke, G. A. (1996). The Adapted-SAD PERSONS: A suicide assessment scale designed for use with children. *Elementary School Guidance and Counseling, 30*, 252–258.

Kazdin, A. E. (1996). Combined and multimodal treatments in child and adolescent psychotherapy: Issues, challenges, and research directions. *Clinical Psychology: Science and Practice, 3*, 69–100.

Kazdin, A. E. (2003). Problem-solving skills training and parent management training for conduct disorder. In A. E. Kazdin & J. R. Weisz (Eds.), *Evidence-based psychotherapies for children and adolescents* (pp. 241–262). New York: Guilford Press.

Keats, E. (2001). *Louie's search*. New York: Scholastic.

Kehoe, P., & Deach, C. (1987). *Something happened and I'm scared to tell: A book for young victims of abuse*. Seattle, WA: Parenting Press.

Kenny, M. C. (2007). Web-based training in child maltreatment for future mandated reporters. *Child Abuse and Neglect, 31*, 671–678.

Kerr, M. M. (2009). *School crisis prevention and intervention*. Upper Saddle River, NJ: Prentice Hall.

KidsCount Databank. (2014). Children in single-parent families. Retrieved from http://datacenter.kidscount.org/data/tables/106-children-in-single-parent-families#detailed/1/any/false/36,868,867,133,38/any/429,430

Kimonis, E. R., Frick, P. J., & McMahon, R. J. (2014). Conduct and oppositional defiant disorders. In E. J. Mash & R. A. Barkley (Eds.), *Child psychopathology* (3rd ed., pp. 145–179). New York: Guilford Press.

Kissane, D., & Bloch, S. (2002). *Family focused grief therapy: A model of family-centered care during palliative care and bereavement*. Maidenhead: Open University Press.

Kovacs, M. (1985). The children's depression inventory (CDI). *Psychopharmocology Bulletin, 21*, 995–1124.

Kübler-Ross, E. (1969). *On death and dying*. New York: Macmillan.

Lahey, B. B., Loeber, R., Burke, J. D., & Rathouz, P. J. (2002). Adolescent outcomes of childhood conduct disorder among clinic-referred boys: Predictors of improvement. *Journal of Abnormal Child Psychology, 30*, 333–348.

Lane, P. S., & McWhirter, J. J. (1992). A peer mediation model: Conflict resolution for elementary and middle school children. *Elementary School Guidance and Counseling, 27*, 15–24.

Lane, P. S., & McWhirter, J. J. (1996). Creating a peaceful school community: Reconciliation operationalized. *Catholic School Studies, 69*, 31–34.

Leeb, R. T., Lewis, T., & Zolotor, A. J. (2011). A review of physical and mental health consequences of child abuse and neglect and implications for practice. *American Journal of Lifestyle Medicine, 5*(5), 454–468. doi:10.1177/1559827611410266

Leeb, R. T., Paulozzi, L. J., Melanson, C., Simon, T. R., & Arias, I. (2008). *Child maltreatment surveillance: Uniform definitions for public health and recommended data elements*. Atlanta, GA: Centers for Disease Control and Prevention. Retrieved from http://www.cdc.gov/violenceprevention/childmaltreatment/definitions.html

Lev-Wiesel, R. (2008). Child sexual abuse: A critical review of intervention and treatment modalities. *Children & Youth Services Review, 30*(6), 665–673.

London, K., Bruck, M., Wright, D. B., & Ceci, S. J. (2008). Review of the contemporary literature on how children report sexual abuse to others: Findings, methodological issues, and implications for forensic interviewers. *Memory, 16*, 29–47.

Lyons-Ruth, K., Zeanah, C. H., & Benoit, D. (2003). Disorder and risk for disorder during infancy and toddlerhood. In E. J. Mash & R. A. Barkley (Eds.), *Child psychopathology* (2nd ed., pp. 589–631). New York: Guilford Press.

MacFarland, W., & Tollerud, T. (2009). Counseling children and adolescents with special needs. In A. Vernon (Ed.), *Counseling children and adolescents* (4th ed., pp. 287–334). Denver, CO: Love.

Mash, E. J., & Wolfe, D. A. (2013). *Abnormal child psychology* (5th ed.). Belmont, CA: Wadsworth.

McMahon, R. J., & Forehand, R. L. (2003). *Helping the noncompliant child: Family-based treatment for oppositional behavior* (2nd ed.). New York: Guilford Press.

McPherson, K., Greene, A., & Li, S. (2010). *Fourth national incidence study of child abuse and neglect (NIS-4): Report to Congress.* Washington, DC: U.S. Department of Health and Human Services, Administration for Children and Families.

McWhirter, B. T., & Burrow-Sanchez, J. J. (2006). Preventing and treating depression and bipolar disorders in children and adolescents. In D. Capuzzi & D. R. Gross (Eds.), *Youth at risk: A prevention resources for counselors, teachers, and parents* (4th ed., pp. 117–142). Alexandria, VA: American Counseling Association and Upper Saddle River, NJ: Merrill.

McWhirter, J. J., McWhirter, B. T., McWhirter, E. H., & McWhirter, R. J. (2012). *At-risk youth: A comprehensive response* (5th ed.). Belmont, CA: Brooks/Cole.

Miller-Perrin, C. L. (2001). Child maltreatment: Treatment of child and adolescent victims. In E. R. Welfel & R. E. Ingersoll (Eds.), *The mental health desk reference* (pp. 169–176). New York: John Wiley & Sons.

Moe, J., Johnson, J. L., & Wade, W. (2007). Resilience in children of substance users: In their own words. *Substance Use & Misuse, 42,* 381–398.

Moore, M., & Carr, A. (2000). Depression and grief. In A. Carr (Ed.), *What works with children and adolescents? A critical review of psychological interventions with children, adolescents and their families* (pp. 203–232). Philadelphia, PA: Brunner-Routledge.

National Association of School Psychologists. (n.d.). Recommended books for children coping with loss and trauma. Retrieved from www.nasponline.net

National Center for Health Statistics. (2014). *National marriage and divorce trends.* Retrieved from http://www.cdc.gov/nchs/nvss/marriage_divorce_tables.htm

National Center for Missing and Exploited Children. (2014). *Laws concerning the sexual exploitation of children.* Retrieved from http://www.missingkids.com/LegalResources/Exploitation

National Institute of Mental Health. (2014). Major depression among adolescents. Retrieved from http://www.nimh.nih.gov/health/statistics/prevalence/major-depression-among-adolescents.shtml.

Office of Planning, Research and Evaluation. (n.d.). *National survey of child and adolescent well-being (NSCAW), 1997–2014.* Retrieved from http://www.acf.hhs.gov/programs/opre/research/project/national-survey-of-child-and-adolescent-well-being-nscaw

O'Rourke, K. (1990). Recapturing hope: Elementary school support groups for children of alcoholics. *Elementary School Guidance and Counseling, 25,* 107–115.

O'Rourke, K., & Worzbyt, J. (1996). *Support groups for children.* Washington, DC: Accelerated Development.

Olweus, D. (1993). *Bullying at School: What we know and what we can do.* Oxford: Blackwell Publishers.

Olweus, D. (2001). *Olweus' core program against bullying and antisocial behavior: A teacher handbook.* Bergen, Norway: HEMIL-senteret, Universitetet i Bergen.

Olweus, D. (2002) A profile of bullying at school. *Educational Leadership, 60,* pp. 12–17.

Olweus, D. (2004). Bullying at school: Prevalence estimation, a useful evaluation design, and a new national initiative in Norway. *Association for Child Psychology and Psychiatry Occasional Papers, 23,* pp. 5–17.

Olweus, D., Limber, S., & Mihalic, S. F. (1999). *Blueprints for violence prevention: Book 9. Bullying prevention program.* Boulder, CO: Center for the Study and Prevention of Violence.

Papilia, D., Feldman, R., & Martorell, G. (2014). *Experience human development* (13th ed.). New York: McGraw-Hill.

Papernow, P. (1995). What's going on here? Separating (and weaving together) step and clinical issues in remarried families. In D.Huntley (Ed.), *Understanding stepfamilies: Implications for assessment and treatment. The family psychology and counseling series* (pp. 3–24). Alexandria, VA: American Counseling Association.

Pasley, K., & Garneau, C. (2011). Remarriage and stepfamily life. In F. Walsh (Ed.), *Normal family processes: Growing diversity and complexity* (4th ed., pp. 149–171). New York: Guilford Press.

Pidcock, B., Fischer, J. L., Forthun, L. F., & West, S. (2000). Hispanic and Anglo college women's risk factors for substance use and eating disorders. *Addictive Behaviors: An International Journal, 25,* 705–723.

Powell, M., & Wilson, C. (2012). *Guide to interviewing children: Essential skills for counsellors, social workers, police and lawyers.* New York: Taylor and Francis.

Price, A. W., & Emshoff, J. G. (1997). Breaking the cycle of addiction: Prevention and intervention with children of alcoholics. *Alcohol Health and Research World, 21,* 241–246.

Pryce, C. R., Azzinnari, D., Spinelli, S., Seifritz, E., Tegethoff, M., & Meinlschmidt, G. (2011). Helplessness: A systematic translational review of theory and evidence for its relevance to understanding and treating depression. *Pharmacology & Therapeutics, 132*(3), 242–267. doi:10.1016/j.pharmthera.2011.06.006

Rainbow House. (1989). *The Rainbow Game.* Houston, TX: Rainbow House Children's Resource Center.

Reynolds, W. M. (1987). *RCDS manual.* Odessa, FL: Psychological Assessment Resources.

Reynolds, W. M. (1988). *The Suicide Ideation Questionnaire.* Odessa, FL: Psychological Assessment Resources.

Reynolds, W. M. (1989). *RADS manual.* Odessa, FL: Psychological Assessment Resources.

Roth, B., & Striepling-Goldstein, S. (2003). School-based aggression replacement training. *Reclaiming Children and Youth, 12,* 138–141.

Sacks, V., Murphey, D., & Moore, K. (2014). Adverse childhood experiences: National and state level prevalence. Retrieved from www.childtrends.org

Salek, E. C., & Ginsburg, K. R. (2014). How children understand death. Retrieved from http://www.healthychildren.org/English/healthy-living/emotional-wellness/Building-Resilience/Pages/How-Children-Understand-Death-What-You-Should-Say.aspx

Salmon, S. (2003). Teaching empathy: The PEACE curriculum. *Reclaiming Children and Youth, 12,* 167–173.

Santrock, J. W. (2012). *Life-span development* (14th ed.). New York: McGraw-Hill.

Schellenbach, C. J. (1998). Child maltreatment: A critical review of research on treatment for physically abusive parents. In P. K. Trickett & C. J. Schellenbach (Eds.), *Violence against children in the family and the community* (pp. 251–268). Washington, DC: American Psychological Association.

Sciarra, D. T. (2004). *School counseling: Foundations and contemporary issues.* Belmont, CA: Brooks/Cole.

Seligman, M. (1998). *Learned optimism.* New York: Simon & Schuster.

Shapiro, J. P., Friedberg, R. D., & Bardenstein, K. K. (2006). *Child and adolescent therapy: Science and art.* Hoboken, NJ: Wiley.

Sheller, B., & Watts, G. B. (1999). *Helping your child cope with grief. Faith home for parents.* Nashville, TN: Abingdon Press.

Shura, M. F. (1988). *The Sunday doll.* New York: Dodd Mead.

Siegel, D. J. (1999). *The developing mind*. New York: Guilford Press.

Sommers-Flanagan, J., & Campbell, D. G. (2009). Psychotherapy and (or) medications for depression in youth? An evidence-based review with recommendations for treatment. *Journal of Contemporary Psychotherapy, 39*, 111–120.

Springer, K. W., Sheridan, J., Kuo, D., & Carnes, M. (2007). Long-term physical and mental health consequences of childhood physical abuse. Results from a large population-based sample of men and women. *Child Abuse & Neglect, 31*, 517–530.

Stark, K. D., Streusand, W., Krumholz, L. S., & Patel, P. (2010). Cognitive-behavioral therapy for depression: The ACTION treatment program for girls. In A. E. Kazdin & J. R. Weisz (Eds.), *Evidence-based psychotherapies for children and adolescents* (2nd ed., pp. 93–109). New York: The Guilford Press.

Stice, E., Shaw, H., Bohon, C., Marti, C. N., & Rohde, P. (2009). A meta-analytic review of depression prevention programs for children and adolescents: Factors that predict magnitude of intervention effects. *Journal of Consulting and Clinical Psychology, 77*, 486–503.

Stien, P. T., & Kendall, J. C. (2004). *Psychological trauma and the developing brain*. New York: Routledge.

Straussner, S. L. A., & Fewell, C. H. (2011). *Children of substance-abusing parents: Dynamics and treatment*. New York: Springer.

Substance Abuse and Mental Health Services Administration (SAMSHA). (2009). *The NSDUH Report: Children living with substance-dependent or substance abusing parents: 2002 to 2007*. Retrieved from http://oas.samhsa.gov/2k9/SAparents/SAparents.cfm

Szumilas, M., & Kutcher, S. (2011). Post-suicide intervention programs: A systematic review. *Canadian Journal of Public Health/Revue Canadienne De Sante'e Publique, 102*(1), 18–29.

Thomas, D., & Gibbons, M. (2009). Narrative theory: A career counseling approach for adolescents of divorce. *Professional School Counseling, 12*, 223–229.

Thomas, P. (1999). *My family's changing*. Hauppauge, NY: Barrons Ed. Series.

Thompson, E. A., & Eggert, L. L. (1999). Using the suicide risk screen to identify suicidal adolescents among potential high school dropouts. *Journal of the American Academy of Child and Adolescent Psychiatry, 38*, 1506–1514.

Timmer, S., & Urquiza, A. J. (2014). *Evidence-based approaches for the treatment of maltreated children: Considering core components and treatment effectiveness*. Dordrecht: Springer. doi:10.1007/978-94-007-7404-9

Timmer, S., Urquiza, A., Zebell, N., & McGrath, J. (2005). Parent-child interaction therapy: Application to physically abusive parent-child dyads. *Child Abuse and Neglect, 29*, 825–842.

UNICEF. (2013). *Protecting children from violence, exploitation and abuse*. Retrieved from http://www.unicef.org/protection/57929_57972.html

U.S. Department of Health and Human Services (USDHHS). (2001). *Youth violence: A report of the Surgeon General*. Rockville, MD: Author.

U.S. Department of Health and Human Services (USDHHS), Administration for Children and Families, Children's Bureau. (2013). *Child maltreatment: 2012*. Retrieved from http://www.acf.hhs.gov/programs/cb/resource/child-maltreatment-2012

Valle, L. A., & Lutzker, J. R. (2006). Child physical abuse. In J. E. Fisher & W. T. O'Donohue (Eds.), *Practitioners' guide to evidence-based psychotherapy*. New York: Springer

Wagner, W. G. (2008). *Counseling, psychology, and children* (2nd ed.). Upper Saddle River, NJ: Merrill.

Wallerstein, J. (2008). Divorce. In M. M. Haith & J. B. Benson (Eds.), *Encyclopedia of infancy and early childhood*. Oxford, UK: Elsevier.

Wallerstein, J., & Blakeslee, S. (2003). *What about the kids?* New York: Hyperion.

Wallerstein, J., & Lewis, J. (2007). Disparate parenting and step-parenting with siblings in the post-divorce family: Report from a 10-year longitudinal study. *Journal of Family Studies*, *13*(2), 224–235.

Webb, N. B. (2002). Counseling and therapy for the bereaved child. In B. Webb (Ed.), *Helping bereaved children: A handbook for practitioners* (3rd ed., pp. 247–264). New York: Guilford Press.

Webb, N. B. (2007). *Play therapy with children in crisis: Individual, group, and family treatment*. New York: Guilford Press.

Webb, N. B. (Ed.). (2011). *Helping bereaved children*. New York: Guilford.

Webster-Stratton, C., & Reid, M. J. (2003). The incredible years parents, teachers, and children training series: A multifaceted treatment approach for young children with conduct problems. In A. E. Kazdin & J. R. Weisz (Eds.), *Evidence-based psychotherapies for children and adolescents* (pp. 224–240). New York: Guilford Press.

Weersing, V. R., & Brent, D. A. (2010). Treating depression in adolescents using individual cognitive-behavioral therapy. In A. E. Kazdin & J. R. Weisz (Eds.), *Evidence-based psychotherapies for children and adolescents* (2nd ed., pp. 126–139). New York: Guilford Press.

Weitz, E., Hollon, S. D., Kerkhof, A., & Cuijpers, P. (2014). Do depression treatments reduce suicidal ideation? The effects of CBT, IPT, pharmacotherapy, and placebo on suicidality. *Journal of Affective Disorders*, *167*, 98–103. doi:10.1016/j.jad.2014.05.036

Wen, M. (2008). Family structure and children's health and behavior: Data from the 1999 national survey of America's families. *Journal of Family Issues*, *29*, 1492–1519.

Willis, C. A. (2002). The grieving process in children: Strategies for understanding, educating, and reconciling children's perceptions of death. *Early Childhood Education Journal*, *29*, 221–226.

Wolfelt, A. (2004). *A child's view of grief: A guide for parents, teachers and counselors*. Bishop, CA: Companion Press.

Worchel, D., & Gearing, R. E. (2010). *Suicide assessment and treatment: Empirical and evidence-based practices*. New York: Springer.

Yasui, M., & Dishion, T. J. (2007). The ethnic context of child and adolescent problem behavior: Implications for child and family interventions. *Clinical Child and Family Psychology Review*, *10*, 137–179.

CHAPTER 20

Counseling with Children with Disabilities

The miracle is not that we do this work, but that we are happy to do it.
—MOTHER TERESA

THE SITUATION

Children with disabilities are different in some way from their peers. They deviate from what is considered to be normal or average in physical appearance, learning abilities, or behavior. They may have a mild, moderate, or severe special need. Educators, parents, and other professionals emphasize meeting these children's physical, psychological, and educational needs in the least restrictive environment (LRE) and providing support for the families through groups, associations, and legislation.

After reading this chapter, you should be able to:

▶ Outline the history of special education in the United States
▶ Explain the categories of disabilities
▶ Discuss the procedures for IDEA and Section 504 in the schools
▶ Describe some counseling strategies for children with special needs
▶ Explain ways of working with the families of children with disabilities

HISTORY

Children with special needs can become accepted, productive members of society. Berns (2013) classified four stages of attitudes toward people with disabilities. In the pre-Christian world they tended to be banished, neglected, or mistreated. As Christianity spread, they were protected and pitied. During the 18th and 19th centuries, they were educated in separate institutions. In the latter part of the 20th century, acceptance of people with disabilities and integration into the mainstream of society became more common.

The 1880s saw the first steps toward recognizing the needs of persons with disabilities with the establishment of the first schools for the deaf and the blind. In the mid-1930s, Congress passed the Crippled Children Act, authorizing financial aid to families of people with orthopedic handicaps. President Franklin D. Roosevelt, a victim of polio that caused him to be disabled, undoubtedly gave impetus to this legislation. President John F. Kennedy, who had a sister with intellectual disability, urged that attention be given to children's developmental disabilities, including intellectual disability and learning disabilities. In 1961, a President's Panel on Intellectual Disability was established, and in 1963, a National Institute of Child Health and Human Development was founded. The child advocacy movement of the late 1960s and early 1970s resulted in the formation of the National Center for Child Advocacy. During the 1970s and 1980s, legislative appropriations and federal committees and agencies increased. In 1975, President Ford signed the Education for All Handicapped Children Act, Public Law 94-142. This law had four purposes which are (1) to mandate the availability of a free appropriate public education (FAPE) for all children with disabilities, with services designed to meet their unique needs; (2) to protect the rights of those children and their parents; (3) to help states in providing education for all children with disabilities; and (4) to assess the effectiveness of the education. The law profoundly changed the educational opportunities for special needs children.

In 1977, the Education of the Handicapped Act was amended to define *learning disabilities*, and in 1978, the Gifted and Talented Children's Education Act provided money to states for planning, training, program development, and research. Amendments in 1983 extended the act to provide additional services to secondary school students and children from birth to 3 years old. The Education for All Handicapped Children Act was renamed Individuals with Disabilities Act (IDEA) in 1990 and was reauthorized in 2004 as the Individuals with Disabilities Education Improvement Act, which is still called IDEA. This bill outlines the way to refer, assess, identify, place, and teach students who have eligible handicapping conditions. The last major changes in the IDEA law occurred in 2006 and included specifics about the qualifications of teachers, teaching methods, transitional services, evaluation and identification of special needs students, as well as some of the components of the Individualized Educational Plan (IEP).

Some students with mental and physical disabilities do not qualify as disabled under IDEA but may need accommodations to be successful in schools. In 1990, President George H. Bush extended the 1973 Rehabilitation Act (Section 504), which prohibited discrimination against qualified individuals in federally funded programs and protected the rights of students with disabilities to free and appropriate public education, by signing the Americans with Disabilities Act (ADA), which prohibits discrimination against persons with disabilities in employment, transportation, public services, public accommodations, and telecommunications, regardless of federal funding (Rock & Leff, 2011). On September 25, 2008, President George W. Bush signed the Americans with Disabilities Act Amendments Act of 2008 (ADAAA). The act, effective January 1, 2009, expands the definition of disability, stating it should be construed in favor of broad coverage of individuals to the maximum extent permitted by the terms of the ADA. Section 504 and the ADAAA (www.wrightslaw

.com/info/sec504.adaaa.htm) provide the "right to accommodations" to qualified persons regardless of whether they need special education. The Disability Rights Education & Defense Fund (http://dredf.org/advocacy/comparison.html) and Henderson (2001) compare the purpose, eligibility requirements, educational implications, due process, placement, and evaluation procedures for the federal acts related to children with disabilities. Rock and Leff explain IDEA focuses on educational remediation and Section 504 focuses on preventing discrimination of students whose disabilities require accommodations to be successful in schools.

CATEGORIES OF DISABILITIES

Berns (2013) explains some important terms. A disability means a reduction or absence of functioning in a particular body part or organ. An impairment implies the loss or limitation of physical, mental, or sensory functions permanently or for the long term. Handicaps are disadvantages or hindrances that interfere with a person's life. Children with a disability have been evaluated as having an impairment that requires special education and related services. *Disability* and *impairment* are terms most often used to reduce the negative stereotypes of the word *handicap*. The United Nations, Convention on the Rights of Persons with Disabilities (2006) states:

> Persons with disabilities include those who have long-term physical, mental, intellectual or sensory impairments, which in interaction with various barriers may hinder their full and effective participation in society on an equal basis with others (Article 1).

The World Health Organization emphasizes that most people will have some degree of disability at some time in life. Therefore, its classification focuses on the child's abilities and strengths and not just impairments and limitations, shifting the focus from the causes of disabilities to their impact.

The National Center for Education Statistics (NCES) (2014) reports that in 2011–2012, children between the ages of 3 and 21 receiving special education services numbered 6.4 million or about 13 percent of all public school students. In IDEA, *children with disabilities* refers to young people who have permanent or temporary mental, physical, or emotional disabilities that adversely affect their education. That federal law requires that school districts provide a free appropriate public education (also called FAPE) in the least restrictive environment (LRE). Accordingly, those school-aged children receive special education and related services through their school systems so that the children can develop, learn, and succeed in school and elsewhere. Categories of disabilities have been defined in IDEA under which a person would be eligible to receive services. A summary of the current definition of disabilities based on information provided by the United States Department of Education (2014) follows:

1. *Autism:* a developmental disability that significantly affects verbal and nonverbal communication and social interaction. Autism is generally evident before the age of 3. Other common characteristics are engaging in restricted and/or repetitive behavior, stereotyped movements, resistance to change, and unusual reactions to sensory experiences.

2. *Deaf-blindness:* the combination of hearing and visual impairments that causes severe communication and other developmental and educational problems.

3. *Deafness:* a hearing impairment so severe that the young person is impaired in processing information through hearing, with or without amplification, and that adversely affects a child's educational performance.

4. *Developmental delay:* a delay in one or more of these areas: physical development; cognitive development; communication; social or emotional development; or behavioral development.

5. *Emotional disturbance:* this is a condition that includes exhibiting one or more of the following over a long period of time and to a marked degree that adversely affects educational performance:
   a. An inability to learn that cannot be explained by intellectual, sensory, or health factors.
   b. An inability to build or maintain satisfactory interpersonal relationships with peers and teachers.
   c. Inappropriate behavior or feelings under normal circumstances.
   d. A general pervasive mood of unhappiness or depression.
   e. A tendency to develop physical symptoms or fears associated with personal or school problems.

6. *Hearing impaired:* an impairment in hearing, either permanent or fluctuating, that adversely affects educational performance but is not included under the definition of deafness.

7. *Intellectual disability:* significantly subaverage general intellectual functioning, existing simultaneously with deficits in adaptive behavior and manifested during the developmental period, that adversely affects a child's educational performance.

8. *Multiple disabilities:* simultaneous impairments such as intellectual disability-blindness, the combination of which causes such severe educational needs that they cannot be addressed in a special education program solely for one of the impairments.

9. *Orthopedic impairment:* severe orthopedic impairment that adversely affects a child's educational performance. The category includes impairments caused by congenital anomaly, by disease (e.g., polio, bone tuberculosis), and from other causes (e.g., cerebral palsy, amputations).

10. *Other health impairment:* means having limited strength, vitality, or alertness, including a heightened alertness to environmental stimuli, that results in limited alertness to the educational environment. The condition may be due to chronic or acute health problems; examples of such health problems are asthma, attention deficit disorder or attention deficit hyperactivity disorder, diabetes, epilepsy, heart conditions, hemophilia, lead poisoning, leukemia, nephritis, rheumatic fever, sickle cell anemia, Tourette syndrome.

11. *Specific learning disability:* disorder in one or more of the psychological processes involved in understanding or in using language that causes difficulties in listening, thinking, speaking, reading, writing, spelling, or doing mathematical calculations.

12. *Speech or language impairment:* communication disorder such as stuttering, impaired articulation, or voice impairment.

13. *Traumatic brain injury:* an acquired injury to the brain caused by an external physical force that results in total or partial functional and/or psychosocial impairment.

14. *Visual impairment including blindness:* impairment in vision that even with correction adversely affects educational performance. The term includes both partial sight and blindness (National Dissemination Center for Children with Disabilities (NICHCY), 2012, pp. 1–3).

The Individuals with Disabilities Education Act (IDEA) provides federal money to states and agencies to educate children with disabilities. In 2004, that act was altered to conform to the requirement of the No Child Left behind Act. Those changes addressed parent choice, transition to post-school options, and accountability for student progress. Each state has criteria and evaluation procedures for eligibility and services (Berns, 2013).

Tarver-Behring and Spagna (2009) explain Section 504 of the Rehabilitation Act of 1973 (Public Law 93-112). Under Section 504, a qualified person with disabilities has a physical or mental impairment that limits one or more major life activities (such as learning), has had the impairment for some time, and is currently exhibiting the impairment. Physical or mental impairment means either a physiological disorder or condition loss affecting one or more body systems or any psychological disorder. Major life activities mean functions of caring for self, performing tasks, walking, seeing, hearing, speaking, breathing, learning, and working. Children may be physically disabled but educationally able. One example would be a typically achieving young person with asthma. That child would probably be qualified under Section 504. To establish whether someone is protected by Section 504, existing records are reviewed and evaluations completed to determine what accommodations and support are needed. A 504 plan describes the services the student receives as well as the accommodations the student needs. Rock and Leff (2011) list impairments most frequently resulting in eligibility under Section 504 of the Rehabilitation Act of 1973: ADHD, temporary medical conditions, physical impairments, behavioral or emotional disorders, addictions, communicable diseases, chronic medical conditions, and dyslexia. The educational modifications may be reduced or adapted assignments, different testing arrangements, having a teacher's aide, and many others.

Discussing each area of exceptionality is beyond the scope of this chapter; therefore, this chapter includes a general discussion of children who have intellectual disability, learning disabilities, physical handicaps, or behavioral-emotional disorders, as well as ADHD. These conditions appear to be those counselors are most apt to encounter daily. Counselors, parents, teachers, and children may need clarification on the process that is followed to identify children who may need special education and related services. Those steps follow:

1. The child is referred as possibly needing services.
2. The child is evaluated in all areas related to the suspected disability.
3. A group of qualified professionals and the parents consider the results of the evaluation and determine whether the child is eligible for services.
4. If the child is found eligible, within 30 calendar days, a team meets to write an individualized educational plan (IEP) for the child.
5. The IEP meeting is scheduled. Parents are invited.

6. The IEP meeting is held and the IEP is written. The plan includes accommodations, modifications, and supports to be provided to the child. Parents must consent to services and placement.
7. Services are provided. The school monitors the plan to determine whether it is being implemented as written.
8. Progress is measured and reported to the parents.
9. The IEP is reviewed at least once a year.
10. The child is re-evaluated at least every 3 years (Center for Parent Information and Resources, 2014, pp. 1–3).

IDEA requires a nondiscriminatory evaluation that is appropriate to a child's cultural and linguistic background. The goal of the act is that children are guaranteed a FAPE in the LRE. The IEP is the primary means of achieving that goal. It is a communication tool between the school and family and is written by a team of those responsible for the child's education—parents, teachers, and other applicable school personnel. Any child eligible for special education services must have an IEP, which is commonly composed at the beginning of each school year and reviewed at the end. Some IEPs can be extended over 3 years if long-term planning is more appropriate. Formats for IEPs are different, but according to Berns (2013), these are always included:

1. A description of the child's current levels of educational performance.
2. A list of the annual goals, including short-term objectives.
3. A statement of the specific services to be provided to the child and the extent of the child's participation in the regular education environments. Dates and duration of services are stated.
4. The required transition services from school to work or to continued education.
5. Objective criteria, evaluation procedures, and schedules for determining if the educational objectives are being achieved.

We have defined *counseling* as a therapeutic relationship, a problem-solving process, a re-education procedure, and a method for changing behavior. We have also discussed counseling as a method for helping children cope with developmental problems and as a preventive process. Children with special needs may be faced with rejection and failure. They may need an accepting relationship, someone to listen, assistance in setting present and future goals, guidance for improving interpersonal relationships, and perhaps most important, help in building a strong self-concept and confidence. Counseling with the exceptional child requires no magic formula; however, it does require counselor's dedication to the philosophy that all individuals are unique and capable of growth to reach their potential.

WORKING WITH CHILDREN WHO HAVE DISABILITIES

Counselors who work with children who have disabilities must begin by examining their own attitudes. One belief that will interfere is providing counseling based on preconceived ideas related to the label which may lead to seeing the child primarily on a single dimension related to the disability. Counselors may then dismiss other attributes of the child such as healthy personality characteristics, social skills, interests, and other parts of life. Each child has potential and should not be limited by any label. Children with disabilities do not need pity. Counselors who see these children as victims are likely to overlook the child's strengths and capabilities, therefore setting counseling goals too low, again limiting the child's potential. Counselors may also reject the child due to revulsion for the particular disability (Thurneck, Warner, & Cobb, 2007). Counselors should examine their attitudes, educate themselves about various disabilities, engage in supervision, and learn to use an assistive technology in working with children who have disabilities.

COUNSELING METHODS WITH CHILDREN WHO HAVE SPECIAL NEEDS

In all therapeutic relationships, helping strategies should be incorporated into a positive, accepting counseling relationship. To understand the world of the exceptional child, counselors need to have a basic knowledge of the disabling condition. What are the symptoms and general characteristics of a child with this exceptionality? What are the child's limitations? What are the child's strengths and potentials? All children have some developmental and psychological needs in common, but are there other needs specific to the exceptional condition that must be considered? The counselor does not need to become an expert in the techniques of special education, but knowledge of the needs and characteristics of these children is necessary for effective counseling.

Counselors should ask themselves if they have taken the time to get to know the child as an individual—not as a "child with a disability." The following questions are helpful:

Has my counseling assisted the child to develop good relationships with his or her classmates?

Has my counseling focused on assisting the child to solve his or her own problems?

Has my counseling helped the child to feel better about himself or herself?

Has my counseling with the parents and teachers of the child helped them to find ways of interacting that enhance the child's self-esteem and feelings of self-sufficiency?

In the professional's attempts to diagnose and find help for a child with special problems, the child as a person is sometimes forgotten in the proliferation of testing, diagnosing, and planning. These procedures that are designed to aid the child may, unfortunately, increase self-doubts and fears and may make it more difficult to build a strong relationship in which the child feels free to express fears, doubts, and insecurities. Thurneck et al. (2007) recommend that counselors have information about the disability—what it is and what it is not. Knowing a child may be afraid to ask questions, counselors may invite conversation by saying something like "Children who have ADHD sometimes ask…." That statement helps children talk about fears and helps them know others have similar concerns. The perceptions children have about their disabilities have a large impact on their self-concept, and counselors who provide an environment in which the child feels respected by the listening, caring counselor contributes to a process of developing or restoring a more positive self-evaluation. Building a better self-concept includes helping children see themselves as people who can and do perform and accomplish goals.

Thurneck et al. (2007) suggest having children list their characteristics in "I am" categories to focus on their emotional adjustment and self-esteem, and on "I can" to concentrate on competence and control. Carmichael (2006) talks about adapting toys for work with children who have disabilities. Her ideas include taping paint brushes to hands, using Velcro on gloves, and using beanbags instead of balls. Thurneck et al. (2007) explain that role-playing and behavioral rehearsal would be most appropriate to help children with disabilities reach their treatment goals. As with all children, having skills in social interactions are particularly important.

Concerns of children with disabilities that often emerge in counseling include the following: self–other relationships, maladaptive behavior, self-conflict, and a need for career counseling. All children have these concerns, but children with disabilities face more frustrations, misunderstandings, and difficulties believing in themselves than others (Thurneck et al., 2007). Counselors can focus on helping children accept their disability and see themselves as capable. Group counseling provides opportunities for helping them use relationship skills and develop a feeling of not being alone. Self-conflicts include anxiety, frustration, lack of motivation, and depression. Counselors may be able to help children with disabilities understand some of the information they have been given, to demystify big words and abstract concepts. Counselors can use relaxation and behavioral techniques to teach skills for coping. Counselors who help children develop realistic goals and recognize their strengths and capacities as well as their limitations, promote their abilities to manage their lives (Karvonen, Test, Wood, Browder, & Algozzine, 2004). Children with disabilities also need to learn decision-making skills, particularly those related to career choices. Although these directions for counseling apply to all children, young people with disabilities may need their counselors to grasp quickly the barriers they face and help them work optimistically toward a life in which the child is connected to friends, school, and a positive future.

CHILDREN WITH EMOTIONAL DISTURBANCE

Children feel and express a range of emotions. Across that variety of emotions, children hopefully learn to control emotions—they have the capacity to restrain, tolerate, and endure their emotional states, a process of regulation that develops over time. Unfortunately some children do not master that type of regulation and suffer with emotional disturbances that interfere with children's life in school, career, and friendships. A broad range of emotional disorders affect children and adolescents between 5 and 10 percent of children and young people affected at any time. Under IDEA criteria the term *emotional disturbance* is associated with mental health or severe behavior issues. The condition must have been present to a marked extent over a period of time and must substantially interfere with the child's educational achievement. Six types of emotional disturbances that have been named are anxiety disorders, bipolar disorder, conduct disorders, eating disorders, obsessive-compulsive disorder (OCD), and psychotic disorders; however, that list is not all-inclusive.

Children with emotional disturbances may exhibit the following ranges of behaviors:

- Hyperactivity (short attention span, impulsiveness)
- Aggression or self-injurious behavior (acting out, fighting)
- Withdrawal (not interacting socially with others, excessive fear or anxiety)
- Immaturity (inappropriate crying, temper tantrums, poor coping skills)
- Learning difficulties (academically performing below grade level)

Young people with the most serious emotional troubles may have distortions in their thinking, extreme anxiety, strange behaviors, and unusual mood swings. Some of these characteristics may also be displayed with typical children. Those with emotional disturbances exhibit these behaviors over long periods of time and the behaviors significantly interfere with their learning, relationships and they may have a lessened ability to cope with the ordinary demands of life (National Alliance on Mental Illness, 2010).

In the 2010–2011 school year, 389,000 children with an emotional disturbance received services in the public schools (NCES, 2014). Rudy and Levinson (2008) state that children with emotional disturbance have the least favorable outcomes of any other group of children with disabilities. Those authors conclude that to increase the possibilities of success for these children (and all others), schools and parents need to allow more time for young people to develop relationship; increase community, parent, and administration participation; and build a school climate of nurturing.

Assessment of emotional disturbances refers to a systematic collection of relevant information used to sort everyday problems from more significant psychopathology as well as then classifying and taking care of people who have the identified disorders (Parritz & Troy, 2014). Rudy and Levinson (2008) outline the practices of multidisciplinary assessment of emotional disturbance. Those evaluations are conducted systematically and include a team of people and the child in order to determine the best treatment course and menu of services. Assessment techniques may include interviews, standardized tests, observations, and other procedures. Descriptions of some emotional disturbances follow.

Anxiety Disorders

Parritz and Troy (2014) explain the difference between fears—anxieties in the presence of something specific—and worries—anxieties about future events. When those fears and worries are excessive, persistent, seemingly uncontrollable, and overwhelming, the child may have an anxiety disorder. That umbrella term refers to separate disabilities that have the core characteristic of irrational fear such as generalized anxiety disorder, obsessive-compulsive disorder, panic disorder, post-traumatic stress disorder, social anxiety disorder, and specific phobias (NIMH, 2014).

According to an adolescent mental health report about 8 percent of adolescents between the ages of 13 and 18 have an anxiety disorder with symptoms emerging around the age of 6 (NIMH). The Anxiety Disorders Association of America (2010) identifies anxiety disorders as the most common psychiatric illnesses diagnosed in children, adolescents, and adults. Treatment for anxiety disorders includes medications, cognitive-behavioral therapy (CBT), exposure therapy, and mindfulness training among other therapies. Higa-McMillan, Francis, and Chorpita (2014) out-line the characteristics, treatment options, and current research on anxiety disorders in children.

Bipolar Disorder

Young people with bipolar disorder, also known as manic-depressive disorder, have dramatic, unusual mood swings that range from very high to very sad and hopeless. Their moods shift from overly joyful or overexcited (manic episode) to despondent (depressive episode) with periods of normality in between. Their energy, activity levels, and ability to function in day-to-day tasks also change with the mood shift. These mood shifts are drastic changes from the person's usual mood and behavior (NIMH, 2014).

According to a literature review conducted by Birmaher (2013), the diagnosis of bipolar disorder in children and adolescents presents significant challenges. He calls for more explicit diagnostic criteria specific to children and adolescents. Particularly troubling is the increased risk of suicidal attempts in children and adolescents with bipolar disorder (Goldstein et al., 2005). Adults must never ignore threats of suicide in any young person but particularly those who are depressed.

While there is no cure for bipolar disorder, treatment with medications, talk therapy, or both may help people recover from their episodes, and may help to pre-vent future episodes (McClellan, Kowatch, & Findling, 2007). Youngstrom and Algorta (2014) review current approaches to treating children with bipolar disorder.

Conduct Disorder

Conduct disorder refers to a group of behavior and emotional problems that are frequent, severe, and lasts for at least 6 months. This incorporates a persistent pat-tern of disruptive and violent behaviors that breach the basic rights of others or the social norms or rules (SAMSHA, 2014).These young people have great difficulty following rules and do not act in socially acceptable ways. Some of the following behaviors may indicate conduct disorder:

- Aggression to people and animals
- Destruction of property
- Deceitfulness, lying, or stealing
- Truancy or other serious violations of rules (American Academy of Child and Adolescent Psychiatry, 2013)

About 8.5 percent of children meet the criteria for conduct disorder at some point in their lives (SAMSHA, 2104). Conduct disorder can be difficult to treat, but the American Academy of Child and Adolescent Psychiatry (2013) suggests the fol-lowing as the beneficial range of services for young people with this problem:

- Training for parents on how to handle child or adolescent behavior
- Family therapy
- Training in problem-solving skills for children or adolescents
- Community-based services that focus on the young person within the context of family and community influences

More specific information can be found in a useful chapter by Kimonis, Frick, and McMahon (2014).

Eating Disorders

Characterized by extremes in eating behavior or feelings of extreme distress about body weight and shape, eating disorders refer to patterns of behaviors around unhealthy eating and dangerous weight management practices. These illnesses may have life-threatening consequences. Three types of eating disorders are *anorexia nervosa*, *bulimia*, and *binge eating*. *Anorexia nervosa* refers to very restricted food intake and a dramatic loss of weight. *Bulimia* involves a cycle of overeating followed by vomiting or other purging behaviors which are used to compensate for the excessive food intake. Both of these disorders require immediate, intensive interventions to prevent death. *Binge eating* is also characterized by eating excessive amounts of food and feeling out of control about how much or what is consumed. People with this disorder do not purge after the binge. Around half a million adolescents struggle with disordered eating (Swanson, Crow, Le Grange, Swendsen, & Merikangas, 2011).

According to the National Eating Disorders Association (2014), the most effective treatment for eating disorders combines counseling, medical attention, and nutritional guidance. In addition, Von Ranson and Wallace (2014) provide an excellent overview of the complexities of eating disorders in children and adolescents.

Obsessive-Compulsive Spectrum Disorder

Obsessive-compulsive spectrum disorders can be considered an anxiety disorder that is characterized by recurrent, unwanted thoughts or obsessions and/or repetitive behaviors or compulsions. Behaviors like hand washing, counting, checking, or cleaning may be repeated with the hope of eliminating an obsessive thought. Those rituals may provide some temporary relief. Not performing those rituals creates increased anxiety. This debilitating disorder affects around 1 in 100 children and adolescents (Marsden & Chowdhury, 2009).

According to the International OCD Foundation (2014) and Piacentini, Chang, Snorrason, and Woods (2014), treatment should include these components:

- Cognitive-behavioral therapy (CBT)
- Exposure and response prevention (ERP)
- Medication (usually an antidepressant)

Piacentini and his colleagues have amassed other very useful information related to this disorder.

Psychotic Disorders

The term *psychotic disorders* refers to severe mental illnesses that cause abnormal thinking and perceptions. The main symptoms include delusions and hallucinations. Delusions can be defined as false beliefs, such as thinking you have been abducted by a space alien. Hallucinations are false perceptions such as seeing, hearing, or believing something that is not present. Generally, psychotic disorders are demonstrated through severe impairment of mental functioning and disturbances in reality testing. One type of psychotic disorder is schizophrenia, but there are others.

The treatment for psychotic disorders must be tailored for each person and specific disorder. Generally a combination of medication, individual therapy, family therapy, and specialized programs are necessary (American Academy of Child and Adolescent Psychiatry, 2014).

Children with emotional disturbances need love and understanding, and they need a counselor who can provide security and stability. The counselor who is effective with children who exhibit emotional disturbances can detect and reflect the feelings and frustrations of the children, discuss these feelings, and decide how to manage them effectively. Much of the success achieved from working with the emotionally disturbed child has been due to the relationship between an adult and the child, as well as the technique used. These children often have experienced inconsistency in their relationships and may be suspicious of adults because of past experiences with hurtful people. The counselor needs to be strong enough to place consistent limits on the children and require them to assume responsibility for their behavior. To bring consistency and stability to the life of the child with behavioral-emotional disorders, the counselor can discuss expected and appropriate behaviors with the child. Writing out what is considered inappropriate and the consequences of this behavior is often helpful.

Cognitive-behavioral therapy (CBT) is an effective treatment for anxiety disorders. The cognitive part supports people as they modify the thinking patterns that support their fears, and the behavioral part allows people to change the way they react to anxiety-provoking situations. The counselor can define expected behaviors by such methods as contracting. The counselor, parents, teachers, and all significant people in the child's life must be willing to set limits and consistently maintain the rules. Behavior modification techniques emphasizing positive reinforcement have been effective. Relaxation exercises, talking therapy, physical activities, writing, drawing, or games may be scheduled into the child's day to provide outlets for tension and other emotions. Changes in the environment, expectations, stimulation, and conflicts should be as minimal as possible.

Some strategies help all children, and the information below could be effective with many populations. Tarver-Behring and Spagna (2009) suggest that counselors help teachers with social skills strategies and classroom programs on problem solving, conflict resolutions, anger management, and making friends. Peer groups can be effective models for appropriate behavior.

The tasks of the counselor with children who have emotional disturbance can be summarized as follows:

1. Forming a counseling relationship with the child that includes well-defined responsibilities and limits
2. Working to change the child's image and expectations through counseling and consultation with family and other significant people in the child's world
3. Conducting individual and group counseling to deal with feelings and behaviors, to teach social skills, and to improve academic performance

4. Assisting parents and teachers in structuring the child's physical environment and schedule, establishing rules for behavior, and providing encouragement, reinforcement, and logical consequences for misbehavior

School programs for children with emotional disturbance include not only academics but also attention to the emotional and behavioral support they need. Developing social skills, building self-awareness, and increasing self-control should be incorporated. These children and others benefit from the positive behavioral support (PBS) program, a whole-school approach to discipline that minimizes problem behaviors and fosters positive, appropriate behaviors (Curtis, Van Horne, Robertson, & Karvonen, 2010). In school students who are eligible for services under the emotional disturbances category should have IEPs that include positive behavior interventions and supports and may have IEPs that include counseling services. Coordinating care for the child with emotional disturbances between home, school, and community enhances the possibilities of learning and growth for the child.

CHILDREN WITH SPECIFIC LEARNING DISABILITIES

The National Center for Education Statistics (2014) figures indicate that 36 percent of the school population served under IDEA have an identified learning disability (LD). Specific learning disability is a general term for different kinds of learning problems, most often skills related to reading, writing, listening, speaking, reasoning, and doing math. The DSM-V (APA, 2013) refers to learning disorders as interfering with the acquisition and use of one or more of the following academic skills: oral language, reading, written language, mathematics. These disorders affect individuals who otherwise demonstrate at least average abilities essential for thinking or reasoning. Therefore, Specific Learning Disorders is a classification distinct from Intellectual Developmental Disorders. This DSM-V definition states that the diagnostic criteria do not depend upon comparisons with overall IQ and are consistent with the changes in the United States' reauthorized IDEA regulations (2004), which state that "the criteria adopted by each State must not require the use of a severe discrepancy between intellectual ability and achievement for determining whether a child has a specific learning disability" (Silver, 2014). Types of learning disabilities are identified by the specific processing problem. The difficulties might relate "to getting information into the brain (**Input**), making sense of this information (**Organization**), storing and later retrieving this information (**Memory**), or getting this information back out (**Output**). Thus, the specific types of processing problems that result in LD might be in one or more of these four areas" (http://www.ldaamerica.us).

The Learning Disabilities Association of America (2014) discusses learning disabilities as an umbrella term that covers the following conditions:

- *Dyslexia:* a language and reading disability
- *Dyscalculia:* problems with arithmetic and math concepts
- *Dysgraphia:* a writing disorder resulting in illegibility
- *Dyspraxia (sensory integration disorder):* problems with motor coordination
- *Central auditory processing disorder:* difficulty processing and remembering language-related tasks

- *Nonverbal learning disorders:* trouble with nonverbal cues, for example, body language, poor coordination, clumsy
- *Visual perceptual/visual motor deficit:* reverses letters, cannot copy accurately, eyes hurt and itch, loses place, struggles with cutting
- *Language disorders (aphasia/dysphasia):* trouble understanding spoken language, poor reading comprehension

Current ways to assess learning disabilities involve large-scale screenings and supportive instruction for all students with more intensive interventions for those who do not learn on a typical timeline (Fletcher & Vaughn, 2009). The goals of this approach are to prevent disabilities as well as enhance education for all students. Butterworth, Varma, and Laurillard (2011) describe an adaptive software package that illustrates the innovations aimed at those with learning disabilities.

As in counseling with other children, the counselor begins by recognizing and reflecting the feelings of the young person with a learning disability. McEachern (2004) explains their possible fear of failure and of learning reflected in their comments such as "I can't do this," "I don't know how," or "I'll never learn this."

Some children with learning disabilities lack social perception and skills and perform poorly in social situations (Lewandowski & Lovett, 2014). They may have trouble making friends and forming good relationships in their families. Indeed Thurneck et al. (2007) state that the lack of social skills is the biggest concern for these children. Activities for building a positive body image and self-perception, sensitivity to other people, social maturity and skills, self-esteem, and emotional well-being may enhance these areas of concern. Cognitive-behavioral, behavioral, and psychoeducational interventions are the treatment choices (Kaffenberger, 2011). Group therapy is advantageous for these children so they can learn skills from their peers. Shechtman and Pastor (2005) found both cognitive-behavioral treatment groups and humanistic group therapy effective for children with learning disabilities. Those groups helped the children look at both their social and emotional problems. The group participants also increased their academic motivation.

Thompson and Littrell (1998) suggest brief solution-oriented counseling for adolescents with learning disabilities. Their four-step model involves building rapport and then helping the student identify, describe, and define a specific problem or concern. In Step 2, the counselor and student consider what had been tried previously, what had worked, and any new possible solutions. During Step 3, the counselor helps the student decide on a specific, concrete, measurable, and attainable goal. Often, this step includes using the miracle question, "Suppose a miracle happened and the problem was solved. What would be different?" The fourth step is the generation of a specific task to help the student reach a goal. The counselors checked with the student 3 and 4 weeks later. These authors report success in 90 percent of the research participants.

Counseling goals for children with learning disabilities would include enhancing social skills, helping overcome a sense of failure, and promoting a positive attitude toward learning. McEachern (2004) recommends play techniques, art, music, and expressive writing to evoke expressions of feelings toward the disability, school, peers, and family. Cognitive-behavioral techniques to teach skills and coping strategies are suggested for older elementary and adolescent students. Brown (2005) states that music therapy that focuses on rhythm, order, and beat helps students who have cognitive disabilities. Reis and Colbert (2004) report that college students who have been identified as gifted or as learning disabled suffered negative experiences in their earlier school experiences. Reis and Colbert advocate for attention to the personal, social, and career development needs of this population. Durodoye, Combes, and Bryant (2004) echo that need for African American students with learning disabilities.

Durodoye et al. (2004) suggest several multidisciplinary strategies for children with learning disabilities—self-motivation, self-control of academic progress, self-reinforcement of academic effort, progress and success, teaching adaptive skills, self-management for reducing problem behaviors, and teaching academic success behaviors. They stress that balancing information about children with special needs requires counseling skills that are flexible and appropriate culturally. Thurneck et al. (2007) recommend brief sessions that are structured and include activity-oriented material. Counselors must realize that children with learning disabilities have difficulties with attention span, concept formation, motor control, and communication skills. All those may impact the counseling process and require the counselor's patience and understanding.

Brown (2009) reminds adults to help these students understand their difficulties, give realistic positive reinforcement, acknowledge the problems in their lives, and talk to them about their behavior. In a 20-year longitudinal study of the attributes that might predict life success for children with learning disabilities, the Frostig Center identifies six life success attributes: self-awareness, proactivity, perseverance, goal-setting, presence, and use of support systems and emotional coping strategies.

More information on that comprehensive study and information about strategies to build those attributes can be found on the Learning Disabilities Association of America's Web site (http://www.ldaamerica.us).

CHILDREN WITH ATTENTION DEFICIT/HYPERACTIVITY DISORDER AND ATTENTION DEFICIT DISORDER

The cluster of problems known as ADHD forms an extremely complex childhood problem and elicits the most frequent referrals for professional help, according to Erk (2008). Approximately 11 percent (6.4 million) of children between the ages of 4 and 17 have been diagnosed with ADHD as of 2011 (http://www.cdc.gov/ncbddd/adhd/data.html). The DSM-V criteria for ADHD follow:

People with ADHD show a persistent pattern of inattention and/or hyperactivity-impulsivity that interferes with functioning or development:

1. *Inattention:* Six or more symptoms of inattention for children up to age 16, or five or more for adolescents 17 and older and adults; symptoms of inattention have been present for at least 6 months, and they are inappropriate for developmental level:
   - Often fails to give close attention to details or makes careless mistakes in schoolwork, at work, or with other activities
   - Often has trouble holding attention on tasks or play activities

- Often does not seem to listen when spoken to directly
- Often does not follow through on instructions and fails to finish schoolwork, chores, or duties in the workplace (e.g., loses focus, sidetracked)
- Often has trouble organizing tasks and activities
- Often avoids, dislikes, or is reluctant to do tasks that require mental effort over a long period of time (such as schoolwork or homework)
- Often loses things necessary for tasks and activities (e.g., school materials, pencils, books, tools, wallets, keys, paperwork, eyeglasses, mobile telephones)
- Is often easily distracted
- Is often forgetful in daily activities

2. *Hyperactivity and impulsivity:* Six or more symptoms of hyperactivity-impulsivity for children up to age 16, or five or more for adolescents 17 and older and adults; symptoms of hyperactivity-impulsivity have been present for at least 6 months to an extent that is disruptive and inappropriate for the person's developmental level:
- Often fidgets with or taps hands or feet, or squirms in seat.
- Often leaves seat in situations when remaining seated is expected.
- Often runs about or climbs in situations where it is not appropriate (adolescents or adults may be limited to feeling restless)
- Often unable to play or take part in leisure activities quietly
- Is often "on the go," acting as if "driven by a motor"
- Often talks excessively
- Often blurts out an answer before a question has been completed
- Often has trouble waiting his/her turn
- Often interrupts or intrudes on others (e.g., butts into conversations or games)

In addition, the following conditions must be met:

- Several inattentive or hyperactive-impulsive symptoms were present before the age of 12 years.
- Several symptoms are present in two or more settings (e.g., at home, school, or work; with friends or relatives; in other activities).
- There is clear evidence that the symptoms interfere with, or reduce the quality of, social, school, or work functioning.
- The symptoms do not happen only during the course of schizophrenia or another psychotic disorder. The symptoms are not better explained by another mental disorder (e.g., mood disorder, anxiety disorder, dissociative disorder, or a personality disorder).

Based on the types of symptoms, three kinds (presentations) of ADHD can occur:

Combined presentation: if enough symptoms of both criteria inattention and hyperactivity-impulsivity were present for the past 6 months

Predominantly inattentive presentation: if enough symptoms of inattention, but not hyperactivity-impulsivity, were present for the past 6 months

Predominantly hyperactive-impulsive presentation: if enough symptoms of hyperactivity-impulsivity, but not inattention, were present for the past 6 months.

These symptoms can change over time. Therefore, the presentation may change over time as well (http://www.cdc.gov/ncbddd/adhd/diagnosis.html; APA, 2013).

Smith and Luckasson (1995) state that the condition is confusing. Not all children diagnosed as having attention deficit disorders (ADDs) are in special education programs; some are diagnosed as learning disabled, and others may be classified as having behavioral disorders, emotional disturbance, or other disabilities. Erk (2008) discusses neuroanatomical abnormalities that may accompany ADHD, as well as educational and social conditions that may also be present.

A national nonprofit organization, Children with Attention Deficit Disorders, has reported that children might have ADD if they fidget, squirm, or seem restless; have trouble remaining seated, playing quietly, waiting their turn, following instructions, or sustaining attention; talk excessively; are easily distracted; blurt out answers; shift from one uncompleted task to another; interrupt others; do not seem to listen; often lose things; frequently engage in dangerous behavior; act without thinking; have low self-esteem; have frequent, unpredictable mood swings; and get angry and lose their temper easily (Parritz & Troy, 2014). However, many of these characteristics may be normal behaviors for a child's particular developmental level, or they could be characteristics of other problems. One must consider the intensity and duration of the symptoms, as well as how they fit into the child's overall developmental pattern.

An assessment of ADHD requires a comprehensive evaluation that includes a medical examination and interviews or other information from teachers, parents, and other adults. The symptoms must be present in more than one setting. Some of the instruments used as scales for assessment of ADHD are the following:

- *The NICHQ Vanderbilt Assessment Scale* (http://www.nichq.org/childrens-health/adhd/resources/vanderbilt-assessment-scales)
- *Behavior Assessment System for Children (BASC)* (Reynolds & Kamphaus, 2004)
- *Child Behavior Checklist/Teacher Report Form* (Achenbach & Rescorla, 2001)

Working with children who have ADHD requires a multidisciplinary, multitreatment model. Usually, such teams are composed of professionals such as physicians, psychologists, psychiatrists, counselors, and speech and other educational specialists. Generally, the treatment will include behavioral intervention strategies, parent training, medications, and school accommodations. According to the Center of Disease Control (2014), several different types of medications may be used to treat ADHD. One type of medication is stimulants, the most widely used medication with between 70 and 80 percent of children with ADHD responding positively to those medications. Nonstimulants have also been approved to treat ADHD and have fewer side effects than stimulants.

Teachers, parents, and other adults who work with children taking medication must be aware of the treatment to provide feedback about its effects. Counselors can serve as coordinators of the many professionals working with the child during the assessment and intervention stages. In addition, they can develop referral lists that include physicians and other helping professionals familiar with ADHD, as well as local groups offering parenting classes or support groups.

Parents will find help with some bibliotherapy sources such as those prepared by Barkley (2013) and Laver-Bradbury (2010). In addition, support groups, a parent education group, and family counseling may be helpful especially during the initial assessment period and while the parent is dealing with his or her feelings about the child's condition. Kottman et al. (1995) recommend a parent training program that includes general information about ADHD, its causes, and possible treatment plans; self-esteem development suggestions; training in parent listening and encouragement skills; dealing with parent stress; suggestions for working with the child's school; and suggested means of social support for parents. Barkley (2005) and Carter, Erford, and Orsi (2004) also provide extensive, helpful suggestions for adults working with children with ADHD.

Erk (2008) reviews a collaborative multimodal study of children with ADHD (MTA Study). Children in the study were assigned to four experimental groups. The findings of that research support the integration of parent training, school intervention, child treatment, and medication management for children with ADHD. Resnick (2000) recommends a treatment menu for individual counseling with children and adolescents. The choices may include things such as understanding the diagnosis and how it can have a positive effect on a person's life, dealing with the reaction to the diagnosis, dealing with stress, dealing with lost opportunities and relationships, and coping with grief and suffering that may have been a part of their lives.

Children with ADHD often need to learn how to interact with others. Counselors may want to respond to this common problem by providing training in effective interpersonal behaviors. Social skills training should target specific skills instead of global ones. These children need to know making-friends skills, like smiling, complimenting others, cooperative behaviors, and genuine interest in others. The training should focus on behaviors that are relevant to social interaction success with both peers and adults. Basic interaction skills, like eye contact, voice level or tone, taking turns, and slowing down are some important behaviors. Counselors should talk about poor self-concept that may have resulted from the rejection of peers. Getting along skills, like polite language, following rules, helping others, and honoring the personal space and privacy of others are needed behaviors. Social skills training goals should be centered on establishing and maintaining appropriate behavior in addition to changing and reducing inappropriate behaviors. Social coping skills like reacting appropriately when someone says no, coping effectively with frustration or anger, responding to a hurtful person, and understanding that things do not always go well are behaviors to build (Erk, 2008; Thurneck et al., 2007).

Cognitive restructuring techniques may teach the child more positive ways of thinking, as well as self-monitoring of behavior. Thurneck et al. (2007) suggest that cognitive-behavioral therapy appeals to children with ADHD because it gives them some control in problem solving and monitoring their behavior. Those authors discussed that typical behavior management programs may be seen as threats to independence. Group counseling to teach more effective social skills may be helpful at some point during treatment; however, counselors must carefully assess the child's readiness to benefit from this interaction and to function as a group member.

Erk (2008) recommends parent training and counseling, teacher education, individual counseling, group counseling, behavioral interventions, and self-esteem and social skills education. The services provided from different agencies and people need to be coordinated with follow-up to refresh parents on behavior management, as well as to update school plans.

THE CHILD WITH INTELLECTUAL DISABILITY DISORDER

The American Association on Intellectual and Developmental Disabilities (AAIDD, 2014) defines intellectual disability as a disability of significant limitations both in intellectual functioning and in adaptive behavior. *Intellectual functioning* refers to general mental capacity, such as learning, reasoning, and problem solving. One measurement of intellectual functioning is an IQ test. Generally, an IQ test score of around 70 or as high as 75 indicates a limitation in intellectual functioning. Standardized tests can also determine limitations in *adaptive behavior,* which includes three sets of skills:

- Conceptual skills—language and literacy; concepts of money, time, and number; and self-direction
- Social skills—interpersonal skills, social responsibility, self-esteem, gullibility, social problem solving, and the ability to follow rules/obey laws and to avoid being victimized
- Practical skills—activities of daily living (personal care), occupational skills, health care, travel/transportation, schedules/routines, safety, use of money, use of the telephone

The American Association on Intellectual and Developmental Disabilities (AAIDD) definition takes into account the person's intellectual abilities within the environment that is typical for the person's peers and culture. Furthermore, professionals are admonished to recognize that a person's limitations coexist with strengths, and that a person's level of functioning will improve with appropriate personalized supports over a sustained period.

The AAIDD suggest the subgroups of intellectual disability classified according to a person's strengths and weaknesses in four areas: intellectual functioning and adaptive skills; psychological and emotional functioning; physical functioning and health; and the person's current environment and the optimal environment. The profile of the classification indicates the level of support needed by the person: intermittent or "as needed"; limited; extensive or pervasive (Mash & Wolfe, 2010).

Other systems classify intellectual disability by level of severity—mild, moderate, severe, and profound. That system refers to the degree of impairment in adaptive functioning (Parritz & Troy, 2014). Mild intellectual disability, an estimated 85 percent of people with intellectual disability, is defined as having IQ levels of 55 to 70. The below average intellectual functioning exists with deficits in adaptive behavior as well as adverse effects on the child's educational performance. Moderate intellectual disability is an IQ level of 40 to 54; severe is IQ of 25 to 39; and profound intellectual disability refers to an IQ level below 20 or 25. People with profound intellectual disability require pervasive, lifelong care.

Services and support are based on the level of intensity of need. Hardman, Drew, Egan, and Wolf (1993) suggest that the child may need help with adaptive skills such as coping in school, developing interpersonal relationships, developing language skills, coping with emotional concerns, and taking care of personal needs.

The causes of intellectual disability vary, and the characteristics of the children also differ. Parritz and Troy (2014) summarize the various factors in these categories: prenatal, perinatal, and postnatal causes. Prenatal causes include chromosome disorders (Down syndrome), syndrome disorders (Tuberous sclerosis), metabolism errors (Phenylketonuria), developmental disorders (spina bifida), malnutrition (fetal alcohol syndrome), and other unknown causes. Perinatal causes include things like premature birth and intracranial hemorrhage. Some causes of intellectual disabilities that occur after birth include head injuries, infections, degenerative disorders, seizure disorders, toxic disorders such as lead exposure, malnutrition, and environmental deprivations.

The counseling techniques in this section are geared toward those children categorized as intermittent or limited, the groups most likely to face societal problems and pressures. These children have physical and psychological needs similar to those of other children, but the added handicap of their exceptionality interferes with their adjustment. The AAIDD (2014) definition suggests that children may need help in ten "adaptive skill" areas: communication (understanding and expression), self-care, home living, social interactions, understanding the community, self-direction (making choices), health and safety, obtaining functional academic skills (reading, writing, everyday mathematics), effectively using leisure time, and developing employment skills (Mash & Wolfe, 2010).

Counseling goals include improving social interactions, enhancing skills, developing interpersonal relationships, and promoting a positive self-image. Peer feedback and modeling can be highly effective counseling techniques. Group counseling can help the child learn and rehearse effective ways of behaving. Behavior modification techniques, such as the token system or contingency contracting, have been found to work effectively with individuals who have intellectual disability (Kaffenberger, 2011). The counselor will want to use the same effective practices for all children—be clear and concise in communications, limit the number of directions, display respect, and provide encouragement.

Wicks-Nelson and Israel (2014) cite behavioral techniques that help shape and strengthen adaptive skills and weaken ineffective behavior. Those authors support social skills training and functional communication training for children with intellectual disability. The authors encourage counselors to be direct and set specific goals with this population. Counselors should use concrete, clear language and have short, frequent meetings with children with intellectual disability. Mash and Wolfe (2010) state that interventions should begin in preschool and be matched to the individual child and integrated into the family, school, and community environment. Those authors recommend behaviorally based training and specific skill training for children with intellectual disabilities. Parritz and Troy (2014) cite behavioral treatments, cognitive treatments, socioemotional programs, and family, educational, and vocational planning as effective mental health interventions with children who have intellectual disabilities. Counselors will need to work with the parents and other significant people in the child's life to help them understand and encourage the child's abilities. Special attention should be on teaching the child independent living skills, as well as personal and social skills. The child and parents also need guidance and assistance in planning for the child's educational and vocational future.

THE CHILD WITH A PHYSICAL DISABILITY

Under IDEA 2004 physical disabilities refers to *orthopedic impairments*. These students have difficulty with the structure or the functioning of their bodies. Physical disability includes conditions that may be congenital, accidental, or related to disease that cause physical limitations. The two major groups of physical disabilities are neuromotor impairments, conditions caused by damage to the central nervous system, and muscular/skeletal impairments, conditions that affect the limbs or muscles. To meet IDEA diagnostic criteria, the impairment must interfere with school attendance or learning to the extent that special services, training, equipment, or materials are required. These impairments may be caused by a congenital anomaly (e.g., clubfoot, absence of some member, among others), impairments caused by disease (e.g., poliomyelitis, bone tuberculosis, and others), and impairments from other causes (e.g., cerebral palsy, amputations, and fractures or burns that cause contractures) (NICHCY, 2012).

Other health impairments is the term used to describe conditions and diseases that require special health care needs. The two types of health disabilities are chronic illnesses and infectious diseases. The conditions cause limited strength, vitality, or alertness, including a heightened alertness to environmental stimuli, that results in limited alertness with respect to the educational environment that (1) is due to chronic or acute health problems such as asthma, ADD or ADHD, diabetes, epilepsy, a heart condition, hemophilia, lead poisoning, leukemia, nephritis, rheumatic fever, and sickle cell anemia; and (2) adversely affects a child's educational performance. They may include cerebral palsy, spina bifida, spinal cord injuries, amputations, muscular dystrophy, cystic fibrosis, sickle cell anemia, adolescent pregnancy, and cocaine addiction (NICHCY, 2012).

Many children have more than one disability, and some conditions have overlapping symptoms. Children with physical disabilities make up a heterogeneous group. They may or may not have average intelligence. Some have adapted to their physical concerns while others have not. Knowing the characteristics, physical problems, symptoms, and prognosis of the child with a physical disability helps counselors understand the child's world. Counselors also want to know the child's strengths. Lack of knowledge and fear of the unknown can make the counselor apprehensive, which the child can sense. The children's needs vary according to the type of disability; some may need help with basic functioning and others may need help in building relationships and dealing with ridicule. Thurneck et al. (2007) recommends counselors take care to see each child in relation to the specific condition and to use a counseling approach focused on strengths and coping strategies corresponding to the disability.

The child may have anxiety, shame, or other negative feelings because of his or her disability. The children's perceptions of self and their abilities are also determined by the child's age at the time the disabling condition occurred and the severity of the condition. These reactions may reflect how the child has been treated by others, especially family. Cognitive-behavioral counseling, play therapy, art therapy, bibliotherapy, and sand play are recommended (Thurneck et al., 2007).

The demands for energy, time, and financial resources may add a heavy burden of stress to families. Families of children with severe physical and health problems may experience fatigue and low vitality, a restricted social life, financial setbacks, and career interruptions, and can become preoccupied with the child's illness. Thurneck et al. (2007) cite the benefits of interventions with children with physical disabilities and their families.

GENERAL IDEAS

Teachers may feel unprepared to work with children with special needs in the classroom. Often they may request help with classroom management techniques. Because teachers' attitudes are critical to the success of children with disabilities, counselors should be prepared to work with them in a consultative manner to alleviate their personal concerns and anxieties about teaching children with disabilities and assist them in developing whatever skills are needed. Some resources for staff development include those found at The Person-Centered Planning Education Site (http://www.personcenteredplanning.org/) and The Self-Determination Synthesis Project (www.uncc.edu/sdsp).

Counselors will also want to understand the ways teachers can design their curriculum for all students. Burgstahler (2008) explains the principles and applications of universal design in education (UDE). She talks about education courses, technology, and student services normally being designed for the range of characteristics of the average student. UDE expands that range for people with disabilities to make all parts of the educational experience accessible. The principles of UDE are equitable, flexible, simple, and intuitive use for all products and environments. Other principles include information that can be perceived in many ways, a tolerance for error, low physical effort, and size and space for approach and use. Her article provides examples of UDE application in physical space, information technology, instruction, and student services. By instruction she refers to using multiple means of representation or giving learners many ways to get information and knowledge. Her term "multiple means of expression" indicates that learners have alternatives for showing what they know. Finally, she encourages multiple means of engagement to tap learners' interests, offer appropriate challenges, and build motivation.

More specifically, Strangman, Hall, and Meyer (2004) explain three sets of teaching methods to support recognition, strategies, and affect. To support different recognition networks, teachers should give many examples, highlight critical features, have various media and formats, and support background context. Teachers and counselors can build different strategic networks by giving flexible models of skilled performance, having opportunities to practice with supports, provide ongoing, relevant feedback, and offer flexible opportunities for demonstrating a skill. As the third UDE, teachers and counselors can support motivation by offering choices of learning context, content and tools, having adjustable levels of challenge, and offering choices of rewards. The National Center on Accessing the General Curriculum Web site (www.cast.org) has a toolkit for UDE.

The counselor who works with children who have disabilities needs to be able to work with all agencies, professionals, parents, and other significant persons in the child's life. Coordinating services, rearranging physical environments, removing barriers and inconveniences, and securing special equipment and materials may be only the first step to meeting the needs of those with physical disabilities. Counselors can advocate for all services needed to help children with disabilities reach their full potential (Tarver-Behring & Spagna, 2004).

As with many other child clients, counselors would focus the goals of counseling on helping the student identify his or her strengths and encouraging the student to become a self-advocate. Counselors should focus on building feelings of self-worth and healthy attitudes. The child may need encouragement to express and recognize his or her feelings toward the disability, help to learn social or personal skills, counsel in the area of independent living, and assistance in making vocational plans for the future. Adlerian counseling (see Chapter 11) may help a child recognize strengths. More important than the physical limitation is that each child is a unique individual who has capabilities and potential; the counselor's role is to facilitate growth toward reaching this potential.

Several years ago Deck, Scarborough, Sferrazza, and Estill (1999) recount some of the issues of school counselors working with students with disabilities that continue to be useful guidelines. They discuss using small-group counseling, classroom guidance, individual counseling, after-school counseling, and collaboration with teachers and parents. Another summary of the tasks of the counselor working with any type of exceptional child might include the following:

1. Recognize that the child is a *person* first.
2. Work toward an understanding of the child's specific exceptionality and the unique social, learning, or behavioral problems that may accompany this exceptionality.
3. Counsel to enhance self-concept.
4. Facilitate adjustment to exceptionality.
5. Coordinate the services of other professionals or agencies working with the exceptional child.
6. Help the significant people in the child's life (parents and teachers especially) understand the child's exceptionality, strengths and limitations, and special problems.
7. Assist in the development of effective, independent living skills.
8. Encourage recreational skills and hobbies.
9. Teach personal and social skills.
10. Assist in educational planning and possibly securing needed educational aids and equipment for the child.
11. Counsel with the parents.
12. Acquire a knowledge of and working relationship with professional and referral agencies.

COUNSELING WITH PARENTS OF EXCEPTIONAL CHILDREN

Taub (2006) provides a useful overview of the concerns of parents of students with disabilities. Many parents are able to accept and adjust to their child's condition in a healthy manner; others, even though they love their child, may have trouble dealing with their feelings and the situation. Parents may experience a range of emotions: grief, shock, and disbelief; fear and anxiety about the child's future; helplessness because they cannot change the condition; and disappointment because theirs is not the perfect child they expected. They may resent the burdens the child's disability places on the family. Taub categorizes the reactions as grief and loss as well as safety concerns and overprotectiveness. Whatever the feelings, the counselor needs to help the parents work through them. Parents are the child's main support system, and they must be free to accept and support the child in his or her growth and development.

Counseling tasks for the counselor working with the parents of exceptional children include the following:

1. Encourage and help parents to gain knowledge about their child's exceptionality, prognosis, strengths, and limitations.
2. Assist the parents in working through feelings and attitudes that may inhibit the child's progress.
3. Advise parents concerning state, federal, or community resources available for educational, medical, emotional, or financial assistance.
4. Assist the parents in setting realistic expectations for their child.
5. Encourage the parents to view their child as a unique individual with rights and potentials and the ability to make choices about his or her own life.

Of the excellent books available to help both children and parents understand the characteristics of an exceptionality and the future of children with a particular exceptionality, those of R. A. Gardner contain a section written to parents about the disability and a section written for children to explain the disability in terms they can understand. The publications of the Center for Parent Information and Resources (NICHCY's new home) have current, valuable information for parents, children, and professionals.

The Centers for Disease Control and Prevention (2014) produced a booklet for practitioners that addressed the components of parent training programs to determine those associated with more effective programs. Better parent outcomes on acquiring parenting skills and behaviors were correlated with two content areas and one program delivery model. The content areas that were effective included teaching parents emotional communication skills and positive parent–child interaction skills. Requiring parents to practice with their child during the program sessions was also associated with more effective training. This practice contrasted with programs in which no practice happened or where parents role-played skills.

Other positive outcomes in the parent training programs reviewed (Centers for Disease Control and Prevention, 2014) were decreases in children's externalizing behaviors of aggression, noncompliance, or hyperactivity. The significant content areas were teaching parents the correct ways to use time-out, teaching parents to interact positively with their child, and instructing parents to respond consistently to their child. Again, the program practice that led to success was requiring parents to practice with their child during program sessions.

Parent groups are probably a good way of helping parents of exceptional youngsters. Through sharing, the parents learn that others have the feelings and problems they are experiencing. They realize they are not alone in their plight; many other parents have children who are different. Parents not only share their feelings in groups but also share methods for problem solving. Others may have lived through the particular crisis one set of parents is facing, and solutions can be discussed. Parent groups provide an atmosphere of understanding, acceptance, and support; they reassure troubled parents that they are not alone and that others care.

Counselors also may want to explore the possibilities of family therapy. Family sessions could explore feelings of anger, frustration, and shame; tendencies to scapegoat, exclude, or overprotect; communication styles or blocks; and effective and ineffective interactions and other problems of families not functioning effectively.

SUMMARY

Children with special needs can learn, enjoy life, be independent and productive, and fulfill their individual potential just as surely as all other children can. They have the same rights to respect and growth as other children, and they have the same needs. Counselors must understand the complexities of different types of disabilities, the provision of special education services, and the many ways counselors may contribute to these children's lives, which include all of these typical services:

Advocacy: supporting the child's rights

Assessment: identifying areas of need

Career counseling: assisting with the development of a career path

Case management: coordinating delivery of services

Clinical support: providing supervision to trained assistants

Collaboration: working with other team members

Crisis intervention: intervening in urgent situations such as suicide risk and panic

Decision making: contributing to team determinations of services and supports

Dropout prevention: working with high-risk students

Direct services: providing counseling

IEP development: help in designing individual educational plans

IEP team membership

Parent counseling and training: helping families

Positive behavioral support: participating in system of prevention and intervention

Referral: to multidisciplinary special education team

Safekeeping of confidential records

Self-determination training: aiding students' acquisition of skills needed to direct their lives

Transition program planning: development and implementation

Counselors who help children with special needs celebrate their strengths and move successfully into their future roles will be richly rewarded.

WEB SITES FOR COUNSELING WITH EXCEPTIONAL CHILDREN

Internet addresses frequently change. To find the sites listed here, visit www.cengage .com/counseling/henderson for an updated list of Internet addresses and direct links to relevant sites.

American Association on Intellectual and Developmental Disabilities (AAIDD)

Center for Parent Information and Resources

Children and Adults with Attention Deficit Disorders (CHADD)

Office of Special Education Programs (OSEP)

REFERENCES

Achenbach, T. M., & Rescorla, L. A. (2001). *Manual for the ASEBA school-age forms & profiles*. Burlington, VT: University of Vermont, Research Center for Children, Youth, and Families.

American Academy of Child and Adolescent Psychiatry. (2013). Conduct disorder. Retrieved from http://www.aacap.org/AACAP/Families_and_Youth/Facts_for_Families/Facts_for _Families_Pages/Conduct_Disorder_33.aspx

American Association on Intellectual and Developmental Disabilities (AAIDD). (2014). *Definition of intellectual disability*. Retrieved from http://aaidd.org/intellectual-disability /definition#.VJSezP8HAo

American Psychiatric Association (APA). DSM-5 Task Force. (2013). *Diagnostic and statistical manual of mental disorders: DSM-5*. Washington, D. C: American Psychiatric Association.

Anxiety Disorders Association of America. (2010). *Understanding anxiety*. Retrieved from http://www.adaa.org/understanding-anxiety

Barkley, R. A. (2005). *Attention-deficit hyperactivity disorder: A handbook for diagnosis and treatment* (3rd ed.). New York: Guilford Press.

Barkley, R. (2013). *Taking charge of ADHD: The complete, authoritative guide for parents* (3rd ed.). New York: The Guilford Press.

Berns, R. M. (2013). *Child, family, school, community: Socialization and support* (9th ed.). Belmont, CA: Wadsworth.

Birmaher, B. (2013). Bipolar disorder in children and adolescents. *Child and Adolescent Mental Health, 18*(3), 140–148. doi:10.1111/camh.12021

Brown, S. (2005). Art therapy urged for inclusion under IDEA: Advocates tout its effectiveness for students with disabilities. *Education Daily, 38*, 2.

Brown, D. (2009). Counseling students with learning disabilities on social skills. Retrieved from http://www.ldanatl.org

Burgstahler, S. (2008). Universal design in education: Principles and applications. Retrieved from http://www.washington.edu/doit/Brochures/Academics/ud_edu.html

Butterworth, B., Varma, S., & Laurillard, D. (2011). Dyscalculia: From brain to education. *Science, 332*, 1049–1053.

Carmichael, K. D. (2006). *Play therapy: An introduction.* Upper Saddle River, NJ: Pearson.

Carter, D. J., Erford, B. T., & Orsi, R. (2004). Helping students with attention-deficit /hyperactivity disorder (AD/HD). In B. T. Erford (Ed.), *Professional school counseling: A handbook* (pp. 485–494). Austin, TX: ProEd.

Center for Parent Information and Resources. (2014). *Emotional disturbance.* Newark, NJ: Author.

Center for Parent Information and Resources. (2014). The ten basic steps in special education. Retrieved from http://www.parentcenterhub.org/repository/steps/

Centers for Disease Control and Prevention. (2014). Parent training programs: Insights for practitioners. Retrieved from http://www.cdc.gov/violenceprevention/pub/parenting _meta-analysis.html.

Curtis, R., Van Horne, J. W., Robertson, P., & Karvonen, M. (2010). Outcomes of a school-wide positive behavioral support program. *Professional School Counseling, 13* (3), 159–164. doi:10.5330/PSC.n.2010-13.159

Deck, M., Scarborough, J. L., Sferrazza, M. S., & Estill, D. M. (1999). Serving students with disabilities: Perspectives of three school counselors. *Intervention in School and Clinic, 34,* 150–156.

Durodoye, B. A., Combes, B. H., & Bryant, R. M. (2004). Counselor intervention in the post-secondary planning of African American students with learning disabilities. *Professional School Counseling, 7,* 133–140.

Erk, R. R. (2008). Attention-deficit/hyperactivity disorder in children and adolescents. In R. R. Erk (Ed.), *Counseling treatment for children and adolescents with DSM-IV-TR disorders* (pp. 114–162). Upper Saddle River, NJ: Merrill.

Fletcher, J. M., & Vaughn, S. (2009). Response to intervention: Preventing and remediating academic difficulties. *Child Development Perspectives, 3,* 30–37.

Goldstein, T. R., Birmaher, B., Axelson, D., Ryan, N. D., Strober, M. A., Gill, M. K., et al. (2005). History of suicide attempts in pediatric bipolar disorder: Factors associated with increased risk. *Bipolar Disorders, 7*(6), 525–535.

Hardman, M., Drew, C., Egan, M., & Wolf, B. (1993). *Human exceptionality: Society, school and family.* Boston: Allyn & Bacon.

Henderson, K. (2001). An overview of ADA, IDEA, and Section 504: Update 2001. *ERIC clearinghouse on disabilities and gifted education, ERIC EC Digest #E606.* Arlington, VA: ERIC.

Higa-McMillan, C. K., Francis, S. E., & Chorpita, B. F. (2014). Anxiety disorders. In E. J. Mash & R. A. Barkley (Eds.), *Child psychopathology* (3rd ed., pp. 345–428). New York: The Guilford Press.

International OCD Foundation. (2014). About treatment. Retrieved from http://iocdf.org /about-ocd/treatment/

Kaffenberger, C. J. (2011). Helping students with mental and emotional disorders. In B. T. Erford (Ed.), *Transforming the school counseling profession* (3rd ed., pp. 342–370). Upper Saddle River, NJ: Pearson.

Karvonen, M., Test, D. W., Wood, W. M., Browder, D., & Algozzine, B. (2004). Putting self-determination into practice. *Exceptional Children, 71,* 23–41.

Kimonis, E. R., Frick, P. J., & McMahon, R. J. (2014). Conduct and oppositional defiant disorders. In E. J. Mash & R. A. Barkley (Eds.), *Child psychopathology* (3rd ed., pp. 145–179). New York: The Guilford Press.

Kottman, T., Robert, R., & Baker, D. (1995). Parental perspectives on attention deficit/hyperactivity disorder: How school counselors can help. *The School Counselor, 43,* 142–150.

Laver-Bradbury, C. (2010). *Step by step help for children with ADHD: A self-help manual for parents.* Philadelphia, PA: Jessica Kingsley Publishers.

Learning Disabilities Association of America. (2014). Specific learning disabilities. Retrieved from http://ldaamerica.org/educators/

Lewandowski, L. J., & Lovett, B. J. (2014). Learning disabilities. In E. J. Mash & R. A. Barkley (Eds.), *Child psychopathology* (3rd ed., pp. 625–672). New York: The Guilford Press.

Marsden, A., & Chowdhury, U. (2009). Child and adolescent OCD: Obsessive compulsive disorder (OCD) in children and adolescents. *Community Practitioner, 82*(11), 42–44.

Mash, E. J., & Wolfe, D. A. (2010). *Abnormal child psychology* (4th ed.). Belmont, CA: Wadsworth.

McClellan, J., Kowatch, R., & Findling, R. L. (2007). Practice parameter for the assessment and treatment of children and adolescents with bipolar disorder. *Journal of the American Academy of Child and Adolescent Psychiatry, 46*(1), 107–125.

McEachern, A. G. (2004). Students with learning disabilities: Counseling issues and strategies. In B. T. Erford (Ed.), *Professional school counseling: A handbook* (pp. 591–600). Austin, TX: ProEd.

National Alliance on Mental Illness. (2010). *What is mental illness: Mental illness facts.* Retrieved from http://tinyurl.com/3ew3d

National Center for Educational Statistics (NCES). (2014). How many students with disabilities receive services? Retrieved from http://nces.ed.gov/programs/coe/indicator_cgg.asp

National Center for Learning Disabilities. (2014). *The state of learning disabilities: Facts, trends and emerging issues* (3rd ed.). Retrieved from http://www.ncld.org/types-learning-disabilities/what-is-ld/state-of-learning-disabilities

National Dissemination Center for Children with Disabilities (NICHCY). (2012). *Categories of disability under IDEA.* Retrieved from www.parentcenterhub.org/wp-content/uploads/repo_items/gr3.pdf

National Eating Disorders Association (2014). *Learn.* Retrieved from http://www.nationaleatingdisorders.org/general-information

NIMH. (2014). *Anxiety disorders.* Retrieved from http://www.nimh.nih.gov/health/topics/anxiety-disorders/index.shtml

Parritz, R. H., & Troy, M. F. (2014). *Disorders of childhood: Development and psychopathology* (2nd ed.). Belmont, CA: Cengage.

Piacentini, J., Chang, S., Snorrason, I., & Woods, D. W. (2014). Obsessive-compulsive spectrum disorders. In E. J. Mash & R. A. Barkley (Eds.), *Child psychopathology* (3rd ed., pp. 429–475). New York: The Guilford Press.

Reis, S. M., & Colbert, R. (2004). Counseling needs of academically talented students with learning disabilities. *Professional School Counseling, 8,* 156–167.

Resnick, R. J. (2000). *The hidden disorder: A clinician's guide to Attention-Deficit/Hyperactivity Disorder in adults.* Washington, DC: American Psychological Association.

Reynolds, C. R., & Kamphaus, R. W. (2004). *BASC-2: Behavior assessment system for children, second edition manual.* Circle Pines, MN: American Guidance Service.

Rock, E., & Leff, E. H. (2011). The professional school counselor and students with disabilities. In B. T. Erford (Ed.), *Transforming the school counseling profession* (3rd ed., pp. 314–341). Upper Saddle River, NJ: Pearson.

Rudy, H. L., & Levinson, E. M. (2008). Best practices in the multidisciplinary assessment of emotional disturbances: A primer for counselors. *Journal of Counseling and Development, 86,* 494–504.

SAMSHA. (2014). Mental disorders. Retrieved from http://www.samhsa.gov/disorders/mental

Shechtman, Z., & Pastor, R. (2005). Cognitive-behavioral and humanistic group treatment for children with learning disabilities: A comparison of outcomes and process. *Journal of Counseling Psychology, 52*, 322–336.

Silver, L. B. (2014). Changes in DSM 5 and its impact on individuals with learning disabilities. Retrieved from http://ldaamerica.org/dsm-v-do-the-changes-impact-individuals-with-learning-disabilities/

Smith, D., & Luckasson, R. (1995). *Introduction to special education: Teaching in an age of challenge.* Needham Heights, MA: Allyn & Bacon.

Strangman, N., Hall, T., & Meyer, A. (2004). *Background knowledge with UDL.* Wakefield, MA: National Center on Accessing the General Curriculum. Retrieved from http://www.cast.org/publications/ncac/ncac_backknowledgeudl.html

Swanson, S. A., Crow, S. J., Le Grange, D., Swendsen, J., & Merikangas, K. R. (2011). Prevalence and correlates of eating disorders in adolescents. Results from the national comorbidity survey replication adolescent supplement. *Archives of General Psychiatry, 68*(7), 714–723. doi:10.1001/archgenpsychiatry.2011.22

Tarver-Behring, S., & Spagna, M. E. (2009). Counseling with exceptional children. In A. Vernon (Ed.), *Counseling children and adolescents* (pp. 203–254). Denver, CO: Love Publishing.

Taub, D. J. (2006). Understanding the concerns of parents of students with disabilities: Challenges and roles for school counselors. *Professional School Counseling, 10*(1), 52–57.

Thompson, R., & Littrell, J. M. (1998). Brief counseling for students with learning disabilities. *Professional School Counseling, 2*, 60–68.

Thurneck, D. A., Warner, P. J., & Cobb, H. C. (2007). Children and adolescents with disabilities and health care needs: Implications for intervention. In H. T. Prout & D. T. Brown (Eds.), *Counseling and psychotherapy with children and adolescents: Theory and practice for school and clinical settings* (4th ed., pp. 419–453). Hoboken, NJ: Wiley.

United Nations, Convention on the Rights of Persons with Disabilities, United Nations, New York. (2006). Retrieved from http://www.un.org/disabilities/convention/conventionfull.shtml

United States Department of Education. (2014). Building the legacy: IDEA 2004. Retrieved from http://idea.ed.gov/explore/view/p/,root,regs,300,A,300%252E8

Von Ranson, K. M., & Wallace, L. M. (2014). Eating disorders. In E. J. Mash & R. A. Barkley (Eds.), *Child psychopathology* (3rd ed., pp. 801–847). New York: The Guilford Press.

Wicks-Nelson, R., & Israel, A. C. (2014). *Abnormal child and adolescent psychology* (8th ed.). Upper Saddle River, NJ: Prentice Hall.

Youngstrom, E. A., & Algorta, G. P. (2014). Pediatric bipolar disorder. In E. J. Mash & R. A. Barkley (Eds.), *Child psychopathology* (3rd ed., pp. 264–316). New York: The Guilford Press.

Name Index

Subject Index